Psychiatric-Mental Health Nursing

Integrating the Behavioral and Biological Sciences

Psychiatric-Mental Health Nursing

Integrating the Behavioral and Biological Sciences

ANGELA BARRON MCBRIDE, PHD, RN, FAAN

Distinguished Professor and University Dean, Indiana University
School of Nursing

JOAN KESSNER AUSTIN, DNS, RN, FAAN

Professor, Department of Psychiatric–Mental Health Nursing,
Indiana University School of Nursing

W.B. SAUNDERS COMPANY

A Division of Harcourt Brace & Company

Philadelphia   London   Toronto   Montreal   Sydney   Tokyo

W.B. SAUNDERS COMPANY

A Division of Harcourt Brace & Company

The Curtis Center
Independence Square West
Philadelphia, Pennsylvania 19106

Library of Congress Cataloging-in-Publication Data

Psychiatric–mental health nursing : integrating the behavioral and
    biological sciences / [edited by] Angela Barron McBride, Joan
    Kessner Austin. — 1st ed.
        p.   cm.
    Includes bibliographical references.
    ISBN 0–7216–4038–9
    1. Psychiatric nursing.   I. McBride, Angela Barron.   II. Austin,
Joan Kessner.
    [DNLM: 1. Mental Disorders—nursing.   2. Psychiatric Nursing.   WY
160 P97206 1996]
RC440.P734   1996
610.73'68—dc20
DNLM/DLC
                                                                            95-10059

PSYCHIATRIC–MENTAL HEALTH NURSING: ISBN   0–7216–4038–9
INTEGRATING THE BEHAVIORAL AND BIOLOGICAL SCIENCES

Printed in the United States of America

Last digit is the print number: 9   8   7   6   5   4   3   2   1

To Angela's Father
JOHN STANLEY BARRON

AND

To Joan's Mother
DOROTHY ZIEGELGRUBER KESSNER

CONTRIBUTORS

JOAN KESSNER AUSTIN, DNS, RN, FAAN

Professor, Department of Psychiatric–Mental Health Nursing, Indiana University School of Nursing; Adjunct Professor, Department of Psychiatry, Indiana University School of Medicine, and Department of Psychology, Purdue University School of Science, Indianapolis, Indiana

Behavior Problems in Children with Epilepsy; Integrating the Behavioral and Biological Sciences: Implications for Practice, Education, and Research

LINDA S. BEEBER, PhD, RN, CS

Professor, Syracuse University College of Nursing, Syracuse, New York
Depression in Women

CYNTHIA FRAME BONGARTEN, PhD

Associate Professor, Department of Psychology, University of Georgia, Athens, Georgia
Caring for Depressed Children and Adolescents

MARY ANN BOYD, PhD, DNS, RN, CS

Professor, Southern Illinois University at Edwardsville, Edwardsville, Illinois; Clinical Associate Professor of Psychiatry, University of Missouri School of Medicine, Columbia, Missouri, and Missouri Institute of Mental Health, St. Louis, Missouri
Fluid Imbalance and Water Intoxication: The Elusive Syndrome

KATHLEEN COEN BUCKWALTER, PhD, RN, FAAN

Professor, University of Iowa College of Nursing, and Associate Director, Office of Nursing Research, University of Iowa Hospitals and Clinics, Iowa City, Iowa
Alzheimer's Disease

ANN W. BURGESS, DNSc, RN, CS

Van Ameringen Professor of Psychiatric–Mental Health Nursing, University of Pennsylvania School of Nursing, Philadelphia, Pennsylvania
Rape Trauma and Posttraumatic Stress Disorder

JEANNE C. FOX, PhD, RN, FAAN

Professor, School of Nursing, Professor, Psychiatric Medicine, School of Medicine, and Director, Southeastern Rural Mental Health Research Center, University of Virginia, Charlottesville, Virginia
Information Processing Deficits in Schizophrenia

MARY R. HAACK, PhD, RN, FAAN

Senior Research Scientist, Center for Health Policy Research, and Associate Research Professor, Department of Psychiatry and Behavioral Sciences, The George Washington University, Washington, D.C.
Drugs, Children, and Families

GERI RICHARDS HALL, PhD(c), ARNP, CS

Gerontology Clinical Nurse Specialist, University of Iowa Hospitals and Clinics, Iowa City, Iowa
Alzheimer's Disease

SALLY BROSZ HARDIN, PhD, RN, FAAN

Professor and Director of the PhD Nursing Program, University of Massachusetts School of Nursing, Amherst, Massachusetts
Catastrophic Stress

CAROL R. HARTMAN, DNSc, RN, CS

Professor of Psychiatric–Mental Health Nursing, Boston College School of Nursing, Chesnut Hill, Massachusetts
Rape Trauma and Posttraumatic Stress Disorder

ARLENE D. HOULDIN, PhD, RN, CS

Assistant Professor of Psychosocial Oncology Nursing, University of Pennsylvania School of Nursing; Psychosocial Oncology Consultant, University of Pennsylvania Cancer Center, Philadelphia, Pennsylvania
From Stressor to Illness: The Psychological-Biological Connections

CATHERINE F. KANE, PhD, RN

Associate Professor, School of Nursing, Associate Professor, Psychiatric Medicine, School of Medicine, and Director, Division of Psychiatric–Mental Health Nursing and Aging, University of Virgina, Charlottesville, Virginia
Information Processing Deficits in Schizophrenia

MAUREEN REED KILLEEN, PhD, RN, FAAN

Professor, Department of Mental Health and Psychiatric Nursing, Medical College of Georgia School of Nursing, Athens, Georgia
Caring for Depressed Children and Adolescents

ERNEST D. LAPIERRE, DSN, RN, CS, CNAA

Director, Consulting and Services Development, Potomac Home Support, Rockville, Maryland; Director, Clinical Operations, Dupont Therapy and Counseling Center, Washington, D.C.
Fluid Imbalance and Water Intoxication: The Elusive Syndrome

MICHELE T. LARAIA, MSN, RN

Assistant Professor, Department of Psychiatry and Behavioral Sciences, College of Medicine, Medical University of South Carolina, Charleston, South Carolina
Panic Disorder with Agoraphobia

BARBARA J. LOWERY, EdD, RN, FAAN

Independence Foundation Professor of Nursing, University of Pennsylvania School of Nursing, Philadelphia, Pennsylvania

From Stressor to Illness: The Psychological-Biological Connections

ANGELA BARRON McBRIDE, PhD, RN, FAAN

Distinguished Professor and University Dean, Indiana University School of Nursing; Adjunct Professor, Department of Psychiatry, Indiana University School of Medicine, and Department of Psychology, Purdue University School of Science, Indianapolis, Indiana

Psychiatric–Mental Health Nursing in the Twenty-first Century; Integrating the Behavioral and Biological Sciences: Implications for Practice, Education, and Research; A Final Word About Career Development

HELEN NAKAGAWA-KOGAN, PhD, RN, FAAN

Professor of Psychosocial Nursing, University of Washington School of Nursing, Seattle, Washington

Using the Brain to Manage the Body

SUSAN SIMMONS-ALLING, MSN, RN, CS

Consultant Lecturer, Biological Psychiatric Nursing, Rockville, Maryland; Advanced Practice Nurse, Eisenstein Associates, Red Bank, New Jersey

Bipolar Mood Disorders: Brain, Behavior, and Nursing

GAIL W. STUART, PhD, RN, CS, FAAN

Professor, College of Nursing, Associate Professor, College of Medicine, and Administrator, Institute of Psychiatry, Medical University of South Carolina, Charleston, South Carolina

Panic Disorder with Agoraphobia

JANE HOWARTH WHITE, DNSc, RN, CS

Associate Professor, Catholic University of America School of Nursing, Washington, D.C.

Bulimia Nervosa

PREFACE

Psychiatric–Mental Health Nursing: Integrating the Behavioral and Biological Sciences builds on the keynote address that I presented in 1989 at a landmark conference on "Biological Psychiatry and the Future of Psychiatric Nursing" sponsored by the Mental Health and Alcohol Nursing Service of the Clinical Center at the National Institutes of Health, as well as the National Institute of Mental Health, the National Institute of Alcohol Abuse and Alcoholism, and the Upjohn Company. The paper was published by W. B. Saunders Company in its journal *Archives of Psychiatric Nursing* (McBride, 1990) and eventually provided the impetus for this book with the same publisher. The original paper was entitled "Psychiatric Nursing in the 1990's," and the first chapter of this book reprises the central tenets of that glance at the decade ahead: the specialty must integrate the behavioral and biological sciences and become fundamentally realigned with the basics of nursing care.

This book highlights exemplary work under way in which psychiatric nurses are addressing those themes. Chapters 2 to 15 each describe how those issues play out in a specific area, and Chapters 16 and 17 analyze the agenda that these individual chapters collectively suggest for practice, education, and research in psychiatric–mental health nursing. This book provides a historical perspective, showing the richness of the phenomena of concern to psychiatric nurses, while articulating the challenge for the decades ahead.

The contributors were selected because they all have actively conducted research in their focus areas. Lowery and Houldin's consideration of the progression "From Stressor to Illness" and its corresponding activation of the central nervous system and subsequent changes in immune phenotype and function builds on their ongoing investigation of stress reactions in subjects who are physically ill and their relationship to adaptational strategies, attributional thinking, and denial. Nakagawa-Kogan uses her pioneering work in biofeedback training to pursue the concept of illness as dysregulation and the role of the nurse as self-management trainer with the aim of restoration of regulation. Burgess and Hartman extend previous discussions of the consequences of hyperarousal by sharing their experience in addressing rape trauma, a form of posttraumatic stress disorder. Hardin draws from her research on the consequences of an outbreak of botulism in Illinois and of Hurricane Hugo in South Carolina to explore catastrophic stress.

Austin uses her knowledge of epilepsy in children as a paradigmatic area for the development of a practice-research agenda that makes use of both behavioral and biological theoretical frameworks. She examines the extent to which psychological variables may account for behavioral problems, although research has traditionally emphasized the importance of biological variables. Haack draws from her study of

---

McBride, A. B. (1990). Psychiatric nursing in the 1990's. *Archives of Psychiatric Nursing, 4,* 21–28.

drug-exposed infants and their families to propose a comprehensive model of care that weaves together individual and family considerations along with service delivery policies. Similarly, White provides an analysis of bulimia nervosa that embeds psychobiological concerns within a context replete with complex societal pressures.

Killeen and Bongarten explore depression in children and adolescents, while Beeber considers depression in women. Both chapters focus more on symptoms than on medical diagnosis per se and are concerned with correcting dysregulation (be it hormonal, neurochemical, or rhythm disrupting) and restoring self-worth. Simmons-Alling explores the importance of monitoring and managing mood changes through the strategic use of psychotropic medications and other means of restoring appropriate chronobiological rhythms. Stuart and Laraia extend the discourse on hyperarousal in their consideration of the symptoms characteristic of phobic behavior.

Fox and Kane discuss schizophrenia in terms of information processing deficits and point the way to the use of midrange theories in developing interventions that are mindful of specific incapacities. In a similar vein, Buckwalter and Hall show how the Progressively Lowered Stress Threshold Model can be used to create a therapeutic environment that encourages routine, minimizes stimuli and excess demands, and is sensitive to physical stressors and fatigue. Boyd and Lapierre demonstrate how care of water intoxication syndrome remains inadequate if it does not respect complex behavioral and biological considerations.

Taken as a whole, these 14 commissioned chapters point the way to a reconceptualization of psychiatric–mental health nursing that projects the specialty beyond the mere application of communication skills to psychological problems and psychiatric disorders. In recent years the specialty has often been criticized for being out of the mainstream of nursing. This book is intended to counteract that perception by providing in-depth examples of how some psychiatric nurses are addressing key clinical concerns through research-based practice (all commissioned chapters were subjected to extensive blind review to encourage a state-of-the-science approach). Although the chapters are not intended to represent the full breadth of the specialty, they are illustrative of how psychiatric–mental health nursing is not separate from overall heath care research and of how it advances a program of study that complements other discussions of how the health care professions are bridging the gap between the behavioral and biological sciences in the provision of care.

The concluding chapters weave together key themes and point the way to the future in setting a practice research agenda for careerists to achieve. They make clear that a renaissance is taking place in this important and extensive specialty area that is bound to have an energizing effect on the field as a whole as it assumes leadership for symptom management, self-care training, and maximizing patients' functional strengths in the face of some disability. The book acknowledges the extent to which the hyper/hypo arousal that is part of the stress system influences emotional tone, the retrievability and use of information, and the initiation of specific action. In the process, the work articulates a vision for nursing that does much more than bring the behavioral and biological sciences together in linear fashion; it binds psychiatric and mental health nursing through a common commitment to facilitating dynamic self-regulation in patients with actual or potential problems.

ANGELA BARRON MCBRIDE

ACKNOWLEDGMENTS

Many people have contributed to the development of this book over the course of its four years in the making—our students, our colleagues, the other authors, and the reviewers of each chapter. There are several who deserve particular recognition. Robyn Gibboney is chief among them; she carefully coordinated the project in its final stages, making sure that there was uniformity across chapters. Marilyn Pesci facilitated that effort, as did Jeanne Critchfield. To our editor at Saunders, Dan Ruth, goes the credit for envisioning this book in the first place and for never failing to be encouraging. We salute our husbands, William Leon McBride and David Ross Austin, for their support of this project but even more so for their support over the years. Finally, we both wish to acknowledge the extent to which Hildegard Peplau has contributed to our separate and shared professional development.

ANGELA BARRON MCBRIDE
JOAN KESSNER AUSTIN

CONTENTS

CHAPTER

1

PSYCHIATRIC–MENTAL HEALTH NURSING IN THE TWENTY-FIRST CENTURY

Angela Barron McBride, PhD, RN, FAAN

ABSTRACT
This chapter reviews the accomplishments of psychiatric–mental health nursing—theory development, advanced practitioner roles, family-centered care—and notes some limitations—a projected shortage of psychiatric nurses, devaluation of biological knowledge, a preference for addressing mental health rather than psychiatric care. The challenges ahead are described with a focus on the tremendous need to integrate the behavioral and biological sciences in the practice of psychiatric–mental health nursing. At a time when psychiatry is realigning itself with medical practice, it is important that psychiatric–mental health nursing become reassociated with what are considered the fundamentals of nursing care.

There was a strong sense from the 1950s through the 1970s that psychiatric–mental health nursing was a specialty in the ascendancy (Aiken, 1987). This was a period when graduate programs proliferated, and Dr. Rhetaugh Graves Dumas became the first nurse Deputy Director of the National Institute of Mental Health (NIMH). Many other nurses in national leadership positions also came from that clinical background, and they were able to demonstrate that their interpersonal skills and systems orientation were useful in being effective deans and directors. In addition, many of the leading nurse theorists, particularly those designated as interaction theorists—for example, Orlando (1961), Paterson and Zderad (1976), Peplau (1952), Travelbee (1971)—were also prime movers in the development of psychiatric–mental health nursing.

Psychiatric nurses contributed significantly to the development both of practice theory (Wald & Leonard, 1964) and of clinical research, especially in studies of the effects of mental health nursing on the course of threatening events (Diers, 1970; Dumas & Leonard, 1963; Elms & Leonard, 1966; Johnson, 1972; McBride, 1967). One could even argue that the concern with health in the last quarter century in both psychology and sociology has been partially due to collaboration between social scientists and psychiatric nurses as they explored what nursing research might encom-

---

This chapter is an updated revision of the author's article "Psychiatric Nursing in the 1990s," which appeared in *Archives of Psychiatric Nursing*, Vol. IV, No. 1, February 1990, pp. 21–28.

pass, for example, the collaboration between Jean Johnson and Howard Leventhal (Johnson & Leventhal, 1974; McBride, 1994).

Psychiatric nurses drew attention to the importance of process issues as a basic ingredient of effective nursing, for example, eloquently discussing therapeutic use of self (Krauss, 1987); they incorporated interpersonal relations skills into the overall undergraduate curriculum and developed liaison psychiatric nursing, thereby becoming consultants to medical-surgical nurses on behavior problems or stress and anxiety (Fagin, 1981). The specialty took the lead in the development of the clinical nurse specialist role with its emphasis on independent practice, certification, and third-party reimbursement for services rendered (Hocking, Hassanein, & Bahr, 1976), and was largely responsible for encouraging the profession as a whole to emphasize family-centered care (Mereness, 1968). While nursing was often seen as only an allied health profession in many forums, it has long been viewed at the NIMH as one of the four core health professions, along with psychiatry, psychology, and psychiatric social work, thus encouraging psychiatric nurses to be regarded as co-equal with their colleagues in other fields in principle if not always in practice.

By the 1980s, however, the sense of the specialty's being in the ascendancy had dissipated (Martin, 1985; Mitsunaga, 1982; Robinson, 1986; Slavinsky, 1984; Thomas, 1986). An acute shortage of psychiatric–mental health nurses was projected (Kramer, 1986). Undergraduate nursing programs had become organized around unifying nursing theories rather than specialized content (Carter, 1986), so caring for schizophrenic patients tended to be discussed less than the communication skills all effective nurses are expected to demonstrate. To the extent that the specialty's primary domain was equated with the interpersonal skills needed to allay stress and anxiety generally, the incorporation of this material into the generic curriculum seemed to leave psychiatric–mental health nursing without an articulated focus. Since new graduates were regularly encouraged to get at least a year of experience in medical-surgical nursing before specializing, few had much exposure to the opportunities in psychiatric nursing, and thus there was no feeder system encouraging nurses to specialize in this area.

Related to the question of what is distinctive about the specialty was the comparative reluctance of nurse researchers to study the most differentiated patient population, the severely and persistently mentally ill. The specialty's emphasis on mental health rather than on psychiatric care per se may have been prompted by the wish of practitioners to identify with nursing's health-oriented perspective rather than with the medical model. Nonetheless, it had the effect of making psychiatric nursing seem relatively more concerned with the worried well than with serious problems and somewhat oblivious to the realities that concerned the general public and the present disease-oriented system, for example, the devastating effects of drug addiction and the number of homeless hallucinating in public places.

The relationship of psychiatric disorders to mental health has been a general problem for the specialty (Sills, 1977) and is reflected in the various names used to describe the area. Is it psychiatric *and* mental health nursing (any program of study is concerned with both illness and health), psychiatric/mental health nursing (with the slash indicating either/or in a program of study), psychosocial nursing (a name that makes physiological issues invisible), or some other combination (McBride, 1986)? The name problem was itself connected with existing conceptualizations both of whether mental illness and mental health exist on the same continuum and of whether psychiatric nurses have a distinct role in the treatment of brain disorders.

The sense of a specialty in decline had been further accentuated by the concomitant plummeting of clinical traineeships for study in psychiatric nursing at the

NIMH and the development of the National Center for Nursing Research (NCNR) within the National Institutes of Health (NIH). As NIMH's primary mission became research, nurses became less of a presence there because their orientation had traditionally been to clinical training rather than to research training. In 1976–1977, NIMH awarded nurses 1,252 stipends at a cost of $8.1 million; a decade later, NIMH awarded only 97 stipends at a cost of $1.2 million (Chamberlain, 1986). When the NCNR (now the National *Institute* for Nursing Research) first became a presence within the NIH, psychiatric nurses also felt excluded there because studies bearing on psychiatric disorders were then not even part of the NIH's mission, although they now are with the formal incorporation of the NIMH, the National Institute of Alcohol Abuse and Alcoholism (NIAAA), and the National Institute of Drug Abuse (NIDA) into the NIH structure. The notion that psychiatric nurses may not be in the mainstream can be summarized in the remarks of one nurse leader who was overheard to say at a meeting: "You psychiatric nurses are behind the times. Everyone else is getting sophisticated about research, but you keep doing *therapy,* and that is not nursing as I know it."

The previous quote suggests that psychiatric nursing is derivative and not vital, but one only has to look at developments since the late 1980s to argue that the field is again on the upswing. Some indicators of progress include: the debut of new journals—*Archives of Psychiatric Nursing,* the *Journal of Child and Adolescent Psychiatric and Mental Health Nursing,* and *Capsules & Comments in Psychiatric Nursing;* record-breaking attendance at annual professional meetings (Southeastern Regional Conference for Clinical Specialists in Psychiatric–Mental Health Nursing and meetings of the Society for Education and Research in Psychiatric Nursing, Association of Child and Adolescent Psychiatric Nurses, and the American Psychiatric Nurses Association); establishment of the Coalition of Psychiatric Nursing Organizations (COPNO) so the field can present a united front around common concerns; acknowledgment of the specialty's interventions (e.g., music therapy, group psychotherapy, assertiveness training) as basic to nursing (Bulechek & McCloskey, 1985); development of a classification system for psychiatric–mental health nursing (Loomis et al., 1987); willingness on the part of the Division of Nursing to award training monies for educational programs in psychiatric nursing along with all other specialities; the involvement of nurses in developing a plan for research on child and adolescent mental disorders (McBride, 1992); implementation of the recommendations of a Task Force on Nursing to examine ways of increasing the participation of nurses in the NIMH (McBride, 1993; McBride, Friedenberg, Babich, & Bush, 1992); and efforts to develop psychogeriatrics as an important subspecialty (Abraham, Buckwalter, Harper, & Hight, 1994; Harper & Grau, 1994).

Along with infrastructure development, there is also a host of personal triumphs that can be put forth as evidence of progress, for example, the establishment of the Hildegard Peplau Award within the American Nurses Association to celebrate psychiatric nurses of distinction; the leadership of Dr. Grayce Sills in assessing Ohio's implementation of the Mental Health Act of 1988 (Study Committee on Mental Health Services, 1993); Dr. Joan Austin's becoming in 1993 the first nurse to receive a clinical investigator award from the American Epilepsy Society in recognition of her research on childhood-onset seizures and their effects on family adaptation; the appointment of Dr. Gail Stuart as administrator of the Institute of Psychiatry at the Medical University of South Carolina.

These indicators of a revitalized specialty have left the field poised for a new leap forward. Psychiatric nurses are prepared to greet the future with a proud history, standards, credentials, advanced powers of observation, and communication skills. But coming years will only be a renaissance for the specialty if psychiatric nurses can state clearly their own agenda for practice, education, and research. And setting such an extensive agenda will necessitate two major adjustments: (1) revaluing biological knowledge and (2) becoming fundamentally reassociated with the essentials of nursing care.

VALUING BIOLOGICAL KNOWLEDGE

There is a tremendous need to integrate the biological sciences—neurobiology, genetics, and immunology—and behavioral sciences in the practice of psychiatric–mental health nursing. The pressure for this move is coming from three separate, but interrelated, directions. First of all, there is a general concern within the profession that "in recoiling from the male-dominated, reductionistic, disease-oriented biomedical model, nursing science has (perhaps unintentionally) narrowed its scope primarily to the study of the social and behavioral sciences" (Drew, 1988, p. 25). This devaluation of biological knowledge is regarded as dangerous at the present time when increasingly sick patients require complex care that is equally mindful of the influence of physiology *and* environment. Reemphasizing the biological sciences can have several benefits (Drew, 1988): (a) reminding other behavioral scientists and health care professionals that psychiatric nurses are prepared to provide a special perspective because they are schooled to proceed from a biopsychosocial model (Christman, 1987); (b) providing the promise of finding discernible biological markers to estimate systemic change, for example, pigmentation of the skin that is indicative of low levels of melatonin hormone may be associated with seasonal affective disorder (Restak, 1989); and (c) narrowing the gap between nursing research—largely peopled by social scientists—and practice, which is so often oriented to providing physical care and administering medications.

The second push to value biological knowledge is coming from consumer advocacy groups who argue that disorders of the mind cannot be diagnosed and treated without regard to the brain. The National Alliance for the Mentally Ill (NAMI) is so committed to the notion that mental illness is a disease of the brain that it has established a separate research foundation to study the biological basis of the major mental illnesses and has vigorously lobbied Congress to support brain research at NIMH. Theirs is a view that differentiates sharply between adjustment problems and mental illness: "It [NAMI] does not agree that there is a continuum of difficulty from childhood upset to major psychosis in adulthood, or that treating the child will prevent mental illness. Prevention will become possible when we understand how brain chemistry goes awry" (Hatfield, 1987, p. 82). By redefining mental illness as a biological disorder and decrying some social scientists' predilection to blame the family for the illness (e.g., the notion that a schizophrenic child has necessarily had a schizophrenogenic mother), NAMI and similar groups have demanded a paradigm shift in the conceptualization of psychiatric disorders away from largely holding stricken families responsible for creating their problems. They prefer to describe schizophrenics as ill and the stressed as responding to environmental demands; the former require medical treatment, while the latter need guidance. One might reasonably argue, however, that both groups need psychiatric–mental health nursing!

The third influence deserving attention is the shift away from the behavioral sciences to the neurosciences in the organizing frameworks of psychiatry. The last decade has been a period of major breakthroughs in genetics, immunology, and brain function. Imaging techniques now permit looking into the living human brain to identify structural defects in specific regions, thus making differential diagnosis truly possible. New drugs are being developed to correct biochemical imbalances, and their effectiveness is increasingly being monitored by blood titers. The study of genetics is moving away from a focus on rare disorders to common ones, for example, schizophrenia and the affective disorders. Recent developments indicating the importance of bright light in resetting circadian rhythms (Czeisler et al., 1989) have implications in the treatment repertoire for everything from jet lag and shift-work dyssomnia to disrupted sleep in the elderly and seasonal depression.

An emphasis on brain dysfunction has led to a reconceptualization of diagnosis and treatment strategies in no area more than schizophrenia, which has definitely ceased to be regarded as a unitary illness. As a complex, variable picture of brain dysfunction has emerged (including ventricular enlargement, cerebral atrophy, and disturbances of cerebral mechanisms), treatment approaches have become more differentiated. For example, documented brain damage requires treatment with a greater emphasis on social rehabilitation and environmental manipulation than on psychotherapy (Seidman, 1983) because keeping the patient's frustration level low to promote maximal functioning is likely to be more successful than expecting to promote insights beyond the individual's capabilities. The NIMH report (National Advisory Mental Health Council, 1988) to Congress on the decade of the brain provides an elegant summary of the range of gains made in knowledge regarding the epidemiology, diagnosis, treatment, and prevention of the major mental illnesses and of research questions that should be addressed as the twenty-first century approaches.

Psychiatric nurses have not been oblivious to the biomedicalization of psychiatry. In a survey of *Journal of Psychosocial Nursing* readers (What Are Your Feelings, 1988), questions regarding this trend elicited responses that applauded resulting roles for the nurse (e.g., in assessment of medication side effects and in treating depression in patients with sleep apnea with continuous positive air pressure) but warned against any assumption that biological advances will ever replace the need to teach clients interpersonal skills and more adaptive ways of responding to stressful events. That warning was not unlike the one issued at a meeting on the "Next Steps That Will Revolutionize Psychiatry in the 21st Century" (Barnes, 1988), where participants were reminded not to go from psychiatry's being brainless to its becoming mindless. The task ahead is to combine information about brain function with the psychological, social, cultural, and environmental factors that also influence human behavior.

Revaluing biological knowledge does not mean giving up the basic tenets of the psychosocial orientation in nursing; what it means is truly integrating nature and nurture (Church, 1987). Psychiatric nurses should clearly take responsibility for the interface between the behavioral and the biological sciences in the maintenance of mental health and the prevention/limitation of psychiatric dysfunction through the provision of care to individuals, families, and communities (Pothier, Stuart, Puskar, & Babich, 1990; Wilson, 1994). To date, this mission has involved nurses in a range of exciting efforts: identifying, then managing akinesia and akathisia (Michaels & Mumford, 1989; Whall, Engle, Edwards, Bobel, & Haberland, 1983); monitoring mood states and circadian rhythms (Harris, 1989; Ryan, Montgomery, & Meyers, 1987; Simmons-Alling, 1987); understanding the eating problems caused by Parkinson's disease with and without dementia (Athlin et al., 1989).

When one is dealing with any interaction between neuronal loss and subsequent impairment in memory storage and recall, resulting nursing care must take into account both the extent of damage and what can be done to promote optimal functioning within existing limitations. The preparation one needs to be effective has specific consequences for a reintegration of neurological nursing and psychiatric–mental health nursing because both specialties are broadly concerned with understanding central nervous system impairment and fostering maximal adjustment. This is not unlike Green's (1993) call for cognitive remediation in schizophrenia that takes advantage of what is already known about the rehabilitation of brain-injured patients.

CARE AND CARING

Psychiatric nurses played a pioneer role in the movement to regard nurses as therapeutic. They did this, in part, by emphasizing that clinical nurse specialists, who were assumed to have obtained educational preparation at the master's level, could function as interchangeable members of mental health center teams, along with psychiatrists, psychologists, and psychiatric social workers (McBride, 1988). That conceptualization, however, had the effect of weakening their identification with nursing because it tended to emphasize similarities across the core disciplines in providing episodic care, rather than what could be accomplished by having a nonsegmented view (i.e., 24-hour caregiving responsibility), which has traditionally been the special province of nursing. That conceptualization had the added consequence of rendering invisible the role of the nurse who is without graduate preparation and plays a general role in a specialty setting.

The landmark monograph *Psychiatric Nursing 1946 to 1974: A Report on the State of the Art* (Huey, 1975) described the entire specialty in terms of accomplishments in the therapies favored by all mental health professionals—individual therapy, group therapy, family therapy, and milieu therapy. The emphasis on psychiatric nursing's expertise with key treatment modalities served the important historical purpose of aligning nurses with being therapeutic, but the publication of *Nursing: A Social Policy Statement* (ANA, 1980), with its emphasis on the nursing process, declared that determining how behavior can be treated is secondary to assessing the phenomena under study. This shift made doing therapy (especially when that got translated into 50-minute hours) seem removed from the nursing mainstream, which was focusing on the nursing process rather than on being a physician substitute.

One can make a strong case for the fact that the process of convincing Congress to support establishment of an NIH institute for nursing research provided opportunities for nurse scientists to highlight what they are positioned to study (McBride, 1987). The testimony, arguing that our nation's research agenda needs to be broadened from a focus on biomedical cure to one that addresses care priorities, led Representative Edward R. Madigan (1986) to state that nursing research is particularly needed to find answers to questions that concern the public as they consider the limits of technological advancements and begin to address care for people with continuing health problems. One might add that psychiatric nursing research should be particularly concerned with how to care for the persistently mentally ill, given the limited number of psychiatric cures and the consequent extent of continuing mental health problems. By design, NIMH's Task Force on Nursing (1987) defined psychiatric nursing research as encompassing three general areas that paralleled the caregiving divisions of the NCNR (Merritt, 1986): (a) fostering mental health, preventing mental illness, and improving the understanding, treatment, and rehabilitation of the mentally ill; (b) facilitating care of persons who are acutely or chronically mentally ill; and (c) improving the delivery of mental health nursing services.

The American Academy of Nursing co-sponsored a conference on "Knowledge about Care and Caring" with Sigma Theta Tau International and several universities to elaborate on what nursing's overall care agenda might include (Stevenson & Tripp-Reimer, 1990). The ensuing discussion considered caring in three separate but related ways, all of which bear on psychiatric-mental health nursing as much as any other specialty (McBride, 1989). Caring refers to: (a) a way of being for people that is responsive rather than judgmental or hierarchical; (b) a range of nurturing and protective acts devoted to assessing, monitoring, and responding to patient conditions; and (c) a health care system that truly encourages health care and not just disease management. To be concerned about care is to be involved at the macro level (e.g., social values, policies, and organizational structures) as well as at a more micro level (e.g., interpersonal processes and symptom management).

If one applies these points to describing psychiatric–mental health nursing's purview, its subject matter should be minimally concerned with (1) the structure of discrete caregiving acts (e.g., managing instances of aggressive behavior, hallucinations, or wandering); (2) whole programs of caregiving involving a series of acts (e.g., case management of patients with Alzheimer's disease or discharge planning for patients on lithium); and (3) the structural components of a system that encourages caring (e.g., models of interdisciplinary collaboration or cost-effective organization of quality services).

Biological advances have increased the demands placed on caregivers to provide high-quality care. New knowledge has meant more to incorporate in developing patient education strategies. Alleviating distress and discomfort becomes even more important when patients are subjected to a battery of biological tests and procedures. Even if schizophrenia is cured tomorrow, millions of individuals will need social rehabilitation and environmental manipulation to handle the deficits that remain after the disease process has been reversed. Prevention activities will also have to be mobilized to protect future generations. As McGue wisely argued, "The issue properly framed is not so much nature *versus* nurture as it is nature *via* nurture" (1989, p. 508). For example, current data make clear that the expression of schizophrenia depends upon both an inherited genetic predisposition *and* exposure to environmental stressors (McGue & Gottesman, 1989).

Psychiatric–mental health nursing can play a leadership role in explicating nature via nurture because it has been traditionally concerned with the person-environment fit (a feature of all nursing theories). Psychiatric–mental health nurses believe that high-quality care presupposes an understanding of how an individual's disease process and recuperative powers are affected by contextual factors (e.g., social support of a material, emotional, and/or informational nature). Nursing's commitment to examining what facilitates or limits individuals in their activities of daily living requires an appreciation not only of the complicated forces creating a problem (e.g., psychosocial factors influencing anorexia nervosa) and responsible for sustaining a problem (e.g., physiological changes that accompany starvation and frenetic exercise) but also of the varied actions necessary to effect change over time (e.g., dealing with interactions between the psychosocial and physiological).

LOOKING FORWARD

The chapters that follow all recount current research that aims to integrate the behavioral and biological sciences in the conceptualization and provision of care. Each chapter focuses on a different topic, but all strive to outline how that integration is proceeding and how it is setting the stage for new directions in practice, education, and research. These chapters are meant to provide concrete examples of how particular areas of psychiatric–mental health nursing are being reconceptualized, but they also raise some general issues that are discussed in the concluding chapters. Collectively, these chapters demonstrate that addressing the interface between the behavioral and the biological sciences has relevance to a broad range of phenomena.

REFERENCES

Abraham, I. L., Buckwalter, K. C., Harper, M. S., & Hight, V. A. (1994). Geropsychiatric nursing: Bringing advances in practice and research to education. *Journal of Psychosocial Nursing, 32*(4), 5.

Aiken, L. H. (1987). Unmet needs of the chronically mentally ill: Will nursing respond? *Image: Journal of Nursing Scholarship, 19,* 121–125.

American Nurses Association. (1980). *Nursing: A social policy statement.* Kansas City, MO: Author.

Athlin, E., Norberg, A., Axelsson, K., Moller, A., & Nordstrom, G. (1989). Aberrant eating behavior in elderly Parkinsonian patients with and without dementia: Analysis of video-recorded meals. *Research in Nursing and Health, 12,* 41–51.

Barnes, D. M. (1988). Psychiatrists psych out the future. *Science, 242,* 1013–1014.

Bulechek, G. M., & McCloskey, J. C. (Eds.). (1985). *Nursing interventions. Treatments for nursing diagnoses.* Philadelphia: W. B. Saunders.

Carter, E. W. (1986). Psychiatric nursing: 1986. *Journal of Psychosocial Nursing, 24*(6), 26–30.

Chamberlain, J. G. (1986). An up-date on psychiatric mental health nursing education at the federal level. In *Psychiatric-mental health nursing: Proceedings of a conference defining the discipline for the year 2000* (pp. 3–19). Rockville, MD: National Institute of Mental Health.

Christman, L. (1987). Psychiatric nurses and the practice of psychotherapy: Current status and future possibilities. *American Journal of Psychotherapy, 41,* 384–390.

Church, O. M. (1987). From custody to community in psychiatric nursing. *Nursing Research, 36,* 48–55.

Czeisler, C. A., Kronauer, R. E., Allan, J. S., Duffy, J. F., Jewett, M. E., Brown, E. N., & Ronda, J. M. (1989). Bright light induction of strong (type o) resetting of the human circadian pacemaker. *Science, 244,* 1328–1333.

Diers, D. (1970). Faculty research development at Yale. *Nursing Research, 19*(1), 64–71.

Drew, B. J. (1988). Devaluation of biological knowledge. *Image: Journal of Nursing Scholarship, 20,* 25–27.

Dumas, R. G., & Leonard, R. C. (1963). The effect of nursing on the incidence of postoperative vomiting. *Nursing Research, 12*(1), 12–15.

Elms, R. R., & Leonard, R. C. (1966). Effects of nursing approaches during admission. *Nursing Research, 15,* 39–48.

Fagin, C. M. (1981). Psychiatric nursing at the crossroads: Quo vadis. *Perspectives in Psychiatric Care, 19*(3), 99–l06.

Green, M. F. (1993). Cognitive remediation in schizophrenia: Is it time yet? *American Journal of Psychiatry, 150,* 178–187.

Harper, M., & Grau, L. (1994). State of the art in geropsychiatric nursing. *Journal of Psychosocial Nursing, 32*(4), 7–12.

Harris, E. (1989). Lithium: In a class by itself. *American Journal of Nursing, 89,* 190–195.

Hatfield, A. B. (1987). The National Alliance for the Mentally Ill: The meaning of a movement. *International Journal of Mental Health, 15*(4), 79–93.

Hocking, I. L., Hassanein, R. S., & Bahr, R. T. (1976). Willingness of psychiatric nurses to assume the extended role. *Nursing Research, 25,* 44–48.

Huey, F. L. (Ed.). (1975). *Psychiatric nursing 1946 to 1974: A report on the state of the art.* New York: American Journal of Nursing Company.

Johnson, J. E. (1972). Effects of structuring patients' expectations on their reaction to threatening events. *Nursing Research, 21,* 499–504.

Johnson, J. E., & Leventhal, H. (1974). The effects of accurate expectations and behavioral instructions on reactions during a noxious medical examination. *Journal of Personality and Social Psychology, 29,* 710–718.

Kramer, M. (1986). Target-populations for psychiatric-mental health nursing 1980–2005. In *Psychiatric–mental health nursing: Proceedings of two conferences on future directions* (pp. 4–27),

DHHS Publication No. (ADM) 86-1449. Rockville, MD: National Institute of Mental Health.

Krauss, J. B. (1987). Nursing, madness, and mental health. *Archives of Psychiatric Nursing, 1,* 3–15.

Loomis, M. E., O'Toole, A. W., Brown, M. S., Pothier, P., West, P., & Wilson, H. S. (1987). Development of a classification system for psychiatric/mental health nursing: Individual response class. *Archives of Psychiatric Nursing, 1,* 16–24.

Madigan, E. R. (1986). Nursing research to take its rightful place [Editorial]. *Nursing and Health Care, 7,* 3.

Martin, E. J. (1985). A specialty in decline? Psychiatric–mental health nursing, past, present and future. *Journal of Professional Nursing, 1*(1), 48–53.

McBride, A. B. (1967). Nursing approach, pain, and relief: An exploratory experiment. *Nursing Research, 16*(4), 337–341.

McBride, A. B. (1986). Theory and research. Present issues and future perspectives of psychosocial nursing. *Journal of Psychosocial Nursing, 24*(9), 27–32.

McBride, A. B. (1987). The National Center for Nursing Research. *Social Policy Report* [a publication of the Society for Research in Child Development], 2(2), 1–11.

McBride, A. B. (1988). Coming of age: Child psychiatric nursing. *Archives of Psychiatric Nursing, 2,* 57–64.

McBride, A. B. (1989). Knowledge about care and caring: State of the art and future development. *Reflections, 15*(2), 5–7.

McBride, A. B. (1992). Nurses develop a plan for research on child and adolescent mental disorders. *Journal of Child and Adolescent Psychiatric and Mental Health Nursing, 5,* 41–43.

McBride, A. B. (1993). Psychiatric nursing: Coming of age at NIMH. *Hospital and Community Psychiatry, 44*(1), 11–12, 15.

McBride, A. B. (1994). President's message. A tribute to Jean E. Johnson. *Nursing Outlook, 42,* 39–42.

McBride, A. B., Friedenberg, E. C., Babich, K., & Bush, C. (1992). Nursing research at NIMH: An update. *Archives of Psychiatric Nursing, 6,* 138–141.

McGue, M. (1989). Nature-nurture and intelligence. *Nature, 340,* 507–508.

McGue, M., & Gottesman, I. I. (1989). Genetic linkage in schizophrenia: Perspectives from genetic epidemiology. *Schizophrenia Bulletin, 15,* 453–464.

Mereness, D. A. (1968). Family therapy: An evolving role for the psychiatric nurse. *Perspectives in Psychiatric Care, 6,* 256–259.

Merritt, D. H. (1986). The National Center for Nursing Research. *Image: Journal of Nursing Scholarship, 18,* 84–85.

Michaels, R. A., & Mumford, K. (1989). Identifying akinesia and akathisia: The relationship between patients' self-report and nurse's assessment. *Archives of Psychiatric Nursing, 3,* 97–101.

Mitsunaga, B. K. (1982). Designing psychiatric/mental health nursing for the future: Problems and prospects. *Journal of Psychosocial Nursing, 20*(12), 15–21.

National Advisory Mental Health Council. (1988). *Approaching the 21st century: Opportunities for NIMH neuroscience research* [a report to Congress on the decade of the brain]. Rockville, MD: National Institute of Mental Health.

National Institute of Mental Health. (1987). *Report of the task force on nursing.* Rockville, MD: Author.

Orlando, I. J. (1961). *The dynamic nurse-patient relationship.* New York: G. P. Putnam's Sons.

Paterson, J. G., & Zderad, L. T. (1976). *Humanistic nursing.* New York: John Wiley & Sons.

Peplau, H. (1952). *Interpersonal relations in nursing.* New York: G. P. Putnam's Sons.

Pothier, P. C., Stuart, G. W., Puskar, K., & Babich, K. (1990). Dilemmas and directions for psychiatric nursing in the 1990s. *Archives of Psychiatric Nursing, 4,* 284–291.

Restak, R. M. (1989). The brain, depression and the immune system. *Journal of Clinical Psychiatry, 50*(5, suppl.), 23–25.

Robinson, L. (1986). The future of psychiatric/mental health nursing. *Nursing Clinics of North America, 21,* 537–543.

Ryan, L., Montgomery, A., & Meyers, S. (1987). Impact of circadian rhythm research on approaches to affective illness. *Archives of Psychiatric Nursing, 1,* 236–240.

Seidman, L. J. (1983). Schizophrenia and brain dysfunction: An integration of recent neurodi-agnostic findings. *Psychological Bulletin, 94,* 195–238.

Sills, G. M. (1977). Research in the field of psychiatric nursing 1952-1977. *Nursing Research, 26,* 201–206.

Simmons-Alling, S. (1987). New approaches to managing affective disorders. *Archives of Psychiatric Nursing, 1,* 219–224.

Slavinsky, A. T. (1984). Psychiatric nursing in the year 2000: From a nonsystem of care to a caring system. *Image: Journal of Nursing Scholarship, 16*(1), 17–20.

Stevenson, J. S., & Tripp-Reimer, T. (Eds.). (1990). *Knowledge about care and caring. State of the art and future development.* Kansas City, MO: American Academy of Nursing.

Study Committee on Mental Health Services. (1993). *The results of reform: Assessing implementation of the Mental Health Act of 1988.* Columbus, OH: Ohio Department of Mental Health.

Thomas, S. P. (1986). Mental health nursing clinical specialization: Extinction or adaptation. *Issues in Mental Health Nursing, 8*(1), 1–13.

Travelbee, J. (1971). *Interpersonal aspects of nursing* (2nd ed.). Philadelphia: F. A. Davis.

Wald, F. S., & Leonard, R. C. (1964). Towards development of nursing practice theory. *Nursing Research, 13,* 309–313.

Whall, A. L., Engle, V., Edwards, A., Bobel, L., & Haberland, C. (1983). Development of a screening program for tardive dyskinesia: Feasibility issues. *Nursing Research, 32,* 151–156.

What are your feelings about the trend toward the biomedicalization of psychiatry? (1988). *Journal of Psychosocial Nursing, 26*(l), 40–41.

Wilson, H. S. (1994). Special feature. Psychobiological knowledge update for "the decade of the brain." *Capsules & Comments in Psychiatric Nursing, 1*(1), 4–8.

CHAPTER

2

FROM STRESSOR TO ILLNESS
THE PSYCHOLOGICAL-BIOLOGICAL CONNECTIONS

Barbara J. Lowery, EdD, RN, FAAN, and Arlene D. Houldin, PhD, RN, CS

ABSTRACT

This chapter reviews the biological and psychosocial literature related to the connections among activators/stressors, reactions, consequences, and mediators. It notes the limitations of research design and conflicting results concerning the association of chronic stress reactions to the development and exacerbation of health problems (e.g., the common cold and myocardial infarction) and suggests that new techniques make it possible to measure the involvement of neuroendocrine and immune systems in the stressor-to-illness-to-outcome chain. While the expected correlations have not always been found, combining behavioral and biomolecular measurement offers an opportunity to bring more sophistication and conceptual richness to the extant research on which behaviors and attitudes—such as personality types and adaptational strategies—most strongly affect outcomes of illness. In examining both psychological and biological factors in intervention research, efforts are being made to determine whether the intervention has a positive effect in terms of patient outcomes and what mechanisms might account for such outcomes. This biopsychosocial focus, in turn, has implications for nursing education and nursing's clinical and research agendas.

The word *stress* has generally had two separate but related meanings. It has been used as a term for a stimulus that upsets the organism's homeostasis or as the organism's response to that stimulus. In this chapter the word *stressor* will refer to the stimulus that creates upset in the individual. It is used in a general sense to refer to any stimulus that creates such upset, including general life stressors and those associated with illness. Stress with the latter definition is the primary focus. The major emphasis is on the psychological and biological reactions of the individual to a stressor (or activator) and the consequences of those reactions with respect to physical illness.

Because physiological reactions and psychological reactions to a stressor may be complex and interactive, the term stress as employed within this chapter is global. It is meant to include emotions such as anxiety, fear, anger, depression, or a combina-

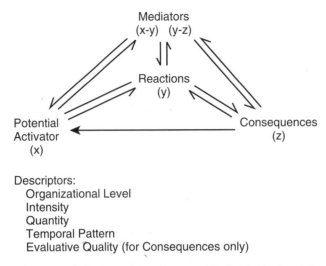

Descriptors:
  Organizational Level
  Intensity
  Quantity
  Temporal Pattern
  Evaluative Quality (for Consequences only)

FIGURE 2–1. A framework for interactions between the individual and the environment. (From Elliott, G., & Eisdorfer, C. [Eds.]. [1982]. *Stress and human health* [p. 19]. New York: Springer Publishing Company.)

tion of these, as well as myriad physiological reactions that may occur in the neuroendocrine or immune system.

The clearest framework for examination of the psychological/biological connections in stress research is the model reported by the Institute of Medicine study of *Stress and human health* (Elliot & Eisdorfer, 1982) (see Fig. 2–1). There are three primary elements in the model: the activators/stressors, the reactions, and the consequences. These can be referred to as the x-y-z sequence (Elliot & Eisdorfer, 1982). *Activators/stressors* may be internal or external events or conditions that are sufficiently intense or frequent to evoke some change in the individual, for example, a serious illness or death in the family. *Reactions,* which are the focus of the present chapter, include both the biological and psychosocial responses that occur in response to the activator/stressor. Because of recent advances in psychoneuroimmunology, these reactions—for example, depression, anxiety, or alterations in catecholamines or the immune system and their connections—will increasingly comprise the core of stress research. *Consequences* are the prolonged and cumulative effects of the aforementioned reactions, for example, physical illness. The model attends to individual differences and variations throughout the sequence through its conceptualization of mediators, which are the filters and modifiers in the sequence (Elliot & Eisdorfer, 1982). This model suggests a dynamic, interactive process across the stress continuum between an individual and the environment (Lowery, 1987).

Attention to all aspects of this model in detail is far beyond the scope of this chapter. (For an in-depth discussion of the model and the research that led to its conceptualization, the reader is referred to the original work.) Instead, the authors' research and the related work of others will provide examples of psychological and biological reactions to an activator/stressor, their potential interconnectedness, and their consequences in terms of physical illness. Some examples of individual difference mediators will also be provided, as well as examples of interventions that may be used to reduce the effects of potential activators/stressors, their reactions, and consequences. Finally, the chapter discusses the basic biological sciences in nursing's clinical and research agendas on stress assessment and intervention among the physically ill.

STRESS AND ILLNESS CONSEQUENCES

The word stress is used widely in our culture, and the idea that it can be harmful to health is commonly accepted. As a result, stress reduction is big business today, as are do-it-yourself books on stress reduction. Psychiatric nurses, psychiatric liaison nurses, and their nurse colleagues in general hospitals and in the community are also attuned to the harmful effects of stress. In fact, it is hard to imagine a nursing textbook or a clinical nursing course that does not address the subject of stress, its potential for exacerbating illness, the mechanisms that patients use to reduce distress, and nursing interventions that might help in stress reduction.

Aristotle hypothesized a link among stress, susceptibility to disease, and recovery (Hall, 1989). However, most nurses need not refer back to Aristotle to find support for the notion that stress can trigger illness or compromise recovery from it. They can document many examples of this link from their practice with patients and, indeed, from their own experiences. Unfortunately, documentation through scientific study of the phenomenon is still very limited, despite growing interest, and the results to date are contradictory.

There is evidence, albeit somewhat conflicting, that chronic stress reactions are associated with the development and exacerbation of health problems. In both physical and mental illnesses, it has long been thought that prolonged exposure of susceptible individuals to a stressor can produce chronic neuroendocrine reactions with biological consequences such as schizophrenia, depression, gastrointestinal disorders, heart disease, pulmonary disease, rheumatoid arthritis, and cancer (Chiappelli, 1988; Elliott & Eisdorfer, 1982; Nowak, 1991). In fact, psychological and neuroendocrine reactions are also thought to be associated with outcomes once an illness has developed.

Stress has been a major topic in nursing research for the past 30 years. A few recent examples that support the stressor-reaction-consequence link are the studies of Leidy (1990), which links perceived distress and symptomatic experience in patients with chronic obstructive pulmonary disease, and of Maio-Esteves (1990), in which daily stress was a predictor of perceived health status in adolescent girls. As with stress research in other disciplines, some nursing research examples do not support such a link. Gurklis and Menke (1988), for example, did not find a direct association between perceived stress and length of time on hemodialysis. Similarly, Norbeck and Anderson (1989) did not find the expected relationship between stress and pregnancy outcomes in low-income women. Sorting out the actual association of stress reactions with illness will undoubtedly continue to comprise a major portion of nursing research. However, several changes will be necessary as this work proceeds.

Design issues comprise a major limitation in the stress research to date. By and large, retrospective designs have been used to examine the stressor-to-illness link, so most studies have all the potential sampling and measurement problems associated with such designs. In addition, most studies look for associations between stressors and disease or disease outcomes (e.g., mortality), a pattern that provides important but limited information. As is indicated in the model presented earlier, individual difference mediators may influence the development and progression of illness following exposure to a stressor. Sociodemographic variables such as age, income, and education; the adaptational strategies employed by individuals to deal with stressors; variables such as severity in those who are ill—all these may have some effect on consequences. The important thing at this time is that investigators of the stressor-to-illness question should begin to employ prospective designs and to sort out those variables which may independently contribute to the risk of illness or to the risk of subsequent morbidity and mortality following diagnosis of illness. Following are two good examples of the kind of research that is required to link stressors to the development of illness and to illness outcomes.

It has long been thought that stress reactions play a part in the development of the common cold. However, the evidence collected through research over the years has been relatively weak. In their recent prospective study of the relationship of psychological stress and susceptibility to colds, Cohen, Tyrrell, and Smith (1991) used a stress-index measure derived from scores related to stressful life events in the past year, current perceived stress, and current affect. They controlled for several potential confounders and examined other possible stress-illness mediators. While the effect size was small, they found that respiratory infection rates and colds increased with increased levels of psychological stress.

Research on the relation of stress to morbidity and mortality following myocardial infarction provides another example of the value of prospective and longitudinal designs in studying the consequences of stress. In this research, investigators examined stress reactions during hospitalization (Garrity & Klein, 1975) and life stress and isolation during convalescence (Ruberman, Weinblatt, Goldberg, & Chadhary, 1984), then followed patients over time. The results suggest that stress reactions during hospitalization and perceived stress and isolation in convalescence can make independent contributions to the prediction of morbidity and mortality beyond those made by illness variables.

Research design issues comprise only one of the problems with the stressor/illness research to date. Another problem, and the one that will comprise a major focus of this paper, is that many studies, including those nursing studies mentioned above, study consequences of psychological reactions to potential stressors. Very little research addresses the link from psychological upset to illness effects. While it has generally been accepted that the neuroendocrine and immune systems are involved in the stressor-to-illness-to-outcome chain, research that sorts out that involvement has been slow to develop. Moreover, much of what we know about these central systems comes from general work in the biological sciences and not from research designed to study the stressor/illness link (Elliott & Eisdorfer, 1982). Some studies, however, provide a basis for discussing how that association might be studied.

PSYCHOLOGICAL AND PHYSIOLOGICAL REACTIONS TO STRESSORS

The mechanisms by which stress might be linked to illness or compromised recovery have not been fully explicated. However, it is becoming increasingly clear that the psychological reactions that occur in response to a stressor and the related alterations in the neuroendocrine and immune system might affect illness outcomes (Elliott & Eisdorfer, 1982). For example, if psychological upset is associated with a reduction in natural killer cells, then such upset might logically be linked to the development of cancer and to recovery problems. If psychological distress is associated with an increase in catecholamines, which may produce an increase in arrhythmias, such distress might be associated with reinfarction and even mortality in patients with myocardial infarction.

Together, Cannon's (1914) description of the "fight or flight" response and Selye's (1956) ideas about the "general adaptation syndrome" provided considerable insight into the biological and molecular reactions to stressors in the sympathetic nervous system, the pituitary-adrenocortical axis, and the immune system. Although these ideas were met with much skepticism in the past, over the past 20 years there has been a growing number of believers in the links these early scientists proposed, albeit with modifications (Mason, 1975; McEwen & Stellar, 1993). Interest in the study of the physiological and pathological responses to stressors is no doubt heightened by developments in neuroscience, immunology, and technology in recent years. These new developments allow for better measurement of reactions in both the neuroendocrine and immune systems. The following examples are of research that employs developing technology in the study of physiological and psychological stress response associations.

NEUROENDOCRINE RESPONSES TO PSYCHOLOGICAL DISTRESS

There have been attempts in the past to measure the reactions in the neuroendocrine system to psychological influences. Early research on the body's reactivity to stressors centered on measurement of responses such as blood pressure, heart rate, galvanic skin response, and other reactions in the end-organs (Mills & Dimsdale, 1988). Perhaps because these responses are such indirect indicators of sympathetic nervous system activity, the research was largely inconclusive. As new techniques became increasingly available, other more direct indicators of neuroendocrine arousal—such as measures of urinary and salivary cortisols—were used. Although these indicators, too, have limitations (Mills & Dimsdale, 1988), research into their change as a response to stressors has been informative. For example, in their comparison of physiological responses to laboratory and real-life stressors, van Doornen and van Blokland (1992) found that urinary catecholamine levels were increased under both situations. However, the reactions during the laboratory task were not correlated with those under real-life stress conditions. Perhaps more important, under real-life stress, catecholamine responses were significantly related to systolic and diastolic blood pressure levels.

As measures of plasma levels of catecholamines, cortisols, and other indicators of acute arousal have become more sophisticated, they have increasingly become the measures of choice for understanding such neuroendocrine arousal. While much of this research is still being carried out in laboratories, a growing number of clinical studies has successfully linked reports of anxiety and depression with plasma indicators of changes in the neuroendocrine system. Davis, Dunlop, Shea, Brittain, and Hendrie (1985), for example, linked baseline differences in serotonin levels to high and low trait anxiety in students. In addition, they found that these levels increased for all students as their reported stress levels increased. Similarly, Fell et al. (1985) found that anxiety, as measured by a visual analog scale, increased along with plasma adrenalin in presurgical patients. Jacobs et al. (1986) found that high levels of depression and anxiety were positively correlated with prolactin response in individuals facing a stressful situation.

However, not all attempts to link psychological and biological measurements of stress have been successful. Matthew, Beng, Taylor, and Semchuk (1981), for example, did not find the expected relationships between anxiety and catecholamines or dopamine beta hydroxylase. This same failure to find correlations between psychological stress and sympathetic activation has occurred with studies examining urinary-free cortisol (Jacobs, Mason, Kostin, Brown & Ostfeld, 1984) and growth hormone responses (Kosten, Jacobs, & Mason, 1984).

Such negative results have led some investigators to conclude that clinical anxiety and biochemical arousal may be entirely different concepts and that study of them may need to proceed along different lines (Matthew et al., 1981). On the other hand, such negative results may be a function of: (a) different reactions to stress in different parts of the psychoneuroendocrine system (Jacobs et al., 1986) and (b) the problems inherent in the measurement of both psychological and biological markers of distress. Despite these shortcomings, there is no doubt that most scientists are beginning to see promise in the search for behavioral correlates to responses in the neuroendocrine system.

While linking emotions to measurement of arousal of the neuroendocrine system is a key step in the process of untangling stress-illness mechanisms, it does not provide the total picture. In a relatively new area, investigators interested in psychophysiologic research are beginning to study receptors that link catecholamine responses to end-organ changes such as increased heart rate or elevated blood pressure (Mills & Dimsdale, 1988). Graafsma et al. (1987) noted that mental stress has been associated with increases in catecholamines but that its effects on adrenoreceptor density had never been studied. They examined changes in catecholamine levels and receptor density of normotensive volunteers undergoing a mental arithmetic test in a laboratory situation. They found an immediate increase in plasma catecholamines, the expected increase in beta-receptor density, and a small increase in affinity of receptors following the test. This brief laboratory situation suggests that the chain of events from acute stressor to cardiac changes might involve an up-regulation of receptor numbers and their affinity. However, study of receptor changes also holds promise for study of chronic stress reactions.

Chronic stress undoubtedly plays a major role in illness outcomes because the psychological and physiological reactions to chronic stress are much more subtle and thus not likely to be noticed. In situations of defined chronic stress, there is chronic but not necessarily constant arousal of the neuroendocrine system. Thus, plasma indicators of arousal may provide an incomplete and perhaps inaccurate estimate of the extent of distress experienced over time. Receptor research may provide important insights in this regard. In several studies, for example, it has been shown that prolonged or repetitive stimulation of receptors by agonists such as catecholamines results in a reduction or down-regulation of beta-adrenoreceptor density (Maki, Kontula, & Harkonen, 1990). This number may be a useful measure of chronic arousal, which can be studied for its relationship to chronic psychological arousal and illness consequences. Current research by one of the authors on lymphocyte beta-adrenergic receptor changes and their association with stress levels and denial following myocardial infarction is an example of how receptor research may help nurses find more definitive answers about the efficacy of certain coping strategies for patients, then design interventions based on those answers.

THE EMOTION–IMMUNE RESPONSE LINK

A number of studies suggest that psychological factors are also linked to changes in immunity through activation of both the sympathetic adrenal-medullary (SAM) system and the hypothalamic-pituitary-adrenocortical (HPAC) system. It is believed that the most common neuroendocrine link between emotions and immune changes is through activation of the HPAC system and release of corticosteroids, which can alter immunity in a number of ways (O'Leary, 1990). However, demonstration of this link has been hampered by problems in measurement of HPAC chronic arousal. Plasma levels of cortisols can be measured, but they are indicative of acute activation of the HPAC system and cannot provide a clear picture of chronic activation. Moreover, indirect measures such as urinary cortisols are easily confounded by variables such as diet and urinary output (O'Leary, 1990).

Despite the lack of data establishing the associations between neuroendocrine activation and immunological changes, the association of stress with changes in the immune system has been the subject of a growing number of studies. Two recent papers (O'Leary, 1990; Vollhardt, 1991) provide excellent overviews of the research to date.

As is the case with research on the emotion-neuroendocrine association, the research into immunity changes as a result of stress is limited and mixed in terms of its outcomes. For example, in their research on exam stress, Kiecolt-Glaser, Garner, Speicher, Penn, and Glaser (1984) found that natural killer (NK) cell activity was reduced under such stress, but total plasma IgA was increased. In their research on immune responses to stress in caregivers, Kiecolt-Glaser et al. (1987) found that caregivers had lower helper-to-suppressor T-cell ratios and higher antibody titers to Epstein-Barr virus than a matched control group. However, there were no differences in NK cell percentages. Last, Fittschen et al. (1990) evaluated the effects of exam stress over a 2-month period. They found stress-related shifts in the cell volume of immunocytes and decreased urinary-neopterin concentration in students who perceived the exam as highly challenging.

There are several criticisms of the stress–immune response research to date. First, it might be argued that the physiological changes that accompany distress— for example, loss of appetite, sleeplessness—explain the immune responses and not psychological upset (O'Leary, 1990). While some investigators have taken such variables into account, others have not. Another criticism is that investigators have not studied potential neuroendocrine mediators of immunological changes so that the pathways from distress to neuroendocrine arousal to immunological changes can be better specified. As indicated earlier, this problem is methodological to some extent, since accurate measurement of chronic arousal of the HPAC system is difficult to accomplish. Finally, and perhaps most important, it has been argued that, unless immunological changes can be linked to some illness consequences, their clinical significance may be limited (O'Leary, 1990; Swartz, 1991).

An example of a program of research that addresses these stress-illness linkages by examining central arousal, immune changes, and clinical outcomes, albeit with different populations, is the work of Levy and colleagues. In a series of studies, Levy et al. (1985, 1987) found that breast cancer patients who were rated as less well-adjusted to their illness—that is, expressing more distress—had higher levels of NK activity than patients who were less distressed. Moreover, lower NK activity was associated with cancer spread to the axillary lymph nodes. In a sample of healthy individuals (Levy et al., 1991), younger subjects (18 to 29 years of age) who reported more perceived stress were more likely to have lower NK activity and lower levels of plasma beta endorphins; they also reported more infectious morbidity. While this is a promising beginning, establishing stress-illness linkages will require continuing research using prospective, longitudinal designs that attend to the neuroendocrine and immunological alterations that occur in the stressor-to-illness chain.

MEASUREMENT ISSUES

There are both behavioral and biomolecular measurement issues in the research that attempts to link psychological and physiological stress reactions. With respect to behavioral measurement, it has been noted (Lowery, 1987) that two common ways of measuring psychological reactions to stressful events—observation and self-report—have both positive and negative attributes. Both are limited by social desirability considerations, since individuals may not want to show or say that they are upset. Observational measures may be complicated by the patient's symptoms; self-report, by the patient's ability to describe stress reactions.

Despite these limitations, a number of valid and reliable measures can be used to gather such data. While they may not correlate with one another, it seems important to use both observation and self-report measures in this early phase of the study of both biological and behavioral stress reactions.

Another issue is the choice of measures specific to anxiety, depression, or hostility, or those measuring a combination of stress reactions. Investigators studying the association of stress with neuroendocrine and immunological changes have tended to employ one measure, usually an anxiety measure. However, there are limited data on the association of particular psychological reactions to physiological changes. Thus, the use of one measure of one construct might reduce the chances of finding correlations between behavioral and biomolecular markers of stress.

Measurement of arousal of the neuroendocrine and immunological systems is similarly problematic. Measured levels in these systems can be altered by the illness itself, the drugs employed to treat the illness, physical activity, diet, and myriad other potential confounders. Some biological markers that may correlate with activation may not be appropriate with certain populations. For example, the study of beta$_2$-adrenergic receptors as a marker of chronic stress would be inappropriate with patients with heart disease who are on beta-blocking agents known to block beta$_2$-receptor uptake. The study of immune phenotype and function may be problematic in cancer patients who are receiving therapy known to affect the immune system. Careful consideration of the potential confounders is critical in the selection of the activation marker.

In addition, we know very little about which markers in the neuroendocrine or immune systems might be affected by different psychological stress reactions, for example, anxiety, depression, or hostility. Recent research on depression confirms the long-suspected link between cortisol levels and severe clinical depression (Nowak, 1991). However, whether severe clinical depression and depressed mood in nondiagnosed individuals have the same neuroendocrine marker has yet to be established. Thus, regardless of the responses of interest, it will be valuable to study more than one marker as research into these associations and their consequences for illness and recovery proceeds.

MEDIATORS OF THE STRESSOR-ILLNESS LINK: SOME EXAMPLES

The study of the association of psychological distress and changes in the neuroendocrine and immune systems is clearly a critical part of the stress research agenda for the future. However, as is indicated in the stress framework, it should not proceed without some attention to the person within whom such reactions are occurring. In both laboratory and clinical studies, investigators must recognize that individuals may respond to a stressor in different but characteristic ways and that such responses can mediate the results of research into the chain of events from stressor to consequences.

The notion that behavioral characteristics and adaptive behaviors can affect the outcomes of illness has long been held. Despite conflicting findings, behaviorists continue to try to sort out which behaviors and attitudes most strongly affect such outcomes. There is a substantial body of research, for example, on how persons with different personality styles—for example, introvert/extrovert, Type A/Type C, internal/external, to name only a few—react to stressors. Research into the efficacy of specific adaptational strategies, both attentional and avoidant, in stressful situations is also substantial. However, by and large, nurses and other investigators have tended to test the association of potential mediator variables with psychological reactions or with end-organ changes or consequences. If physiological indicators of arousal are measured, they are very indirect indicators, as mentioned earlier.

In a sense then, the technology for measurement of activation in the neuroendocrine and immune system offers an opportunity to bring more sophistication and conceptual richness to research on the efficacy of different personality styles and particular adaptational strategies in illness situations. It also provides a mechanism for arriving at conclusions with more confidence and then proceeding to design interventions for individuals who are ill.

Research that can provide definitive answers to the myriad of questions about the biobehavioral precursors to illness and its outcomes is just beginning. A nursing research agenda that attends to state-of-the-art physiological measurement in future attempts to answer these questions will serve both patients and the nursing profession well. Several examples of how this research has proceeded and how it might progress follow.

PERSONALITY

Probably the most studied personality is Type A. While the research findings are mixed, Type A behavior is generally thought to be associated with risk of heart disease, and nurses are among the many investigators to test this association. Meininger, Hayman, Coates, and Gallagher (1988), for example, are attempting to sort out the heritability of Type A behavior and its association with cardiovascular risk factors in children. While they did not find a link between cardiovascular risk factors and Type A behavior, they recommended continued rigorous investigation of the potential link between personality type and risk factors. Since emotional reactivity is thought to be a central feature of Type A personality, some evidence that these individuals are easily centrally aroused will provide greater support for the theory than has occurred thus far.

Another promising area for linking psychobehavioral and physiologic research is oncology. The notion that immune system changes might alter the course of cancer development, progression, and treatment is becoming more acceptable to scientists, clinicians, and the public (Spiegel, 1993). In fact, a number of well-designed studies examine positive mental attitudes to determine their outcomes for cancer patients (Greer & Watson, 1985: Temoshok, 1985). For a comprehensive overview of the research to date and future directions, see Redd et al. (1991). For purposes of this discussion, a set of personality factors called Type C will serve as an example of the proposed links.

Type C, which is said to be the opposite of Type A personality, has been linked with poor outcomes after cancer diagnosis. The literature suggests that Type C individuals respond to stress with feelings of helplessness, depression, and emotional suppression (Temoshok, 1987) and with conformity-compliance, unassertiveness, and patience (Greer & Watson, 1985). Some research indicates that breast cancer patients with these traits have poorer outcomes at both 5 years (Greer, Morris, & Pettingale, 1979) and 10 years (Greer, Pettingale, Morris, & Haybittle, 1985). In addition, Type C patients with malignant melanoma were shown by Temoshok (1985) to have more rapid tumor growth and invasion than non–Type C individuals.

It has been suggested that the repression of anger and action that occurs with Type C personality is associated with increased neuroendocrine arousal and that this arousal leads to negative outcomes for patients exhibiting those characteristics. No research to date compares levels of distress and neuroendocrine arousal in Type C and non–Type C individuals following diagnosis of cancer. However, the research by Levy, Herberman, Lippman, and d'Angelo (1987), which has associated psychological distress with changes in immune status in cancer patients, suggests that studying these links for those with Type C personality characteristics might be promising in explaining the negative outcomes that have been reported.

Until the links among personality characteristics, psychological stress reactions, neuroendocrine activation, alterations in the immune system, and outcomes are more fully explicated, conclusions about Type C personality research and its danger to patients are, at best, quite weak. In new research, in addition to characterizing cancer patients as Type C or non–Type C, investigators could follow patients over time and systematically measure their psychological stress levels, a physiological indicator of central arousal, changes in immune phenotype and function, and morbidity and mortality outcomes.

With respect to personality types it is important to note that conclusions about their positive or negative consequences will not necessarily directly lead to intervention strategies. The association of different personality styles to illness and its outcomes has long been of interest to nurse investigators because the understanding of which styles eventuate in poor outcomes helps nurses to predict problems and intervene accordingly. With Type A behavior, for example, research has proceeded from examination of the overall construct to sorting out which trait or behavior exhibited accounts for the most variance in prediction equations. Hence, much of the work that is currently underway focuses on the anger and hostility typical of the Type A personality (Strube, 1991). The same kind of research will probably be necessary if the Type C personality construct is found to be associated with psychological and biological arousal and negative outcomes for patients. Once such data become available, then interventions to alter these characteristics could be tested.

Adaptational Strategies

In contrast to personality research, the research about adaptational strategies that patients use following diagnosis of illness might be more readily applied. For example, if denial following a heart attack were found to be associated with decreased psychological and physiological distress and with better outcomes for patients, then nursing interventions that encourage denial and discourage too much attention to the illness and its potential outcomes could be readily applied and tested for their efficacy in altering outcomes.

Thus, a promising line of research would bring physiological measures into the study of different adaptational strategies employed by patients. While many adaptational strategies might mediate psychological and biological reactions to illness and its consequences, two will serve as examples here: denial (a defensive, avoidant strategy) and causal thinking (a coping, attentional strategy). Both denial and causal attributions have received considerable study for their association with illness and its outcomes, and they seem particularly appropriate for discussion here.

Causal Attributions

Heider's (1958) view that individuals attribute causes to events to make sense of and gain control over their lives serves as the basis for attributional theory. Causal thinking—that is, asking, "Why did this happen?"—is the underlying cognitive activity. The basic assumptions about such causal thinking are that (1) individuals search for causes to interpret new information; (2) causal thinking is the first step in coping with novel or unexpected life events (Weiner, 1985); and (3) affect, expectations, and actions will be based on the causes generated (Weiner, 1979). Since Heider's early work, many investigators have studied the effects of causal thinking on responses to different life events, and in general the tenets of the theory have received support.

In recent years a series of studies has been conducted that attempted to determine to what extent patients' causal explanations for the origin of their illness explain their adaptation to that illness. (For an excellent overview of this work see Michela and Wood [1986], and for a review of the studies that focus on life-threatening illnesses, see Turnquist, Harvey, and Andersen [1988].) Such research obviously holds promise for interventions if the theory holds with patients. If it were shown, for example, that causal thinking is the first step in adjustment, then interventions that encourage such thinking would clearly follow. Moreover, if particular causes were found to be associated with better adjustment, encouraging patients to posit such causes would also follow.

However, while some research in illness situations supports the theoretical propositions noted above, many studies do not lend support to those ideas. For example, there is research that indicates some individuals do not engage in causal thinking in the face of an illness, although illness represents the kind of event that should elicit such thinking. For example, in one study 54% of chronically ill individuals and 58% of patients newly diagnosed with myocardial infarction said they had not wondered, "Why me?" (Lowery, Jacobsen, & McCauley, 1987). In addition, Taylor, Lichtman, and Wood (1984) found that 35% of cancer patients had not developed a "hunch or theory" about why they became ill, and Affleck, Allen, Tennen, McGrade, and Ratzan (1985) reported that 14.7% of mothers with insulin-dependent children had not asked themselves, "Why me?"

The question remains whether those who do not engage in causal thinking are worse off than those who do, as would be predicted by the theory. Interestingly, in most research, differences in affect, adjustment, or outcomes for those who have or have not thought about the why of their illness are not studied. Moreover, in the few studies that examine this relationship (Lowery et al., 1987; Silver & Wortman, 1983), patients who had not asked themselves about a cause were better off in terms of their affect and outlook than those who had, the opposite of what might be predicted.

Research into the relationships between particular causes posited by patients and psychological adjustment also bring into question the propositions of attributional theory. Although causes and adjustment are hypothesized to be correlated (Weiner, 1979), many studies have not found a link between the controllability (controllable or uncontrollable) or locus of the cause (internal or external) and affect, and many have not found the stability of the cause (changeable or unchangeable) to be associated with future expectations (Michela & Wood, 1986). Research with cancer patients by Lowery, Jacobsen, and DuCette (1993) and by Taylor et al. (1984) also shows little relationship between particular causes and affect or adjustment.

The current state of affairs with respect to attributions in illness situations clearly suggests a need for more and better research to sort out the value of such thinking for patients. First, most of the research, including that of the authors, is not linked to morbidity and mortality consequences but rather to psychological reactions. Second, none of the work that the authors located used a measure of physiological upset in addition to psychological measures. As is the case with the other examples given, study of the chain of events—from causal thinking to particular attributions to psychological reactions and central arousal to outcomes for patients—will best inform caregivers about the efficacy of causal thinking and particular causes in illness situations.

DENIAL

Denial has been defined in various ways, but it is most commonly thought of as a mechanism by which individuals repudiate their illness or its outcomes to avoid psychological upset. While denial has been suggested as one of the more primitive adaptational mechanisms (Vaillant, 1971), there is no doubt that it is widely employed in illness situations, particularly those which might be life-threatening. However, the results of research into the efficacy of denial in reducing distress and the negative outcomes that might be associated with it are, at best, conflicting.

The illness situation in which denial has received the most study is recovery from myocardial infarction. For an overview of that research, see Lowery (1991). In addition, many other studies examine the value of avoidant strategies such as denial and attentional strategies such as causal thinking. For an overview of earlier work and a meta-analysis on outcomes, see Mullen and Suls (1982).

Despite denial's presumed value in reducing distress, research results thus far do not clearly show that patients who deny have less psychological stress. Hackett, Cassem, and Wishnie (1968) found no significant relationship between denial and affect—as judged by observation, nursing notes, relatives' reports, or patient self-report of denial—to psychological status during hospitalization, although in the posthospital follow-up none of the deniers presented with infarct-related depression or anxiety. Similarly, Gentry, Foster, and Haney (1972) reported that deniers had significantly less state anxiety than nondeniers on all but 1 day of the 5-day study period. However, there were no significant differences in self-report of depression in the two groups. Froese, Hackett, Cassem, and Silverberg (1974) reported that over six different study periods, the mean anxiety scores of deniers and nondeniers were significantly different at only one time point; they found no significant differences in depression of deniers and nondeniers over the study period.

In more recent research, Havik and Maeland (1988) also found only partial support for the hypothesis that denial reduces distress. They found that denial of the illness was unrelated to emotional upset throughout the 5-year study period. However, denial of the impact of the illness was associated with less reported anxiety, depression, and irritability. The work of Levine et al. (1987) also provides some support for the high denial/low distress link; they found a small but significant negative correlation between denial and anxiety/depression/general distress.

There is only one small pilot study of 10 patients that examined the link between patient report of denial, distress, and a physiological marker of central arousal. Miller and Rosenfeld (1975) studied patients in coronary care on measures of denial, anxiety, and suppression of affect for their relationship to plasma catecholamine levels. They developed an 11-point denial scale, which was completed by the investigators and the nurses, and a 7-point anxiety rating scale for patients in the study to use. Although they provided no information on the relationship of denial to anxiety, they did find that anxiety was significantly correlated with epinephrine levels, an indicator of arousal, and that denial was not related to the physiological measures of distress. However, they also found a significant difference in the denial ratings of the investigators and the nurses caring for patients, suggesting that the denial measure was susceptible to observer bias. Thus, it may not have provided a sufficient test of the association of denial and the physiological distress marker.

To date, only one study has systematically examined the extent to which denial contributes to the prediction of morbidity and mortality following myocardial infarction. Havik and Maeland (1988) reported that low denial of illness (which, as indicated above, was unrelated to emotional upset) was associated with higher mortality in a survival analysis of heart attack patients, even after control for many potential confounders. However, high denial of the impact of the illness (which was associated with less anxiety, depression, and irritability) was also weakly associated with higher mortality, suggesting that denial of illness alone may be protective in terms of outcome. Other research on denial and outcomes is much less systematic in examining how, taken together, demographic variables, illness variables, and denial contribute to outcomes. However, in general, the research supports the notion that high denial might be associated with lower morbidity and mortality following heart attack, although not necessarily through its association with lower levels of distress. How then does it influence outcomes, if indeed it does?

The authors have posited that the link between psychological distress and central arousal may be harmful for patients. Perhaps in the situation of denial this is not the case. The relative lack of association of denial with psychological distress and the possible association of denial with illness outcomes afford investigators a unique opportunity to see whether denial has an influence on central arousal without influencing psychological arousal. While it seems quite unlikely that denial does have such an influence, well-designed prospective research that examines the association of denial to psychological and central activation mediators and outcomes could prove quite useful to health professionals.

While Type A, Type C, denial, and causal thinking provide only a few examples of how little is known about the mediation of these psychologic variables on the stress response and about the efficacy of certain personality styles and adaptational strategies, they are prototypic of the field. Despite paying careful attention to the extant research, nurses will find no easy answers to guide nursing intervention that might help patients to better adapt. The excitement at this time lies in the possibility for finding such answers.

STRESS AND PSYCHOLOGICAL INTERVENTIONS

Although the focus in this chapter is on psychological and physiological reactions to stressors, these same reactions are important in studying the effectiveness of stress-reducing interventions. Over the years, an increasing number of studies has used a range of psychological interventions that show reduced distress and enhanced well-being for patients (Holland, 1991). It is becoming increasingly common to examine both psychological and biological factors in intervention research in an effort to determine: (1) whether an intervention has a positive effect in terms of patient outcomes and (2) what mechanisms might account for such outcomes. The following examples serve to highlight the issues.

There are those who believe that interventions to reduce stress reactions have a positive effect on the immune system. Enhanced cellular and humoral immune functioning has been demonstrated after relaxation training for a geriatric population (Kiecolt-Glaser et al., 1985) and for healthy college students (Green & Green, 1987; Green, Green, & Santoro, 1988; Jasnoski & Kugler, 1985; Kiecolt-Glaser et al., 1984; Kiecolt-Glaser et al., 1986). Pennebaker, Kiecolt-Glaser, and Glaser (1988) reported that having a sample of healthy college students write about traumatic experiences had a significantly positive effect on the response of T lymphocytes to two mitogens, phytohemagglutinin (PHA) and concanavalin (ConA).

Still others believe that positive responses in the immune system will alter outcomes for patients with certain illnesses. For example, Fawzy, Cousins, Fawzy, Elashoff, and Morton (1990) examined the immediate and long-term effects of a structured psychiatric intervention for cancer patients. The intervention group showed significant increases in the percentage of large granular lymphocytes and

NK cells, along with an increase in NK cytotoxic activity and a small decrease in the percentage of helper/inducer T cells at the 6-month assessment point. They also found a reduction in levels of psychological distress and greater use of active coping methods for the intervention group. However, whether reduced distress, active coping strategies, and immune changes alter patient outcomes has yet to be established.

Other research examines a stress intervention and its association with receptor number. Arguing that transcendental meditation might be effective in reducing chronic stress through its effect on adrenergic receptors, Mills, Schneider, Hill, Walton, and Wallace (1990) presented preliminary findings indicating that neither catecholamines or beta adrenergic receptors were different for meditation subjects and controls. However, meditation subjects did have fewer receptors in the high-affinity state, indicating that their sensitivity to potentially damaging stress hormones was somewhat less than for controls.

Despite these early promising results linking some stress-reducing interventions with biological change, the state of the research is such that there are no clear-cut answers to guide clinical practice. Unfortunately, popular readings today cite some of these mind-body studies as proof that development of the right attitude cures all sorts of serious diseases (Bower, 1991) and that interventions should focus on encouraging positive thinking and active coping. Because of increasing public information and the potential for misuse of these data, it is important that nursing professionals have a firm knowledge base from which to advise patients and their families about the mind-body interactions and about the potential advantages of a variety of interventions.

Patients should be informed about the contradictory and preliminary state of research on the mind-body connections, and they should know that the available data do not support notions about one best intervention or one right attitude. The current state of the science suggests there may be many healthy ways of coping with illness, and patients should be given permission to use whatever strategies work for them. Each patient's unique style of coping should be understood and respected, and an individualized plan of support should be developed to address particular needs. In general, patients will be comforted to know the following:

- Periods of distress normally accompany illness.
- There is no need to remain continually hopeful and positive.
- There is no need to fit into a particular pattern for the proper management of feelings.
- Preillness skills and resources, including support systems, can be used in a flexible manner to cope with the often changing demands of illness and treatment.

Moreover, as research proceeds, patients should be offered a variety of supportive interventions, such as relaxation training and support groups, and should be encouraged to use the forms of psychological support that they find most helpful (Houldin & Lowery, 1992).

THE AGENDA FOR NURSING

A major change in the study of the association of psychological factors and illness outcomes is underway. Increasingly sophisticated biomolecular technology is available for examining the links among psychological distress, activation of the central nervous system, and changes in immune phenotype and function. Study of these links and of their association with personality and adaptational strategies holds promise for rapidly expanding understanding of illness and its outcomes. Moreover, such research can provide more definitive data on which to base interventions.

The agenda proposed here is one to which nursing must attend if it is to bring itself into the current research linking behavior and biology. Such research is new to all disciplines, so despite the fact that nursing is a relative newcomer to research in general, it is not behind with respect to biobehavioral research. In fact, nursing's emphasis on behavior makes it one of the disciplines well poised to capitalize on the technological advances that hold promise for linking clinical work with the biological. However, nurses must confront several issues if they are to keep pace with the opportunities for advancing biobehavioral science.

First, the longitudinal studies, which are necessary and which Elliott and Eisdorfer (1982) called for more than 10 years ago, are expensive. Adding laboratory research to nurses' characteristically psychological work will also be an expense. Thus, the budget for well-designed studies to accomplish the proposed agenda is going to be quite high. Unless such research becomes a nursing priority and funds are set aside for the work, other fields will undoubtedly take the lead in answering questions that are clearly within the domain and interest of nursing.

Developing the cadre of investigators interested in such research is also an important issue for the future. Despite the claim that nursing is interested in the biopsychosocial nature of patients, for the most part, nurses have focused on the psychosocial in their education and research. To keep pace with the emerging field of psychoneuroimmunology, nurses need to begin educating students at both the undergraduate and graduate level in its basics.

The current curriculum in undergraduate studies generally includes some attention to neuroendocrine and immunological functioning, and there is usually ample attention to distress and how it might be involved in the development and course of an illness. In the future, however, it will be critical for educators to see that these two areas of the curriculum—distress and physiological change at the central level—are linked. At the very least, the hypothesized links should be taught, and as research begins to confirm these links, findings should also become part of the curriculum. Psychiatric–mental health nursing courses are the logical place to present and study the chain of events from stressors to outcomes. This curriculum would provide students the opportunity to see that, with respect to stress, mental illness and physical illness are more similar than different in both their etiology and progression.

While this chapter has not focused on stress and mental illness, it might well have done so. Some of the most important breakthroughs in research into mental illness are occurring through the examination of problems in the neuroendocrine response to stressors. Graduate students who will practice in psychiatric settings must be educated in current thinking about the etiology and course of mental illness and their association with distress. While most current students are probably learning about the stress-diathesis theory, attention to the physiology that might link stress to mental illness and its outcomes would clearly strengthen that learning.

For those students who intend to practice as psychiatric liaison nurses, the curriculum should include considerable attention to the association of distress with the development and course of physical illness for each of the major illnesses. At the very least, they should learn about the proposed neuroendocrine and immunological links from stress to physical illness and its outcomes. The limitations of the personality and adaptational research in guiding practice should also be a major part of the curriculum for these nurses. That is, while stress reduction will need to be an essential part of their practice, liaison nurses need to know that study of those individual strategies which reduce central arousal have yet to be accomplished.

Finally, for whatever reason, nursing has tended to train its doctoral students in fields other than the basic biological sciences; therefore, most are not prepared to conduct the laboratory research essential to participation in research that links the behavioral and biological. There is no doubt that nursing and its research agenda would be well served by a more balanced approach to the study of patients and by similarly balanced doctoral preparation. However, the research proposed in this chapter can also be accomplished through collaboration with basic scientists, and nurses should be encouraged to seek out such collaboration. In the near future these links will be critical if the necessary rigor in the design and implementation of laboratory approaches is to be accomplished.

The opportunities and challenges for nursing to keep pace with these new developments for integrating behavioral and biological science to better understand stress and illness associations are clear. Nursing's attention to them is in the nurses' best interest and in the best interest of the patients for whom they care.

REFERENCES

Affleck, G., Allen, D. A., Tennen, H., McGrade, B. J., & Ratzan, S. (1985). Causal and control cognitions in parent coping with a chronically ill child. *Journal of Social and Clinical Psychology, 3,* 367–377.

Bower, B. (1991). Questions of mind over immunity. *Science News, 139,* 216–217.

Cannon, W. B. (1914). The interrelations of emotions as suggested by recent physiological researchers. *American Journal of Psychology, 25,* 256–282.

Chiappelli, F. (1988). The "stress analogy" in the context of psychoneuroimmunology. *Schizophrenia Bulletin, 14*(2), 135–137.

Cohen, S., Tyrrell, D. A., & Smith, A. P. (1991). Psychological stress and susceptibility to the common cold. *The New England Journal of Medicine, 325*(9), 606–612.

Davis, D., Dunlop, S., Shea, P., Brittain, H., & Hendrie, H. (1985). Biological stress responses in high and low trait anxious students. *Biological Psychiatry, 20,* 843–851.

Elliott, G. R., & Eisdorfer, C. (1982). *Stress and human health.* New York: Springer.

Fawzy, F. I., Cousins, N., Fawzy, N., Elashoff, R., & Morton, D. (1990). A structured psychiatric intervention for cancer patients: 2. Changes over time in immunological measures. *Archives of General Psychiatry, 47*(8), 729–735.

Fell, D., Derbyshire, D., Maile, C., Larsson, I., Ellis, R., Achola, K., & Smith, G. (1985). Measurement of plasma catecholamine concentrations: An assessment of anxiety. *British Journal of Anaesthesia, 57,* 770–774.

Fittschen, K., Schulz, K. H., Schulz, H., Raedler, A., & Kerekjarto, M.V. (1990). Changes of immunological parameters in healthy subjects under examination stress. *International Journal of Neuroscience, 51,* 241–242.

Froese, A., Hackett, T. P., Cassem, N. H., & Silverberg, E. L. (1974). Trajectories of anxiety and depression in denying and nondenying acute myocardial infarction patients during hospitalization. *Journal of Psychosomatic Research, 18,* 413–420.

Garrity, T. F., & Klein, R. F. (1975). Emotional response and clinical severity as early determinants of six-month mortality after myocardial infarction. *Heart and Lung, 4*(5), 730–737.

Gentry, W. D., Foster, S., & Haney, T. (1972). Denial as a determinant of anxiety and perceived health status in the coronary care unit. *Psychosomatic Medicine, 34*(1), 39–44.

Graafsma, S. J., van Tits, B., Westerhof, R., Lenders, J. W., Rodrigues de Miranda, J. F., & Thien, T. (1987). Adrenoreceptor density on human blood cells and plasma catecholamines after mental arithmetic in normotensive volunteers. *Journal of Cardiovascular Pharmacology, 10*(Suppl. 4), 107–109.

Green, M. L., Green, R. G., & Santoro, W. (1988). Daily relaxation modifies serum and salivary immunoglobulins and psychophysiologic symptom severity. *Biofeedback and Self-Regulation, 13*(3), 187–198.

Green, R. G., & Green, M. L. (1987). Relaxation increases salivary immunoglobulin A. *Psychological Reports, 61,* 623–629.

Greer, S., & Watson, M. (1985). Towards a psychobiological model of cancer: Psychological considerations. *Social Science and Medicine, 20,* 773–777.

Greer, S., Pettingale, K. W., Morris, T., & Haybittle, J. (1985). Mental attitudes to cancer: An additional prognostic factor. *Lancet, 1,* 750.

Greer, S., Morris, T., & Pettingale, K. W. (1979). Psychological response to breast cancer: Effect on outcome. *Lancet, 2,* 785–787.

Gurklis, J. A., & Menke, E. M. (1988). Identification of stressors and use of coping methods in chronic hemodialysis patients. *Nursing Research, 37*(4), 236–239.

Hackett, T., Cassem, N., & Wishnie, H. (1968). The coronary-care unit: An appraisal of its psychologic hazards. *The New England Journal of Medicine, 279*(25), 1365–1370.

Hall, S. S. (1989). A molecular code links emotions, mind and health. *Smithsonian, 20*(3), 62–71.

Havik, O., & Maeland, J. G. (1988). Verbal denial and outcome in myocardial infarction patients. *Journal of Psychosomatic Research, 32*(2), 145–157.

Heider, F. (1958). *The psychology of interpersonal relations.* New York: Wiley.

Holland, J. C. (1991, October). *Psychosocial variables: Are they factors in cancer risk or survival?* Presented at "Current Concepts in Psycho-Oncology" Conference, New York.

Houldin, A. D., & Lowery, B. J. (1992). Emotional distress in breast cancer patients. *Med-Surg Nursing Quarterly, 1*(2), 1–28.

Jacobs, S., Brown, S., Mason, J., Wahby, V., Kasl, S., & Ostfeld, A. (1986). Psychological distress, depression and prolactin response in stressed persons. *Journal of Human Stress, 12*(3), 113–118.

Jacobs, S., Mason, J., Kostin, T., Brown, S., & Ostfeld, A. (1984). Urinary-free cortisol excretion in relation to age in acutely stressed persons with depressive symptoms. *Psychosomatic Medicine, 46,* 213–221.

Jasnoski, M. L., & Kugler, J. (1985). Relaxation, imagery and neuroimmunomodulation. *Annals of the New York Academy of Sciences, 496,* 722–730.

Kiecolt-Glaser, J. K., Garner, W., Speicher, C. E., Penn, G., & Glaser, R. (1984). Psychosocial modifiers of immunocompetence in medical students. *Psychosomatic Medicine, 46,* 7–14.

Kiecolt-Glaser, J. K., Glaser, R., Shuttleworth, E. C., Dyer, C. S., Ogrocki, P., & Speicher, C. E. (1987). Chronic stress and immunity in family caregivers of Alzheimer's disease victims. *Psychosomatic Medicine, 49,* 523–535.

Kiecolt-Glaser, J. K., Glaser, R., Strain, E. C., Stout, J. C., Tarr, K. L., Holliday, J. E., & Speicher, C. E. (1986). Modulation of cellular immunity in medical students. *Journal of Behavioral Medicine, 9,* 5–21.

Kiecolt-Glaser, J. K., Glaser, R., Williger, D., Stout, J., Messick, G., Sheppard, S., Ricker, D., Romisher, S. C., & Briner, W. (1985). Psychosocial enhancement of immunocompetence in a geriatric population. *Health Psychology, 4,* 25–41.

Kosten, T., Jacobs, S., & Mason, J. (1984). Psychological correlates of growth hormone response to stress. *Psychosomatic Medicine, 46,* 49–58.

Leidy, N. K. (1990). A structural model of stress, psychosocial resources, and symptomatic experience in COPD patients. *Nursing Research, 39*(4), 230–236.

Levy, S. M., Fernstrom, J., Herberman, R. B., Whiteside, T., Lee, J., Ward, M., & Massoudi, M. (1991). Persistently low natural killer cell activity and circulating levels of plasma beta endorphin: Risk factors for infectious disease. *Life Sciences, 48,* 107–116.

Levy, S. M., Herberman, R. B., Lippman, M., & d'Angelo, T. (1987). Correlation of stress factors with sustained depression of natural killer cell activity and predicted prognosis in patients with breast cancer. *Journal of Clinical Oncology, 5,* 348–353.

Levy, S., Herberman, R., Maluish, A., Schlien, B., & Lippman, M. (1985). Prognostic risk assessment in primary breast cancer by behavioral and immunological parameters. *Health Psychology, 4,* 99–113.

Levine, J., Warrenburg, S., Kerns, R., Schwartz, G., Delaney, R., Fontana, A., Gradman, A., Smith, S., Allen, S., & Cascione, R. (1987). The role of denial in recovery from coronary heart disease. *Psychosomatic Medicine, 49,* 109–117.

Lowery, B. J. (1991). Psychological stress, denial, and myocardial infarction outcomes. *Image, 23*(1), 51–53.

Lowery, B. J. (1987). Stress research: Some theoretical and methodological issues. *Image, 19*(1), 42–46.

Lowery, B. J., Jacobsen, B., & DuCette, J. (1993). Attributions, control and adjustment to breast cancer. *Psychosocial Oncology, 10*(4), 37–53.

Lowery, B., Jacobsen, B., & McCauley, K. (1987). On the prevalence of causal search in illness situations. *Nursing Research, 36,* 88–93.

Maio-Esteves, M. (1990). Mediators of daily stress and perceived health status in adolescent girls. *Nursing Research, 39*(6), 360–364.

Maki, T., Kontula, K., & Harkonen, M. (1990). The beta-adrenergic system in man: Physiological and pathophysiological response. *Scandinavian Journal of Clinical Laboratory Investigation, 50*(Suppl. 201), 25–43.

Mason, J. W. (1975). A historical view of the stress field. *Journal of Human Stress, 1*(1), Part II, 22–36.

Matthew, R., Beng, T., Taylor, D., & Semchuk, K. (1981). Catecholamine and dopamine-B-hydroxylase in anxiety. *Journal of Psychosomatic Research, 25,* 449–504.

McEwen, B. S., & Stellar, E. (1993). Stress and the individual. *Archives of General Medicine, 153,* 2093–2101.

Meininger, J. C., Hayman, L., Coates, P., & Gallagher, P. (1988). Genetics or environment? Type A behavior and cardiovascular risk factors in twin children. *Nursing Research, 37*(6), 341–346.

Michela, J., & Wood, J. (1986). Causal attributions in health and illness. *Advances in Cognitive-Behavioral Research and Therapy, 5,* 179–235.

Miller, W. B., & Rosenfeld, R. (1975). A psychophysiological study of denial following acute myocardial infarction. *Journal of Psychosomatic Research, 19,* 43–54.

Mills, P. J., & Dimsdale, J. F. (1988). The promise of receptor studies in psychophysiologic research. *Psychosomatic Medicine, 50,* 555–566.

Mills, P. J., Schneider, R. H., Hill, D., Walton, K. G., & Wallace, R. K. (1990). Beta-adrenergic receptor sensitivity in subjects practicing Transcendental Meditation. *Journal of Psychosomatic Research, 34*(1), 29–33.

Mullen, B., & Suls, J. (1982). The effectiveness of attention and rejection as coping styles: A meta-analysis of temporal differences. *Journal of Psychosomatic Research, 26*(1), 43–49.

Norbeck, J. S., & Anderson, J. N. (1989). Psychosocial predictors of pregnancy outcomes in low-income black, hispanic, and white women. *Nursing Research, 38*(4), 204–209.

Nowak, R. (1991). Windows on the brain: Cortisol secretion and depression. *The Journal of NIH Research, 3*(11), 62–67.

O'Leary, A. (1990). Stress, emotion, and human immune function. *Psychological Bulletin, 108*(3), 363–382.

Pennebaker, J. W., Kiecolt-Glaser, J. K., & Glaser, R. (1988). Disclosure of traumas and immune function: Health implications for psychotherapy. *Journal of Consulting and Clinical Psychology, 56*(2), 239–245.

Redd, W. H., Silberfarb, P. M., Andersen, B. L., Andrykowski, M. A., Bovbjerg, D. H., Burnish, T. G., Carpenter, P., Cleeland, C., Dolgin, M., Levy, S., Mitnick, L., Morrow, G., Schover, L., Spiegel, D., & Stevens, J. (1991). Physiologic and psychobehavioral research in oncology. *Cancer, 67,* 813–822.

Ruberman, W., Weinblatt, E., Goldberg, J., & Chadhary, B. (1984). Psychosocial influences on mortality after myocardial infarction. *The New England Journal of Medicine, 311,* 552–559.

Selye, H. (1956). *The stress of life.* New York: McGraw-Hill.

Silver, R., & Wortman, C. (1983). *The search for meaning among the recently disabled.* Unpublished Manuscript, University of Waterloo, Department of Psychology, Waterloo, Ontario, Canada.

Spiegel, D. (1993). Psychosocial intervention in cancer. *Journal of the National Cancer Institute, 85*(15), 1198–1205.

Strube, M. J. (Ed.). (1991). *Type A behavior.* Newbury Park: Sage.

Swartz, M. N. (1991). Stress and the common cold. *The New England Journal of Medicine, 325*(9), 654–656.

Taylor, S., Lichtman, R., & Wood, J. (1984). Attributions, beliefs about control, and adjustment to breast cancer. *Journal of Personality and Social Psychology, 46,* 489–502.

Temoshok, L. (1987). Personality coping style, emotion and cancer. Towards an integrative model. *Cancer Surveys, 6,* 545–567.

Temoshok, L. (1985). Biopsychosocial studies on cutaneous malignant melanoma: Psychosocial factors associated with prognostic indicators, progression, psychophysiology, and tumor-host response. *Social Science Medicine, 20,* 833–840.

Turnquist, D. C., Harvey, J. H., & Andersen, B. L. (1988). Attributions and adjustment to life-threatening illness. *British Journal of Clinical Psychology, 27,* 55–65.

Vaillant, G. E. (1971). Theoretical hierarchy of adaptive ego mechanisms. *Archives of General Psychiatry, 24,* 107–117.

van Doornen, L. J. P., & van Blokland, R. W. (1992). The relationship between cardiovascular and catecholamine reactions to laboratory and real-life stress. *Psychophysiology, 29*(2), 173–181.

Vollhardt, L. (1991). Psychoneuroimmunology: A literature review. *American Journal of Orthopsychiatry, 61*(1), 35–47.

Weiner, B. (1985). An attributional theory of achievement motivation and emotion. *Psychological Review, 42,* 548–573.

Weiner, B. (1979). A theory of motivation for some classroom experiences. *Journal of Educational Psychology, 71,* 3–25.

CHAPTER

3

Using the Brain
to Manage the Body

Helen Nakagawa-Kogan, PhD, RN, FAAN

ABSTRACT

This chapter considers how the newfound knowledge about the working of the brain can extend psychosocial nursing practice in a way that integrates care for the mind and care for the body. It focuses particularly on the role of self-management training for somatizing patients and the power of the brain on bodily processes in situations where clients are experiencing psychophysiologic hyperactivity, chronic disease, or increased vulnerability to accompanying disorders (e.g., AIDS). Indeed, if one thinks of illness as dysregulation (e.g., behavioral, cognitive, emotional, or psychophysiological), then self-management is a logical method of restoring regulation; the challenge is not for nurses to manage minds and bodies but to teach patients to manage their own, thereby achieving personal control over their cognitive/affective and physiological processes. A programmatic approach using self-monitoring and biofeedback is discussed, using hyperventilation as an illustration of the way in which emotions, perceptions, bodily arousal, and biochemical outcomes have an impact on a patient's symptomatology and general state of health and illness.

Challenging the boundaries of the present-day practice of psychiatric mental health is an important step. Nurses sense the need to make changes in response to new and important theories about the brain as they approach the midpoint in the decade of the brain. Undoubtedly, nurses will also want to change in response to important shifts in thinking about the way health care is delivered. The boundaries are appropriate concerns for the psychiatric nursing specialty for the remainder of the century.

This chapter addresses the issues of both the widening knowledge base and of the boundaries of nursing practice. Newfound knowledge about the working of the brain will extend psychosocial nursing practice in a way that closes the ranks between health care workers who care for the mind and those who care for the body. Once the rationale is fully developed for interfacing mind and body health care, one small step may point the way to a giant leap into a new health care that no longer separates mental illness from physical disorders.

This chapter therefore is about treatment of the brain. Nurses have found that persons can self-manage the mind and, with it, the body. Fritz Perls (Gestalt Therapy Verbatim, public source unknown) notes that:

> What is first to be considered is that the organism always works as a whole. We *have* not a liver or a heart. We *are* liver and heart and brain and so on, and even this is wrong. We are not a summation of parts, but a *coordination*—a very subtle coordination of all these different bits that go into making of the organism.

The body and mind act as a whole. Furthermore, if it were necessary to name the master control, it would have to be said that the brain is master. The integrative functions managed by the brain produce the dynamic homeostatic activity of the body, be it a pathologic homeostasis or a positive, healthy, functioning process. We need to be concerned with the study of the brain mechanisms that control the body's homeostatic processes during disease states and with emotional and bodily habits that trigger these brain mechanisms.

BRAIN-BODY INTERFACE
PSYCHOPHYSIOLOGIC PROCESSES

Not new, but newly discovered, is the power of the brain on bodily processes. Day by day, new findings emerge about the effects of brain functioning on health and illness. For example, alterations in immunocompetence during stress can be depicted by leukocyte inhibition. This neural mediation of immune responses, seen in the trajectory of illnesses such as cancer, depression, and autoimmune diseases, highlights the way in which brain processes interfere with immune action (Cohen, Tyrrell, & Smith, 1991; Eysenck, 1988; Glaser, Rice, Stout, & Kiecolt-Glaser, 1986; Levy, Herberman, & Lippman, 1991; Nerozzi et al., 1989). Additionally, in-depth study of cardiovascular activity now helps us to realize the effect of cortical functioning and sympathetic action upon cardiac output and, consequently, hypertension and left ventricular hypertrophy (Corea et al., 1984; Esler et al., 1986; Ferrara et al., 1989; Henry, 1986; Hollenberg, 1990).

Such findings serve to highlight the importance of human dynamic function and the way in which the brain manages the body. They also suggest how we might traverse the chasm between the two (mental and physical) health care systems by intervening with high-risk populations such as the bereaved who are prone to physical illnesses. Another population, one used as an example for this chapter, is patients showing evidence of stress responses, such as somatizing patients who the primary care health professionals seem to sense are "making themselves physically ill" or whose symptoms are stress related. We can directly intercede with these populations through behavioral intervention, thereby mitigating the neglect we have heretofore perpetuated while observing traditional boundaries of practice.

Certainly, we were not totally neglectful, but as psychiatric nurse specialists we have tended to focus on only one of two pathways by which the brain affects health. The pathway familiar to us is traced via cognitive-behavioral processes, wherein stressors produce dysfunctional emotions and ineffective coping behaviors. We have behavioral interventions for just such responses, such as crisis intervention and brief solution-focused treatment. However, this chapter addresses the need for extending nursing practice to incorporate the other major pathway of stress responses—the psychophysiologic processes. Steptoe (1991) suggests that under psychosocial stress at least three distinct processes can be outlined:

1. Psychophysiologic hyperreactivity, in which neuroendocrine arousal, sympathetic overactivity, and destabilized organ response depict a patterned, established disorder, such as in hypertension;
2. An impact upon chronic disease, influencing the disease stability or progression in an undesirable direction, as seen in the lability of diabetes or arthritis; and
3. Increased vulnerability of the host, making a stressed person more susceptible to other accompanying disorders, as seen in AIDS patients.

The suggestion is that these processes override the homeostatic pattern achieved through prior adaptation. This override produces a tenuous and dysfunctional pattern of psychophysiologic stress reaction and, over a prolonged time, generates chronic disease. Much of the literature about the psychophysiologic stress response traces the stressors-stress response paradigm as if it were etiologic. These studies examine coping, emotional reactions, and psychophysiologic responses as if they were direct effects of stressors, neglecting the chronic paradigm in which this dysfunctional state itself produces a neurally mediated pathophysiologic process, now a step removed from the implicated stressors. Thus, in most chronic major illnesses, it is possible to trace a configuration of symptoms that are neurally mediated, overlying and interacting with a pathophysiologic process (Johnson, Kalmilaris, Chrousos, & Gold, 1992).

This understanding of processes of the brain indicates that the brain contains the central adaptive resources for recovery from illnesses or from stress responses. Drugs and surgical intervention can intercede to alter pathologies that are derivatives of illnesses or stress responses. Psychotropic drugs, for example, can alter the biochemical environment in the neurally mediated depression that overlies physical disease. Although drugs can be plugged into this mechanical model of pathology, it does not finally get at the psychosocial cause of disease. New interventions will necessitate regard and consideration beyond the initial symptomatology and focus upon the behavioral and emotional changes that we believe will alter the psychopathophysiologic processes.

Louis Pasteur's germ theory guided a century of medical research, invoking a focus on the microorganism as the etiologic factor in disease. Yet Pasteur himself questioned, along with his contemporary, Claude Bernard, whether the microorganism or the body's equilibrium was more central to the disease trajectory. Together, they wondered if the terrain, the body environment, did not more crucially determine the outcome of infectious disease (Ornstein & Sobel, 1987). Now that infectious diseases no longer top the list of causes of mortality, we can see with clarity that the psychoneural regulation of the body and its biochemical and physiological substrate is the major factor in disease progression. This view reflects the new dawning of the kinds of disorders that we face—diseases of dysregulation. Patterns of dysregulation reflect the catabolic state of the brain, one in which self-regulatory mechanisms have failed in their compensatory neuroregulation.

Bergland (1985) has developed the concept of the brain as the most prolific gland in the human body. While a full inventory of the secretions is yet to be completed, several hundred have been identified so far. They perform everything from modulating pain (endorphins) to altering the immune function (gamma globulin and interferon). Other secretions nurture human development. But most remarkable of all is that these brain secretions can be stimulated or diminished by thought, behavior, and environment (Cousins, 1981). William James (1948) wrote: The greatest revolution of our generation is the discovery that human beings, by changing the inner attitudes of their minds, can change the outer aspects of their lives.

Self-Management Training

This litany of psychophysiologic theory suggests that many ill persons lack guidance in countering their own predilections for dysfunctional psychophysiologic processes. In sudden cardiac arrest, for example, after one event the likelihood of a second arrest is greatly enhanced due to the predisposition of the person for triggering a ventricular fibrillation. The staging for sudden cardiac arrest is set initially by cortical interference, leading to a marked imbalance of the sympathetic and parasympathetic drives. The resulting electrophysiologic instability in the cardiac muscle perpetrates ventricular fibrillation and sudden cardiac arrest (Lown, deSilva, & Lenson, 1978; Lown & Verrier, 1976; Skinner & Verrier, 1982). Subsequently, the predisposition for a second event of sudden cardiac arrest is recognized by indicators in heart-rate variability that show that the parasympathetic tone remains low and quite out of balance with the high sympathetic arousal that is manifested following the first event.

Self-management training consists of training the person to increase the parasympathetic tone, while recognizing at the same time how cortical processes enter into the sympathetic-parasympathetic imbalance. This training is achieved by focusing upon a bodily action that is under voluntary control, in this instance, breathing. Tracings of breathing by the pneumograph can reflect emotional status. Breathing is achieved not only by musculoskeletal activity but also by neural control. In turn, breathing impacts upon the respiratory sinus arrhythmia, an indicator of parasympathetic tone. The crux of self-management training for sudden cardiac arrest is, therefore, the fact that individuals can be trained to control their breathing. This can be done both through showing pneumographic feedback and by enhancing cognitive status, thereby training parasympathetic tone and heart-rate variability. In shaping interventions, it is important to recall that the psychophysiologic process belongs to the person, not to the disease. Hence, each patient's cognitive-neural-physiologic responses must be traced to establish the framework for treatment. Present intervention research on sudden cardiac arrest is derived from the belief that we can offer self-management training to change this risk factor (Cowan, Nakagawa-Kogan, Burr, Hendershot, & Buchanan, 1991).

Results of self-management research findings lie at the crux of nursing's dynamic future. In the psychiatric-psychosocial nursing field, we are in a key leadership position if we will absorb this mind-body nexus. Heretofore, we lacked understanding of the processes and nursing techniques by which to manage this unity. Now we have the theory and the skills (Nakagawa-Kogan & Beaton, 1982; Nakagawa-Kogan & Betrus, 1984; Nakagawa-Kogan, Garber, Egan, Jarrett, & Hendershot, 1988). Training patients to self-manage their bodily processes is a well-researched means of restoring health. If one thinks of illness as dysregulation, self-management is a logical method for restoring regulation. Dysregulation may be: (a) at a behavioral level, as in the dysfunctional coping of borderline personality disorder; (b) cognitive, as in schizophrenia; (c) emotional, as in depression; or (d) psychophysiological, as in hypertension. The goal of a self-management training program is to assist the individual in developing self-regulating skills as a self-healing effort. Nurses, regarded as facilitators of health, have embraced holistic health philosophically. As the professional caregivers who are closest to the patient, we must treat the mind and body together.

The theory and strategies for self-management training do not suggest we should manage minds and bodies; rather, we should teach patients to manage their own processes. An intervention of self-management training of cognitive/affective and physiologic processes provides a means for patients to achieve personal control over their bodies and health. In a classic article, Sterling and Eyer (1981) trace the treatment of chronic disease (e.g., hypertension) not only at the physiologic level but also the behavioral and the neocortical levels. The restoration of the health condition to its original state, Sterling and Eyer conclude, ultimately must rest upon the brain's delicate and rich system of control. "The interlocking, mutually reinforcing mechanisms by which the brain controls the body are "asked to achieve a great deal in mitigating the arousal generated from forces which are powerfully and deeply ingrained in our social structure and culture (Sterling & Eyer, 1981).

Self-management training programs need not use physiologic symptomatology as their only focus. Indeed, self-management training is gaining a strong foothold in care of psychiatric disorders, and it requires only one more step to expand the treatment mode to other patients. As a philosophic approach to the chronically mentally ill, self-management training was derived initially from the written experiences of patients with long-term schizophrenia who had learned to manage their symptoms and live long periods with symptom control (Lovejoy, 1984; Leete, 1989). Recently, considerable effort has been expended to develop reliable tools for measuring symptom management and to inaugurate programs for symptom self-management (Birchwood et al., 1989; Breier & Strauss, 1983; Carr, 1988; Clarke, Lewinsohn, & Hops, 1990; Cohen & Berk, 1985; Greenfield, Strauss, Bowers, & Mandelkorn, 1989; Herz, Glazer, Mirza, Mostert, & Hafez, 1989; Liberman, 1988; McCandless-Glimcher et al., 1986; Murphy & Moller, 1993; O'Connor, 1991; Schepp, 1992a, 1992b; Strauss, 1989; Tarell, 1989). Even here the bodily connection is not lost when teaching self-monitoring, since a window to the cognitive and mood status is opened by evaluating bodily tensions and strain as a way of recognizing cognitive disarray.

Research by Schepp makes elegant use of the family structure to teach psychotically ill adolescents a symptom self-management program (Schepp, 1992a, 1992b). The program aims to:

1. Increase the adolescents' awareness of their symptoms;
2. Increase their range of coping strategies for managing their symptoms;
3. Increase their ability to manage or control their symptoms;
4. Decrease the occurrence and severity of symptoms;
5. Increase their sense of control over their illnesses; and
6. Increase their level of functioning as they experience fewer and less severe symptoms in their illnesses. (Schepp, 1992a)

By training groups of families together with the affected adolescents, these researchers use the total family unit to teach self-management strategies and to prevent a downward trajectory of recidivism and chronicity of young psychotic adolescents. This program, while not in the domain of the psychophysiologic theme of this chapter, illustrates the span of activities in self-management programming.

Psychosocial nurses ought to take up the gauntlet of offering self-management training to patients who fall between the cracks of physical and psychiatric–mental health care services. Psychosocial nurses could serve a large array of patients who visit primary care providers with somatoform complaints and have emotional distress as a dominant problem. A practice could also include many patients with emotionally laden chronic diseases, among whom the lack of personal control is clearly demonstrated in somatization. Personal control, which is badly wanting in this sector of the population, can be repossessed. Indeed, the expanded practice could close the gap between physical and psychiatric care.

CONCEPTUAL THREADS IN SELF-MANAGEMENT TRAINING

At the heart of self-management training is the concept that the mind-body interface is a self-regulatory system, cycling through adaptive and maladaptive states. Maladaptation creates the conditions necessitating self-regulatory strategies, which have adaptation as their goal. A cogent paradigm by which to examine self-management is the work of Epstein (1983), who conceived of the natural healing processes of the mind as a way of placing adaptive-maladaptive processes into a longer-term perspective. Once it can be understood that novel experiences provide the background for adaptive mechanisms in subsequent encounters, the paradigm can be useful for thinking about intervening with persons suffering from chronic dysregulation.

Epstein lists three neural adaptive systems that persons use as a means for coping with each novel encounter: learning, regulation of arousal, and maintenance of an organized conceptual system. Each life encounter demands regulatory action by all of these neural adaptive systems, that is, acquisition of cognitive content. Completeness of cognitive content permits smooth interaction of the present encounter with successive ones, with automatic appraisal and adaptive emotional response, thus preventing the triggering of catecholamines and stimulation of the autonomic nervous system. Automatic reframing of a conceptual orientation maintains meaning and perspective.

The meaning of these neural adaptive systems is best illustrated through recognizing chronic maladaptive states, such as faulty learning, dysregulation through poor management of arousal, and disorder from threats to the integrity of the individual's conceptual system. An example of a chronic disorder of faulty learning is attention deficit disorder, wherein the inability to attend leads to inability to learn and to achieve in school. Chronic dysregulation in arousal can be seen in panic disorders, in which anxiety and subsequent surges of catecholamines elicit the generalized behavior of flight. Disorder of the conceptual system is evident in thought process disorders such as schizophrenic reactions.

Tracing the process of acquiring reregulation in each disorder exemplifies how self-management training plans are generated. Targets of self-management training are:

- Social-environmental events
- Personal control
- Cognitive appraisal
- Social support
- Central nervous system functions
- Limbic system functions
- Information-processing feedback
- Emotional responses
- Behavioral and end-organ responses
- Neurally mediated physical responses
- Coping with perceived stressors

To describe self-management training fully demands an iteration of the concept of self-management. Afterwards, examples of reregulation using these target foci will expand the practice strategies.

CONCEPTION OF SELF-MANAGEMENT TRAINING

Self-management training for clients has multiple roots. Drawn predominantly from social learning and cognitive theories, it is buttressed by psychophysiologic research and spurred by the insatiable desire of the new consumerism to participate in health care. While it is a philosophy of care in one sense, self-management training is also a specified group of intervention techniques that are compatible with that care philosophy.

SELF-REGULATION

The dominant umbrella concept of self-management training interventions is self-regulation. Self-regulation is an automatic feedback system that runs effectively until novel input requires a feed-forward effort. Left unabated, a negative sign or symptom that is fed forward may force the body to achieve a reregulated state, sometimes a pathologic equilibrium. The stress response is an example. Henry (1992) notes that while a challenge perceived as easy to manage will elicit an initial active coping response and accompanying release of norepinephrine, difficulties in managing the task will change the neuroendocrine parameters. In the animal model, the path toward pathologic reregulation begins with threat. As anxiety rises, the norepinephrine-epinephrine ratio decreases; as distress grows, cortisol levels rise and a passive mode of coping is observable. Further, the ratio of catecholamines to corticoids decreases as frustration and uncertainty grow. Finally, the model of posttraumatic stress syndrome emerges, with repression and denial expressed in impaired attachment and increased irritability. The corticoids paradoxically return to normal, but lasting emotional trauma remains. Such reregulation is abundant in the patient populations treated by this author, but the model also fits for the less traumatized. When anxiety, anger, and depression are dominant features, intervention by self-management training could aptly apply.

PERSONAL CONTROL

Personal control is the cornerstone in the goal orientation of self-management training. In a dysregulated condition, the threat of lack of control is great. In the face of a sense of loss of personal control, predictability of adaptation is tenuous. It reflects upon self-competence. Pennebaker, Burnam, Schaeffer, and Harper (1977), very early in their series of studies of somatic complaints, found a relationship between perception of control and the incidence of physical complaints. The mechanism of symptomatology, furthermore, seems to be unrelated to physiologic functioning but related to understanding of events, prediction, and control (Pennebaker et al., 1977; Tetrick & LaRocco, 1987).

A signal that self-management training is a success is restoration of personal control. Indeed, an operational analysis of personal control suggests that one can measure indicators such as the following: behavioral control in ability to influence or modify events; cognitive control by processing information so as to reduce the cost of adaptation; and decision control through taking opportunities to choose from a number of courses of action. Personal control is clearly a matter of central focus in self-management training.

BIOFEEDBACK

Biofeedback is a basic health care tool, although it is not always labeled as such, or used to its maximum advantage. Clinicians feed weight, temperature, and blood pressure measures back to patients. Just as we use photos, mirrors, or audiovisual tapes to inform persons of their health status, we could use biofeedback for patients with eating disorders, depression, or anxiety states, but more formal biofeedback has made little linkage with the everyday tools at our fingertips. Instead, it has relied on psychophysiologic feedback—for which much instrumentation to measure digital temperature, electromyograph readings, and skin conductance has been developed—with little consideration of the meaning of feedback to holistic health or illness.

Much of the success in biofeedback treatment has to do with the conceptual approach to the training. The roots of biofeedback training are in operant conditioning theory, embracing a limited concept of neural training without recognizing the cognitive-affective components critical to present-day theory. Tursky (1982) notes that biofeedback training is more than merely physiologic training of neural pathways. Rather, it is a cognitive event, that is, information processing of biological signals. Feedback enables the subject to become conscious of the interface among bodily status, environmental events, and internal cognitive information and provides behavioral strategies to alter physiologic activity (Tursky, 1982; Schwartz, 1982).

Biofeedback training that employs self-management training fits easily into the nursing domain. Principles include placing the burden of responsibility for change upon the patient, but offering ways to document his/her changes in status and strategies for achieving change (Kanfer, 1991; Nakagawa-Kogan & Betrus, 1984). Brener (1982) maintains that most biofeedback is practiced using a calibration mode, that is, feedback is compared to baseline status and only changes in biological signals receive attention. Unfortunately, this calibration mode is only oriented to the afferent stimuli arising from the peripheral system and directed *toward* the central nervous system, whereas it is also important to focus on the mechanisms arising from afferent activity that alter the biological signals, that is, the central cortical, limbic, and autonomic nervous system activity directed *away from* the central organ.

If biological signals are to be used, the more specific, immediate, and continuous they are, the more effectively one can examine the neural-metabolic mechanisms. For example, in hypertension self-management–biofeedback training, we focus on heart-rate training as a reflection of cardiovascular activity due to sympathetic arousal. The plethysmograph is used as feedback of heart rate, and the training uses abdominal respiratory training (with pneumograph feedback) to alter respiratory sinus arrhythmia, thus affecting heart rate. However, the critical feature is the use of self-management training strategies to alter cognitive-affective events and sympathetic arousal. In this way a holistic approach to hypertension is achieved.

KANFER'S PROGRAMMATIC APPROACH

It may be saying the obvious to suggest that a programmatic approach is imperative in establishing a contract with a client. In a change program where modification of behavior is desired, Kanfer (1991) notes that inherent in the elements of the program are the processes to be acquired by the self-managing client. They consist of the following:

1. A self-monitoring or self-observation period wherein the client must define the behavior to be measured or altered, count the frequency, and note circumstances of the occurrence;
2. Establishment of a set of criteria or standards by which to develop goals and to measure success;
3. Acquisition of self-awareness and discrimination of functional levels for self-evaluation, based on careful feedback and documentation of changes in behavior; and
4. Administration of self-reinforcement, with rewards based on successful changes in behavior and prior establishment of extrinsic rewards to help bolster the intrinsic reward derived from behavior modification.

EXAMPLES OF DISORDERS TREATABLE IN EXPANDED PSYCHOSOCIAL NURSING PRACTICES

Somatization is the broad term used to describe the numerous physical symptoms generated or augmented by emotions such as depression, anxiety, or anger. In this section, the term somatization is defined, and the syndrome of hyperventilation is used to illustrate how psychosocial nursing can make both physiologic and psychosocial interventions.

SOMATIZATION

Somatization is the tendency to experience discomfort in physical form in response to psychosocial distress. In any week, 80% of healthy individuals experience somatic symptoms (Pennebaker, Burman, Schaeffer, & Harper, 1977). The more affected persons, those with recurring or enduring bodily complaints, visit general practitioners (from 10 to 30% of visits) who substantiate no detectable physical cause (Kellner, 1986, 1990). This does not mean that no physical pathology concurrently exists; it simply means the physical pathology is not directly causally linked.

Somatization, neither a disorder nor a diagnostic category in its more transient form, is a process that subsumes a wide range of clinical phenomena such as depression, anxiety, and panic states. It may signal a more severe disease entity as a precursor of a developing psychiatric illness, or it may be an early-stage chronic disorder such as systemic lupus erythematosus or multiple sclerosis (Lipowski, 1987).

The clinical picture of a somatizing patient is one who has multiple complaints in multiple organ systems. The complaints are vague, not coherently related, and often generalized, including fatigue, dizziness, shortness of breath, palpitations, insomnia, and pain (Rasmussen & Avant, 1989). A common component is overt emotionality, an expression of distress not in proportion to the illness complaints (Katon, Kleinman, & Rosen, 1982). More often, symptoms cluster in one body system, giving rise to chronic states of somatoform disorders, such as mitral valve prolapse, irritable bowel syndrome, and fibromyalgia. However, it is unwise to negate the physiologic component of somatization, even though symptoms associate poorly with physiologic conditions. As in hyperventilation, some physiologic or biochemical changes may indeed explain some of the symptomatology (Fried, 1987; Kellner, 1990).

One reason treatment of these extended somatic complaints ought to be relevant for nurses with a psychosocial bent is the association of this display with manifestations of depression and anxiety. Somatoform pain is almost consistently associated with depression. Pain is one of the most manifest complaints in a general practice, and its consistent positive correlation with depression is striking (Cadoret, Widmer, & Troughton, 1980; Katon, Kleinman, & Rosen, 1982; Kellner, 1986, 1990, 1991). In fact, some authors describe somatization as an equivalent of masked depression (Katon, Kleinman, & Rosen, 1982). Anxiety is also described as a component of somatic complaints. Somatic complaints are invariably more numerous in persons with anxiety disorders than in normal subjects. Chest pain, palpitations, dyspepsia, headaches, dizziness, fainting, and dyspnea are common presenting complaints when anxiety is somatized (Lipowski, 1987).

The somatizing expression of disorders that are essentially of emotional origin is a dilemma for primary care practitioners whose orientation and structure of practice do not easily fit behavioral approaches to care. Perceptual or emotional responses accompanying somatic complaints are rarely managed and are difficult to change when primary care practitioners do attempt such alteration (Mabe, Jones, &

Riley, 1990). Yet it is the primary care practitioner who usually manages somatization phenomena. Still, many primary care professionals would prefer not to manage these phenomena; for them, the goal in self-management of preventing reinforcement of symptoms or altering coping strategies is counterintuitive to their usual orientation of aiming toward removal of symptoms (Purcell, 1991; Morrison, 1990).

A natural intermediary is a nurse who accepts self-management training as his or her talent, thereby helping patients to self-manage their somatic symptoms. The theoretic underpinnings of self-management intervention—which incorporate an integrated psychopathophysiologic theory, cognitive-affective theory, and biological feedback—can serve as the foundation for nursing practice.

EXAMPLE: THE PSYCHOPATHOPHYSIOLOGY OF HYPERVENTILATION

The psychopathophysiology of hyperventilation is outlined here as an illustration of the way in which emotions, perceptions, bodily arousal, and biochemical outcomes have an impact on the symptomatology and general state of health and illness. Hyperventilation exemplifies how maladaptive respirations as a consequence of anxiety can upset the body's homeostatic balance. Hyperventilation, a complex breathing activity triggered by anxiety, involves shallow thoracic breathing that is irregular in rhythm and cycles that contain sighing, gasps, and overbreathing. These produce the hyperventilation challenge, that is, a body response composed of dizziness, faintness, vertigo, tachycardia, chest pains, syncope, and even tetany. While hyperventilation breathing might be observable in some patients, the dysrhythmic breathing in chronic hyperventilation is more often subtle, and the clinical state is more often suspected on the basis of a broader clinical pattern with accompanying emotional distress. In fact, Fried (1987, 1993) notes that more often fainting and vague cardiovascular symptoms rather than dyspnea or exaggerated breathing signal hyperventilation. An excellent validation method is examination of the gas composition of end-tidal air. If $PaCO_2$ is low (below 37 mm Hg), the hyperventilation diagnosis can be verified (Bass & Gardner, 1985). Hyperventilation presents not only patterned somatic complaints such as palpitations, chest pain, and dizziness but also an outcome of metabolic acid-base imbalance.

Hyperventilation provides an illustration, par excellence, for demonstrating that a focus on changing a physical habit can correct the pathophysiology and even allay the anxiety that may have produced the dysregulation in the first place. But somatic symptoms do interfere with attending to emotional distress. They absorb all the focus and can lock the primary health practitioner into that focus as well. The skill in self-management training is to break that deadlock and engage the patient in self-managing the appropriate problem—in this case, anxiety.

The psychophysiology of hyperventilation illuminates the somatization process in a way that allows us to link psychophysiology with self-management training. The fact that breathing is a process that is readily brought under voluntary control simplifies this illustration. Somatization is less readily traceable in, for example, the gastrointestinal and neurologic systems. Nonetheless, it is an important concept for practitioners who attend to symptom patterns that bridge the psychophysiologic interface.

A self-management training program extrapolates the behavior, cognitions, emotional responses, and physical signs that will be the targets for self-regulation. The training protocol makes clear the changes that must be made. It further stipulates the activities that must be undertaken and skills that must be acquired to reduce the disorder and reproduce the reregulated state (Nakagawa-Kogan & Beaton,

1982). For hyperventilation, the ultimate focus of self-management is management of anxiety, which is easily demonstrated by psychophysiologic indices such as skin conductance. Learning to make skin conductance decrease demands that sensitization to anxiety habits be recognized and that methods of countering anxiety be instituted. Even without biofeedback, consciousness of habit patterns can be developed, and instituting bodily methods to reduce arousal can be a strategic measure. Relaxation methods such as autogenic training, the quieting response, or deep breathing are all aimed at lowering arousal, thus reducing anxiety. Small targets can be readily extracted and micromanaged in an attempt to obtain holistic self-management.

Behavioral habits are fundamental focal issues in all self-management training interventions. Basic to self-management training is self-monitoring. Often, self-monitoring not only provides a baseline but also heightens self-awareness. Having the baseline awareness of the frequency of habits or symptoms offers a client definable measures by which to determine change and success. Such psychometric indicators as anxiety, depression, and interpersonal sensitivity serve as psychological assessments of change. Additionally, some physiologic indicators (electromyograph readings, skin conductance, digital temperature levels, weight, blood pressure, and heart rate, for example) offer feedback for amount of change in a client's physical status. If unavailable, however, they are unnecessary. Behavioral guidance consists of counseling using emotion desensitization, cognitive change techniques, and training for physiologic control. The latter may include such diverse feedback as blood pressure, temperature, heart rate, weight, mirror images, and even photos.

APPLYING A PROGRAMMATIC APPROACH

A programmatic approach to hyperventilation involves a contractual agreement of a goal to be achieved within a time frame. The contractual agreement might encompass not only developing self-awareness of responses to social encounters but also possibly changing the social circumstances themselves. A program might consist of the following:

1. Contractual agreement of self-change:
   a. Taking baseline measure of quality of breathing patterns every hour of the day, to change to increased depth and decreased rate
   b. Changing life-style to alter types of social situations encountered
   c. Altering life-style to include some aerobic exercise
   d. Learning problem solving to reduce anxiety state
2. A self-monitoring program and recording system to observe breathing pattern hourly throughout the training period
3. Criteria for measuring success in altering anxiety, that is, changes in psychophysiologic reduction of arousal, breathing pattern, and exercise
4. Self-awareness of style of abdominal breathing, sighing, holding breath, and shallow upper chest respirations
5. Therapeutic approach combining cognitive-affective strategies with problem-solving skills and psychophysiologic feedback
6. Gauging a self-reward system that promotes self-esteem, such as promising oneself a new piece of clothing that can be worn as a reminder of success

The targets of change for hyperventilation are the following:

1. Achieving personal control through changing physiologic behavior
2. Changing appraisals of threat by reframing situations to be nonthreatening
3. Strengthening social support by learning reciprocal networking

4. Biofeedback training of breathing patterns using abdominal and chest pneumography; use of capnograph to measure end-stage CO_2 and oxygenation (if technology is available)
5. Changing anxiety levels and/or autonomic nervous system arousal (using digital temperature or skin conductance)
6. Learning problem solving by promoting alternative views to offer choices of action

In developing an intervention in self-management training, it is clear that unless the client is dedicated to setting goals and taking responsibility for achieving them, success cannot be achieved. Therefore, as much as possible is put into writing. Not only does this achieve the end of having the client self-monitor but it also records changes in concrete terms. As much as possible is quantified, even though these symptoms and emotions are subjective. Appendix 3-1 includes a number of examples of paper work, including a self-contract, three examples of various symptoms and emotions to be monitored, an exercise in the quieting response, and progress notes for use by the therapist.

Outcome measures are of paramount importance in this type of approach, since success in self-management training is in part demonstrated through outcome changes that indicate an increase of personal control and reduction of symptoms. Appendix 3-2 includes the Symptoms of Stress Inventory for pre- and postevaluation developed by Maxine Leckie and Elaine Thompson at their Management of Stress Response Clinic. This inventory has been widely and successfully used in research around the world, having been translated, to date, into five languages. Validation and reliability studies demonstrate that it taps the emotions highly correlated to those in the Symptom Check List-90R. The scale is useful in that it additionally taps the physical symptoms evident in stress-response disorders. The scale has 10 subscales: peripheral manifestations, cardiopulmonary symptoms of arousal, central neurological symptoms, gastrointestinal symptoms, muscle tension, habitual patterns, depression, anxiety/fear, anger, and cognitive disorganization. The items have been shown to be quite reliable to reflect change as a result of self-management interventions.

A cumulative record of personal control, important to this training, is not supplied here for copyright reasons, but many are capable of serving this purpose. Indeed, nothing is so impelling as a chart that records the progressive changes in physiologic measures, if these measures are included in the self-management training program.

Finally, it is important for a clinic to have ongoing evaluation of its therapy sessions. To accomplish this, an evaluation of a treatment session—filled out by the client and given to the secretary—can be kept separate from the clinical chart and not accessible to the therapist. An example of the evaluation and summary developed by Dr. Patricia Betrus appears in Appendix 3-3.

SUMMARY

Somatizing patients are prime candidates for self-management training. The rationale for using such training with somatic responses is fairly straightforward and readily acknowledged. Dysregulatory stress patterns such as hyperventilation; chronic head, neck, and back pain; migraines; hypertension; ambulatory urinary incontinence; and the mood disorders mentioned already all have significantly successful self-management training protocols. Protocols for schizophrenia, posttraumatic stress syndrome, attention deficit disorder, labile diabetes, and irritable bowel syndrome are still being developed. Although research has not demonstrated that clients have much conscious control of their mechanisms and symptoms, these conditions hold promise of responding to self-management programs.

What nurses know about the brain in action, combined with extending their practice arena, will clearly position them for a new health care delivery approach, particularly should it involve managed care. Nurses must join in as the new health care delivery model emerges, keeping their eyes on the critical feature of the mind-body interface.

REFERENCES

Bass, C., & Gardner, W. N. (1985). Respiratory and psychiatric abnormalities in chronic symptomatic hyperventilation. *British Medical Journal, 290,* 1387–1390.

Bergland, R. (1985). *The fabric of the mind.* Middlesex, England: Viking Penguin.

Birchwood, M., Smith, J., MacMillan, F., Hogg, B., Prasad, R., Harvey, C., & Bering, S. (1989). Predicting relapse in schizophrenia: The development and implementation of an early signs monitoring system using patients and families as observers—A preliminary investigation. *Psychological Medicine, 19,* 649–656.

Breier, A., & Strauss, J. (1983). Self-control in psychotic disorders. *Archives of General Psychiatry, 40,* 1141–1145.

Brener, J. M. (1982). Psychobiologic mechanisms in biofeedback. In L. White & B. Tursky (Eds.), *Clinical biofeedback: Efficacy and mechanisms* (pp. 24–48). New York: Guilford.

Cadoret, R. J., Widmer, R. B., & Troughton, E. P. (1980). Somatic complaints—Harbinger of depression in primary care. *Journal of Affective Disorders, 2,* 61–70.

Carr, V. (1988). Patients' techniques for coping with schizophrenia: An exploratory study. *British Journal of Medical Psychology, 61,* 339–352.

Clarke, G., Lewinsohn, P., & Hops, H. (1990). *Adolescents coping with depression course.* Eugene, OR: Castalia.

Cohen, C., & Berk, L. (1985). Personal coping styles of schizophrenic outpatients. *Hospital and Community Psychiatry, 36,* 407–410.

Cohen, S., Tyrrell, D. A., & Smith, A. P. (1991). Psychological stress and susceptibility to the common cold. *The New England Journal of Medicine, 325*(9), 606–612.

Corea, L., Bentivoglio, M., Verdecchia, P., & Montolese, M. (1984). Plasma norepinephrine and left ventricular hypertrophy in systemic hypertension. *American Journal of Cardiology, 53,* 441–445.

Cousins, N. (1981). *Human options.* New York: Norton.

Cowan, M. J., Nakagawa-Kogan, H., Burr, R., Hendershot, S., & Buchanan, L. (1991). Power spectral analysis of heart rate variability after biofeedback training. *Journal of Electrocardiology, 23*(Suppl.), 85–94.

Epstein, S. (1983). Natural healing processes of the mind: Graded stress inoculation as an inherent coping mechanism. In D. Meichenbaum & M. Jamerko (Eds.), *Stress reduction and prevention* (pp. 39–66). New York: Plenum.

Esler, M., Jennings, G., Biviano, B., Lambert, G., & Hasking, G. (1986). Mechanism of elevated plasma noradrenaline in the course of essential hypertension. *Journal of Cardiovascular Pharmacology, 8*(Suppl. 5), S39–S43.

Eysenck, H. J. (1988). Personality, stress and cancer. *British Journal of Medical Psychology, 61,* 57–75.

Ferrara, L. A., Mancini, M., de Simone, G., Pisanti, N., Capone, D., Fasono, M. L., & Mancini, M. (1989). Adrenergic nervous system and left ventricular mass in primary hypertension. *European Heart Journal, 10,* 1036–1040.

Fried, R. (1987). *The hyperventilation syndrome.* Baltimore and London: The Johns Hopkins University Press.

Fried, R. (1993). The role of respiration in stress and stress control: Toward a theory of stress as a hypoxic phenomenon. In P. Lehrer & R. Woolfolk (Eds.), *Principles and practice of stress management* (2nd ed.) (pp. 301–332). New York: Guilford.

Glaser, R., Rice, J., Stout, J. C., & Kiecolt-Glaser, J. K. (1986). Stress depresses interferon production by leucocytes concomitant with a decrease in natural killer cell activity. *Behavioral Neuroscience, 100,* 675–678.

Greenfield, D., Strauss, J., Bowers, M., & Mandelkorn, M. (1989). Insight and interpretation of illness in recovery from psychosis. *Schizophrenic Bulletin, 15,* 245–252.

Herz, M., Glazer, W., Mirza, M., Mostert, M., & Hafez, H. (1989). Treating prodromal episodes to prevent relapse in schizophrenia. *British Journal of Psychiatry, 155*(5), 123–127.

Henry, J. P. (1992). Biological basis of the stress response. *Integrative Physiological and Behavioral Science, 27*(1), 66–83.

Henry, J. P. (1986). Mechanisms by which stress can lead to coronary heart disease. *Post Graduate Medical Journal, 62,* 687–693.

Hollenberg, N. K. (1990). Management of hypertension: Considerations involving cardiovascular risk reduction. *Journal of Cardiovascular Pharmacology, 15*(Suppl. 5), S73–S78.

James, W. (1948). *Psychology.* New York: World Publishing.

Johnson, E. O., Kalmilaris, T. C., Chrousos, G. P., & Gold, P. W. (1992). Mechanisms of stress: A dynamic overview of hormonal and behavioral homeostasis. *Neuroscience and Biobehavioral Reviews, 16,* 115–130.

Kanfer, F. H. (1991). Self-management methods. In F. H. Kanfer & A. P. Goldstein (Eds.), *Helping people change* (pp. 305–360). New York: Pergamon.

Katon, E. S., Kleinman, A., & Rosen G. (1982). Depression and somatization: A review, part I. *American Journal of Medicine, 72,* 127–135.

Kellner, R. (1991). *Psychosomatic syndromes and somatic symptoms.* Washington, DC: American Psychiatric Press.

Kellner, R. (1986). *Somatization and hypochondriasis.* New York: Praeger-Greenwood.

Kellner, R. (1990). Somatization: The most costly comorbidity? In J. D. Maser & C. R. Cloninger (Eds.), *Comorbidity of mood and anxiety disorders* (pp. 239–252). Washington, DC: American Psychiatric Press.

Leete, E. (1989). How I perceive and manage my illness. *Schizophrenia Bulletin, 15*(2), 197–200.

Levy, S. M., Herberman, R. B., & Lippman, M. (1991). Immunological and psychological predictors of disease recurrence in patients with early-stage breast cancer. *Behavioral Medicine, 17*(2), 67–75.

Liberman, R. (1988). Coping with chronic mental disorders: A framework for hope. In R. Liberman (Ed.), *Psychiatric rehabilitation of chronic mental patients* (pp. 2–28). Washington, DC: American Psychiatric Press.

Lipowski, Z. J. (1987). Somatization: The experience and communication of psychological distress as somatic symptoms. *Psychotherapy and Psychosomatics, 47,* 160–167.

Lovejoy, M. (1984). Recovery from schizophrenia: A personal odyssey. *Hospital and Community Psychiatry, 35,* 809–812.

Lown, B., deSilva, R. A., & Lenson, R. (1978). Roles of psychologic stress and autonomic nervous system changes in provocation of ventricular premature complexes. *American Journal of Cardiology, 41,* 979–985.

Lown, B., & Verrier, R. (1976). Neural activity and ventricular fibrillation. *The New England Journal of Medicine, 294,* 1165–1170.

Mabe, P. A., Jones, L. R., & Riley, W. T. (1990). Managing somatization phenomena in primary care. *Psychiatric Medicine, 8*(4), 117–127.

McCandless-Glimcher, L., McKnight, S., Hamera, E., Smith, B., Peterson, K., & Plumlee, A. (1986). Use of symptoms by schizophrenics to monitor and regulate their illness. *Hospital and Community Psychiatry, 37,* 929–933.

Morrison, J. (1990). Managing somatization disorder. *Disease of the Month, 36*(10), 542–591.

Murphy, M., & Moller, M. (1993). Relapse management in neurobiological disorders: The Moller-Murphy Symptom Management Assessment. *Archives of Psychiatric Nursing, 7,* 226–235.

Nakagawa-Kogan, H., & Beaton, R. (1982). Blending of a conceptual model and nursing practice. In *From accommodation to self-determination: Nursing's role in the development of health care policy* (pp. 28–67). Kansas City, KS: Academy of Nursing.

Nakagawa-Kogan, H., & Betrus, P. (1984). Self-management: A nursing mode of therapeutic influence. *Advances in Nursing Science, 6*(4), 55–73.

Nakagawa-Kogan, H., Garber, A., Egan, K., Jarrett, M., & Hendershot, S. (1988). Hypertension self-regulation: Predictors of success in diastolic blood pressure reduction. *Research in Nursing and Health, 11,* 105–115.

Nerozzi, D., Santoni, A., Bersani, G., Magnani, A., Bressan, A., Pasini, A., Antonozzi, I., & Grajese, G. (1989). Reduced natural killer cell activity in major depression: Neuroendocrine implications. *Psychoneuroendocrinology, 14,* 295–301.

O'Connor, R. (1991). Symptom monitoring for relapse prevention in schizophrenia. *Archives in Psychiatric Nursing, 5*(4), 193–201.

Ornstein, R., & Sobel, D. (1987). *The healing brain.* New York: Simon & Schuster.

Pennebaker, J. W., Burnam, M. A., Schaeffer, M. A., & Harper, D. C. (1977). Lack of control as a determinant of perceived physical symptoms. *Journal of Personality and Social Psychology, 35*(3), 167–174.

Purcell, T. B. (1991). The somatic patient: Psychiatric aspects of emergency medicine. *Emergency Medical Clinics of North America, 9*(1), 137–159.

Rasmussen, N. H., & Avant, R. F. (1989). Somatization disorder in family practice. *Association of Family Practice Practical Therapeutics, 40*(2), 206–214.

Schepp, K. G. (1992a). A symptom management program for adolescents with psychotic illnesses: Theoretical basis. *Journal of Child and Adolescent Psychiatirc and Mental Health Nursing, 5*(4), 7–12.

Schepp, K. G. (1992b). A symptom management program for psychotically ill adolescents and their families: Preliminary clinical outcomes. *Journal of Child and Adolescent Psychiatric and Mental Health Nursing, 5*(4), 13–17.

Schwartz, G. (1982). Testing the biopsychosocial model: The ultimate challenge. *Journal of Consulting and Clinical Psychology, 50,* 1040–1053.

Skinner, J. E., & Verrier, R. L. (1982). Task force report on sudden cardiac death and arrhythmias. In O. Smith, R. Galosy, & S. Weiss (Eds.), *Circulation, neurobiology and behavior* (pp. 309–316). New York: Elsevier Science.

Steptoe, A. (1991). The links between stress and illness. *Journal of Psychosomatic Research, 35*(6), 633–644.

Sterling, P., & Eyer, J. (1981). Biological basis of stress-related mortality. *Social Science and Medicine, 15,* 1–42.

Strauss, J. (1989). Mediating processes in schizophrenia. *British Journal of Psychiatry, 155*(5), 22–28.

Tarell, J. (1989). Self-regulation of symptoms in schizophrenia: Psychoeducational interventions for clients and families. In J. Maurin (Ed.), *Chronic mental illness: Coping strategies* (pp. 151–186). Thorofare, NJ: Slack.

Tetrick, L. E., & LaRocco, J. M. (1987). Understanding, prediction and control as moderators of the relationships between perceived stress, satisfaction and psychological well-being. *Journal of Applied Psychology, 72*(4), 538–543.

Tursky, B. (1982). An engineering approach to biofeedback. In L. White & B. Tursky (Eds.), *Clinical biofeedback: Efficacy and mechanisms* (pp. 108–126). New York: Guilford.

3-1

PROGRESS NOTES

Client # _____   Date _____

Session # _____   Training Modality _____

1. SUBJECTIVE - Symptom Activity - Client's Description

2. OBJECTIVE - Psychophysiologic Data - Trainer's Observations

3. ASSESSMENT - Postsession (Client and/or Trainer)

4. PLAN - Summary and Recommendations

Clinician Signature: _____
_____
Courtesy Helen Nakagawa-Kogan.

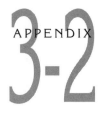

APPENDIX

3-2

SYMPTOMS OF STRESS INVENTORY
A SELF-ASSESSMENT

This questionnaire is designed to measure the different ways people respond to stressful situations. The questions deal with various physical, psychological, and behavioral responses. We are particularly interested in the frequency with which you may have experienced these stress-related symptoms during the past week.

Check one: [ ] Screening   [ ] Exit   [ ] 6 Month   [ ] 1 Year

Please circle the most appropriate response to each question.

Sometimes people under stress experience a variety of physical responses. During the designated period have you been bothered by:	NEVER	INFREQUENTLY	SOMETIMES	OFTEN	VERY FREQUENTLY
1. Flushing of your face	0	1	2	3	4
2. Sweating excessively even in cold weather	0	1	2	3	4
3. Severe itching	0	1	2	3	4
4. Skin rashes	0	1	2	3	4
5. Breaking out in cold sweats	0	1	2	3	4
6. Cold hands or feet	0	1	2	3	4
7. Hot or cold spells	0	1	2	3	4
Have you noticed any of the following symptoms when not exercising:					
8. Pains in your heart or chest	0	1	2	3	4
9. Thumping of your heart	0	1	2	3	4
10. Rapid or racing heart beats	0	1	2	3	4
11. Irregular heart beats	0	1	2	3	4
12. Rapid breathing	0	1	2	3	4
13. Difficult breathing	0	1	2	3	4
14. A dry mouth	0	1	2	3	4

Courtesy Maxine S. Leckie and Elaine Thompson.

	NEVER	INFREQUENTLY	SOMETIMES	OFTEN	VERY FREQUENTLY

Have you experienced:

	NEVER	INFREQUENTLY	SOMETIMES	OFTEN	VERY FREQUENTLY
15. Having to clear your throat often	0	1	2	3	4
16. A choking lump in your throat	0	1	2	3	4
17. Hoarseness	0	1	2	3	4
18. Nasal stuffiness	0	1	2	3	4
19. Colds	0	1	2	3	4
20. Colds with complications (e.g., bronchitis)	0	1	2	3	4
21. Increased asthma attacks	0	1	2	3	4
22. Sinus headaches	0	1	2	3	4

Have you experienced:

	NEVER	INFREQUENTLY	SOMETIMES	OFTEN	VERY FREQUENTLY
23. Spells of severe dizziness	0	1	2	3	4
24. Feeling faint	0	1	2	3	4
25. Blurring of your vision	0	1	2	3	4
26. Migraine headaches	0	1	2	3	4
27. Increased seizures (convulsions)	0	1	2	3	4

Have you been bothered by:

	NEVER	INFREQUENTLY	SOMETIMES	OFTEN	VERY FREQUENTLY
28. Indigestion	0	1	2	3	4
29. Nausea	0	1	2	3	4
30. Severe pains in your stomach	0	1	2	3	4
31. Increased appetite	0	1	2	3	4
32. Poor appetite	0	1	2	3	4
33. Loose bowel movements or diarrhea	0	1	2	3	4
34. Heartburn	0	1	2	3	4
35. Constipation	0	1	2	3	4

Muscle tension is a common way of experiencing stress. Have you noticed excessive tension, stiffness, soreness, or cramping of the muscles in your:

	NEVER	INFREQUENTLY	SOMETIMES	OFTEN	VERY FREQUENTLY
36. Abdomen or stomach	0	1	2	3	4
37. Neck	0	1	2	3	4
38. Jaw	0	1	2	3	4
39. Forehead	0	1	2	3	4
40. Eyes	0	1	2	3	4
41. Back	0	1	2	3	4
42. Shoulders	0	1	2	3	4
43. Hands or arms	0	1	2	3	4

	NEVER	INFREQUENTLY	SOMETIMES	OFTEN	VERY FREQUENTLY
44. Legs	0	1	2	3	4
45. Tension headaches	0	1	2	3	4

In your day-to-day activities, have you noticed symptoms of anxiety or restlessness, such as:

	NEVER	INFREQUENTLY	SOMETIMES	OFTEN	VERY FREQUENTLY
46. Fidgeting with your hands	0	1	2	3	4
47. Pacing	0	1	2	3	4
48. Chewing on your lips	0	1	2	3	4
49. Difficulty sitting still	0	1	2	3	4
50. Increased eating	0	1	2	3	4
51. Increased smoking	0	1	2	3	4
52. Biting your nails	0	1	2	3	4
53. Having to urinate frequently	0	1	2	3	4
54. Having to get up at night to urinate	0	1	2	3	4
55. Difficulty in falling asleep	0	1	2	3	4
56. Difficulty in staying asleep at night	0	1	2	3	4
57. Early morning awakening	0	1	2	3	4
58. Changes in your sexual relationship	0	1	2	3	4
59. Working tires you out completely	0	1	2	3	4
60. Severe aches and pain make it difficult for you to do your work	0	1	2	3	4

Stress is often accompanied by a variety of emotions. During the designated period have you felt:

	NEVER	INFREQUENTLY	SOMETIMES	OFTEN	VERY FREQUENTLY
61. Alone and sad	0	1	2	3	4
62. Unhappy and depressed	0	1	2	3	4
63. Like crying easily	0	1	2	3	4
64. Like life is entirely hopeless	0	1	2	3	4
65. That you wished you were dead	0	1	2	3	4
66. That worrying gets you down	0	1	2	3	4
67. You get up tired and exhausted in the morning even with your usual amount of sleep	0	1	2	3	4
68. You suffer from severe nervous exhaustion	0	1	2	3	4

Have you noticed:

	NEVER	INFREQUENTLY	SOMETIMES	OFTEN	VERY FREQUENTLY
69. Worrying about your health	0	1	2	3	4
70. Stuttering or stammering	0	1	2	3	4
71. Shaking or trembling	0	1	2	3	4

	NEVER	INFREQUENTLY	SOMETIMES	OFTEN	VERY FREQUENTLY
72. Being keyed up and jittery	0	1	2	3	4
73. Feeling weak and faint	0	1	2	3	4
74. Frightening dreams	0	1	2	3	4
75. Being uneasy and apprehensive	0	1	2	3	4
76. You get nervous or shaky when approached by a superior	0	1	2	3	4
77. You become so afraid you can't move	0	1	2	3	4
78. You are fearful of strangers and/or strange places make you afraid	0	1	2	3	4
79. Sudden noises make you jump or shake	0	1	2	3	4

Does it seem:

	NEVER	INFREQUENTLY	SOMETIMES	OFTEN	VERY FREQUENTLY
80. That little things get on your nerves	0	1	2	3	4
81. You are easily annoyed and irritated	0	1	2	3	4
82. When you feel angry, you act angrily toward most everything	0	1	2	3	4
83. Angry thoughts about an irritating event keep bothering you	0	1	2	3	4
84. You become mad or angry easily	0	1	2	3	4
85. Your anger is so great that you want to strike something	0	1	2	3	4
86. You let little annoyances build up until you just explode	0	1	2	3	4
87. You become so upset that you hit something	0	1	2	3	4

In your day-to-day living do you find:

	NEVER	INFREQUENTLY	SOMETIMES	OFTEN	VERY FREQUENTLY
88. Your thinking gets completely mixed up when you have to do things quickly	0	1	2	3	4
89. You must do things very slowly to do them without mistakes	0	1	2	3	4
90. You get directions and orders wrong	0	1	2	3	4
91. You are unable to keep thoughts from running through your mind	0	1	2	3	4
92. Frightening thoughts keep coming back	0	1	2	3	4
93. You become suddenly frightened for no good reason	0	1	2	3	4
94. You have difficulty in concentrating	0	1	2	3	4

95. What other ways do you experience stress, tension, or anxiety?_____

_____

_____

The following section is for WOMEN ONLY:

Around the time of your period do you feel:

	NEVER	INFREQUENTLY	SOMETIMES	OFTEN	VERY FREQUENTLY
96. Tense or jumpy	0	1	2	3	4
97. Mildly depressed	0	1	2	3	4
98. Moderately depressed	0	1	2	3	4
99. Severely depressed	0	1	2	3	4
100. Have you been pregnant within the last year?	yes		no		
101. Did you experience any complications during this pregnancy?	yes		no		
102. Did you experience any complications during or after delivery?	yes		no		
103. Have you had a hysterectomy?	yes		no		
104. Have you had both ovaries removed?	yes		no		
105. In the last year have you experienced any symptoms due to this surgery?	yes		no		
106. Have you experienced menopause?	yes		no		
107. In the last year have you experienced any symptoms related to menopause?	yes		no		

This questionnaire is adapted in part from the Cornell Medical Index, 1949. It may not be copied or reproduced without first obtaining permission from Maxine S. Leckie or Elaine Thompson.

Department of Psychosocial Nursing, SC-76, University of Washington, Seattle, Washington 98195.

APPENDIX 3-3

EVALUATION OF TREATMENT SESSION*

Client # _____

Date _____

Session # _____

SECTION I

1. How do you feel about the treatment session you have just completed?

1	2	3	4	5
very good	good	satisfied	unsatisfied	disappointed

2. How much progress do you feel you made in this session in dealing with your symptoms?

1	2	3	4	5
considerable progress	moderate progress	minimal progress	no progress	things have gotten worse

3. Do you feel you gained useful skills and/or knowledge in this session which can be used in daily living?

1	2	3	4	5
a great deal	a moderate gain	some gain	slight gains	no gain

4. How much involvement in the treatment session did you experience today?

1	2	3	4	5
actively involved	moderately involved	minimally involved	not involved	excluded

5. How much confidence do you have that the treatment you received in this session will help you deal with existing and future problems?

1	2	3	4	5
extremely confident	very confident	confident	unsure	not at all confident

*University of Washington Clinical Program in the Management of Stress Response.
Courtesy Patricia A. Betrus.

SECTION II

Check those statements that seemed to apply to your reactions today.

_____ 1. I could trust my therapist.

_____ 2. My therapist often did not seem to understand me.

_____ 3. My therapist seemed to know what s/he was doing.

_____ 4. My therapist was too passive.

_____ 5. The things my therapist said or suggested seemed helpful.

_____ 6. My therapist talks too much

_____ 7. My therapist really seemed to understand me.

_____ 8. My therapist didn't give me enough of a chance to express myself.

SESSION NUMBER	SATIS-FACTION	PROGRESS	GAINS	INVOLVE-MENT	CONFI-DENCE	SECTION I TOTAL	SECTION II TOTAL*
1							
2							
3							
4							
5							
6							
7							
8							
9							
10							
11							
12							
1 Mo FU							
3 Mo FU							

---

*Section II is tabulated by adding the number of positive and negative responses.
Questions 1, 3, 5, 7 are positive responses.
Questions 2, 4, 6, 8 are negative responses.
Range of possible responses is –4 to +4.

CHAPTER

4

RAPE TRAUMA AND POSTTRAUMATIC STRESS DISORDER

Ann W. Burgess, DNSc, RN, CS, and Carol R. Hartman, DNSc, RN, CS

ABSTRACT

   This chapter combines a case study and discussion with information on a neuropsychosocial model of information processing that has been used in developing interventions for rape trauma and posttraumatic stress disorder (PTSD). The chapter relates the symptoms associated with PTSD to the biological and structural changes in complex neurological systems that may occur when the system is overwhelmed during a traumatic experience such as rape, emphasizing especially the limbic system, which is the primary system for coding information and is linked to memory retrieval and recall. Topics include the victim's acute and long-term reactions to rape and the social response; instruments commonly used in assessment; the characteristics of PTSD; the dimensions of rape and the phases of rape trauma (pretrauma, assault, disclosure, and postdisclosure); and victims' coping and survival strategies. Nursing problems in diagnosing and treating rape trauma are presented and four models of therapy described, with emphasis on the multidimensional model. Finally, implications for nursing education and research are suggested.

CASE STUDY

   A 19-year-old college coed, pseudonym Lynn, seeks consultation because of "persistent thoughts about men chasing her in a graveyard, inability to concentrate, and declining self-confidence." The youngest of three children, with two older brothers, Lynn grew up in a traditional, intact family in a suburban home environment. Both parents worked, mother as a psychiatric nurse and father as a chemist. She attended boarding school prior to starting college. Teacher reports noted Lynn to be conscientious, creative, warm, popular, and intelligent. She participated in school activities, had positive and substantive interpersonal relationships with parents, siblings, teachers, classmates, and friends.

   During the consultation, Lynn described how a year ago, she was reading stories from a book she received as a birthday gift while sitting by a quiet, secluded brook near a cemetery. She saw a brown car with three men driving and remembers hearing them yell, "Stay here, honey, and we'll come back." She left the area. The next thing she remembers is being grabbed, falling backwards, and a man holding her arms. As she talks, she gets very cold. Then, she reports, she returned to campus, took a shower, and went to dinner at the college dining hall. She did not eat but sat with friends and her boyfriend. She was shaking and unable to respond when friends asked what was wrong. Later, when alone with her boyfriend, she told him about the men in the graveyard chasing her. She asked her boyfriend to stay the night.

During the consultation, Lynn acknowledges that something abusive may have happened, but she is unable to remember any details. She agrees to seek treatment to help with memory recall.

This chapter describes a neuropsychosocial model of information processing of rape trauma that emphasizes the limbic system as the primary system for coding information. This encoding relates to the process of memory retrieval and recall. When the limbic system is overwhelmed by incoming information, as it is when a person is violated, there is an initial altering response that, if unsuccessful in managing and responding to the information, becomes the survival response of numbing (dissociation). This response of hyperarousal followed by dissociation can lead to disruption of the interconnections of key processes operant in the construction of memory and in associative learning. The case example of Lynn will be discussed in some detail following an overview of rape trauma that will include applicable behavioral and biomedical knowledge, nursing assessment and diagnosis, key nursing problems, and care interventions. Finally, some recommendations regarding nursing education and research will be made.

RAPE TRAUMA AND SEXUAL ASSAULT

Rape is a serious public health problem (Kilpatrick, Edmunds, & Seymour, 1992). Since 1977, the rate of forcible rape has increased by 21%, the largest increase in all violent crimes. In 1990, three separate reporting units described the incidence of rape: FBI Uniform Crime Report cited 102,560 cases of forcible rape to females of consenting age; the U.S. Department of Justice, Bureau of Justice Statistics (NCS) reported 130,000 forcible rapes; and the National Women's Study estimated 683,000 cases of forcible rape (Kilpatrick et al., 1992).

What is forcible rape? Although states and jurisdictions legally define rape differently, three criteria are generally present: an event that occurs without the individual's consent, that involves the use of force or threat of force, and sexual penetration of the victim's vagina, mouth, or rectum.

Sexual assault refers to a wider range of forced or pressured sexual contact—specifically, child sexual assault, incest, acquaintance rape, and marital rape. Also, there are situations involving relationships of unequal power where the person in authority violates the normal bounds of the relationship and abuses and sexually pressures or forces the subordinate. Such abusive relationships include husband/wife, doctor/patient, nurse/patient, parent/child, teacher/student, and employer/employee.

Why are rape trauma and sexual assault of concern to psychiatric nurses? First, they affect the lives of hundreds of thousands of women and their families and partners each year; second, they play a major role in health and mental health problems; and third, rape is a crime on the upswing. To understand its presentation clinically, nurses need to recognize the behavioral and biopsychosocial nature of rape and the resulting treatment implications. The behavioral knowledge with which nurses should be familiar includes the acute reaction to rape, the long-term reaction, the social response, and the interaction of these variables for the resolution or continuation of symptoms.

ACUTE REACTION TO RAPE

A behavioral assessment of an acute reaction to rape includes the type of rape, the modus operandi of the victimizer, and whether the rape was a blitz–sudden attack or one in which the confidence of the victim was betrayed (Burgess & Holmstrom, 1974). The victim-offender interaction and the coping and survival behaviors employed by the victim are also important trauma variables in this phase.

Research on coping and survival strategies during the rape has focused primarily on what the victim did vis-à-vis the offender. A wide variety of reported behaviors emerge: verbal strategies, physical action as a way to escape attack, and verbal negotiations (Burgess & Holmstrom, 1976). Recent investigations of coping strategies and the response of the rapist to them indicate that some of the violence toward the victim may be a function of how the rapist interprets any struggle. Of particular importance is the investigation by Hazelwood, Reboussin, and Warren (1989), who studied 41 serial rapists. Ten of these rapists reported an increased pleasure and an increase in violence toward their victims when the victims fought back. Another study that examined the amount of injury to the victim indicated that there are rapists who will inflict more harm if a strategy used by victims is to defend themselves (Prentky, Burgess, & Carter, 1986).

LONG-TERM REACTION

Clinical research indicates that there are victims who withstand the assault, the immediate aftermath, and within 3 to 6 months return to social integration. A small portion, 17 to 25%, are reported to be symptom-free 1 year postrape without any intervention (Burgess & Holmstrom, 1978; Veronen & Kilpatrick, 1983). However, the majority report some fear and anxiety symptoms above prerape functioning (Kilpatrick, Resick, & Veronen, 1981). Sales, Baum, and Shore (1984) suggest that there is an uneven course of recovery, with the acute phase subsiding within a 6-month period only to exacerbate at a later period, perhaps to a less intense degree than immediate postassault, but nevertheless with intensity. Their data suggest that there is never a return to a preassault state. This view is supported by several studies that indicate rape victims experience significant long-term problems in the areas of psychological functioning (e.g., fear/anxiety, depression), social adjustment, and sexual behavior (Ellis, 1983; Holmes & St. Lawrence, 1983; Steketee & Foa, 1987). Further, being a victim of rape may be associated with an increased risk of suicide (Kilpatrick, Best, Veronen, et al., 1985; Kilpatrick et al., 1987). In fact, the results of one study indicated that 19.2% of rape victims had attempted suicide, a rate 8.7 times higher than the rate for nonvictims (Kilpatrick, Best, Veronen, et al., 1985), and Resnick (1987) suggests it is impossible to know how many victims kill themselves as a function of crime-induced trauma. In a study by Katz and Burt (1988), self-blame was correlated with a longer recovery; that is, the more victims blamed themselves for the rape, the greater the likelihood that they had been psychiatrically hospitalized, the more suicidal they had been, and the lower their self-esteem. In a large national representative survey of 2,626 adult Americans, both men and women who had a history of childhood sexual abuse involving penetration were likely to report a disrupted marriage, dissatisfaction in sexual relationships, and a tendency to be a religious non-practitioner (Finkelhor, Hotaling, Lewis, & Smith, 1989).

The impact of rape on self-esteem has been reported to extend at least over a 2-year period after the rape (Murphy et al., 1988), and where a victim has had a prior history of sexual abuse, symptoms may extend over an even longer period (Marhofer-Devorak, Resick, Hutter, & Girelli, 1988).

Social Response

Social support has been found to be an important factor in determining outcome. It is important not only to identify, characterize, and estimate the strength of the victim's social network support system but also to understand how a victim's responses interact to influence the response of the system over time, and how this interaction affects symptoms and recovery. The strength of this variable is most evident if the treatment includes family members. Family members influence the amount of talk that surrounds the event, and their patterns of expectations often reflect anxiety over the prolonged effects the trauma will have on all concerned. Personal guilt of family members, combined with avoidance patterns, can greatly influence the victim's response.

A differential response to social support has been noted by Sales, Baum, and Shore (1984) at various stages of recovery, in that victims with close family ties had a greater amount of distress during the acute phase, with diminution of symptoms on a long-term basis. This finding may support a different interpretation of what is initially termed symptoms. As suggested in the work of Horowitz (1976), the manifestation of intrusive thoughts may, in fact, be a necessary process in organizing traumatic experiences into long-term memory. There is evidence that the quality of the social support of the victim has a differential influence on psychological disruption over time.

Newly emerging as an area of concern both for the victim and her family are the medical consequences of rape (Cunningham, Pearce, & Pearce, 1988). Victims are increasingly raising questions and concerns regarding sexually transmitted diseases, in particular AIDS, because fear of having become HIV positive is a long-term concern that cannot be resolved for months (Baker, Burgess, Davis, & Brickman, 1990; Murphy, Kitchen, Harris, & Forster, 1989).

Biological Knowledge of PTSD

The brain, a complex, living organ, reflects the complexity of the multifaceted functions of neurons, that is, the building blocks for brain processes and mental functions. Both the central nervous system (CNS) and the autonomic nervous system (ANS) are continually responding to stimuli—from the external environment, a constant source of stimulation to our senses, as well as internal systems of appraisal and meaning. Traumatic life events, however, force the issues of how we learn, what we learn, and how we remember. Therefore, a review of the brain as the regulating system for all functions of the human organism and of its adaptive processes (within itself and within the body as a whole) is a basis for understanding the biology of psychological trauma.

Characteristics of PTSD

The intricate connection between behaviors following traumatic life events and the CNS is supported by clinical studies and biological studies of a variety of trauma populations (Bremmer, Southwick, Johnson, Yehuda, & Charney, 1993; Putnam, 1984; Mason, Giller, Kosten, Ostroff, & Podd, 1986). The most definitive biological studies of PTSD have been carried out on Vietnam veterans (Giller, 1990). Furthermore, the basis of biological studies of stress response in humans is driven by an important body of animal research that leads to a deeper understanding not only of how key aspects of the CNS are affected by high levels of stress but also of how the neurochemistry and morphology of the brain are altered (McEwen & Mendelson, 1993).

The astute observations of early clinicians working with nonveteran trauma populations supported the constellation of symptoms that are similar to those found in combat veterans (Burgess & Holmstrom, 1974; Herman, 1981; Walker, 1984). These works, and many other clinical writings since, support the official diagnostic category of posttraumatic stress disorder in the DSM-IV (American Psychiatric Association, 1994) across numerous traumatic events such as rape (Burgess & Holmstrom, 1974; Kilpatrick, Veronen, & Best, 1985); kidnapping (Terr, 1983); natural disasters (Shore, Tatum, & Vollmer, 1986); accidents (Wilkinson, 1983); and torture and/or imprisonment (Agger & Jensen, 1993).

Three broad categories of symptoms are the hallmark of PTSD. First are symptoms of persistent re-experiencing of the traumatic event by recurrent and intrusive distressing recollections of the event. In children it is found in repetitive play patterns that simulate the traumatic event. The second category includes symptoms of persistent avoidance of situations and stimuli that are associated with the trauma or a general numbing of responsiveness to stimuli and reminders (van der Kolk, Pitman, Orr, & Greenberg, 1989). The third category's symptoms are those of persistent, increased arousal that was not present before the trauma, including exaggerated startle response (Perry, Southwick, Yehuda, & Giller, 1990), physiological reactivity to stimuli that is either neutral or associated in some manner with the traumatic event, difficulty concentrating, hyperalertness, vigilance, and irritability. Disrupted sleep is also a major symptom (Ross, Ball, Sullivan, & Caroff, 1989; van Kammen, Christiansen, van Kammen, & Reynolds, 1990).

While these are the key symptoms outlined in the DSM-IV, clinicians must be sensitive to additional variations in behavioral presentations over time. Somatic symptoms, problems related to sexuality and sexual functioning, and problems in the areas of identity and gender orientation, as well as qualities in type and/or styles and patterns of interpersonal relationships are now being linked with the long-term sequelae of PTSD (Burgess et al., 1984; Herman, Perry, & van der Kolk, 1989; Herman, 1992; Sandford, 1990).

This constellation of symptoms and limiting personal traits demonstrates problems in arousal, numbing (dissociation), memory, sleep, and psychosomatic reactions. All of these phenomena have been linked with limbic system alterations and effective modulation of noradrenergic and seotonergic pathways via the brain stem (van der Kolk & Saporta, 1993). Further, these disruptions are ultimately realized in the social attachment and social behaviors that compromise adjustment to life (van der Kolk, 1987).

BIOLOGICAL RESPONSE TO STRESS AND PSYCHOLOGICAL TRAUMA

In a variety of human research programs, PTSD appears to be associated with a complex array of abnormalities in several biological systems of the ANS and the CNS. Distinctive physiological, neuropharmacological, and neuroendocrinological alterations have been exhibited in the PTSD patients studied, mainly in Vietnam veterans (Friedman, 1993). In addition, several animal models may be directly applicable to PTSD: learned helplessness, conditioned fear, and inescapable shock (van der Kolk, Greenberg, Boyd, & Krystal, 1985; Hemingway & Reigle, 1985; Kolb, 1988).

Studies of physiological and neurohumoral/neuroendocrinological alterations in PTSD point to shifts in ANS and CNS functioning wherein the excitatory and in-

TABLE 4–1. PHYSIOLOGICAL AND ENDOCRINE ALTERATIONS ASSOCIATED WITH PTSD

Physiological Alterations

Sympathetic hyperarousal: a complex interface of the hippocampus and the HPA involving interaction of glucocorticoids, benzodiazepine receptors and serotonin receptors, and neuro pathways to the cortex (McEwen & Mendelson, 1993)

Tonic - resetting of the homeostasis at a higher level

Episodic - in response to neutral and traumatic stimuli

Excessive startle reflex: early trauma experience on the development of limbic and cortical circuits (Bremner et al., 1992; Teicher, Glod, Surrey, & Swett, 1993)

Lowered threshold

Increased amplitude

Sleep Physiology Alterations

Sleep latency versus sleep time movements, awakenings

Disturbance in sleep architecture

Traumatic nightmares

Endocrine Alterations

Increased circulating catecholamine: hyperadrenergic state (Korf, 1976; Kosten, Mason, Giller, Ostroff, & Harkness, 1987)

Urinary catecholamine levels

Down-regulation of alpha-2 and beta receptors

Hypothalamic-pituitary-adrenocortical (HPA) axis: (hypo functioning: Mason, Giller, Kosten, & Yehuda, 1990)

Urinary - free cortisol levels

Blunted ACTH response to cortical releasing hormone (CRH)

Opioid system dysregulation (van der Kolk, Greenberg, Boyd, & Krystal, 1985; Pitman, van der Kolk, Orr, & Greenberg, 1990)

Pain threshold at rest

Stress-induced analgesia elicited by traumatic stimuli

Beta-endorphin levels

From Friedman, M. J. (1993). Psychobiological and pharmacological approaches to treatment. In J. P. Wilson and B. Raphael (Eds.), *International handbook of traumatic stress syndrome.* New York: Plenum Press.

hibitory mechanisms for both systems are set at a level of higher arousal. This resetting suggests alterations in the systems involved with the inhibition of behavioral responses. For example, there may be elevated blood pressure and pulse rate at a resting state in those with PTSD, and there is evidence of greater cardiovascular arousal following exposure to either a neutral stimulus (white noise) or to trauma stimuli. Disturbance in sleep and sleep architecture (insomnia, movement disorders, activity during REM, night terrors, nightmares, and vivid dreams of the trauma) are also common (Kolb, 1987; Pitman, Orr, Forgue, de Jong, & Claiborn, 1987). These findings and data from other studies support the DSM-IV for the symptoms of hyperarousal, startle, and disturbed sleep (Friedman, 1988; Lavie, Hefez, Halperin, & Enoch, 1979). Systems that appear to be involved in persistent biological abnormalities in trauma research are identified in Table 4–1.

GENERAL ADAPTATION SYNDROME (GAS) AND TRAUMATIC STRESS

Basically, three key circuits are activated when a person is confronted with a traumatic stressor (see Table 4–2). First is the preparatory circuit, which mobilizes the body for an emergency. The anatomical core of the physiological processes for this

TABLE 4–2. CIRCUITS ACTIVATED DURING TRAUMA

CIRCUIT	NEUROSTRUCTURE

1. The preparatory circuit: regulates hormones that prepare for emergency	Locus coeruleus
	  • Noradrenergic arousal
	Raphe nuclei
	  • Serotonin modulations
	  • Decreased serotonin from LC activation

2. The stress-response circuit: regulates the stress-response hormones	Limbic system
	Adrenergic system
	Hypothalamic-pituitary-adrenocortical axis
	  • Catecholamines released
	  • Behavior-facilitating system (BFS)
	  • Increased norepinephrine
	  • Decreased cortisol

3. The blunting circuit: provides hormones that have an analgesic effect to control response to pain and/or immobilize	Opioid-benzodiazepine system
	  • Locus coeruleus
	  • Hypothalamus
	  • Amygdala
	  • Behavior-inhibiting system (BIS)
	  • Decreased K^+

preparatory circuit, as outlined by Friedman (1993), starts in the locus coeruleus (LC). Located in the brain stem, the LC is the CNS's main source of noradrenaline (NE), the substance that triggers the principal neurotransmitters responsible for delivering messages—about the need to prepare for emergencies—to various parts of the limbic system and the rest of the CNS. Two major routes innervating the brain from the LC are those that go to the hypothalamic mechanisms (controlling defensive reactions) and those that go to the septohippocampal system, that is, the part of the limbic system involved in the evaluation of incoming stimuli. Arousal levels of ions and hormones alter these systems and prepare them for immediate action, if necessary. There are also connections with the amygdala. In addition, the LC contains corticotropin-releasing hormone (CRH) and opioid neurons, both of which play a role in PTSD.

Parallel to the role of the LC is the raphe nuclei, also located in the brain stem. The raphe nuclei is a primary source of serotonin and has important serotonergic pathways that innervate the septohippocampal system as well as the cortex. If the initial signals being processed via the LC, the hypothalamic-pituitary-adrenocortical (HPA) axis, and the septohippocampal system indicate that punishment is imminent, two related systems are activated. One is the behavioral facilitating system, which prepares for the emergency fight or flight; the other is an opposing process, the behavioral inhibition system, which prevents initiation of emergency responses until it is clear they will be useful (van der Kolk & Saporta, 1993; Friedman, 1993; Tortora & Grabowski, 1993). Low levels of serotonin or depletion of serotonin in the brain stem are thought to result in an excess of LC activity, the primary source of hyperarousal found in PTSD.

The second circuit, the stress response circuit, is innervated by the adrenergic system and is known to increase the secretion of the corticotropin-releasing factor (CRF) and, in some cases, cortisol. This hormone, one of the main ones mobilizing the body to fight/flight (handling the emergency), is regulated by key structures in the limbic system, where the pituitary gland responsible for CRF interacts with the hypothalamus (part of the limbic structure). Because there is an increase in norepinephrine and a decrease in cortisol in PTSD, the ratio of norepinephrine/cortisol is a biological benchmark for this condition.

The hypothalamus, which receives hormonal signals and sensory input from the viscera, controls and integrates activities of the ANS. The principal link between endocrine and nervous systems, it regulates the pituitary gland; secretes hypothalamic-regulating hormones; functions in rage and aggression; controls normal body temperature, food intake, and thirst; and helps maintain the waking state and sleep.

The limbic system surrounds the brain stem and contains innervations to the cerebral cortex, the dominant tissue of the cerebrum. During embryonic development, this gray matter enlarges much faster than the white matter of the cerebrum and plays an important role in connecting the left and right hemispheres of the brain. The left hemisphere, containing billions of neurons, is the seat of intelligence; it is primary in reading, writing, speaking, making calculations, abstract thinking, and problem solving. The right hemisphere is responsible for creative works, such as composing music, insight, and spatial comparisons; it also has an important role in the processes of learning and memory.

In particular, the limbic system, with the amygdala and hippocampus, functions in the emotional aspects of learning and survival behaviors. The hippocampus is especially important to memory and learning (Squire, Weinberger, Lynch, & McGaugh, 1991), and the amygdala, which has been strongly implicated in the control of aggressive and sexual behaviors, plays a role in emotional learning. The amygdala is also one of the most sensitive structures in the brain for the emergence of kindling, that is, when repeated intermittent stimulation produces greater and greater alteration in neuronal excitability (Moriata, Okamoto, Seki, & Wada, 1985).

After Circuit I has been activated and a person has moved into Circuit 2, the release of CRF can lead to an increase in plasma cortisol, which leads to an increase in tryptophan hydroxylase, a neuroactivator that activates seratonin circuits. Sustained stress and trauma, however, decrease serotonin, resulting in a decrease in its modulating effects and, hence, to an unchecked excretion of noradrenalin from the LC. This is just one example of dysregulation. There can also be dysregulation in the HPA axis or between the opioid system and the noradrenergic system.

The third circuit, the blunting circuit, is regulated by hormones secreted from the opioid-benzodiazepine system. The stress response circuit (Circuit 2) interacts with this third circuit and accounts not only for fight and avoidance responses but also for symptoms such as detachment, dissociation, and apathy. In short, this third circuit blunts the feeling of pain. It includes the LC, hypothalamus, and amygdala, where strong emotion is registered.

In many situations the resistance stage is generally successful in seeing us through a stressful episode, and our bodies then return to normal by virtue of the behavioral inhibitory actions of the systems that involve the hippocampus and serotonergic pathways. If, however, the demands are in excess of the resistance phase, then the general adaptation syndrome (GAS) moves into the stage of exhaustion. Exhaustion is mainly a function of the loss of K^+, which is partly responsible for controlling the water concentration of the cytosol. When the mineralocorticoids (aldosterone) stimulate the kidneys to retain NA^+, the kidneys trade off K^+ and H^+. As the cells lose more and more K^+, they function less and less effectively, until finally, they start to die. Unless the K^+ loss is rapidly reversed, vital organs cease to function, and the person dies.

Another cause of exhaustion is depletion of the adrenal glucocorticoids. The sudden loss of blood glucose does not allow the brain and other organs to get the needed nutrition to survive. Weakening of organs contributes to death because the person can no longer withstand the demands of the stressor.

When long-term action is necessary (as in the resistance reaction phase), CRH, growth hormone–releasing hormone (GHRH), and thyrotropin-releasing hormone (TRH) are activated in the anterior pituitary gland, via the hypothalamus. Adrenocorticotropic hormone (ACTH) then stimulates the adrenal cortex to secrete more cortisol, which triggers the conversion of a noncarbohydrate into glucose (gluconeogenesis) and protein catabolism. This reaction makes blood vessels more sensitive to stimuli, bringing about their constriction and counteracting a drop in blood pressure, such as that caused by bleeding. Cortisol also reduces inflammation and prevents it from becoming disruptive rather than protective, but the benefits of cortisol are for short-lived responses. Unfortunately, cortisol also discourages formation of new connective tissue, and wound healing is therefore slowed during a prolonged resistance stage. Consequently, when levels remain high, the adaptive function is lost and can lead to tissue damage; on the other hand, lower cortisol levels can interfere with the glucose metabolism essential for brain functioning. While excessively high or low levels of cortisol are associated with depression, the lower cortisol levels associated with PTSD indicate that regulation of the corticosteroids is different from that found in major depression, where cortisol levels may be higher (Yehuda et al., 1990; Yehuda, Boisoneau, Mason, & Giller, 1993a; Yehuda, Resnick, Kahana, & Giller, 1993b; Yehuda et al., 1993c).

GHRH causes the anterior pituitary gland to secrete human growth hormone (HGH), and TRH causes it to secrete thyroid-stimulating hormone (TSH), which stimulates the thyroid (increasing catabolism) to secrete T3 and T4. These in turn stimulate production of adenosine triphosphate (ATP) from glucose (ATP is most responsible for the efficient management of transferring manageable amounts of energy from one molecule to another). These catabolic reactions provide the energy that most anabolic reactions require to proceed.

Similarly, HGH stimulates the catabolism of fats and the conversion of glycogen (within the liver) to glucose (glycogenolysis). The combined actions of TSH and HGH increase catabolism and thereby supply additional ATP for the body and brain. Further, mineralocorticoids allow for the retention of sodium by elimination of H^+ and K^+ ions, resulting in the water retention that compensates for blood loss and keeps blood pressure up.

The second group of corticoids resulting from stimulation of the adrenal cortex are glucocorticoids. This group sets into action gluconeogenesis and protein catabolism. Within the brain, the hippocampus has the highest concentrations of bioactive corticosteroid receptors (Sapolsky, Krey, & McEwen, 1984), and these glucocorticoid receptors play a vital role in modulating the adrenocortical stress response by acting as inhibitors of the hypothalamus. However, excessive norepinephrine—coming to the hippocampus from the LC—and excessive glucocorticoids—destroying cells in the hippocampus and interfering with serotonergic pathways and production—disrupt the behavioral inhibition system (BIS), which is linked to the HPA. An inability to shut off glucocorticoids ensues.

Damage to hippocampus cells may account for the disturbance in memory through cellular damage. In addition, disturbance in memory may occur when the hippocampus is initially sensitized by the excesses of the LC during the short-term phase of stress (McEwen & Mendelson, 1993; van der Kolk & Saporta, 1993). In fact, intrusive imagery (e.g., in the form of flashbacks) and/or dissociative, amnesic responses can now be partially understood by the biological impact at various phases of adapting to the traumatic events: the preparatory first phase (LC) results in sensitization of the amygdala and the hippocampus (van der Kolk, 1987). Furthermore, the anxiogenic, disinhibitory, and neuroendocrine aspects of PTSD can now be considered within the broader concept of some type of disruption to BIS, part of which is now associated with the hippocampus and hypothalamus connection (Sapolsky, Krey, & McEwen, 1984; Sapolsky, Uno, Rebert, & Finch, 1990; McEwen & Mendelson, 1993; Teicher, Glod, Surrey, & Swett, 1993).

People with PTSD generally do not die. However, because of the nature and perceptions of the stressor, the alarm system is overwhelmed, and to preserve the life of the person, counterregulatory processes are set into motion during the resistance phase. This response alters adaptive processes and inhibits a return to the flexible arrangements of the GAS.

Stress and/or trauma have been shown to alter all three key circuits, which interconnect via feedback loops that aim at achieving homeostasis. Rather than these adaptive systems being depleted, they accommodate the imbalance to preserve a protective response as well as homeostasis, but then these accommodations err in that they prime the alarm system to react with less provocation and less capacity to discriminate error. As a result, disordered behaviors are assumed to arise out of the overwhelming of these adaptive systems. They are thrown into states of dysregulation via processes of hyposecretion and/or hypersecretion that occur in the limbic center and regulate life-preserving functions, for example, sleep, memory, attachment, sex, aggression, and self-defense. Stress and trauma are therefore seen to have a significant effect on personal and interpersonal behavior patterns, including actions and thinking.

All three circuits also influence memory. All experience is first remembered at a basic level that some refer to as taxonomic, or primarily categorical, memory. The key aspect of this memory is that it is sensory-motor and not related to time and space. Therefore, it is immediate, as if it is happening in the present. This primary memory system is, in turn, basic to higher-order memory structures. Therefore, when there is dysregulation of sensory input, alterations in primary memory influence the elaboration of secondary memory, that is, when there is interference with basic categorization (discrimination, sorting, etc.), there is disruption in the processing and storing of information on a secondary level. For example, the interpretation of cues that clarify the intentions and motivations of others can be disturbed because of a restricted repertoire of responses that are biased to produce avoidant responses.

In the face of a traumatic event such as a rape, the unremitting release of the catecholamines (noradrenaline, adrenaline, and dopamine)—as well as second messengers derived from these hormones—stimulates phosphyrolation. Further, the proteins that regulate genes within the cell nucleus can change gene expression for hours and days, leading to changes in levels of key enzymes and structural proteins in the nerve cells. The symptoms of PTSD and the behavioral changes suggest that during this initial adaptive process, which prolongs necessary hormonal responses to sustain resistance to a stressor, changes occur that alter the response within these critical biological systems so that they never return to their original restorative states. Instead, hyperconditioning and structural change occur within prior complementary regulatory subsystems of the GAS.

SUMMARY

In the phases of arousal and alarm many of the intrusive, episodic, and chronic symptoms of posttraumatic stress can be understood by biological and structural changes in complex systems. The location of these systems in the brain stem and limbic system further direct us to observable behavior changes that are often perplexing to the person with PTSD and those relating to him/her. Hyperarousal and the numbing experiences accompanied by memory disturbances impact on the person's sense of self. In fact, the sense of division, fragmentation, and discontinuity represents more than psychological efforts to forget unpleasant and terrorizing experiences; these distortions of self contribute to a continuing fragility and vulnerability of the person to ongoing life issues. Such disturbances should, however, be understood as having roots in natural, protective, biological processes. With this understanding, symptoms of dissociation, fragmentation, discontinuity, and split sense of self can be turned around; through medication, relaxation, and grounding strategies, the victim can move from self-recrimination to gaining a personal sense of control. With this control, the individual can then move closer to facing the recallable trauma information and reframing cognitive and emotional responses.

NURSING ASSESSMENT AND DIAGNOSIS

The nurse's careful assessment of a victim leads to a nursing and psychiatric diagnosis, and that diagnosis in turn directs care interventions. This section discusses assessment issues, presents an interview schedule, identifies standardized tests for trauma evaluation, outlines diagnoses for rape trauma, and discusses key nursing problems.

ASSESSMENT OF RAPE TRAUMA

The assessment of a victim includes four major phases defined by time: (a) the pretrauma phase, including dynamic and stable factors of the victim's life and personality prior to the assault; (b) the assault phase, including the rape and its characteristics, the rapist's interaction with the victim, and the victim's survival strategies; (c) the disclosure phase, including the response of the health care system, the social network of the victim, the criminal justice system, and how the rape is cognitively and affectively processed by the victim; and (d) the postdisclosure phase, which is concerned with the demand for integration of the rape experience, the consequences of disclosure, organization of a symptom-free state, and planning for the future.

PRETRAUMA

In addition to a general history assessment of individual and family background, two important areas related to the pretrauma phase of a victim include prior life events and experiences of the victim and personality characteristics. The influence of prior events on recovery is a complex matter, but mastery of prior events may help an individual handle another major stress. Thus, it is important to assess coping behaviors; of particular interest is discerning whether an individual has a particular trait (constellation) of cognitive processes for handling new and traumatic information. There are, however, many difficulties in defining and measuring personality characteristics.

ASSAULT

The critical factors of this phase are the type of rape, circumstances and dimensions of the rape, and the victim's coping and survival response. First, a rape may be classified as blitz or confidence type (Burgess & Holmstrom, 1979). Blitz rape is an assault that occurs out of the blue and has a sudden, anonymous quality to it (the typical example is a victim crossing the path of the predator who is looking for someone to capture and attack). The confidence-style assailant, on the other hand, gains access to the victim under false pretenses by using deceit, followed by betrayal and often violence. Characteristically, in the latter type of rape there is prior acquaintance between the victim and the assailant, however brief. The assailant might know the victim and thus already have developed some kind of relationship with her, or he may establish a nonthreatening interaction as a prelude to attack. The assailant may, for example, attempt to offer protection or help, for example, fix a tire or provide a ride. For this rape type, the elements of force, conning, or betrayal have specific meanings and may affect the rate and degree of recovery.

Type. Questions related to circumstances of the assault include some of the following: When and where was the victim approached? Why was the victim there, and where did the assault occur? Who was the assailant, for example, was he of the same race, and was he a stranger, acquaintance, or relative of the victim? What conversation occurred? What sexual, aggressive, and/or humiliating remarks were made, and what was the victim's response? What methods of control were used in the assault, for example, were there threats, weapons, and/or physical force? What types of sexual acts were demanded and obtained? What additional degrading acts were demanded?

Dimensions. The dimensions of the rape include the following: type of abuse, use of weapon and/or threats, the assailant's characteristics and relationship to the victim, event characteristics, victim characteristics, and response/aftermath. In completing an initial assessment, the nurse should constantly focus on how the victim felt and thought about all details of the rape. To assist in covering all assessment areas, an instrument such as the Dimensions of Rape Interview Schedule (DORIS) (Reed, Burgess, & Hartman, 1991) may be used (see Table 4–3).

Coping and Survival Strategies. Determining how the victim coped with and survived the assault is crucial in a clinical assessment. It is useful to assess the coping strategies to predict future coping strengths, although the assessor should realize that coping behavior may change according to the tasks required in the various phases of the attack. For example, some victims report an early awareness of danger ("I heard a noise in the kitchen and went to investigate.") The coping task at this phase is to react quickly to the warning. In the threat-of-attack phase, victims realize that there is definite danger to life, and the coping task is to try to avoid the danger by various methods. For example, victims try stalling for time, talking their way out of the situation, reasoning with the assailant, trying to change his mind, using flattery, bargaining, feigning helplessness, threatening the assailant, and joking and sarcasm (Burgess & Holmstrom, 1976).

When the victim realizes rape is inevitable, the coping task becomes physical and psychological survival. Coping strategies may be cognitive (mentally focusing attention to a specific thought, remaining calm, memorizing details, recalling advice, praying, concentrating); verbal or affective (talking, yelling, screaming, crying); and/or physical (trying to avoid full sexual penetration or trying to get the assault over with as fast as possible).

Immediately after the rape, the coping task is to escape from the assailant and seek help. Victims cope by trying to alert others, bargaining for freedom, and physically freeing themselves from the scene and the assailant.

DISCLOSURE

The disclosure phase occurs when the victim identifies herself as a victim of rape and socially discloses the event. This can be initiated by the victim or by others (e.g., when the police or a parent comes upon the assault or its aftermath). Important factors in this phase are the reactions of the health care system, the criminal

TABLE 4–3. DIMENSIONS OF RAPE INTERVIEW SCHEDULE

Type of Abuse

A. Physical Acts
1. Hit, punched, or beaten
2. Cut, stabbed, or bitten
3. Tied up or restrained, gagged, or blindfolded
4. Forced to walk or crawl long distance
5. Burned
6. Given drugs or alcohol
7. Other (describe)

B. Sexual Acts
1. Oral penetration by assailant/object (oral sex)
2. Vaginal penetration by assailant/object (sexual intercourse)
3. Anal penetration by assailant/object (anal sex)
4. Assault witnessed by other people
5. Victim witnessed sexual acts of others
6. Pornographic materials used or produced
7. Other (describe)

C. Use of Weapon
1. Gun
2. Knife
3. Other (describe)

D. Threats
1. Threatened with death
2. Threatened with disfigurement or physical injury
3. Threatened with loss of job or income
4. Threatened with harm to loved ones
5. Threatened with repeat rape
6. Other

Assailant Characteristics and Relationship to Victim

A. Verbal Strategies
1. Threats (see above)
2. Orders
3. Ploy used to gain access to victim (confidence line)
4. Personal inquiries of victim
5. Personal revelations by rapist
6. Obscene names/racial epithets
7. Exploitation of victim's forced sexual response ("you like it")
8. Soft-sell departure (apologies, safe return, socializing)
9. Sexual put-downs
10. Possession of victim ("you're mine now")
11. Taking property from another male (partner statements)

B. Relationship of Rapist to Victim
1. Stranger
2. Acquaintance or friend
3. Current or former spouse or cohabitant
4. Date
5. Authority figure (describe)
6. Relative or in-law
7. Other (describe)

C. Assailant(s) Characteristics
1. Gender
2. Approximate age
3. Race/ethnicity
4. Use of alcohol or drugs (describe)

Event Characteristics

A. Characteristics of Rape
1. Multiple rapists
2. Multiple victims
3. Time of day/night, approximate date (month and year)

From Reed, C. R., Burgess, A. W., & Hartman, C. R. (1991). Victim assessment: The dimensions of rape interview schedule (DORIS). In A. W. Burgess (Ed.), *Rape and sexual assault* (Vol. 3, pp. 16–17). New York: Garland.

justice system, and the victim's social network. Although the official reporting agencies indicate an increase in reported rape, it should be remembered that not all victims report a sexual assault. Therefore, nurses should be alert to situations in which the victim does report immediately and those in which there is a delay. Clinical studies have stressed that the callousness of the various persons who come in contact with the victim can greatly compromise the victim, exacerbating symptoms. In the case example, for instance, the victim does not report to authorities until she has full memory.

POSTDISCLOSURE PHASE

Critical factors to be considered during the postdisclosure phase (the period following the event) with regard to evaluating recovery include crisis intervention and treatment, outcome of the criminal justice system, and evaluation of the victim's recovery. In the case example, for instance, the victim notified campus police of the rape after trauma therapy, but nothing further was done.

Nursing Diagnosis of Rape Trauma

Rape trauma syndrome (RTS) is a nursing diagnosis that originated in a scientific paper co-authored by Burgess and Holmstrom and published in the *American Journal of Psychiatry* in 1974. This paper reported on rape victim responses and described an acute, physiologically focused pattern and long-term phase of psychological, cognitive, and behavioral recovery from the assault. It also described a victim's behavior following assault. Behaviors such as remaining calm and composed during and while reporting an assault, failing to report the incident immediately, or falsely claiming not to know the attacker may seem strange to some but may actually not be at all unusual responses to an attack. Rape trauma syndrome has, in fact, been accepted in many courts across the United States.

Expert testimony of RTS is generally offered for two purposes: (a) to prove lack of consent and (b) to explain certain behaviors, such as delay in reporting, that jurors might misconstrue as evidence that the rape did not occur. Meyers and Paxson (1992) provide a legal update on the admissibility of RTS in legal proceedings, reviewing reference to it in over 300 appellate court decisions. The legal definition of rape varies by statute from state to state, but the main issues generally addressed in all statutes include lack of consent, force or threat of force, and sexual penetration by a person who is not the spouse of the other. Within a humanistic context, rape is described by psychiatrist Elaine (Hilberman) Carmen as "the ultimate violation of the self, short of homicide, with the invasion of one's inner and most private space, as well as the loss of autonomy and control" (Carmen, Rieker, & Mills, 1984).

RAPE TRAUMA: IMMEDIATE REPORT

As a clinical term, rape trauma describes a clustering of biopsychosocial and behavioral symptoms exhibited in varying degrees by a victim following a rape. Most victims of forcible rape develop a pattern of moderate to severe symptoms described as RTS; a minority of victims report no or mild symptoms. This syndrome is an acute reaction to an externally imposed, situational crisis (Burgess & Holmstrom, 1974).

There is generally an immediate impact. Victims evidence a wide range of emotions in the hours and days following the rape. The physical and emotional impact may be so intense that the victim feels shock and disbelief. Two styles of emotion are often noted in victims: expressed and controlled. In the expressed style, the victim demonstrates such feelings as anger, fear, and anxiety. The nurse may note this style in the victim's restlessness during an interview, tenseness when certain questions are asked, crying or sobbing when describing specific acts of the assailant, and smiling in an anxious manner when certain issues are stated. In the controlled style, the feelings of the victim are masked or hidden, and a calm, composed, or subdued affect can be noted.

An acute phase of the syndrome includes physical symptoms, especially skeletal muscle tension, gastrointestinal irritability, and genitourinary disturbance. Marked disruption may also be noted in eating and sleeping patterns and in a wide range of emotional reactions.

REORGANIZATION PHASE

The second phase of the syndrome includes increased motor activity. During this phase a search for security may necessitate changes in telephone and place of residence. There may also be an increased need and request for family and social network support. In addition, fears and phobic reactions to the circumstances of the assault are common, as are repeated frightening and disturbing daymares and nightmares. The trauma of the victim results from the person's confrontation with a life-threatening and highly stressful situation. The crisis that results when a person is raped relates to self-preservation, and the victim's reactions to the impending threat to her life are the nucleus around which an adaptive pattern may be noted.

PSYCHIATRIC DIAGNOSIS: PTSD

For many rape victims, responses during and after the rape correspond to the critical symptoms of PTSD. Symptoms of this disorder were noted in the early editions of the Diagnostic and Statistical Manual (DSM) under war neuroses; the DSM-III, DSM-III-R, and DSM-IV include the term under anxiety disorders. PTSD is used as an umbrella term for a variety of major traumatic events, and rape victim responses may be consistent with the DSM-IV (American Psychiatric Association, 1994) diagnostic criteria, outlined below:

A. The person has been exposed to a traumatic event in which both of the following have been present:
   1. the person has experienced, witnessed, or been confronted with an event or events that involve actual or threatened death or serious injury, or a threat to the physical integrity of oneself or others.
   2. the person's response involved intense fear, helplessness, or horror. In children, it may be expressed instead by disorganized or agitated behavior.
B. The traumatic event is persistently reexperienced in at least one of the following ways:
   1. recurrent and intrusive distressing recollection of the event, including images, thoughts, or perceptions. In children, repetitive play may occur in which themes or aspects of the trauma are expressed.
   2. recurrent distressing dreams of the event. In children, there may be frightening dreams without recognizable content.
   3. acting or feeling as if the traumatic event were recurring (includes a sense of reliving the experience, illusions, hallucinations, and dissociative flashback episodes, including those that occur upon awakening or when intoxicated). In children, trauma-specific reenactment may occur.
   4. intense psychological distress at exposure to internal or external cues that symbolize or resemble an aspect of the traumatic event.
   5. physiologic reactivity upon exposure to internal or external cues that symbolize or resemble an aspect of the traumatic event.
C. Persistent avoidance of stimuli associated with the trauma and numbing of general responsiveness not present before the trauma, as indicated by at least three of the following:
   1. efforts to avoid thoughts, feelings, or conversations associated with the trauma.
   2. efforts to avoid activities, places, or people that arouse recollections of the trauma.
   3. inability to recall an important aspect of the trauma.
   4. markedly diminished interest or participation in significant activities.

  5. feeling of detachment or estrangement from others.
  6. restricted range of affect (e.g., unable to have loving feelings).
  7. sense of a foreshortened future (e.g., does not expect to have a career, marriage, children, or a normal life span).
D. Persistent symptoms of increased arousal (not present before the trauma), as indicated by at least two of the following:
  1. difficulty falling or staying asleep.
  2. irritability or outbursts of anger.
  3. difficulty concentrating.
  4. hypervigilance.
  5. exaggerated startle response.
E. Duration of the disturbance (symptoms in B, C, and D) is more than one month.
F. The disturbance causes clinically significant distress or impairment in social, occupational, or other important areas of functioning.

STANDARDIZED INTERVIEWS AND TESTS

Several interview schedules may be used for a general assessment of PTSD. The difficulty with these schedules is that they have been aimed at combat veterans; nevertheless, they are of clinical use with victims of rape and other traumatic events.

The Structured Clinical Interview Diagnostic (SCID) schedule is part of the diagnostic protocol for the DSM-IV (American Psychiatric Association, 1994). In addition, the National Center for PTSD study at the Behavioral Science Unit at the Boston Veterans Hospital, under the direction of Terance Keane and colleagues, developed the Clinician-Administered PTSD Scale (CAPS) for use in a major nationally funded study of veterans. Reliability, validity, and convergent/divergent validity studies are being done on the latter, which has the advantage of not only arriving at a diagnosis but also providing a continuous rating on presenting symptoms. Both of these schedules have been developed for research and clinical purposes and are lengthy to administer. They assess for immediate and chronic PTSD.

Several other instruments used to measure PTSD also have discriminant powers; these have been, and continue to be, used on the evaluation of different trauma populations. Included in this group are the Impact of Event Scale (Horowitz, Wilner, & Alvarez, 1979); the SCL-90R (Derogatis, 1977); the MMPI subscale for PTSD (Keane, Malloy, & Fairbank, 1984) and the Penn Inventory (Hammarberg, 1992).

In addition to these instruments, other measures of fear and physiological arousal are being used in various trauma populations (Pitman & Orr, 1993). Most of these measures, aimed at assessing the acute manifestation of PTSD, attempt to discern trait patterns in the long-term consequences of sexual abuse and early physical trauma. These issues of assessment are being actively debated and explored in the field trial for the DSM-IV. Because of the long-term effects of trauma on psychological functioning and its underassessment in prior psychiatric research, present diagnostic categories are being challenged; most apparent are the Axis II personality disorder groups.

KEY NURSING PROBLEMS

Key nursing problems include (a) symptom management and resolution and (b) forensic nursing responsibilities. Research findings have direct implications for clinical practice and for symptom management and resolution. First, the long-term symptoms of rape and sexual abuse victims have to be understood not only from a psychosocial-political perspective but also from a biological basis. Trauma learning entails alterations in primary and secondary memory processes; that is, learning and memory are a function of both implicit and explicit memory processes (Squire, Weinberger, Lynch, & McGaugh, 1991). Explicit memory refers to the type of brain functioning that deals with the integration and interpretation of stimuli into facts and events. Implicit memory refers to the basic brain structures that are realized in skill habits (typing, driving); priming (categorization of shapes and sizes); simple classical conditioning; and nonassociative learning such as kindling, sensitization, and neurohabitization. Failures of recall, the persistence of bodily and imagery experiences, and persistent sensitivity or numbing come from implicit memory dysregulation that is at the level of the brain stem and limbic system processes (Squire et al., 1991). The search for appropriate biological interventions that can re-establish dysregulation is therefore an optimum outcome. However, the associative damage done via the prolongation of symptoms and the interpersonal violations requires a variety of approaches from self-help support groups to focused psychotherapy.

The aftermath of rape can be prolonged. Victimization of women and children is a public health problem of major importance, given the large number of the population affected. Furthermore, the rate of recovery for rape victims is slower than for victims of other types of crimes (Resnick, 1987), and the increasingly distressing fact is that for some victims, recovery may not be as complete as once thought. Kilpatrick et al. (1987) found 16.5% of assessed rape victims were diagnosed with PTSD an average of 17 years postassault. Although it has been shown that most types of crime have a psychological impact on victims (Kilpatrick et al., 1987), rape and sexual assault have been shown to be particularly deleterious (Burgess & Holmstrom, 1974; Burgess, Hartman, McCausland, & Powers, 1984a; Kilpatrick, Best, Veronen, et al., 1985). Long-term problems in psychological functioning, social adjustment, and sexual behavior have been identified (Ellis, 1983; Holmes & St. Lawrence, 1983; Steketee & Foa, 1987; Finkelhor, Hotaling, Lewis, & Smith, 1989).

CARE INTERVENTIONS
MODELS OF THERAPY

Four major models of treatment have been used with traumatized victims with varying degrees of success. The first, crisis intervention, is successful in the acute phase. Initially employed by paraprofessionals at the rape crisis centers in the early 1970s, it utilizes a strong advocacy framework (Largen, 1985). This model, designed as a counseling and research project and used in the Boston study by Burgess and Holmstrom (1974), applies the tenets of crisis theory to a method of assisting victims. Most crisis counseling efforts have followed, in modified form, this type of programming: outreach, emergency care, and advocacy assistance. The objective is to validate the crisis nature of the event, carefully review the details of the rape, and address issues raised by the crisis. The focus is on the assault and its aftermath, with an emphasis on assisting the person to achieve mastery over the life-threatening anxiety created by the rape. This method also seeks to identify a supportive social network and self-enhancing ways of solving problems related to the rape and any subsequent events.

The second model, a cognitive-behavioral intervention that subscribes to a wide variety of therapeutic techniques, is based upon somewhat different conceptualizations. The techniques cover rational-emotive therapy, cognitive therapy, coping skills therapies, problem-solving therapies, self-instructional training, self-control processes, and interpersonal skills training, to name a few. Among these approaches are various theoretical differences. The theories range from conditioning to cognitive information processing and social learning conceptualizations. Interventions and prescriptions are primarily directed toward interruptions of the cognition-affect-behavior-consequences complex.

Even though these theories and techniques are implemented in a variety of ways (directly, collaboratively, indirectly), they share basic assumptions about style and behavior change. With regard to style, these interventions are usually active, time-limited, and fairly structured. There is a basic assumption that behavior and feeling are largely determined by the way an individual perceives and constructs meaning of the world and self. Therefore, the techniques are designed to enhance the person's awareness and control over cognitions and behavioral responses.

Behavioral change is believed to be an outcome of interrelationships of the person's cognitive structures (schemata, beliefs, programs), internal cognitive processes (automatic thoughts, internal dialogue, images, kinesthetic experiences), internal states (moods, feelings, labeling), and external behaviors, where interpersonal and intrapersonal consequences feed back to the internal processes.

While the cognitive-behavioral model may differ markedly from psychoanalytic approaches in style, it appears that the therapeutic process and client outcomes that result may allow the victim to work through distorted perceptions emanating from unconscious conflicts; therefore, psychoanalytic activities may converge with many of the activities of cognitive-behavioral approaches. Thus the cognitive-behavioral model offers an integrative approach that prioritizes victim content regarding the rape; this permits therapist flexibility in dealing with the multiple facets of behavior and circumstances confronting a rape victim. In addition, it allows for an interpretive scheme of victim behavior that is not grounded in pathology but respects the yet unclarified, natural processes put into play during crises and crisis resolution.

The third model of treatment, traditional psychotherapy, has been less successful. Werner (1972) described a case in which the patient, a graduate student in her twenties, was in the second year of therapy when the attack occurred. Werner conceptualized the attack as an external stress and spoke of the subsequent therapy material as resulting from an "actual tragedy rather than a fantasy." He emphasized how the rape interrupted therapy in several important ways: (a) the pace and content changed, in that it was no longer a leisurely exploration of relationships and fantasies; and (b) new symptoms of insomnia, appetite loss, frequent crying, and fears of being alone gave a clinical picture suggestive of a severe grief reaction.

The fourth model of intervention is multidimensional. The other three models of treatment support the clinical belief that fearful responses can be modified effectively when the structure of the cognitive defense and emotional arousal is addressed and when resource and skill training is provided. The increasing awareness of the impact of trauma on the limbic system (van der Kolk, 1989), however, suggests that many of the symptoms associated with forcible rape represent an overriding of the human alarm system that impacts on memory, sleep, sexual functioning, and attachment. In essence, there has been a type of "trauma learning" that alters sensory, perceptual, cognitive, behavioral, and interpersonal regulatory patterns (Hartman & Burgess, 1988). The resulting vulnerability of the rape victim to subsequent victimization and/or self-limiting underscores the need for a multidimensional approach to treatment.

The resolution of traumatic aftereffects is complicated in the case of rape. Kilpatrick and Veronen (1983) suggest that the amount of disorganization immediately after the attack is too much for the full participation of the victim. Moos and Billings (1982) stress that there is a differential use of coping responses, given the nature of the life stressor; they also indicate that there is a tendency for women to use more avoidant than active coping responses and that these are more highly associated with symptoms and depression.

The work of Horowitz (1976) addressed this question in part. In his research on whether intrusive and repetitive thoughts after experimental stress are characteristic of certain individuals, as opposed to representative of a general stress-response tendency, he concluded that the symptoms of repetitive imagery, thoughts, sounds, and feelings are part of a general stress-response tendency and can be further understood by using a model of information processing. For example, the work of Foa and Kozak (1986) not only addressed the hyperarousal associated with rape but also challenged the negative belief and cognitive patterns that are engendered subsequent to the rape. The flooding and implosion sessions used with veterans to ameliorate flashbacks is another example (Keane, Fairbanks, Caddell, Zimering, & Bender, 1985).

The continued manifestation of intrusive imagery indicates then that the victim, overwhelmed with new information, is attempting to place important information in storage, with the first level of storage being recent memory. It is only relegated to long-term memory when more important information takes its place. Based on Horowitz's (1982) propositions, symptoms can now be understood as parts of a process of cognitive reorganization. Therapeutic techniques that address this process hold promise for victims.

A model that allows for the convergence of techniques that address sensory, perceptual, cognitive, behavioral, and interpersonal patterns is neurolinguistic programming (Bandler & Grinder, 1975; Grinder & Bandler, 1976; Dilts, Grinder, Bandler, Bandler, & DeLosier, 1980). This model, which addresses the structure of subjective experience, is based on the responses of the person, and interventions are devised to disrupt patterns that impede flexibility. A major contribution of this model has been the memory storage of experience. This is particularly important in assessing how the victim processes trauma and how members of the victim's social support system process the trauma (Hartman & Burgess, 1986). Overriding images, internal dialogue, and kinesthetic responses are recognized for their stimulus value, and strategies that address the symptom maintenance aspect of these images and internal dialogue can be devised to reduce the dysfunctional consequences. Because fragments (internal and external) of powerful experiences act as an anchor, they have a signal effect and can trigger unwanted states or desired states. Therefore, techniques (referred to as meta programs) are aimed at (a) broad patterns of the victim's beliefs, presuppositions, and criteria; (b) external behavior; and (c) internal states and processes.

The value of this model is that it does not exclude different theoretical positions regarding causality. Rather, it focuses on accomplishing behavior change through different strategies and on testing changes within the intervention space and then on the outside. If the desired outcome is not achieved, more work can be done. Since the outcome is set in terms of the person seeking assistance, motivation to persist until goals have been achieved is enhanced. This fits with Horowitz's (1976) model of cognitive information processing.

The model develops and demands flexibility on the part of the clinician. If the change to be effected is too hard, then the task is broken down into smaller units. Thus, if the victim is overwhelmed with emotion during an acute state (immediately postassault), the first step is to assist the person in gaining control over feeling states by reducing their intensity in the here and now. This not only establishes a sense of control but begins to address the connection of internal processes—such as images, sounds, and thoughts—with emotional arousal and the arousal potential of the assault.

If the person is numb, cut off from feeling and thoughts, the first step is to build a strong sense of comfort in the present and establish an external cue for the state. Then gradually the patient is moved back in time, using the positive cue to reduce emotional arousal when it is too intense. In this way the person gains personal control in the here and now. As these steps are taken, the emergent beliefs and presuppositions regarding the assault are elicited and their power for symptom maintenance can be scrutinized. Furthermore, as personal control is experienced and increased, the person can focus more on the defensive cognitions and their alterations.

The important point is that therapeutic interventions are not prescribed but tailor-made for the individual. The intervener works actively with the victim. This approach does not exclude the social support system, but it does direct attention to the quality of that system's support. In the case of rape, since the social support network can be equally upset, it is important to note how individuals in the support system cope with the new information and the behavior of the victim.

CASE ANALYSIS

The case of Lynn reviews the course of a structured, time-limited trauma therapy.

SESSION 1: NEGOTIATION FOR TRAUMA THERAPY

A general pretrauma assessment was conducted. This history revealed no prior traumatic experiences. Prior to the graveyard event, Lynn had functioned at a very high level, for example, honor roll student, strong family and social network.

The convergence of the following situations prompted Lynn to take a semester off from college and to enter treatment to try to recover her memory of "the day in the graveyard." The rape had been her first penetrative sexual experience. Three months after the event Lynn began to have repetitive nightmares about men chasing her; she started to feel less confident about herself. She had mood swings and crying spells; she lost weight. She began a sexual relationship with her boyfriend and went on birth control. She began experiencing severe headaches; she had difficulty concentrating; she lost interest in previously enjoyed activities.

One year later, the news media covered a highly publicized rape trial; she dropped a course in order to "think more." She began running again and had a flashback of someone grabbing her shoulder and turning her around. She was disturbed after the run, and her boyfriend asked her what was wrong. She didn't know. The next day she met her boyfriend's parents, and she felt very uncomfortable when she thought the father was looking at her legs. She traveled home for a semester break. She became upset on the airplane and was not able to read. At home in the bathtub she had a flashback of the graveyard. She had planned to visit New York with friends as a birthday present but was unable to leave the house. She had the first cognitive thought that she might have been raped at the graveyard.

She returned to college but was irritable and cranky; the smallest thing upset her. She was unable to resume sex with her boyfriend. She began to worry that she might run into the men from the graveyard, that they might live in the town. She called her mother, and the decision was for her to return home and begin therapy. She agreed to a course of trauma therapy that would be paced for her ability to tolerate distressing affects. The goal of therapy was to recover her memory. She had a 10-week leave from school. Lynn was instructed by the nurse-therapist to keep a daily log of thoughts, feelings, and actions; she also kept a dream diary.

In the first session, the nurse-therapist sought to (1) anchor the patient for safety and (2) provide psychoeducation on the neurobiology of trauma. In the anchoring for safety (sometimes called *grounding* or *centering*), experiences are provided for learning inner relaxation in the here and now. Having first learned inner relaxation in the therapist's office, traumatized persons can transfer the learning outside the office, especially when they feel themselves getting upset. Because of the hyperarousal symptoms of PTSD, relaxation techniques that induce deep relaxation are another strategy in the grounding experience. If practiced frequently for short intervals during the day, they can help alter and manage the hyperarousal. Many times, individuals take a single block of time to practice relaxation, but this intermittent approach helps to reduce the tonic tension consistently throughout the day (Danford, 1994).

The key component of the psychoeducational process in trauma work is connecting the psychological and physiological experiences of the person to the underlying natural response to trauma. This becomes a grounding basis for the individual to understand experiences of fragmentation and other symptoms related to dissociation (e.g., disruptions in a sense of self, loss of time, memory fragments), as well as arousal, flashbacks, and a general sense of fatigue. All these physiological symptoms and manifestations of psychological disorganization now have a framework that help the individual to engage in strategies that are strengthening and healthy, as opposed to hiding these symptoms and using maladaptive coping mechanisms (e.g., substance abuse or entering into abusive, repetitive, disruptive relationships).

SESSION 2: FRAGMENTED MEMORIES AND DISTRESSING AFFECTS

Lynn reported that she had a "bad weekend" after the first session. She remembered a nightmare about a girlfriend who was at a festival and having to hide from a town guy who could kill her.

She described bits of memories, including the following: (1) hiding behind a gravestone, standing up, and being grabbed by the arm and turned around; (2) two men holding her arms; (3) hearing the noise of feet scuffing on a road; (4) bending over and feeling resistance to thigh muscle; (5) feeling a hand on her breast and feeling someone on her stomach; (6) descriptions of two men. She remembered the feel of the men's skin and the screaming in her head.

Environmental cues that triggered memories were identified as to the type of day (warm and sunny), exercising (she had been running that day), and position (lying with head to the side). When thinking of the rape, she felt physically ill and nauseated. Over the 2 weeks she had a bad migraine. She could not remember the middle part of the rape.

SESSION 3: THREE WEEKS LATER

Lynn had a full memory several days after the second session. She felt chilled during the memory. She also had a couple of bad days after the session, but the nightmares and heavy feeling subsided. She reported the full memory as follows:

> I heard their car. One man said, "Hey, baby, stay right there. We'll be right back." I tried to cut across the graveyard, then hid behind a gravestone. The car stopped. I heard the door slam. They got to me, and one said, "Don't worry, honey, we're not going to hurt you." They took me between some hedges. My head hit something. One man held my hands over my head. One man was darker than the others. The blond one pulls my shirt off. His hands were very rough. I felt the ground underneath me. His skin was sweaty. The men laughed. He unbuttons my jeans; stands me up. I think, "God, this is going to happen." I feel tears but don't cry. I close my eyes. He says, "Are you ready, baby?" He pushes me down. Each man holds one arm. I remember the pain and feel his hip bone. He's pressed against me; I can't breathe. He's done. He stands up. They release my knees. He hears something. Someone pulls up my pants. They sit me up. Someone grabs my head and elbow. I close my eyes. I hear another zipper. Someone pries open my mouth. I gag. I feel him ejaculate. He ordered me to swallow it. I had to; I was almost sick. One said, "See you next time." They left.

Session 4: Revisiting the Scene

Lynn made a trip back to college prior to the fourth session. Her goal was to visit the graveyard. It was a warm clear day, and she sat on a bench for 45 minutes near the graveyard. Then she gathered some wildflowers and put them at the location of the rape. She felt at peace. She buried the memory.

She talked with the woman in charge of security at the college. Lynn felt other students should know there had been a rape, but the security official did not agree. Lynn felt frustrated.

Session 5: Linking Memory with Symptoms

This session was spent reviewing symptoms of the first year after the rape. Her boyfriend made some observations. For example, after the rape, Lynn wore only old familiar clothes; she cried a lot about things that didn't make sense; she was moody, dependent, and passive during sex. Lynn reported feeling nauseated with a bad taste in her mouth after having novocaine for the removal of wisdom teeth. She had to bite down on a wet tea bag and remembered something in her mouth made her sick. The thought of tea bags stimulates the bad taste and nausea.

Session 6: Termination

The time-limited therapy enabled Lynn to recover her traumatic memories and reduce symptoms so that she could return to college. She knew there was additional work to be done and planned to recontract for treatment at a later date. At this session Lynn brought her homework, which included drawings of her memories of the rape—five sketches of her memory before and after treatment.

Discussion

The case illustrates several principles. First, the resources for recovering from rape reside in the individual. Second, the victim's personal resources (e.g., coping) are at different levels of development and accessibility. Third, a safe, supportive social network is essential to productive therapy.

The adaptation to trauma exemplified in this case goes through several phases. The first phase of adaptation is suppression; the experience is out of awareness. Lynn does not remember the rape. However, a unique aspect in this case is this young woman's attempts to establish a positive relationship with her boyfriend without being aware on a conscious level of the rape. This speaks to the need for support and ongoing work with developmental stages that can be disrupted via trauma. Lynn teaches us that even though the trauma itself has not been dealt with or integrated, an essential step in being in control is moving on with life activities commensurate with where one is developmentally. The repression and dissociation break through as a distressed affective state. This in part comes about through the support of the boyfriend and parents, who gently suggest that perhaps more went on in the graveyard than she can call into awareness. She demonstrates the capacity for self-observation of internal states but is still unable to connect and resolve the issue. Her distress increases because she is not successful. She then abridges her plans and agrees with the suggestion to see a nurse-therapist. With the support of the therapist and her capacity to use a log and recount her sensations, Lynn moves forward in associating to content; in particular, she recalls bodily sensations. This point is important in the process of trauma therapy. If Lynn had not had the capacity for self-monitoring and self-evaluation, that step would have had to be built in because self-awareness is the structure for discovering resources and using them to tolerate recovery of sensory, affective, and cognitive memory.

The sessions and homework of therapy demonstrate that Lynn has the capacity to keep moving with the material as it presented itself. With the therapist's support and expectations, Lynn can tolerate the intensity of the emotion and the memories. This allows her to pursue the work of uncovering and linking psychological states, physical states, and images stimulated by external and internal cues associated with the rape. Her dream material is accepted as working through efforts in the more direct linkages; therefore, dreaming is not dwelled upon with excessive interpretation or intrusion but is accepted as a statement that her mind is working on making the associative links.

We note further that Lynn has set goals for herself and that there is symptom reduction. She feels better, her headaches have subsided, and she is aware that it has been beneficial to experience what went on and to talk about it. Although she recovers her memory of the rape, there is still some numbing, as noted through her avoidance of sex. Another level of therapy needs to be conducted that leads her toward integration of the experience, for example, recognizing hyperarousal, numbing, and how her defenses are organized. Sometimes secondary factors related to anxiety are also uncovered at this stage of therapy, for example, earlier traumas, earlier fears of sexuality, earlier conflicts that are tied into her development. Therefore, another level of evaluation and negotiation for therapy would occur at this point.

In summary, we do not understand the amount of amnesia with rape, but we do know that neurobiologically, intimidation hinders memory recall. Threat to life floods the noradrenergic system and triggers the opioid system, causing amnesia or a poor encoding of information. Therefore, information is fragmented (i.e., Lynn remembers part of the rape). Even though sensory encoding is always present, it is not linked to the perceptual/cognitive system. In trauma therapy, however, the therapist tries to desensitize the patient to the overwhelming reaction to the information and pull the material together so there is no fragmentation of memory.

Drawings are a key clinical tool in work with traumatized clients because they offer a way of understanding the visual structure of the traumatic memories. Through drawings, we can tap into the kinesthetic, visual, and auditory memory, which enables us to look at how memory is being stored, retrieved, and processed. This includes the interpersonal aspects as well as environmental cue responses. Drawings also allow the expression of conceptualized information, serving as a window to the victim's organization of past experience and her use of it in present efforts to explain what has happened to her. When victims are asked to draw what happened, they must select and focus on some sequence or phase of a complex experience that occurred over time. In their drawings they will retrieve and communicate a variety of details, or they may choose to leave out certain details. While some of these details are elaborations of environmental cues that may be peripheral, others may be representative of a more central issue.

The drawings access the victim's system of retrieval and memory structuring. Some victims draw step-by-step frames. Others deal with what appear to be extraneous antecedent events, such as being threatened or abducted before being taken to a location and raped. They choose color, interject language, and depict themselves and/or the offender. Drawings are also useful in providing victim-initiated descriptions of what happened (Burgess, Hartman, Grant, & Wolbert, 1988).

NURSING EDUCATION

Content on rape is generally found in several areas of undergraduate nursing curricula. In the freshman year content regarding safety and campus life often includes prevention programs. Clinical content on interpersonal violence is generally found in the junior/senior years. In addition, crisis counseling of victims may be part of community health, psychiatric–mental health, and/or emergency nursing. The curriculum for graduate nursing students generally includes content on victimology, the biology of trauma and stress, and trauma therapy. For both undergraduate and graduate programs, however, content should be included on the following: (1) a foundation in the biology of stress and trauma, (2) assessment of trauma and specifically how to manage the acute crisis phase, and (3) introduction to principles of multimodal therapeutic strategies.

Clinical supervision is an essential part of victim treatment. Students should be able to review their experience, especially their reactions and responses to their interpersonal work with victims, in a safe context. It is essential to introduce students to the concepts of countertransference reactions when working with victims, including the student's feelings in listening to the trauma information itself and the complex dynamics that both the victim and student bring to the relationship. Given the limitations of clinical supervisory time in most education programs, we would recommend that attention be focused on the reaction to the trauma material itself and to the defensive pattern of the trauma victim.

Educators should also be sensitive to the fact that students may have had their own experiences with victimization. If academic and clinical content brings forth disclosure, educators need to assess the student's level of recovery from the experience and whether a counseling referral is indicated. While educators have an academic counseling relationship with students, they should not take on the role of therapist.

A new area for inclusion in nursing curricula is forensic nursing principles. Rape and crime-related traumas generally bring the nurse into contact with the legal system. As a result, nursing students must learn about documentation, testifying in court, and the use of expert testimony (Lynch, 1993).

NURSING RESEARCH

While research on rape trauma and its treatment is certainly not the exclusive domain of nursing, nursing's special focus on certain areas can benefit all disciplines in their search for basic and clinical-services knowledge.

BASIC RESEARCH

Because we believe there are biological changes from trauma, there needs to be study on the vulnerability of women and the biology of trauma. The seriousness of RTS speaks to the fact that it deserves as much in-depth biological research as the trauma of male war veterans. In addition to research on the relationship of the biological disruptions to the kinds of cognitive issues that arise postrape, nurse investigators should develop a united approach to research on victims and offenders, including programs of rehabilitation. Obviously, offenders can produce more victims than we can treat; consequently, to somehow reduce their output, either through prevention or curtailment, it is important to address prevention of rape trauma. These programs of research must employ the scientific basis that we know about trauma and behavior.

SERVICE RESEARCH

Another primary need in victim research is developing a better understanding of the nature of the long-term, cognitive-emotional responses associated with assault (Koss, 1990) because victims often seek therapy months, even years, after the event.

Although the response patterns to rape are disruptive to one's life-style, most victims seek only crisis intervention services. Rarely do they initially seek help or utilize individual psychotherapy services (Koss, 1990). Thus, it is suggested that psychiatric nurses be prepared to address the needs of the nonrecent victim.

CLINICAL SERVICES

A broad array of clinical interventions has been used to treat victims of violence, but none of the ones tested has been found sufficiently effective in and of itself. Therefore, clinicians must continue to work on integrating the research information and recognizing the need for a multimodal approach. They also should recognize and address the needs of the entire family, particularly when treating children.

CONCLUSION

In conclusion, there is a great need on the part of nursing to combine clinical and research efforts with other groups studying traumatic events and their consequences. The lack of adequate assessment and treatment interventions heretofore requires that nursing histories focus on past and present traumatic and stressful life events as well as more subtle behaviors associated with trauma. Understanding the biological substrata of trauma and their link with a variety of symptoms and behavioral traits that restrict the functioning of people has challenged the field of mental health and mental illness, and this understanding has important implications for psychiatric–mental health nursing practice. Nurses can, however, take the initiative to develop organized programs of intervention that address various levels of dysfunction and eventual recovery from trauma. The challenge is to create developmentally strategic stages of interventions that move the victim from crisis to recovery.

REFERENCES

Agger, I., & Jensen, S. B. (1993). The psychosexual trauma of torture. In J. P. Wilson & B. Raphael (Eds.), *International handbook of traumatic stress syndromes* (pp. 658–702). New York: Plenum Press.

American Psychiatric Association. (1994). *Diagnostic and statistical manual of mental disorders* (4th ed.). Washington, DC: Author.

Baker ,T., Burgess, A. W., Davis, R. C., & Brickman, E. (1990). Rape victims' concern over possible exposure to HIV. *Journal of Interpersonal Violence, 5*(1), 49–60.

Bandler, R., & Grinder, J. (1975). *The structure of magic* (Vol. 1). Palo Alto, CA: Science and Behavior Books.

Bremner, J. D., Scott, T. M., Seibyl, J. P., Southwick, S. M., & Delaney, R. C. (1992). Neurochemical and neuroanatomical correlates of learning and memory in posttraumatic stress disorder. *American College of Neuropsychopharmacy Abstracts, 31,* 11.

Bremner, J. D., Southwick, S. M., Johnson, E. R., Yehuda, R., & Charney, D. S. (1993). Childhood abuse in combat-related post-traumatic stress disorder. *American Journal of Psychiatry, 150*(2), 235–239.

Bureau of Justice Statistics. (1988). *Report to the nation on crime and justice.* Washington, DC: US GPO.

Burgess, A. W., Hartman, C. R., Grant, C., & Wolbert, W. (1988). The event drawing series. In A. W. Burgess & C. Grant (Eds.), *Sex rings and traumatized children* (pp. 15–23). Arlington, VA: National Center for Missing and Exploited Children.

Burgess, A. W., Hartman, C. R., McCausland, M. P., & Powers, P. (1984). Response patterns in children exploited in sex rings and pornography. *American Journal of Psychiatry, 141*(5), 656–662.

Burgess, A. W., & Holmstrom, L. L. (1974). Rape trauma syndrome. *American Journal of Psychiatry, 131,* 981–986.

Burgess, A. W., & Holmstrom, L. L. (1976). Coping behavior of the rape victim. *American Journal of Psychiatry, 133,* 413–418.

Burgess, A. W., & Holmstrom, L. L. (1978). Recovery from rape and prior life stress. *Research in Nursing and Health, 1*(4),165–174.

Burgess, A. W., & Holmstrom, L. L. (1979). Adaptive strategies and recovery from rape. *American Journal of Psychiatry, 136,* 1278–1282.

Carmen (Hilberman), E., Rieker, P. P., & Mills, T. (1984). Victims of violence and psychiatric illness. *American Journal of Psychiatry, 141*(3), 378–383.

Cunningham, J., Pearce, T., & Pearce, P. (1988). Child sexual abuse and medical complaints in adult women. *Journal of Interpersonal Violence, 3*(2), 131–144.

Danford, D. (1994). Personal communication.

Derogatis, L. R. (1977). *The SCL-90R: Administration, scoring, and procedures manual.* Baltimore: Clinical Psychometrics Research.

Dilts, R., Grinder, J., Bandler, R., Bandler, L., & DeLosier, J. (1980). *The study of the structure of subjective experience, neuro-linguistic programming* (Vol. 1). Cupertino, CA: Meta Publications.

Ellis, E. M. (1983). A review of empirical rape research: Victim reactions and response to treatment. *Clinical Psychology Review, 90,* 263–266.

Federal Bureau of Investigation. (1988). *Crime in the United States: Uniform crime reports.* Washington, DC: US Department of Justice.

Finkelhor, D., Hotaling, G., Lewis, I., & Smith, C. (1989) . Sexual abuse and its relationships to later sexual satisfaction, marital status, religion, and attitudes. *Journal of Interpersonal Violence, 4*(4), 379–399.

Foa, E., & Kozak, M. (1986). Emotional processing of fear: Exposure to corrective information. *Psychological Bulletin, 99,* 20–35.

Friedman, M. J. (1988). Toward rational pharmacotherapy for posttraumatic stress disorder. *American Journal of Psychiatry, 145,* 281–285.

Friedman, M. J. (1993). Psychobiological and pharmacological approaches to treatment. In J. P. Wilson & B. Raphael (Eds.), *International handbook of traumatic stress syndrome.* New York: Plenum Press.

Giller, E. (Ed.). (1990). *Biological assessment and treatment of posttraumatic stress disorder. Progress in psychiatry series.* Washington, DC: American Psychiatric Press.

Grinder, J., & Bandler, R. (1976). *The structure of magic* (Vol. 2). Palo Alto, CA: Science and Behavior Books.

Hammarberg, M. (1992). *Penn inventory.* Philadelphia: University of Pennsylvania.

Hartman, C. R., & Burgess, A. W. (1986). Child sexual assault: Generic roots of the experience. *Psychotherapy and the Family, 22,* 77–87.

Hartman, C. R., & Burgess, A. W. (1988). Information processing of trauma: Case application of a model. *Journal of Interpersonal Violence, 3*(4), 443–457.

Hazelwood, R. R., Reboussin, R., & Warren, J. I. (1989). Serial rape: Correlates of increased aggression and the relationship of offender pleasure to victim resistance. *Journal of Interpersonal Violence, 4*(1), 65–78.

Hemingway, R., & Reigle, T. (1985). Endogenous opiate involvement in learned helplessness and associated changes in brain norepinephrine metabolism. *Society for Neuroscience Abstracts, 11,* 1280.

Herman, J. (1981). *Father-daughter incest.* Cambridge, MA: Harvard University Press.

Herman, J. W. (1992). *Trauma and recovery.* New York: Basic Books.

Herman, J. W., Perry, M., & van der Kolk, B. A. (1989). Childhood trauma in borderline personality disorder. *American Journal of Psychiatry, 146,* 490–495.

Holmes, M. R., & St. Lawrence, J. B. (1983). Treatment of rape-induced trauma: Proposed behavioral conceptualization and review of the literature. *Clinical Psychology Review, 3,* 417–433.

Horowitz, M. (1976). Intrusive and repetitive thoughts after experimental stress. *Archives of General Psychiatry, 32,* 1457–1463.

Horowitz, M. (1982). Stress response syndromes and their treatment. In L. Goldberger & S. Breznitz (Eds.), *Handbook of stress: Theoretical and clinical aspects* (pp. 711–732). New York: The Free Press.

Horowitz, M., Wilner, N., & Alvarez, W. (1979). Impact of event scale: A measure of subjective stress. *Psychosomatic Medicine, 41*(3), 209–218.

Katz, B. L., & Burt, M. R. (1988). Self-blame in recovery from rape. In A. W. Burgess (Ed.), *Rape and sexual assault* (Vol. 2, pp. 151–167). New York: Garland.

Keane, T. M., Fairbanks, J. A., Caddell, J. M., Zimering, R. T., & Bender, M. E. (1985). A behavioral approach to assessing and treating posttraumatic stress disorder in Vietnam veterans. In C. Figley (Ed.), *Trauma and its wake* (pp. 257–294). New York: Brunner/Mazel.

Keane, T. M., Malloy, P. F., & Fairbank, J. A. (1984). Empirical development of an MMPI subscale for the assessment of combat-related posttraumatic stress disorder. *Journal of Consulting and Clinical Psychology, 52*(5), 888–891.

Kilpatrick, D. G., Best, C. L., Veronen, L. J., Amick, A. E., Villeponteaux, A., & Ruff, G. A. (1985). Mental health correlates of criminal victimization: A random community survey. *Journal of Consulting and Clinical Psychology, 53,* 866–873.

Kilpatrick, D. G., Edmunds, C. N., & Seymour, A. (1992). *Rape in America.* Arlington, VA: National Victim Center.

Kilpatrick, D. G., Resick, H., & Veronen, L. J. (1981). Effects of a rape-experience longitudinal study. *Journal of Social Issues, 37*(4), 105–120.

Kilpatrick, D. G., & Veronen, L. J. (1983). Treatment for rape-related problems: Crisis intervention is not enough. In L. H. Cohen, W. Claiborn, & G. Specter (Eds.), *Crisis intervention.* New York: Human Sciences Press.

Kilpatrick, D. G., Veronen, L. J., & Best, C. L. (1985). Factors predicting psychological distress in rape victims. In C. Figley (Ed.), *Trauma and its wake* (pp. 113–141). New York: Brunner/Mazel.

Kilpatrick, D. G., Veronen, L. J., Saunders, B. E., Best, C. L., Amick-McMullen, A., & Paduhovich, J. (1987). *The psychological impact of crime: A study of randomly surveyed crime victims* (Final report). National Institute of Justice, Grant No. 84-IJ-CX-0039.

Kolb, L. C. (1987). A critical survey of hypotheses regarding posttraumatic stress disorders. *American Journal of Psychiatry, 144,* 989–995.

Kolb, L. C. (1988). A critical survey of hypotheses regarding posttraumatic stress disorders in light of recent findings. *Journal of Traumatic Stress, 1,* 291–304.

Korf, J. (1976). Locus coeruleus, noradrenalin metabolism, and stress. In E. Usdin, R. Kvetnansky, & I. Kopin (Eds.), *Catecholamines and stress* (pp. 105–111). New York: Pergamon Press.

Koss, M. P. (1990). The women's mental health research agenda: Violence against women. Paper prepared for NIMH.

Largen, M. A. (1985). The anti-rape movement. In A. W. Burgess (Ed.), *Rape and sexual assault: A research handbook* (Vol. 1, pp. 1–13). New York: Garland.

Lavie, P., Hefez, A., Halperin, G., & Enoch, D. (1979). Long-term effects of traumatic war related events on sleep. *American Journal of Psychiatry, 136*(2), 175–178.

Lynch, V. (1993). Forensic nursing. *Journal of Psychosocial Nursing, 31*(11), 7–13.

Marhoefer-Dvorak, S., Resick, P., Hutter, C., & Girelli, S. (1988). Single versus multiple-incident rape victims: A comparison of psychological reactions to rape. *Journal of Interpersonal Violence, 3*(2), 145–160.

Mason, J. W., Giller, E. L., Kosten, T. R., Ostroff, R. B., & Podd, L. (1986). Urinary-free cortisone levels in posttraumatic stress disorder. *Journal of Nervous and Mental Disease, 174,* 145–149.

Mason, J. W., Giller, E. L., Kosten, T. R., & Yehuda, R. (1990). Psychoendocrine approaches to the diagnosis and pathogenesis of posttraumatic stress disorders. In E. L. Giller (Ed.), *Biological assessment and treatment of posttraumatic stress disorder* (pp. 65–86). Washington, DC: American Psychiatric Press.

McEwen, B. S., & Mendelson, S. (1993). Effects of stress on the neurochemistry and morphology of the brain: Counterregulation versus damage. In L. Goldberger & S. Breznitz (Eds.), *Handbook of stress: Theoretical and clinical aspects* (2nd ed.) (pp. 101–126). New York: MacMillan.

Meyers, J. E. B., & Paxson, J. (1992). Rape trauma syndrome in litigation involving adult victims. In J. Conte (Ed.), *Violence Update* (pp. 2–4). Newbury Park, CA: Sage Publishers.

Moos, R., & Billings A. (1982). Conceptualizing and measuring coping resources and process. In L. Goldberger & S. Breznitz (Eds.), *Handbook of stress: Theoretical and clinical aspects* (pp. 212–230). New York: Macmillan.

Moriata, K., Okamoto, M., Seki, K., & Wada, J.A. (1985). Suppression of amygdala-kindled seizures in the substantia innominata. *Experimental Neurology, 89*, 225–236.

Murphy, S., Amick-McMullen, A., Kilpatrick, D., Haskett, M., Veronen, L., Best, C., & Saunders, B. (1988). Rape victims' self-esteem: A longitudinal analysis. *Journal of Interpersonal Violence, 3*(4), 355–370.

Murphy, S., Kitchen, V., Harris, J. R. W., & Forster, S. M. (1989). Rape and subsequent seroconversion to HIV. *British Medical Journal, 299*, 718.

Perry, B. D., Southwick, S. M., Yehuda, R., & Giller, E. L. (1990). Adrenergic receptor regulation in posttraumatic stress disorder. In E. L. Giller (Ed.), *Biological assessment and treatment of posttraumatic stress disorder* (pp. 87–114). Washington, DC: American Psychiatric Press.

Pitman, R. K., & Orr, S. P. (1993). Psychophysiologic testing for posttraumatic stress disorder: Forensic psychiatric application. *Bulletin of the American Academy of Psychiatry and Law, 21*(1), 37–52.

Pitman, R. K., Orr, S. P., Forgue, D. F., de Jong, J. B., & Claiborn, J. M. (1987). Psychophysiologic assessment of posttraumatic stress disorder imagery in Vietnam combat veterans. *Archives of General Psychiatry, 44*, 970–975.

Prentky, R. A., Burgess, A. W., & Carter, D. (1986). Victim responses by rapist type: An empirical and clinical analysis. *Journal of Interpersonal Violence, 1*(1), 73–98.

Putnam, F. W. (1984). The psychophysiological investigation of multiple personality disorder: A review. *Psychiatric Clinics of North America, 7*, 31–41.

Reed, C. R., Burgess, A. W., & Hartman, C. R. (1991). Victim assessment: The dimensions of rape interview schedule (DORIS). In A. W. Burgess (Ed.), *Rape and sexual assault* (Vol. 3, pp. 13–28). New York: Garland.

Resnick, P. A. (1987). Psychological effects of victimization: Implications for the criminal justice system. *Crime and Delinquency, 33*(4). 468–478.

Ross, R. J., Ball, W. A., Sullivan, K. A., & Caroff, S. N. (1989). Sleep disturbance as the hallmark of posttraumatic stress disorder. *American Journal of Psychiatry, 146*(6), 697–707.

Sales, E., Baum, M., & Shore, B. (1984). Victim readjustment following assault. *Journal of Social Issues, 40*(1), 117–136.

Sandford, L. T. (1990). *Strong at the broken places.* New York: Random House.

Sapolsky, R. M., Krey, L. C., & McEwen, B. S. (1984). Glucocorticoid-sensitive hippocampal neurons are involved in terminating the adrenocortical stress response. *Proceedings of National Academy of Science, 81*, 6174–6177.

Sapolsky, R. M., Uno, H., Rebert, C. S., & Finch, C. E. (1990). Hippocampal damage associated with prolonged glucocorticoid exposure in primates. *Journal of Neuroscience, 10*, 2897–2902.

Shore, J. H., Tatum, E. L., & Vollmer, W. M. (1986). Psychiatric reactions to disaster: The Mount St. Helens experience. *American Journal of Psychiatry, 143*, 590–595.

Squire, L. R., Weinberger, N. M., Lynch, G., & McGaugh, J. L. (1991). *Memory: Organization and locus of change.* New York: Oxford Press.

Steketee, G., & Foa, E. B. (1987). Rape victims: Posttraumatic stress responses and their treatment: A review of the literature. *Journal of Anxiety Disorders, 1*, 69–86.

Teicher, M. H., Glod, C. A., Surrey, J., & Swett, C., Jr. (1993). Early childhood abuse and limbic system ratings in adult psychiatric outpatients. *Journal of Neuropsychiatry and Clinical Neurosciences, 5*, 301–306.

Terr, L. (1983). Chowchilla revisited: The effects of psychic trauma four years after a school bus kidnapping. *American Journal of Psychiatry, 140*, 1543–1550.

Tortora, G. J., & Grabowski, S. R. (1993). *Principles of anatomy and physiology* (7th ed.). New York: Harper Collins.

van der Kolk, B. (1987). *Psychological trauma.* Washington, DC: American Psychiatric Press.

van der Kolk, B. A. (1989). The compulsion to repeat the trauma. *Psychiatric Clinics of North America, 12*(2), 389–407.

van der Kolk, B. A., Greenberg, M., Boyd, H., & Krystal, J. (1985). Inescapable shock, neuro-transmitters, and addiction of trauma: Toward a psychobiology of posttraumatic stress. *Biological Psychiatry, 20,* 314–325.

van der Kolk, B. A., Pitman, R. K., Orr, S. P., & Greenberg, M. S. (1989). Endogenous opioids, stress induced analgesia, and posttraumatic stress disorder. *Psychopharmacology Bulletin, 25,* 417–421.

van der Kolk, B. A., & Saporta, J. (1993). Biological response to psychic trauma. In J. P. Wilson & B. Raphael (Eds.), *International handbook of traumatic stress syndromes* (pp. 25–33). New York: Plenum.

van Kammen, W. B., Christiansen, C., van Kammen, D. P., & Reynolds, J. (1990). Sleep and the POW experience: Forty years later. In E. L. Giller (Ed.), *Biological assessment and treatment of PTSD* (pp. 159–172). Washington, DC: American Psychiatric Press.

Veronen, L., & Kilpatrick, D. (1983). Stress management for rape victims. In D. Meichenbaum & M. E. Jaremko (Eds.), *Stress reduction and prevention* (pp. 341–374). New York: Plenum.

Walker, L. (1984). *The battered woman syndrome.* New York: Springer.

Werner, A. (1972). Rape: Interruption of the therapeutic process by external stress. *Psychotherapy: Theory, Research and Practice, 9,* 349–351.

Wilkinson, C. B. (1983). Aftermath of disaster: Collapse of Hyatt Regency Hotel skywalks. *American Journal of Psychiatry, 140,* 1134–1139.

Yehuda, R., Boisoneau, D., Mason, J. W., & Giller, E. L. (1993a). Glucocorticoid receptor number and cortisol excretion in mood, anxiety, and psychotic disorders. *Biological Psychiatry, 34,* 18–25.

Yehuda, R., Resnick, H., Kahana, B., & Giller, E. L. (1993b). Long-lasting hormonal alterations to extreme stress in humans: Normative or maladaptive? *Psychosomatic Medicine, 55,* 287–297.

Yehuda, R., Southwick, S. M., Krystal, J. H., Bremner, D., Charney, D. S., & Mason, J. W. (1993c). Enhanced suppression of cortisol following dexamethasone administration in posttraumatic stress disorder. *American Journal of Psychiatry, 150,* 83–86.

Yehuda, R., Southwick, S. M., Nussbaum, G., Wahby, V., Giller, E. L., & Mason, J. S. (1990). Low urinary cortisol excretion in patients with posttraumatic stress disorder. *Journal of Nervous and Mental Disease, 178,* 366–369.

CHAPTER

5

CATASTROPHIC STRESS

Sally Brosz Hardin, PhD, RN, FAAN

ABSTRACT

The chapter describes the role of the nurse in addressing the needs of clients—individuals, families, and communities—who are experiencing catastrophic stress from trauma, illness, disaster, or war. The conceptual model for catastrophic stress notes that human responses include the phases of the general adaptation syndrome and psychophysiological effects and depend not only on stressors but also on mediating variables such as demographics, developmental stage, premorbid personality, and subjective appraisal. A client's final adaptation also depends on a host of interactive factors that include the type, duration, and intensity of the catastrophe and the effects of protective factors. For example, coping style may be even more important than the nature and number of stressors in determining eventual adaptation to catastrophic stress. Within this framework the nurse's role involves the use of assessment instruments and nursing interventions. These include educative and supportive individual, group, or family counseling. Interventions in all phases of the recovery trajectory— that is, acute reactions and long-term consequences—focus on protective variables, thereby encouraging healthy coping, fostering self-efficacy, and providing needed support. Finally, the chapter suggests ways that current findings in catastrophic stress might alter nursing curricula and proposes specific questions that nursing research should address.

As the term itself implies, a *catastrophe* is an intense, uncontrollable, situational crisis of major proportions. Although there is debate in the literature concerning the theoretical definition of catastrophe (Solomon, 1989), general agreement is that it involves an extreme traumatic stressor related to actual or threatened death or serious injury of self or a loved one with subsequent fear, helplessness, or horror (American Psychiatric Association, 1994). A catastrophe produces disruption in daily living and psychological and physiological disequilibrium (Cohen & Hardin, 1989; Cowan & Murphy, 1985; Hardin & Cohen, 1988; Murphy, 1984a, 1984b, 1988, 1989a, 1989b; Silver & Wortman, 1980; Solomon, 1989; Tanaka, 1988; Titchener & Kapp, 1976).

Catastrophes may be related to trauma, illness, disaster, or war. In trauma or catastrophic illness the life-threatening event is somewhat limited (American Psychiatric Association, 1994; Hardin & Cohen, 1988). In disaster or war entire populations are exposed to life-threatening situations and massive personal and environmental destruction (Murphy, 1984a, 1984b). The life-threatening stressor may be acute, such as in a technological disaster, or chronic, such as with catastrophic illness.

Nurses must be prepared to assess and attend to clients experiencing catastrophe. This chapter provides a synthesis of multidisciplinary research findings that nurses can use to understand catastrophe and to guide their assessment and interventions. Nursing assessment and interventions should be based on clients' stage of development and phase in the recovery trajectory. It is important to remember that "client" may refer to individuals, families, or whole communities. In no instance of catastrophe—be it from trauma, illness, disaster, or war—does an individual respond in isolation.

Empirical research of catastrophic events was initiated formally in the 1970s. It is therefore in its early stages. Nurses will need to continue to be apprised of this literature.

THEORETICAL UNDERPINNINGS

Figure 5–1 illustrates a conceptual model of catastrophic stress. Primary concepts within this model include stressors, the client, mediating variables, the general adaptation syndrome and psychophysiological responses, the recovery trajectory with acute reactions and long-term consequences, protective variables, and adaptation. Knowledge about catastrophic stress emanates from three primary domains: Selye's (1974) and Folkman and Lazarus's (1984) classic work on stress, empirical studies of individuals' recovery trajectory following catastrophic events, and research on the psychosocial response of humans to catastrophic illness.

STRESSORS

Selye (1974) introduced classic stress theory, explaining that stress was the psychophysiological result of change. The changes inherent in life-threatening trauma, illness, disaster, or war produce many primary and secondary stressors. Although each of these catastrophes may differ in certain respects, they all share certain basic similarities. Selye's early theory has been amplified over the past two decades. Modern theory points out that stressors are additive; both the nature and number of stressors that the client experiences must be taken into account (Gist & Lubin, 1989; Hardin, Carbaugh, Weinrich, Pesut, & Carbaugh, 1992; Solomon, 1989; Weinrich, Hardin, & Johnson, 1990).

THE CLIENT

The client involved in a catastrophic event may be perceived as an individual, a family, or a whole community. Individual clients can include actual victims of the catastrophic event, disaster workers or caretakers who respond to the catastrophic event, or individual family members related to the victim. Miles (1994), Caputa (1993), and Weinrich et al. (1990) have elaborated upon the psychological distress of rescue workers and caregivers when working with victims of catastrophic events.

FAMILY AS CLIENT

Because families operate as systems, a catastrophic event produces extreme stress not only for an individual but also for the entire family (Bolin, 1982). Johansen (1988) found that parents who suffer the death of a child because of a catastrophic illness initially respond with shock, denial, and guilt. McKearn (1988) showed that families of Vietnam veterans with symptoms of posttraumatic stress also were diag-

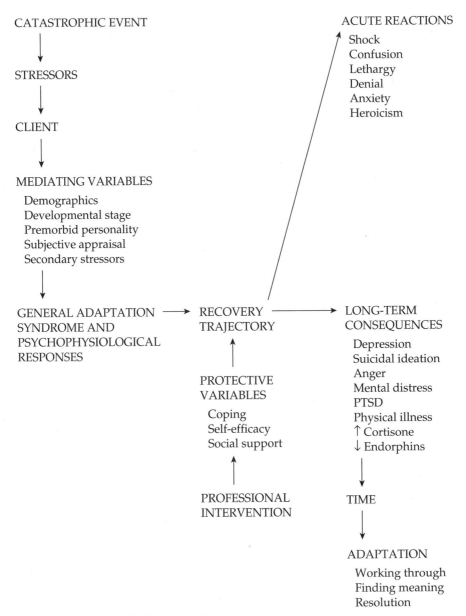

FIGURE 5–1. Model of catastrophic stress.

nosed with posttraumatic stress disorder (PTSD), a specific disorder outlined in the *Diagnostic and Statistical Manual of Mental Disorders* (American Psychiatric Association, 1994). Many studies indicate that parental coping responses are a significant predictor of stress in children (Nir, 1985). However, family members' responses to catastrophic stress do not necessarily parallel clients' responses.

Findings have indicated that families of persons hospitalized with critical illness generally view their critically ill members as sicker than clinical measures indicate (Kreamer, 1989). Hardin and Cohen (1988) found that family members' psychological responses were not like those of patients with catastrophic illness. While patients experienced death anxiety and long-term depression and anger, family members were more likely to suffer only from anxiety, especially early in the hospitalization and then again when patients were discharged. Nevertheless, Hardin and Cohen (1988) concluded that catastrophic illness had a highly negative impact on both patients' and family members' daily life and that the negative psychosocial effects for patients and family members may have persisted because professional psychosocial support was lacking.

The family's ability to adapt to a catastrophic event is contingent upon a variety of factors, for example, the nature of the catastrophe, the coping skills of individual family members, the presence of secondary stressors, the ability of family members to lend each other support, and the general psychological health of the family system. Reider (1989) reported that effective coping strategies and spiritual support were associated with positive familial adjustment to catastrophic illness.

COMMUNITY AS CLIENT

Tierney (1989) described the response of disaster-stricken communities as intense community mobilization, increased community consensus, and organizational adaptation and innovation. Communities that regularly face the threat of catastrophic stressors (e.g., earthquakes) typically are better prepared and able to respond. The recovery of households, businesses, and other social units is, of course, closely linked to community recovery (Perry & Lindell, 1978; Tierney, 1989).

MEDIATING VARIABLES

The way in which the client—whether individual, family, or community—responds to catastrophic stress is mediated by demographic variables, subjective appraisal, developmental stage, and premorbid personality. In catastrophic illness the actual course of the illness and treatment effects also modify response (Morris & Raphael, 1987; Ouslander, 1982).

Demographic variables such as gender, race, economic status, and age are mediating variables of catastrophic stress (Bolin, 1982; Rutter, 1987; Shore, 1986). Mitchell and Hardin (1994) demonstrated that adolescents define stress depending upon the social, economic, and cultural environment in which they live. They also found that poor adolescents rate themselves less mentally healthy than adolescents from higher socioeconomic levels.

A client's stage of development is another variable that affects the course of recovery. Children, adolescents, adults, and the elderly may display unique responses to catastrophe. Personal subjective appraisal is still another mediating variable. In fact, Folkman and Lazarus (1984) argued that subjective appraisal may be a more important mediating variable of catastrophic stress than objective reality. Grant, Hardin, Pesut, and Hardin (in press), for example, showed that adolescents exposed to Hurricane Hugo who were evaluated as having psychological distress did not appraise the impact of the hurricane on their lives. Similarly, another subsample ($n = 195$) of Carolina Adolescent Health Project (CAHP) students did not identify the hurricane as a stressor, even though they described main life stressors as those which threatened their well-being (Hardin et al., 1992). If persons do not appraise a catastrophic event, their final adaptation may be altered.

THE GENERAL ADAPTATION SYNDROME (GAS) AND PSYCHOPHYSIOLOGICAL RESPONSES

Selye (1974) asserted that stress was manifested by a specific, three-phase physiological syndrome, the general adaptation syndrome (GAS). *Phase 1* of the three-phase

TABLE 5–1. SELYE'S MODEL OF CATASTROPHIC STRESS

| | GENERAL ADAPTATION SYNDROME | | |
FACTORS	PHASE 1 ALARM	PHASE 2 RESISTANCE	PHASE 3 EXHAUSTION
Adrenal cortex	↑	↓	
Lymphatic system	↑	↓	Dysfunctional
Glucocorticoids	↑		↓
Mineralocorticoids	↑		↓
Catecholamines	↑		↓

GAS is an alarm reaction characterized by enlargement of the adrenal cortex and the lymphatic system and an increase in serum glucocorticoids, mineralocorticoids, and catecholamines (see Table 5–1). *Phase 2* of the GAS, the stage of resistance, involves shrinkage of the adrenal cortex and a diminishing of the lymph nodes to approximately normal size. *Phase 3*, the stage of exhaustion, includes enlargement and dysfunction of lymphatic structures and an ultimate depletion in the adaptive hormones (glucocorticoids, mineralocorticoids, and catecholamines). A stressed individual may not experience all three stages of the GAS; usually, a significant, acute stressor is characterized only by the first two GAS stages. The last stage, exhaustion, reflects an extreme, sustained stress response that ultimately leads to death (Selye, 1974).

Modern physiological studies on neuroendocrine responses to stress continue to expand Selye's initial model; the role of endorphins and enkephalins especially is being explored. For example, a biochemical explanation of PTSD is that endorphins (endogenous biochemical messengers that mediate pleasurable responses) become depleted with subsequent depletion of opioids (opioid receptors are instrumental in producing pleasurable narcotic-like states) (Hoffman, Watson, Wilson, & Montgomery, 1989). Hoffman et al. (1989) found that veterans with diagnosed PTSD had significantly higher morning serum cortisol levels and lower morning and evening serum betaendorphin levels. The researchers hypothesized that lowered betaendorphin levels resulted in chronic endogenous opioid depletion (Hoffman et al., 1989). They further hypothesized that serum betaendorphin levels could be a diagnostic laboratory test for PTSD (Hoffman et al., 1989).

Kolb (1987) outlined another neuroendocrine theory that may explain the onset of PTSD. He asserted that repeated, high-intensity neuroendocrine bombardment by a stressor that one perceives to be extremely threatening overwhelms the cortical defensive structure, leading to decreased synaptic processes. Subsequent neurochemical changes, and ultimately neuronal death, may occur. The neurons most likely to be affected lie in the temporal-amygdaloid area (Kolb, 1987). Damage to the amygdaloid area is associated with bizarre changes in discriminatory sensations, particularly hearing. This may explain why patients with PTSD are hyperresponsive to low-level auditory stimuli.

Furthermore, hypothalamic structures escape usual adrenocortical inhibition. Therefore cortical perceptual, cognitive, affective, and somatic symptoms associated with the original stressor are reactivated. This ultimately may explain the typical nonspecific sympathetic nervous system response in PTSD sufferers, as well as responses that include rage, irritability, and reliving the traumatic experience (Kolb, 1987).

The research of Harris, Mion, Patterson, and Frengley (1988) concerning catastrophic illness also demonstrated the interrelationship between psychological and physiological variables. Victims of catastrophic illness whose mood improved and depression lessened showed improved physical functioning. Leidy (1990) showed significant interrelationships among psychosocial resources, stress symptoms, and catastrophic illness.

PSYCHOPHYSIOLOGICAL EFFECTS OF CATASTROPHIC STRESS

Researchers consistently have reported a significantly increased incidence of morbidity among the victims of a disaster (Lima, Pai, Caris, & Haro, 1991; Logue, Melick, & Streuning, 1981; Rahe, 1988). Holen (1991) noted significant increases in general morbidity, psychosomatic diagnoses, and accident proneness. Horowitz, Wilner, Kaltreider, and Alvarez (1980) reported increased somatization. Somatic symptoms included gastrointestinal disturbances, sore muscles, hot/cold spells, lower back pain, faintness, dizziness, numbness or tingling in various body parts, heavy feelings in limbs, a lump in the throat, and pains in the chest. These occurred in over 75% of the clients. However, Fairley, Langeluddecke, and Tennant (1985) demonstrated that while physical morbidity was two to three times greater immediately following a natural disaster, it lasted only for a brief 3-month period.

After reviewing the literature on hostages and prisoners of war, Rahe (1988) agreed that catastrophic stress can predict not only mental but also physical health and illness. Blanchard, Kolb, Pallmeyer, and Gerardi (1982) showed significant differences between PTSD combat veterans and controls on measures of heart rate, systolic blood pressure, forehead EMG, and skin conductance level when exposed to combat sounds. Other studies confirmed increased physiological responsiveness in combat veterans (Fairbank, Degood, & Jenkins, 1981; Fairbank & Keane, 1982; Keane & Kaloupek, 1982; McCaffery & Fairbank, 1985).

THE CATASTROPHIC STRESS RECOVERY TRAJECTORY

The Institute of Medicine (1989) and others have documented that all clients (individual, family, and community) may respond to catastrophic stress with a relatively predictable three-phase recovery trajectory consisting of acute reactions, long-term consequences, and eventual adaptation (Cohen & Hardin, 1989; Cohen et al., 1988; Hardin & Cohen, 1988; Weinrich et al., 1990) (See Fig. 5–1).

RESPONSES IN PHASE 1 OF THE RECOVERY TRAJECTORY

Figure 5–1 illustrates that Phase 1, acute reactions to catastrophic stress, often includes early shock, confusion, lethargy, denial, anxiety, and heroics (Cohen et al., 1988; Hardin & Cohen, 1988; Jimerson, 1987; Kinston & Rosser, 1974; Rodriguez, 1985; Schukit, 1983; Shore, Tatum, & Vollmer, 1986; Weinrich et al., 1990). Some researchers (Kinston & Rosser, 1974) also have observed grossly inappropriate or psychotic behavior in this phase. However, Kinzie (1986) found only a 7% incidence of psychosis among Cambodian concentration camp victims. Likewise, Weinrich et al. (1990) did not observe psychotic behavior among victims immediately after Hurricane Hugo.

Anxiety occurs following a catastrophe as a result of feeling vulnerable to life-threatening stressors. In a disaster, stressors and subsequent anxiety are related not only to threats to life but also to property damage and other major life changes that affect large segments of the population (Bolin, 1982, 1985; Demi & Miles, 1982; Institute of Medicine, 1989; Lindy, Grace, & Green, 1981; Lindy, Green, Grace, & Titchener, 1983; Maida, Gordon, Steinberg, & Gordon, 1989; Solomon, 1989; Weinrich et al., 1990). Anxiety may be related to loss of control, role, housing, or employment (Hardin & Cohen, 1988; Shine, 1984). In catastrophic illness, anxiety is related to loss of bodily integrity, uncertainty about the future, or fear of a required treatment regimen (Hardin & Cohen, 1988; Shine, 1984).

RESPONSES IN PHASE 2 OF THE RECOVERY TRAJECTORY

Phase 2 in the recovery trajectory, long-term consequences, is characterized by depression, suicidal ideation, anger, global mental distress, and, possibly, PTSD and physical illness (Cohen & Ahearn, 1980; Dohrenwend & Dohrenwend, 1974; Hardin & Cohen, 1988; Head, Hardin, Pesut, & Gleaton, 1995; Laube, 1973; Horowitz et al., 1986; Murphy, 1984a, 1984b, 1986; Titchener & Kapp, 1976; Weinrich et al., 1990).

Depression develops in response to losses. Murphy (1984a, 1984b) found that Mount St. Helens disaster victims experienced long-term depression and anger related to loss of loved ones, homes, schools, and employment. Similarly, Horowitz et al. (1980) reported high levels of anger and hostility among trauma victims. Laube's (1985) study of the victims of the Xenia, Ohio, tornado reported that their symptoms of subjective distress *increased* over the 2 years following the disaster.

Depression in catastrophic illness occurs in response to loss of control, independence, and bodily functions, as well as the threat of chronic pain or death (Halligan, 1983; Ouslander, 1982). Viney (1984) concluded that life-threatening stressors from catastrophic illness produced anger and uncertainty, whereas stressors related to loss of bodily integrity resulted in anger and feelings of hopelessness and helplessness. Cohen and Hardin (1989; Cohen et al., 1988; Hardin & Cohen, 1988) obtained longitudinal physiological and psychosocial measures on patients and family members involved in the 1983 Illinois catastrophic botulism outbreak and showed that sequelae of depression, anger, and suicide ideation occurred for as long as 3 years postoutbreak.

Catastrophic illness may predispose individuals to psychogenic as well as nonpsychogenic depression. Metabolic and endocrine changes related to physical illness can cause a reduction in feelings of vitality and subsequently result in depression. Additionally, medications such as antihypertensives, corticosteroids, and some sedatives cause iatrogenic depression (Field, 1985).

Loss of independence or body integrity, intolerable pain, or neurological impairment may be related to suicidal ideation (MacKenzie & Popkin, 1987). Cancer, head and spinal cord injuries, Huntington's chorea, and multiple sclerosis are associated epidemiologically with an increased incidence of suicide (MacKenzie & Popkin, 1987). Certain ages appear to be at greater risk for suicide when confronted with a catastrophic illness. Petzel and Riddle (1981) documented that adolescents with a catastrophic illness are at increased risk for suicide if they have a globally negative outlook on life, high emotional reactivity, and a dysfunctional family. Elderly widowed persons with a catastrophic illness also are at greater risk for suicidal behavior than their single, separated, or divorced peers (Conwell, Rotenberg, & Caine, 1990).

Post-trauma response (PTR), a nursing diagnosis approved for testing by the North American Nursing Diagnosis Association (Tanaka, 1988), and PTSD are diagnostic conditions that may occur in Phase 2 of the catastrophic stress recovery trajectory (Peterson, Prout, & Schwarz, 1991; Weinrich et al., 1990). It is important to note that PTR and PTSD are defined as abnormal responses that are not inevitable. These are actual clinical diagnoses, not simply human responses following a catastrophic event.

The psychologically distressing symptoms of PTR and PTSD include sleep difficulties, irritability or outbursts of anger, disturbed concentration, hypervigilance, exaggerated startle response, disturbed interpersonal relationships, and physiological reactivity upon exposure to circumstances symbolizing the traumatic event

(American Psychiatric Association, 1994; Bychowski, 1968; Kolb & Multilipassi, 1982). Tanaka (1988) suggested coping responses in PTR evolve in four stages: (a) immediate survival; (b) oscillating emotional numbness with intrusive recollection; (c) working through the trauma by rationalizing a meaning for the event; and (d) assimilating this meaning into one's worldview.

Empirical studies on the percentage of catastrophic stress victims who sustain PTSD vary. Percentages range from 30 (Gleser, Green, & Winget, 1981; van der Ploeg & Kleijn, 1989) to 40 (Dawes, Tredoux, & Feinstein, 1989; Lima et al., 1991) or 50 (Kinzie, 1986). Many studies do not differentiate between symptoms of posttraumatic stress and the actual clinical diagnosis of PTSD.

RESPONSES IN PHASE 3 OF THE RECOVERY TRAJECTORY

Phase 3, adaptation, is the final phase in the catastrophic stress recovery trajectory. A very intense life experience such as a catastrophic event etches itself into the human memory (Karl, 1989). To heal itself, the mind seeks to accommodate this psychic trauma by incorporating the experience and giving meaning to the event (Horowitz, 1974, 1986). Such incorporation and growth lead to final adaptation to the catastrophe but require time as well as individual strengths and social support. When the catastrophe finally has been worked through and resolved, philosophical and existential meaning is ascribed to the event by its victim (Horowitz, 1974). In catastrophic illness the patient also often must adapt to an altered life-style.

CATASTROPHIC STRESS IN CHILDREN

Empirical findings indicate that children's catastrophic stress response trajectory differs from that of adults. Children appear to be more resilient. Although they often initially complain of posttraumatic-stress-type symptoms, these usually dissipate by 9 to 14 months after the event (Andrews, Tennant, Hewson, & Vaillant, 1978; Nader, Pymoos, Fairbanks, & Frederick, 1990). Nader et al. (1990) measured elementary school children's reactions to the trauma of a sniper attack at their school. Initial acute reactions included reexperiencing the event, emotional detachment, and high states of arousal. However, children with low to moderate exposure (they did not see classmates injured or killed) reappraised the situation and within 14 months no longer perceived it as an extreme stressor. Similar results were found with seventh-grade school bus disaster victims (Milgram, Toubiana, Klingman, Raviv, & Goldstein, 1988) and with British children involved in a ferry disaster (Yule & Williams, 1990).

On the other hand, Kinston and Rosser (1974) proposed that youngsters with a prior history of emotional stress, physical illness, or family problems have a higher risk for psychiatric impairment after a disaster than adults. While youngsters with healthy coping skills and good support reputedly have only a 13% risk for developing psychiatric impairment, children with poor coping and support and high life event stress have a 43% risk of developing serious psychological symptoms following a catastrophic event (Andrews et al., 1978).

Terr (1991) documented that parents underestimate the effect of catastrophic events on their children. Bromet and Shulberg (1986) found that parents believed the Three Mile Island disaster had no effect on their children's mental health 3 years after the event. None of the parents whose children were in the Chowchilla school bus kidnapping sought counseling for their children, and parents consistently downplayed the significance of the event (Terr, 1991). Similarly, parents of children who had been exposed to a blizzard and flood denied the impact of these disasters on their children (Burke et al., 1982). Cambodian survivors of trauma also did not perceive the difficulties that their children had experienced (Sack, Angell, Kinzie, & Rath, 1986).

CATASTROPHIC STRESS IN ADOLESCENTS

Data concerning adolescents' response trajectory are limited. Gleser et al. (1981) found that disaster stress increased from childhood to adolescence and that among teenage victims of the Buffalo Creek disaster, 20% reported anxiety and 30% reported depression. Baum, Fleming, and Singer (1983) showed no sustained psychological distress among teen victims of Three Mile Island, but the data source was parents rather than the teens themselves.

The Carolina Adolescent Health Project (CAHP) compared longitudinal physical and psychological health among high school students ($n = 1685$) who were or were not exposed to Hurricane Hugo (Hardin & Hardin, 1993; Garrison, Weinrich, Hardin, Weinrich, & Wang, 1993; Hardin, Weinrich, Weinrich, Garrison, & Hardin, 1994). Findings showed that on the first anniversary of this natural disaster, adolescents' exposure to Hurricane Hugo was directly related to anxiety, depression, anger, and global mental distress, especially for whites, females, and those with low self-efficacy or social support (Grubbs et al., 1992; Hardin et al., 1994).

Other CAHP findings indicated that these teenagers reported posttraumatic stress symptoms such as reexperiencing the storm (20%), having symptoms of increased arousal (40%), experiencing a numbing of general responsiveness, and avoiding stimuli associated with the hurricane (80%) (Garrison et al., 1993). This is similar to Kinzie's (1986) finding that 50% of adolescent Cambodian refugees demonstrated symptoms of PTSD. In the CAHP study, a total of 4.6% of the females and 1.5% of the males reported all PTSD symptoms (Garrison et al., 1993). Nurse practitioners referred 12% of the total CAHP sample for further psychological evaluation, and about one half of these referred students demonstrated major symptoms of psychological distress (Grant et al., in press; Head et al., 1995).

In terms of long-term consequences of catastrophic stress on adolescents' physical health, Thomas, Shaffner, and Groer (1988) discussed adolescent stressors, and De Maio-Esteves (1990) showed that teenage girls who experienced high levels of stress consequently reported frequent health problems. Greene, Walker, Hickson, and Thompson (1985) had similar findings. Adolescents with chronic pain of unknown etiology and high degrees of behavioral problems reported higher life stress than other teens.

ADOLESCENT COPING WITH CATASTROPHIC STRESS

Abramowitz, Petersen, and Schulenberg (1984) suggested that adolescents avoid major stress by coping with one stressor at a time and responding to proximate stressors, that is, those which have current and immediate effects on their daily lives. LaMontagne (1987) reported that teenagers used a large repertoire of coping skills to deal with the trauma of surgery and that teens who used active versus passive coping mechanisms experienced less distress. Weekes and Savedra (1988) found that adolescent cancer patients coped with pain effectively if they used favored and familiar coping strategies.

Self-efficacy and social support were important protective variables among CAHP teens (Hardin et al., 1994). Concurring with CAHP findings, Kinzie (1986) showed parental support was very important in mediating catastrophic stress among Cambodian refugee adolescents. According to this researcher, 92% of the

Cambodian adolescents without a family member reported symptoms of psychological distress, whereas only 53% of those with a family reported such symptoms.

PROTECTIVE VARIABLES

Protective variables are not only important in helping children and adolescents achieve healthy adaptation but also enhance recovery in adults. Folkman and Lazarus (1984) and others (Institute of Medicine, 1989) have confirmed that coping, self-efficacy, and support are protective variables; they enhance adaptation to catastrophic stress and subsequently diminish its negative effects on health (Bolin, 1982, 1985; Cohen et al., 1988; Demi & Miles, 1982; Hardin & Cohen, 1988; Lindy et al., 1981; Lindy et al., 1983; Murphy, 1984a, 1984b, 1986; Weinrich et al., 1990).

COPING

Weekes and Savedra (1988) defined coping as the effort to manage demand, regardless of the success or failure of the effort. Individuals vary in their ability to cope; factors such as level of maturity and previous experience with managing specific stressors can affect coping (Brown, Stetson, & Beatty, 1989; Hyman & Woog, 1982; Spirito, Overholser, & Stark, 1989). Solomon (1989) suggested that adults have previous life experiences that inoculate them against catastrophe's most deleterious effects. Anecdotal evidence has confirmed that older persons use their past experiences to cope with catastrophic illness (Hardin & Cohen, 1988).

Folkman and Lazarus (1984) explained that while each person copes with stressors in unique ways, all persons use both emotional and cognitive coping strategies. Most studies agree that active, cognitive problem solving is a healthy form of coping (Berlin, Davis, & Orenstein, 1988; Dunn-Geier, McGrath, Rourke, Latter, & D'Astous, 1986; Friedman & Litt, 1987; LaMontagne, 1987; Mindick & Oskamp, 1984; Schneider, Davis, Boxer, Fisher, & Friedman, 1990; Weekes & Savedra, 1988). Atkinson, Atkinson, Smith, and Hilgard (1987) concluded that the personality of stress-resilient persons is characterized by clear cognitive perception, an awareness that change is an opportunity for growth, a commitment to supportive relationships, and an inner sense of competency. However, individuals who are taxed with numerous stressors that have a high degree of intensity can develop maladaptive coping responses resulting in threats to their mental and physical health (Hyman & Woog, 1982). Therefore it is important to note that *coping style may be even more important than the nature and number of stressors in determining eventual adaptation to catastrophic stress.*

Research findings suggest that most individuals who suffer from catastrophic illness (Rodriguez, 1985) or disaster (Murphy, 1987; Weinrich et al., 1990) eventually develop effective coping strategies and adapt. Weinrich et al. (1990) showed that Hurricane Hugo victims coped by talking about their personal experiences and by relying on humor, religion, and altruism. Although these victims also used other, less healthy coping mechanisms (i.e., smoking, abusing alcohol, and compulsive eating), the investigators noted the high caliber and varied repertoire of Hurricane Hugo victims' coping skills (Weinrich et al., 1990). They demonstrated they had the self-efficacy, strength, and resilience that Murphy (1987) found in volcano victims and Gavalya (1987) described among survivors of Mexico City's strongest earthquake.

McCammon and colleagues (McCammon, Durham, Allison, & Williamson, 1988), who investigated disaster workers' coping mechanisms, reported that cognitive understanding and the effort to ascribe meaning to the event were the most frequent coping strategies among police, fire, emergency medical, and hospital personnel.

Hardin and Cohen (1988) showed that victims of catastrophic illness relied on spouses, praying, talking with friends and other victims, and humor to cope. Coping strategies, in turn, may be enhanced by strong, positive social support (Sparks, 1988).

SOCIAL SUPPORT

Social support, or the *belief* that one has interpersonal resources that can help deal with problems, also mediates catastrophic stress (Cook & Bickman, 1990; Dean & Lin, 1977). However, research findings concerning its effects have been less than clear-cut (Coppel, 1980). Tornado victims stated that visits from primary support groups did not ease their disaster stress (Laube, 1973). Solomon and colleagues (Solomon, Smith, Robins, & Fishbach, 1987) showed that for women, in particular, strong social ties were more burdensome than supportive during times of extreme stress. Others concurred, indicating that married subjects have higher rates of PTSD than unmarried persons (Solomon, Mikulincer, Freid, & Wosner, 1987).

On the other hand, Fleming (Fleming, Baum, Gisriel, & Gatchel, 1982) reported the positive influence of social networks for victims at Three Mile Island. Mount St. Helens victims and victims of catastrophic illness also reported that support eased their distress (Murphy, 1987, 1989a; Hardin & Cohen, 1988). Although findings are not entirely consistent, there is sufficient evidence to believe that cognitive coping and social support have the potential to buffer the negative effects of catastrophic stress.

SELF-EFFICACY

Self-efficacy is defined as the belief in one's ability to be successful in meeting goals (Coppel, 1980; Grubbs et al., 1992). Self-efficacy theory espouses that an individual's inner sense of competency, perceptions, and expectations have a profound effect on outcomes (Bandura, 1977). Murphy (1987) showed that self-efficacy was even more significant than social support in buffering Mount St. Helens victims' catastrophic stress. Self-efficacy accounted for 19% of disaster stress variance 1 year postdisaster and for 24% at 3 years postdisaster (Murphy, 1987, 1989a). After the Three Mile Island disaster, victims who perceived themselves as self-efficacious exhibited fewer distress symptoms than those who did not (Baum et al., 1983).

SUMMARY

Human responses to a catastrophic event depend not only on stressors and the client but also on mediating variables. Important mediating variables are demographics, developmental stage, premorbid personality, and subjective appraisal. There is a beginning body of literature that suggests children, adolescents, adults, and elder clients may differ in their responses to a catastrophic event. Clients' final adaptation to a catastrophe also depends on a host of interactive factors that include the type, duration, and intensity of the catastrophe and the effects of protective factors.

NURSING CARE OF PERSONS WITH CATASTROPHIC STRESS

ASSESSMENT

In general the literature reports that nurses are well received and trusted by victims of catastrophic stress. Moreover, nurses are skilled communicators who are prepared to assess and intervene with both physiological and psychological effects. They are comfortable with on-site interventions and accustomed to making critical, decisive, and instantaneous decisions (Durham & Hardin, 1986; Hardin & Cohen, 1988; Weinrich et al., 1990).

The astute clinical practitioner should anticipate the probable psychological and physiological effects of catastrophic stress on individuals, families, and communities. The nurse should assess the client's stage of development, phase in the recovery trajectory, and approximate level of protective variables. Table 5–2 provides a summary of nursing assessment factors and potential diagnostic tools based on a client's phase in the recovery trajectory.

In the acute phase of the recovery trajectory, the nurse determines if a life-threatening emergency exists and assesses the environment to determine the individual's/family's/community's ability to meet basic needs of daily living. The nurse attempts to develop trust and assess general physical and mental health. The nurse may wish to conduct physical examinations of individuals and families.

The nurse should obtain a history of current symptoms of catastrophic stress, noting especially symptoms of shock, confusion, lethargy, denial, or anxiety. At this point, the nurse can also use principles of crisis intervention, that is, identifying the client's primary stressors, providing directives, encouraging catharsis, and offering support (Aguilera & Messick, 1974). The nurse assesses whether the client is using healthy coping mechanisms—such as rationalization, heroicism, or humor—and constructive behaviors such as cleaning up in the wake of a disaster (Weinrich et al., 1990).

In addition to coping mechanisms, the client's sense of self-efficacy and perception of support, such as extended family or helpful neighbors, needs to be determined. In this writer's opinion, directive, structured interviews are the most efficacious method of assessing clients during this early phase in the recovery trajectory.

In the long-term phase of the recovery trajectory, the nurse needs to assess for symptoms of depression, suicidal ideation, anger, global mental distress, and posttraumatic stress. During this phase of recovery, the nurse can, once again, rely on physical examinations or interviews as well as surveys and/or questionnaires to determine clients' status.

CATASTROPHIC STRESS ASSESSMENT INSTRUMENTS

GENERAL HEALTH

Table 5–2 reviews methods for making nursing assessments during each phase of the recovery trajectory. A simple method for assessing clients' health following catastrophic stress is to provide a four-point Likert item that asks: "On a scale of '0' (poor) to '4' (excellent), how do you rate your physical health?" A similar item can assess emotional health. The CAHP (Hardin, Weinrich, Weinrich, Garrison & Hardin, 1990) used these types of items with the adolescent victims of Hurricane Hugo and found they provided a good index of subjective perception of health.

PHYSICAL HEALTH

The nurse can perform a physical examination and take a health history. Another index of physical health that may be used following a catastrophic event is CAHP's physical Health Index (HI). The HI assesses clients' general health state and use of treatment agencies. Another index of physical health is the Demi and Miles Health Change Scale (Miles, 1994). Other tools that assess somatic symptoms, functional health, changes in health perception, and drug and alcohol abuse also may be useful. A thorough assessment of the physical consequences of disasters is one of the weaker aspects of catastrophic stress research. Therefore, there are few published instruments to guide the nurse in this area.

TABLE 5–2. NURSING ASSESSMENT OF CATASTROPHIC STRESS

PHASES	TOOLS
Acute Reactions	
Basic physical needs	Observation
Physical deficits	Nursing exam
Demographic variables	Interview
Shock	Observation/interview
Confusion	
Lethargy	
Denial	
Anxiety	
Heroics	
Protective variables	Observation/interview
Coping	
Self-efficacy	
Support	
Mid Reactions	
Psychological health	Diagnostic Interview Schedule
	Disaster Supplement (DIS)
	Brief Symptom Inventory (BSI)
Coping	Jalowiec Coping Scale (JCS)
	CAHP Adolescent Coping Scale (CAHP-SC)
Self-efficacy	Coppel Self-Efficacy Scale (SES)
Support	Coppel Social Support (CSS)
Physical illness	Nursing Exam
	CAHP Physical Health Index (HI)
	Demi and Miles Health Change Scale
↑ Serum cortisone	Blood work
↓ Serum endorphins	Blood work
Long-term Consequences	
Depression	Brief Symptom Inventory (BSI)
Suicidal ideation	Brief Symptom Inventory (BSI)
	Observation/interview
Anger	Speilberger Anger Expression Scale (AX)
Global mental distress	Brief Symptom Inventory (BSI)
PTSD	Observation/interview

PSYCHOLOGICAL HEALTH

To determine psychological health after a catastrophic event, the Diagnostic Interview Schedule/Disaster Supplement (DIS), a structured interview guide that has been used extensively to assess symptoms of distress following a disaster (Robbins et al., 1982), is effective (see Table 5–2). It is important to note, however, that victims of catastrophic stress report more psychological distress symptoms when interviewed than when surveyed. Nevertheless, the nurse who cannot use a standardized survey instrument may wish to consider using the DIS.

Derogatis's Brief Symptom Inventory (BSI) is an efficacious survey to use following a catastrophic event because of its brevity, readability, validity, reliability, and extensive use in catastrophic research (Derogatis & Spencer, 1982). The BSI is a brief form of the SCL-90-R and Hopkins Symptom Checklist (HSCL). It measures current, point-in-time, symptomatic psychological distress from underlying symptom dimensions that include anxiety, phobic anxiety, depression, hostility, somatization, obsessive-compulsiveness, interpersonal sensitivity, paranoid ideation, and psychoses. In addition, the global mental distress severity index (GSI), a total score of all psychological distress symptoms, provides a useful indicator of overall global mental distress. Hardin et al. (1994) reported Cronbach alpha test results of 0.93 for the total BSI, 0.78 for depression, and 0.66 for anxiety. The tool can be used with adolescents as well as adults. For assessment of children's response to a catastrophic event, Frick offers a variety of play therapy techniques (Frick, 1994).

A useful tool that measures anger, one of the reported long-term consequences of catastrophic stress, is Speilberger's Anger Scale (AX) (Speilberger, 1986; Speilberger et al., 1985; Hardin et al., 1993). The AX is a 24-item self-report questionnaire that yields three subscale scores—anger out, anger in, anger control—plus a total anger score. In testing the AX on 1,114 high school students, Spielberger reported good internal consistency, with alpha coefficients ranging from 0.73 to 0.84. In the CAHP project (Hardin et al., 1994), Cronbach alpha reliability for the AX was 0.76. Like the BSI, the AX can be used with adolescents or adults.

PROTECTIVE VARIABLES

In addition to assessing physical health and the psychological effects of a catastrophic event, the nurse should also assess demographic and protective variables. The Jalowiec Coping Scale (JCS) (Jalowiec, 1988), which is based on Lazarus's coping theory, is a widely used, reliable, and valid instrument to measure coping. A particular benefit of the JCS is its conceptual congruence with the construct of self-efficacy in the catastrophic stress model. Another measure, that particularly addresses coping in adolescents is the Carolina Adolescent Health Project Coping Scale (CAHP-CS) (Hardin, Weinrich, Cheever, Gleaton, & Head, 1995). The CAHP-CS is an expanded and revised version of the original JCS. Revisions were accomplished by generating qualitative, grounded data from a subsample ($n = 195$) of CAHP students, pilot-testing the CAHP-CS with normal high schoolers, and evaluating it with the total CAHP sample (Hardin et al., 1992; Hardin, Weinrich, Cheever et al., 1995). The CAHP-CS provides subscale scores for healthy coping and unhealthy coping, as well as scores for cognitive coping, positive emotional coping, negative emotional coping, and risk-taking coping in adolescents.

Coppel's Self-Efficacy Scale (SES) (1980), originally designed by Coppel for a doctoral dissertation, measures subjects' beliefs about their ability to produce desired outcomes. Typical items include: "I believe I use my skills to the best advantage" or "I am not afraid to make mistakes." The SES was used by Murphy (1987) with Mount St. Helen's victims. Hardin and colleagues used 12 items from the SES to measure self-efficacy and its protective effects in adolescents in the CAHP. For the original scale, Coppel reported an internal consistency reliability of 0.91; in the CAHP it was 0.90 (Grubbs et al., 1992).

The CAHP Social Support Inventory (CAHP-SSI), a modified version of Coppel's (1980) Social Support Inventory, assesses *subjective* perception of social support. Ten items assess perceived social support on a five-point scale ranging from "not at all" to "very much." An example of an item is, "There are people to whom I give and from whom I receive support during difficult periods." Coppel (1980) and Murphy (1987) reported an internal consistency of 0.89 for the Coppel Social Support Inventory, which measured objective and subjective aspects of support. Hardin et al. (1994) found the internal consistency of the CAHP-SSI was 0.90. One also may wish to use a social support instrument with reference to a particular catastrophic event as well as measuring global social support.

INTERVENTIONS

ACUTE RECOVERY PHASE

Therapeutic interventions should be based on findings of the nurse's assessment. Table 5–3 summarizes nursing interventions that can be used over the course of the client's recovery trajectory. Initially, the nurse attempts to decrease stress by attending to physical survival and basic human needs, facilitating activities of daily living, and serving as a liaison between the client and social support agencies. General principles of crisis intervention also will be useful for the nurse to help the client (Weinrich et al., 1990). Throughout all phases of the recovery trajectory, as Figure 5–1 shows, professional interventions are focused on protective variables. The nurse encourages healthy coping, fosters self-efficacy, and provides support. Interventions

TABLE 5–3. NURSING INTERVENTIONS WITH CATASTROPHIC STRESS

PHASES	INTERVENTIONS
Acute Reactions	
Basic physical needs	Provide liaison to social agencies
Physical deficits	Attend to physical emergencies
	Refer to other health care workers as necessary
Psychological effects	One-to-one nurse-patient relationship
Shock	Attentive listening to the disaster story
Confusion	Give nurturing support, permit regression
	Provide libidinal cocoon
Denial	Permit intermittent denial, identify patient's primary concern
Anxiety	Provide structure, consider antianxiety medications
Lethargy/heroics	Encourage sublimation and constructive activity
Protective variables	
Coping	Encourage patient's favored, healthy coping mechanisms; emphasize rationalization, humor, sublimation, and undoing
Self-efficacy	Support patient's previous successes and belief in own abilities; dilute irrational self-doubts; emphasize power of expectations to produce results
Support	Repeople patient's world; provide professional support; advise professional counseling when necessary
Long-term Consequences	
Depression	Provide outpatient individual, group, or family counseling; guide patient in sorting out emotions; encourage cognitive understanding and demonstrate link between depression and traumatic stressors; prescribe physical activity and "homework"
Suicidal ideation	Activate a "no-suicide" contract; consider hospitalization
Anger	Help patient understand normalcy of anger posttrauma; assist patient to recognize anger; provide healthy outlets for anger
Global mental distress	Assess global function every 6 months posttrauma for 3 years (third year should produce adaptation)
PTSD	Provide outpatient individual, group, or family counseling; clarify PTSD symptoms; identify trauma as source of symptoms; encourage cognitive problem solving

include the use of educative and supportive individual, group, or family counseling as well as community interventions (Murphy, Aroian, & Baugher, 1989; Murphy, Laube, & Glittenberg, 1982).

Specific strategies to provide victims with support and catharsis immediately following a disaster have been reported. In the early acute phase of recovery, Hurricane Hugo victims indicated that directive nursing interventions and interventions that encouraged catharsis were most effective (Weinrich et al., 1990). Teams of nurses taught victims very simple, basic principles of physical and mental health, mobilized and directed clients in clearing victims' homes, and provided victims with an opportunity to "tell their Hugo story." This technique may help victims gain cognitive mastery over their catastrophic experience.

Victims of the Iowa plane crash disaster were assigned a one-to-one nurse from point of entry into the emergency room; this nurse allowed the client to repeatedly retell the story of the crash or to withdraw—depending on the *client's* need. Another treatment strategy is the libidinal cocoon, in which victims/relatives are offered protective seclusion and intensive professional emotional support for several days (Black, 1987). Such measures may be effective because they permit victims to regress, regroup, and withdraw from the responsibilities of ordinary daily life.

During this early recovery phase the nurse also might consider using supplemental pharmacologic agents such as antidepressants and antianxiety drugs. Antianxiety drugs of choice could include benzodiazepines or nonbenzodiazepine anxiolytics (Schukit, 1983). However, Kinzie (1986) reported that for some victims with depressive and PTSD symptoms, benzodiazepines and propranolol were not effective, whereas tricyclic antidepressants were. Kinzie (1986) also discussed the efficacy of Clonidine, an alpha 2 adrenergic agonist that reduces opiate withdrawal symptoms and, subsequently, symptoms of PTSD.

LONG-TERM RECOVERY PHASE

Although there is little firm evidence about whether recovery from catastrophe can be expedited or enhanced, many researchers have noted formal interventions' potential to enhance recovery and modify the consequences of catastrophic stress (Hardin, Carbaugh, Stewart, & Walsh, 1991; Hardin & Hardin, 1993; Hardin et al., 1994; Solomon, 1989; Stewart et al., 1992; Walsh & Hardin, 1994). Kinzie (1986) felt that a long-term commitment to a therapeutic relationship with victims of catastrophic stress is necessary. A recent review of research of various treatments for posttraumatic stress indicated that treatment often has a delayed effect that increases over time (Solomon, Gerrity, & Muff, 1992).

In the long-term recovery phase the nurse strives to help clients reduce negative consequences of depression, anger, global mental distress, and posttraumatic stress and continues to enhance protective variables. The nurse might accomplish this through individual, group, family, or community counseling.

Strategies to improve clinical outcomes in family members can include disjoint therapy (in which individual members are treated separately) followed by conjoint therapy (in which all members participate in traditional family therapy) (Rosenheck & Thomson, 1986). Figley (1988) proposed that families be treated with a five-phase program for PTSD that included building commitment to therapeutic objectives, framing and reframing the problem, developing a healing theory, and closure. Referring parents whose child has succumbed to a catastrophic illness to specific support groups such as Candlelighters and Compassionate Friends can help to strengthen their social support and ameliorate their recovery (Johansen, 1988).

CAHP tested group interventions designed to mitigate disaster stress by enhancing healthy coping, self-efficacy, and social support in adolescents (Carbaugh, Hardin, Weinrich, Hardin, & Pesut, 1995; Hardin et al., 1991; Hardin & Hardin, 1993; Hardin et al., 1993; Hardin et al., 1994; Hardin, Weinrich, Garrison et al., 1995; Stewart et al., 1992; Walsh & Hardin, 1994). The teenagers involved in the interventions evaluated them positively, and data showed that adolescents assigned to the CAHP intervention reported significantly less global mental distress than did control adolescents following exposure to Hurricane Hugo (Hardin, Weinrich, Garrison et al., 1995).

EDUCATIONAL ISSUES IN CATASTROPHIC STRESS

Victims of catastrophe—whether in emergency rooms, in-patient physical and psychiatric agencies, or disaster sites—will be cared for by nurses. However, nursing education, in the experience of this author, has given minimal attention to the nurse's role with victims of catastrophe. Usually, undergraduate medical-surgical nursing courses provide only brief reference to disaster victims and the psychosocial effects of catastrophic illness. All too often, psychiatric nursing courses devote little time to the psychosocial aspects of physical illness or to the psychological needs of individuals experiencing trauma.

Nursing undergraduate and graduate curricula should include research-based content about the recovery trajectory of persons experiencing catastrophe. The similarities among victims of a variety of catastrophic events need to be emphasized. In addition to curricular content, creative and less traditional clinical experiences for both undergraduate and graduate nursing students could enhance nurses' skills in working with victims of catastrophe. For example, Weinrich and colleagues (1990) wrote that one of the particular benefits of their naturalistic field study with Hurricane Hugo victims was its incorporation of undergraduate and graduate nursing students. The authors indicated this experience permitted students to appreciate the value of assessment and observation, both clinically and as a research strategy. Moreover, students were exposed at a grass-roots level to the value of research as an essential component, not merely a textbook ideal, of nursing. Students reported that this experience sharpened assessment and critical thinking skills and spurred decisive, goal-directed nursing action (Weinrich et al., 1990).

In the event that nurse scientists and/or faculty can bring groups of students to the site of catastrophic events, it would be beneficial to the victims as well as to the students. An ideal structure would provide teams of baccalaureate nurses, led by master's-prepared medical-surgical-psychiatric nurse specialists. These teams would provide systematic, empirically based interventions designed by nurse scientists/faculty; they could also make careful observations and evaluations that would be reported back to nurse scientists.

RESEARCH ISSUES IN CATASTROPHIC STRESS

There has been minimal testing of theoretical models of catastrophic stress, that is, the relationship among stressors, psychological effects, physiological effects, protective variables, other mediating variables, and various recovery phases. Murphy (1991) noted that although catastrophic research reflects creativity, it is primarily descriptive, with few studies testing linkages among constructs.

Even more obvious is the glaring lack of studies that examine the long-term consequences of catastrophic events. Longitudinal studies are of vital importance, even though they are by their very nature costly and complex to conduct. Melick (1985) and Murphy (1991) noted that research of catastrophic events emphasizes mental rather than physical health consequences. It would seem that nursing science is a particularly relevant profession to investigate the long-term physical health consequences of catastrophe.

Solomon (1989), the coordinator of the Emergency Disaster Research Program at the National Institute of Mental Health (NIMH), noted the importance of examining both immediate reactions and prolonged consequences of catastrophic stress. She advised that research observe not only the quality of human responses but also the phases in the recovery process. To observe immediate human responses to catastrophe is important, but is difficult because of problems in reaching the site, obtaining access to populations, and/or receiving rapid funding. The newly instituted RAPID review program at NIMH should alleviate this latter problem.

Some have argued that stressors and coping mechanisms may be unique to particular types of catastrophic events. Consequently, many recommend that each catastrophic event needs to be studied (Maida et al., 1989; Silver & Wortman, 1980; Titchener & Kapp, 1976). It is also important to point out that some unexpected or positive effects of catastrophic events have been reported, and this area, too, remains entirely open for investigation (Quarantelli & Dynes, 1972, 1973). In addition, there is a glaring lack of replicative studies in all catastrophic events research.

Terr (1991) advised that children experience trauma according to two major types of symptoms. Type I symptoms follow a single, unanticipated event (acute stressors), while Type II symptoms are associated with repeated exposures to extreme events (chronic stressors). The possibility that a similar typology applies to adult and teenage victims of catastrophe needs to be investigated.

Bromet and Shulberg (1986) summarized other persistent methodological flaws in research of catastrophic events. These flaws include the lack of large samples, longitudinal cohorts or control groups, distinct relevant time points in data collection, standardized measures, and differentiation of psychological distress from psychiatric diagnostic conditions. Sampling issues are especially important in catastrophic events research. Often subjects are voluntary, but many victims are reluctant to come forward, especially if there is embarrassment about psychological symptoms. Thus, often these samples may not be representative of the total population.

Combination field and experimental studies that examine the efficacy of interventions with clients are essential. Nursing doctoral students may wish to investigate biobehavioral and psychophysiological variables, including clients' immune response, related to various types of nursing interventions.

Catastrophic stress, a uniquely human experience, may be particularly amenable to qualitative study methods. Murphy (1991) addressed the paradox of nurse scientists' lack of inductive theory development in this area since so many nurse scholars are advocates of grounded theory. On the other hand, disaster research has been criticized for loose research methodologies (Bromet & Shulberg, 1986; Solomon, 1989). Therefore, nurse researchers should consider triangulating both qualitative and quantitative methods to investigate catastrophes. Rapid dissemination of research findings following a catastrophe is critical so that subsequent research methodologies can be modified and future victims helped.

Studies of catastrophic stress that measure psychological status with survey instruments report less psychological distress among victims than studies that use interviews. Therefore, Murphy's (1991) admonition that research use multiple approaches to measure the same construct for enhanced precision and catastrophic theory development is a sound one.

CONCLUSION

As nurses are called upon to assess and intervene with individuals, families, and communities who are experiencing catastrophic stress, nurses' holistic perspective, knowledge of psychophysiological processes, and ability to operationalize theory and take decisive action in emergency situations and field sites are extraordinarily valuable assets. Nursing science can benefit victims of catastrophic events by performing not only brief, descriptive assessments of victims' acute responses but also longitudinal, experimental studies of interventions. Including undergraduate and graduate professional nursing students in such research and then rapidly disseminating research findings will assist both nurses and persons experiencing catastrophic stress.

ACKNOWLEDGEMENT. The author expresses her gratitude to Kerry Cheever, R.N., Ph.D., for her research assistance in completing this article.

REFERENCES

Abramowitz, R., Petersen, A., & Schulenberg, J. (1984). Changes in self-image during early adolescence. *New Directions in Mental Health Services, 22*(6), 19–27.

Aguilera, D. C., & Messick, J. M. (1974). *Crisis intervention.* St. Louis, MO: Mosby.

American Psychiatric Association. (1994). *Diagnostic and statistical manual of mental disorders* (4th ed. [DSM IV]). Washington, DC: Author.

Andrews, G., Tennant, C., Hewson, D. M., & Vaillant, G. E. (1978). Life event stress, social support, coping style and risk of psychological impairment. *Journal of Nervous and Mental Disease, 166,* 307–316.

Atkinson, R. L., Atkinson, R. C., Smith, E. E., & Hilgard, E. R. (1987). *Introduction to psychology.* New York: Harcourt, Brace, Jovanovich.

Bandura, A. (1977). Self-efficacy: Toward a unifying theory of behavioral change. *Psychological Review, 84,* 191–215.

Baum, A., Fleming, R., & Singer, J. E. (1983). Coping with victimization by technological disaster. *Journal of Social Issues, 39*(2), 117–138.

Berlin, R., Davis, R., & Orenstein, A. (1988). Adaptive and reactive distancing among adolescents from alcoholic families. *Adolescence, 23*(91), 577–584.

Black, J. W. (1987). The libidinal cocoon: A nurturing retreat for the families of plane crash victims. *Hospital and Community Psychiatry, 38*(12), 1322–1326.

Blanchard, E. B., Kolb, L. C., Pallmeyer, B. A., & Gerardi, R. J. (1982). A psychophysiological study of post-traumatic stress disorder in Vietnam veterans. *Psychiatric Quarterly, 54*(4), 220–229.

Bolin, R. (1982). *Long-term family recovery from disaster.* Boulder: University of Colorado Institute of Behavioral Science.

Bolin, R. (1985). Disaster characteristics and mental health. In B. Sowder (Ed.), *Disasters and mental health: Selected contemporary perspectives* (DHHS Publication No. 85-1421) (pp. 3–28). Washington, DC: US Government Printing Office.

Bromet, E., & Shulberg, H. C. (1986). The Three Mile Island disaster: A search for high risk groups. In J. H. Shore (Ed.), *Disaster stress studies: New methods and findings.* Washington, DC: American Psychiatric Press.

Brown, S., Stetson, B., & Beatty, P. (1989). Cognitive and behavioral features of adolescent coping in high-risk drinking situations. *Addictive Behaviors, 14,* 43–52.

Burke, J. D., Borus, J. F., Burns, B. J., Millstein, K. H., & Beasley, M. C. (1982). Changes in children's behavior after a natural disaster. *American Journal of Psychiatry, 139,* 1010–1014.

Bychowski, G. (1968). *Evil in man: Anatomy of hate and violence.* New York: Grune & Stratton.

Caputa, J. (1993). Disaster strikes the caregivers. *Caring Magazine,* 60–61.

Carbaugh, L., Hardin, S. B., Weinrich, S., Hardin, T. L., & Pesut, D. (1995). A group protocol to enhance healthy coping in adolescents. Unpublished manuscript, The University of Massachusetts, Amherst.

Cohen, F. L., & Hardin, S. B. (1989). Fatigue in patients with catastrophic illness. In S. G. Funk, E. M. Tornquist, M. T. Champagne, L. A. Copp, & R. A. Wiese (Eds.), *Key aspects of comfort* (pp. 208–216). New York: Springer.

Cohen, F. L., Hardin, S. B., Nehring, W., Keough, M. A., Laurenti, S., McNabb, J., Platis, C., & Weber, C. (1988). Physical and psychosocial health status three years after a catastrophic illness—botulism. *Issues in Mental Health Nursing, 9*, 387–398.

Cohen, R. E., & Ahearn, F. L. (1980). *Handbook for mental health care of disaster victims.* Baltimore: The Johns Hopkins University Press.

Conwell, Y., Rotenberg, M., & Caine, E. D. (1990). Completed suicide at age 50 and over. *Journal of the American Geriatrics Society, 38*(6), 640–644.

Cook, J. D., & Bickman, L. (1990). Social support and psychological symptomatology following a natural disaster. *Journal of Traumatic Stress, 5*(4), 541–556.

Coppel, D. (1980). The relationship of perceived social support and self-efficacy to major and minor stresses. Unpublished doctoral dissertation, University of Washington, Seattle.

Cowan, M., & Murphy, S. (1985). Identification of post-disaster bereavement risk predictors. *Nursing Research, 34*(2), 71–75.

Dawes, A., Tredoux, C., & Feinstein, A. (1989). Political violence in South Africa. *International Journal of Mental Health, 18*(2), 16–43.

Dean, A., & Lin, N. (1977). The stress-buffering role of social support: Problems and prospects for systematic investigation. *Journal of Nervous and Mental Disease, 165*, 403–417.

DeMaio-Esteves, M. (1990). Mediators of daily stress and perceived health status in adolescent girls. *Nursing Research, 39*(6), 360–364.

Demi, A., & Miles, M. (1982). Understanding psychological consequences of disaster. *Journal of Emergency Nursing, 9*(1), 11–16.

Derogatis, L., & Spencer, P. M. (1982). *Administration and procedures: BSI manual I.* Baltimore: The Johns Hopkins University School of Medicine.

Dohrenwend, B., & Dohrenwend, B. (1974). *Stressful life events: Their nature and effects.* New York: Wiley.

Dunn-Geier, B. J., McGrath, P., Rourke, B., Latter, J., & D'Astous, J. (1986). Adolescent chronic pain: The ability to cope. *Pain, 26*(1), 25–32.

Durham, J., & Hardin, S. B. (1986). *The nurse psychotherapist in private practice.* New York: Springer.

Fairbank, J. A., DeGood, D. E., & Jenkins, C. W. (1981). Behavioral treatment of a persistent post-traumatic response. *Journal of Behavioral Therapy and Experimental Psychiatry, 12*(4), 321–324.

Fairbank, J. A., & Keane, T. M. (1982). Flooding for combat-related stress disorders: Assessment of anxiety reduction across traumatic memories. *Behavior Therapy, 13*, 499–510.

Fairley, M., Langeluddecke, P., & Tennant, C. (1985). Psychological and physical morbidity in the aftermath of a cyclone. *Psychological Medicine, 15*(3), 571–576.

Field, W. E. (1985). Physical causes of depression. *Journal of Psychosocial Nursing and Mental Health Services, 23*(10), 7–11.

Figley, C. R. (1988). A five-phase treatment of post-traumatic stress disorder in families. *Journal of Traumatic Stress, 1*(1), 127–141.

Fleming, R., Baum, A., Gisriel, M., & Gatchel, R. (1982). Mediating influences of social support on stress at Three Mile Island. *Journal of Human Stress, 8*, 14–22.

Folkman, S., & Lazarus, R. (1984). *Stress, appraisal, and coping.* New York: Springer.

Friedman, I. M., & Litt, I. F. (1987). Adolescents' compliance with therapeutic regimens: Psychological and social aspects and interventions. *Journal of Adolescent Health Care, 8*, 52–67.

Frick, S. (1994). Play therapy with children exposed to disaster. Unpublished manuscript, The University of South Carolina, Columbia.

Garrison, C. Z., Weinrich, M., Hardin, S. B., Weinrich, S., & Wang, L. (1993). Post-traumatic stress disorder in adolescents after a hurricane. *American Journal of Epidemiology, 138*(7), 522–530.

Gavalya, A. S. (1987). Reactions to the 1985 Mexican earthquake: Case vignettes. *Hospital and Community Psychiatry, 38*(12), 1327–1330.

Gist, R., & Lubin, B. (Eds.). (1989). *Psychosocial aspects of disaster.* New York: Wiley.

Gleser, G. C., Green, B. L., & Winget, C. (1981). *Prolonged psychosocial effects of disaster: A study of Buffalo Creek.* New York: Academic Press.

Grant, S. M., Hardin, S. B., Pesut, D. J., & Hardin, T. (in press). Psychological evaluations, referrals, and follow-up of adolescents after their exposure to Hurricane Hugo. *Journal of Child and Adolescent Psychiatric Nursing.*

Greene, H., Walker, L., Hickson, G., & Thompson, J. (1985). Stressful life events and somatic complaints in adolescents. *Pediatrics, 75*(1), 19–22.

Grubbs, S., Hardin, S. B., Weinrich, S., Weinrich, M., Garrison, C., Pesut, D., & Hardin, T. L. (1992). Self-efficacy in normal adolescents. *Issues in Mental Health Nursing, 13,* 121–128.

Halligan, F. G. (1983). Reactive depression and chronic illness: Counseling patients and their families. *Personnel and Guidance Journal, 61*(7), 401–406.

Hardin, S. B., Carbaugh, L., Stewart, J., & Walsh, S. (1991). A symposium on interventions to mitigate disaster stress in adolescents. *Proceedings of the Southeastern Psychiatric Nursing Conference.* Jacksonville, Florida.

Hardin, S. B., Carbaugh, L., Weinrich, S., Pesut, D., & Carbaugh, C. (1992). Stressors and coping in adolescents exposed to Hurricane Hugo. *Issues in Mental Health Nursing, 13,* 105–119.

Hardin, S. B., & Cohen, F. L. (1988). Psychosocial effects of a catastrophic botulism outbreak. *Archives of Psychiatric Nursing, 2,* 173–185.

Hardin, S. B., & Hardin, T. L. (1993). *Effectiveness of an intervention to increase adolescent coping post-disaster.* Paper presented to the Institute of Psychology, University of Vienna, and to the Jagiellonian University, Krakow, Poland.

Hardin, S. B., Pesut, D., Head, S., Mitchell, J., Stewart, J., & Hardin, T. (1993). An intervention to decrease anger and violence among adolescents. *Proceedings of the Southeastern Psychiatric Nursing Conference.* Charleston, South Carolina.

Hardin, S. B., Weinrich, S., Cheever, K. H., Gleaton, J., & Head, K. M. (1995). The Adolescent Coping Scale (ACS). Unpublished manuscript, The University of Massachusetts, Amherst.

Hardin, S. B., Weinrich, S., Garrison, C., Gleaton, J., Weinrich, M., & Hardin, T. L. (1995). Decreasing global mental distress in adolescents following a disaster: The Carolina Adolescent Health Project intervention. Unpublished manuscript, The University of Massachusetts, Amherst.

Hardin, S. B., Weinrich, M., Weinrich, S., Garrison, C., & Hardin, T. L. (1990). *The Carolina Adolescent Health/Hugo Disaster Project.* Annual Report to the National Institute of Mental Health.

Hardin, S. B., Weinrich, M., Weinrich, S., Garrison, C., & Hardin, T. L. (1994). Psychological distress of adolescents exposed to Hurricane Hugo. *Journal of Traumatic Stress, 7*(3), 427–440.

Harris, R., Mion, L., Patterson, M., & Frengley, J. (1988). Severe illness in older patients: The association between depressive disorders and functional dependency during the recovery phase. *Journal of the American Geriatrics Society, 36*(10), 890–896.

Head, K. M., Hardin, S. B., Pesut, D., & Gleaton, J. (1995). Predicting psychological distress in adolescents: Testing the Carolina Adolescent Health Project (CAHP) model. Unpublished manuscript, The University of South Carolina, Columbia.

Hoffman, L., Watson, P. B., Wilson, G., & Montgomery, J. (1989). Low plasma beta endorphin in post-traumatic stress disorder. *Australian and New Zealand Journal of Psychiatry, 23,* 269–273.

Holen, A. (1991). A longitudinal study of the occurrence and persistence of post-traumatic health problems in disaster survivors. *Stress Medicine, 7*(1), 11–17.

Horowitz, M. J. (1974). Stress response syndrome. *Archives of General Psychiatry, 31,* 768–781.

Horowitz, M. J. (1986). Disaster stress studies: Conclusions. In J. H. Shore (Ed.), *Disaster stress studies: New methods and findings.* Washington, DC: American Psychiatric Press.

Horowitz, M. J., Krupnick, J., Kaltreider, N., Wilner, N., Leong, A., & Marmer, C. (1986). Initial psychological response to parental death. *Archives of General Psychiatry, 38,* 316–323.

Horowitz, M. J., Wilner, N., Kaltreider, N., & Alvarez, M. A. (1980). Signs and symptoms of post-traumatic stress disorder. *Archives of General Psychiatry, 37,* 85–92.

Hyman, R., & Woog, P. (1982). Stressful life events and illness onset: A review of crucial variables. *Research in Nursing and Health, 5,* 155–163.

Institute of Medicine. (1989). *Research on children and adolescents with mental, behavioral, and developmental disorders.* Washington, DC: American Academy Press.

Jalowiec, A. (1988). Analysis of the Jalowiec Coping Scale. In C. F. Waltz & O. Strickland (Eds.), *Measurement of nursing outcomes* (pp. 287–308). New York: Springer.

Jimerson, S. (1987). Post-traumatic stress disorders. In J. Haber, P. Hopkins, A. Leach, & B. Sideleau (Eds.), *Comprehensive psychiatric nursing* (3rd ed.). New York: McGraw-Hill.

Johansen, B. B. (1988). Parental grief over the death of a child. *Loss, Grief, and Care, 2*(3–4), 143–153.

Karl, G. T. (1989). Psychic trauma. *Journal of Psychosocial Nursing, 27*(4), 15–19.

Keane, T. M., & Kaloupek, D. G. (1982). Imaginal flooding in the treatment of a post-traumatic stress disorder. *Journal of Consulting and Clinical Psychology, 550*(1), 138–140.

Kinston, W., & Rosser, R. (1974). Disaster: Effects on mental and physical state. *Journal of Occupational Medicine, 21,* 595–598.

Kinzie, J. D. (1986). Severe post-traumatic stress syndrome among Cambodian refugees: Symptoms, clinical course, and treatment approaches. In J. H. Shore (Ed.), *Disaster stress studies: New methods and findings.* Washington, DC: American Psychiatric Press.

Kolb, L. C. (1987). A neuropsychological hypothesis explaining post-traumatic stress disorder. *American Journal of Psychiatry, 144,* 989–995.

Kolb, L. C., & Multilipassi, L. R. (1982). The conditioned emotional response: A subclass of the chronic and delayed post-traumatic stress disorder. *Psychiatric Annals, 12*(11), 979–987.

Kreamer, C. L. (1989). The relationship of family functioning, family demographics, and severity of illness to family coping with the crisis of critical illness. Dissertation abstracts, The University of Texas at Austin.

LaMontagne, L. (1987). Children's preoperative coping: Replication and extension. *Nursing Research, 36*(3), 163–167.

Laube, J. (1973). Psychological reactions of nurses in disaster. *Nursing Research, 22*(4), 343–347.

Laube, J. (1985). Health care providers as disaster victims. In J. Laube & S. Murphy (Eds.), *Perspectives on disaster recovery.* Norwalk, CT: Appleton-Century-Crofts.

Leidy, N. K. (1990). A structural model of stress, psychosocial resources, and symptomatic experience in chronic physical illness. *Nursing Research, 39*(4), 230–236.

Lima, B. R., Pai, S., Caris, L., & Haro, J. M. (1991). Psychiatric disorders in primary health care clinics one year after a major Latin American disaster. *Stress Medicine, 7,* 25–32.

Lindy, J., Grace, M., & Green, G. (1981). Survivors: Outreach to a reluctant population. *American Journal of Orthopsychiatry, 51,* 468–478.

Lindy, J. D., Green, B. L., Grace, M., & Titchener, J. (1983). Psychotherapy with survivors of the Beverly Hills Supper Club fire. *American Journal of Psychotherapy, 37*(4), 593–610.

Logue, J., Melick, M., & Struening, E. (1981). A study of health and mental health status following a natural disaster. In J. R. Greenley (Ed.), *Research in community mental health: An annual compilation of research* (Vol. 2, pp. 217–274). Greenwich, CT: JAI Press.

MacKenzie, T. R., & Popkin, M. K. (1987). Suicide in the medical patient. *International Journal of Psychiatry in Medicine, 17*(1), 3–23.

McCaffery, R. J., & Fairbank, J. A. (1985). Behavioral assessment and treatment of accident-related post-traumatic stress disorder: Two case studies. *Behavior Therapy, 16,* 406–416.

McCammon, S., Durham, T., Allison, E., & Williamson, J. (1988). Emergency workers' cognitive appraisal and coping with traumatic events. *Journal of Traumatic Stress, 1*(3), 353–372.

McKearn, J. (1988). Post-traumatic stress disorder: Implications for the treatment of family members of alcoholics. *Alcoholism Treatment Quarterly, 5*(1,2), 141–144.

Maida, C. A., Gordon, N. S., Steinberg, A., & Gordon, G. (1989). Psychosocial impact of disasters: Victims of the Baldwin Hills fire. *Journal of Traumatic Stress, 2*(1), 37–49.

Melick, M. E. (1985). The health of post-disaster populations: A review of literature and case study. In J. Laube & S. Murphy (Eds.), *Perspectives on disaster recovery.* Norwalk, CT: Appleton-Century-Crofts.

Miles, M. (1994). The Demi and Miles Health Change Scale. University of North Carolina, Chapel Hill, personal communication.

Milgram, N., Toubiana, Y., Klingman, A., Raviv, A., & Goldstein, I. (1988). Situational exposure and personal loss in children's acute and chronic stress reactions to a school bus disaster. *Journal of Traumatic Stress, 1*(3), 339–352.

Mindick, B., & Oskamp, S. (1984). Individual differences between adolescent contraceptors: Some implications for intervention. In I. R. Stuart & C. F. Wells (Eds.), *Pregnancy in adolescence: Needs, problems, and management* (pp. 140–176). New York: Van Nostrand Reinhold.

Mitchell, J. L., & Hardin, S. B. (1994). Adolescents' perception of psychological health status. *Proceedings of the Southeastern Psychiatric Nursing Conference.* Virginia Beach, Virginia.

Morris, P. L., & Raphael, B. (1987). Depressive disorder associated with physical illness: The impact of stroke. *General Hospital Psychiatry, 9*(5), 324–330.

Murphy, S. A. (1984a). Stress levels and health status of victims of a natural disaster. *Research in Nursing and Health, 7,* 205–215.

Murphy, S. A. (1984b). After Mount St. Helens: Disaster stress research. *Journal of Psychosocial Nursing, 22,* 9–18.

Murphy, S. A. (1986). Health and recovery status of natural disaster victims one and three years later. *Research in Nursing and Health, 9,* 331–340.

Murphy, S. A. (1987). Self-efficacy and social support: Mediators of stress on mental health following a natural disaster. *Western Journal of Nursing Research, 9*(1), 58–86.

Murphy, S. A. (1988). Mediating effects of intrapersonal and social support on mental health one and three years after a natural disaster. *Journal of Traumatic Stress, 1*(2), 155–172.

Murphy, S. (1989a). An explanatory model of recovery from disaster loss. *Research in Nursing and Health, 12,* 67–76.

Murphy, S. A. (1989b). Multiple triangulation: Applications in a program of nursing research. *Nursing Research, 38*(5), 294–297.

Murphy, S. A. (1991). Human responses to catastrophe. In J. J. Fitzpatrick, R. L. Taunton, & A. K. Jacox (Eds.), *Annual Review of Nursing Research, 9,* 57–76.

Murphy, S. A., Aroian, K., & Baugher, R. (1989). A theory-based preventive intervention program for bereaved parents whose children have died in accidents. *Journal of Traumatic Stress, 2*(3), 319–335.

Murphy, S. A., Laube, J., & Glittenberg, J. (1982). Coping with stress following natural disasters: Individual, health care provider, and community responses. *Western Journal of Nursing Research, 4,* 123–125.

Nader, K., Pymoos, R., Fairbanks, L. & Frederick, C. (1990). Children's post-traumatic stress disorder reactions one year after a sniper attack at their school. *American Journal of Psychiatry, 147*(11), 1526–1530.

Nir, Y. (1985). Post-traumatic stress disorder in children with cancer. In S. Eth & R. Pynoos (Eds.), *Post-traumatic stress disorder in children.* Washington, DC: American Psychiatric Press.

Ouslander, J. G. (1982). Physical illness and depression in the elderly. *Journal of the American Geriatrics Society, 30*(9), 593–599.

Perry, R., & Lindell, M. (1978). The psychological consequences of natural disaster: A review of research on American communities. *Mass Emergencies, 3,* 105–115.

Peterson, K. C., Prout, M. F., & Schwarz, R. A. (1991). *Post-traumatic stress disorder.* New York: Plenum.

Petzel, S. V., & Riddle, M. (1981). Adolescent suicide: Psychosocial and cognitive aspects. *Adolescent Psychiatry, 9,* 343–398.

Quarantelli, E. L., & Dynes, R. R. (1972). When disaster strikes. *Psychology Today, 5,* 66–70.

Quarantelli, E. L., & Dynes, R. R. (1973). When disaster strikes. *New Society, 4,* 5–9.

Rahe, R. N. (1988). Anxiety and physical illness. *Journal of Clinical Psychiatry, 49*(Suppl.), 26–29.

Reider, J. A. (1989). The relationship of family needs satisfaction and family coping strategies to family adjustment during the critical illness of a family member. Dissertation abstracts, The Catholic University of America, Washington, DC.

Robbins, L. N., Helzer, J. E., Craughan, J., et al. (1982). *NIMH Diagnostic Interview Schedule (DIS) Wave II.* St. Louis, MO: Washington University School of Medicine.

Rodriguez, R. R. (1985). Psychological crises of the ill and handicapped. *Emotional First Aid: A Journal of Crisis Intervention, 2*(1), 44–50.

Rosenheck, R., & Thomson, J. (1986). "Detoxification" of Vietnam war trauma: A combined family-individual approach. *Family Process, 25*(4), 559–570.

Rutter, M. (1987). Psychosocial resilience and protective mechanisms. *American Journal of Orthopsychiatry, 57*(3), 316–329.

Sack, W. H., Angell, R. H., Kinzie, D., & Rath, B. (1986). The psychiatric effects of massive trauma on Cambodian children: II. The family, the home, and the school. *Journal of the American Academy of Child Psychiatry, 25*(3), 377–383.

Schneider, M. B., Davis, J. G., Boxer, R. A., Fisher, M., & Friedman, S. B. (1990). Marfan Syndrome in adolescents and young adults: Psychosocial functioning and knowledge. *Developmental and Behavioral Pediatrics, 11*(3), 122–127.

Schukit, M. A. (1983). Anxiety related to medical disease. *Journal of Clinical Psychiatry, 44*(11, sect. 2), 31–36.

Selye, H. (1974). *Stress without distress.* New York: Lippincott.

Shine, K. I. (1984). Anxiety in patients with heart disease. *Psychosomatics, 25*(Suppl. 10), 27–31.

Shore, J. H. (Ed.). (1986). *Disaster stress studies: New methods and findings.* Washington, DC: American Psychiatric Press.

Shore, J. H., Tatum, E. L., & Vollmer, W. M. (1986). Evaluation of mental effects of disaster, Mount St. Helen's eruption. *American Journal of Public Health, 76,* 76–83.

Silver, R., & Wortman, C. (1980). Coping with undesirable life events. In J. Barber & M. Seligman (Eds.), *Human helplessness: Theory and applications.* New York: Academic Press.

Solomon, S. D. (1989). Research issues in assessing disaster's effects. In R. Gist & B. Lubin (Eds.), *Psychosocial aspects of disaster* (pp. 308–340). New York: Wiley.

Solomon, S. D., Gerrity, E. T., & Muff, A. M. (1992). Efficacy of treatments for post-traumatic stress disorder. *Journal of the American Medical Association, 268*(5), 633–638.

Solomon, S. D., Smith, E. M., Robins, L. N., & Fishbach, R. L. (1987). Social involvement as a mediator of disaster-induced stress. *Journal of Applied Social Psychology, 17*(12), 1092–1112.

Solomon, Z., Mikulincer, M., Freid, B., & Wosner, Y. (1987). Family characteristics and post-traumatic stress disorder: A follow-up of Israeli combat stress reaction casualties. *Family Process, 26*(3), 383–394.

Sparks, T. F. (1988). Coping with the psychosocial stresses of oncology care. *Journal of Psychosocial Oncology, 5*(1-2), 165–179.

Speilberger, C. D. (1986). *The Anger Expression (AX) scale.* Tampa: The University of South Florida.

Speilberger, C. D., Johnson, E. H., Russell, S. F., Crane, Q. J., Jacobs, G. A., & Worden, T. J. (1985). The experience and expression of anger: Construction and validation of an anger expression scale. In M. A. Chesney & R. A. Rosenman (Eds.), *Anger and cardiovascular and behavioral disorders.* New York: McGraw-Hill.

Spirito, A., Overholser, J., & Stark, L. J. (1989). Common problems and coping strategies: Findings with adolescent suicide attemptors. *Journal of Abnormal Child Psychology, 17*(2), 213–221.

Stewart, J. B., Hardin, S. B., Weinrich, S., McGeorge, S., Lopez, J., & Pesut, D. (1992). A group protocol to mitigate disaster stress and enhance social support in adolescents exposed to Hurricane Hugo. *Issues in Mental Health Nursing, 13,* 105–119.

Tanaka, K. (1988). Development of a tool for assessing post-trauma response. *Archives of Psychiatric Nursing, 2*(6), 350–356.

Terr, L. (1991). Childhood traumas: An outline and overview. *American Journal of Psychiatry, 148*(1), 10–20.

Thomas, S., Shaffner, D., & Groer, M. (1988). Adolescent stress factors: Implications for the nurse practitioner. *Nurse Practitioner, 13*(6), 20–29.

Tierney, K. J. (1989). The social and community contexts of disaster. In R. Gist & B. Lubin (Eds.), *Psychosocial aspects of disaster* (pp. 11–39). New York: Wiley.

Titchener, J., & Kapp, F. (1976). Family and character change at Buffalo Creek. *American Journal of Psychiatry, 33,* 306–312.

van der Ploeg, H. M., & Kleijn, W. C. (1989). Being held hostage in the Netherlands: A study of long-term after-effects. *Journal of Traumatic Stress, 2*(2), 153–159.

Viney, L. L. (1984). Loss of life and loss of bodily integrity: Two different sources of threat for people who are ill. *Omega: Journal of Death and Dying, 15*(3), 207–222.

Walsh, S. M., & Hardin, S. B. (1994). An art intervention to enhance self-efficacy in adolescents. *Child and Adolescent Psychiatric Nursing, 7*(3), 24–34.

Weekes, D., & Savedra, M. (1988). Adolescent cancer: Coping with treatment-related pain. *Journal of Pediatric Nursing, 3*(5), 318–328.

Weinrich, S., Hardin, S. B., & Johnson, M. (1990). Nurses intervene in Hugo disaster stress. *Archives of Psychiatric Nursing, 4,* 195–205.

Yule, W., & Williams, R. M. (1990). Post-traumatic stress reactions in children. *Journal of Traumatic Stress, 3*(2), 279–295.

CHAPTER

6

BEHAVIOR PROBLEMS IN CHILDREN WITH EPILEPSY

Joan Kessner Austin, DNS, RN, FAAN

ABSTRACT

This chapter provides an overview of evolving attitudes toward epilepsy and the mental health problems associated with childhood onset of the disorder, then reviews research related to both biological and psychological risk factors. Biological research has primarily focused on the relationship of behavior in three areas: neurological dysfunction, seizure variables, and the effect of antiepilepsy medications. While associations have been found, very little variance in behavior problems is accounted for by these biological variables, and findings have been limited by research design. Psychological factors—including family environment, parent and child attitudes, and coping strategies—have been even less systematically studied. Still, the complexity of the disorder requires that nurses conduct comprehensive biological and psychological assessments, then develop individualized plans that consider both the child and the family. Assessment instruments and various nursing interventions are reviewed, including ways to reduce seizures and psychological risk factors at cognitive, affective, and behavioral levels. Changes in nursing curricula are proposed, as is a research emphasis on the etiology of epilepsy and interventions that use both biological and behavioral theoretical frameworks to enhance quality of life.

Epilepsy, or recurring seizures, is a common neurological disorder that affects more than 2 million Americans and is one of the most common disorders in childhood (Hauser & Hesdorffer, 1990). In the early part of this century epilepsy was inappropriately considered one of the three major types of mental illness along with schizophrenia and manic-depression (Blummer, 1984). Even though in recent decades epilepsy has come to be considered a major neurological disorder, there appears to be a real association between epilepsy and mental illness. Mental health problems such as depression, anxiety, and psychosis continue to be overrepresented in persons with epilepsy (Perrine, 1991; Robertson & Trimble, 1983). Even though epilepsy occurs in only 1% of the population, approximately 12% of patients treated in inpatient psychiatric facilities have a concomitant diagnosis of epilepsy (Commission for the Control of Epilepsy and Its Consequences, 1979).

Epilepsy, with its dramatic expression of the interface between the brain and behavior, should be seen as a paradigmatic disorder for the direction of research that makes use of both biological and behavioral theoretical frameworks. When epilepsy was considered a mental illness, researchers relied on psychological theories to explain the abnormal behavior. When the use of antiepilepsy medications led to reduced seizures and subsequently a reduction in the most severe psychiatric disturbances associated with epilepsy—"postepileptic insanity" (Blummer, 1984, p. vii)—epilepsy became known as a neurological condition. Since that time, treatment has been carried out almost exclusively by neurologists. Moreover, researchers have focused primarily on seizure variables—for example, location of the underlying epileptogenic lesion in the brain, seizure frequency, seizure type—to explain the psychopathology by understanding which parts of the brain are involved. It is only recently that a multietiological approach, including both biological and psychological variables, has been advocated for understanding behavior problems found in children with epilepsy (Austin, Risinger, & Beckett, 1992; Hermann & Whitman, 1986).

This shift toward a stronger consideration of the environment stands in contrast to current trends with other psychiatric disorders where the shift is toward biological causes and away from psychological ones. If one considers epilepsy as a paradigmatic disorder for research, then a strong message is that focusing exclusively on either psychological or biological theories will not be as fruitful an approach as focusing on both the biological and the behavioral factors.

The focus of this chapter is on the child who has both epilepsy and behavior problems. The psychiatric nurse called upon to provide care to such a child is confronted with a complex situation where both biological and psychological risk factors need to be considered. In this chapter, behavior problems in children with epilepsy are described, as well as the biological and psychological risk factors that are believed to lead to these problems. Following this, key nursing problems are presented, along with strategies for assessment and intervention. Recommendations are made for nursing curriculum changes, and a nursing research agenda is proposed that should lead to nursing practice being more research based.

MENTAL HEALTH PROBLEMS IN CHILDREN WITH EPILEPSY

Most epilepsy has its onset during childhood, frequently in the first decade of life, and children with epilepsy have a higher prevalence of mental health problems than children from the general population. Recent studies of behavior problems in children with epilepsy from clinical populations indicate that approximately one half have behavior problem scores substantially above the norms for the general population on standardized scales (Austin et al., 1992; Hoare & Kerley, 1991). These problems range from minor problems in daily living to psychosis. Most commonly found are poor self-concept, social isolation, depression, and psychiatric disturbances (Austin, 1989a; Hoare, 1984a; Margalit & Heiman, 1983; Matthews, Barabas, & Ferrari, 1982; Rutter, Graham, & Yule, 1970; Scott, 1978).

The mental health problems found in children with epilepsy do not appear to be solely from having a chronic illness because the prevalence rate is higher in children with epilepsy than in children with other chronic conditions. In a major epidemiological study, Rutter, Graham, and Yule (1970) found that for children with idiopathic epilepsy, the prevalence of psychiatric disorders was approximately 29%. In contrast, the prevalence of psychiatric disorders for children with other physical disorders was approximately 12%, while for general population children it was only approximately 6%. Results were similar for Austin (1989a) in a comparison of psychosocial adaptation of school-age children with epilepsy and a similar sample of

TABLE 6–1. RISK FACTORS FOR MENTAL HEALTH PROBLEMS IN CHILDHOOD EPILEPSY

Biological Factors
Early age of onset
More than one seizure type
Severe and frequent seizures
Side effects of antiepilepsy medication
More than one antiepilepsy medication
Neurophysiological deficits

Psychological Factors
Negative family environment
    Increased family strain
    Decreased family adaptive resources
    Decreased satisfaction with family relationships
Negative parental attitudes toward the epilepsy
Negative child attitudes toward having epilepsy
Parental fear about the epilepsy
Maladaptive child coping patterns
Neuropsychological deficits

children with asthma. Austin found children with epilepsy have significantly more behavior problems both at home and at school than children with asthma. When differences in quality of life were compared, children with epilepsy were found to have poorer quality of life in psychological, social, and school domains, even though they were having significantly fewer illness episodes than the children with asthma (Austin, Smith, Risinger, & McNelis, 1994).

Because psychopathology has often been more debilitating than the seizures themselves, there has been a great deal of interest in identifying potential causes of these problems. The many different factors that have been identified as potential causes can be placed into two broad categories: biological and psychological. Descriptions of these risk factors are described below and summarized in Table 6–1.

BIOLOGICAL FACTORS

Most research has focused on studying the relationship between biological variables and behavior problems. The biological factors that are examined here are neurological dysfunction, seizure characteristics (type and frequency), and antiepilepsy medication.

NEUROLOGICAL DYSFUNCTION

A seizure is a sudden, disorderly discharge of cerebral neurons that leads to brief alterations in brain function (Holmes, 1987). Because these changes in brain function can affect thought and behavior, it has been hypothesized that the behavior problems associated with epilepsy are largely a result of central nervous system dysfunctioning, which causes both the seizures and the behavior problems (Hermann & Whitman, 1986). Even though epilepsy is an episodic condition where seizures occur only intermittently, abnormal brain activity does occur between seizures, or interictically. In fact, electroencephalogram (EEG) findings indicate that in the majority of persons with epilepsy, there are abnormalities in brain electrical activity between seizures (Dodrill, 1990). The mental health problems found in children with epilepsy are believed by some to be caused by these abnormal electrical discharges in the brain (Trimble, 1990). For example, abnormal electrical activity in an area of the brain that controls mood would result in changes in mood regardless of whether the changes led to a seizure.

This line of reasoning has focused on the relationship between the abnormal behavior and the location of the abnormal electrical activity in the brain, especially in the limbic system. The limbic system—involved in the memory, sexuality, and affective experience—is thought to control emotional behavior (Steinhausen & Rauss-Mason, 1991). The issue of whether there are specific behavioral traits associated with seizures that originate from the temporal lobe has been greatly debated. For example, Bear and Fedio (1977) identified 18 personality traits associated with temporal lobe epilepsy, including increased aggression, dependence, hypergraphia, emotionality, and irritability. Research investigating the relationship between temporal lobe epilepsy and behavior problems, however, has had inconsistent findings. After an extensive review of the research, Hermann and Whitman (1984) concluded that temporal lobe epilepsy by itself was not a strong predictor of behavior problems and that many other variables contribute to psychological risk in persons with epilepsy. On the other hand, a relationship between dysphoric mood and neuropsychological markers—suggesting associated frontal lobe dysfunction—was found in patients with complex partial seizures originating in the left temporal lobe (Hermann, Seidenberg, Haltiner, & Wyler, 1991). In addition, Leiderman, Csernansky, and Moses (1990) found plasma prolactin to be significantly inversely related to thought disorder in adult males with limbic epilepsy. Devinsky (1991) points out, however, that epilepsy has also been attributed to many positive behaviors, such as moral conviction, creative writing and art ability, and military brilliance; therefore, the a priori assumption that interictally altered behavior is either negative or maladaptive is problematic.

There is also evidence that children with epilepsy who have associated brain damage may be at increased risk for psychopathology (Rutter, 1981). In the epidemiological study by Rutter, Graham, and Yule (1970) the prevalence of behavior problems in children with both epilepsy and associated brain damage, including mental retardation, was substantially higher—50%, compared to the previously noted rate of 29% for children with idiopathic epilepsy. In another comparison—children with epilepsy and normal neuropsychological functioning with a matched group of children with epilepsy and poor neuropsychological functioning—Hermann (1981) found more psychopathology in the children with the poorer neuropsychological performance. Lending further support for this hypothesis are the consistent findings of higher prevalence rates for psychiatric disorder in children with chronic conditions involving the brain than in children with chronic conditions not involving the brain (Austin, 1989a; Breslau, 1985; Rutter, Graham, & Yule, 1970). Furthermore, findings by Hoare (1984a), where children with newly diagnosed epilepsy had a higher rate of psychiatric disturbance than children with newly diagnosed diabetes, support the hypothesis that a neurological dysfunction might have predisposed the children to both the epilepsy and the psychiatric disorder.

Whether seizures per se can also cause the brain damage that then leads to behavior problems is a competing explanation for the link between epilepsy and behavior problems. Again, results of research are inconclusive. Even though a decline in IQ has been found in some children with continued seizures, the effect of seizure frequency and duration cannot be separated from other factors such as an underlying encephalopathic process, educational deprivation, socioeconomic factors, and long-term treatment with antiepilepsy medications (Binnie & Marston, 1992; Hermann & Whitman, 1991; Holmes, 1991; Klein, 1991). There is evidence that prolonged seizures (status epilepticus) can result in cognitive problems and brain damage, such as neuronal necrosis in the hippocampus (Wasterlain, Fujikawa, Penix, & Sankar, 1993). Recent clinical research, however, indicates that status epilepticus in children without other neurological deficits rarely results in cognitive defects (Gross-Tsur & Shinnar, 1993). Nevertheless, Rutter (1993) points out that brain damage that is not observable in a clinical neurological examination can lead to serious psychopathology.

Mental health problems also have been associated with learning disabilities in children with epilepsy (Rausch & Victoroff, 1991; Rutter, 1993; Ziegler, 1985). Moreover, children with epilepsy have long been found to be at risk for cognitive impairment and poor academic achievement (Holdsworth & Whitmore, 1974; Holmes, 1991; Rutter, Tizard, & Whitmore, 1970; Stores, 1978). Distributions of IQ scores for children with epilepsy generally have a slight shift to the left, indicating lower scores than the general population (Holmes, 1987). Dodrill (1992) points out, however, that comparisons of IQ between samples with epilepsy and the general population can be misleading when persons with difficult-to-control seizures are overrepresented in the epilepsy sample. Even in children with IQs above 70, however, there is evidence of more academic problems than in children with other chronic conditions. For example, when Huberty, Austin, Risinger, and McNelis (1992) studied a sample of children with epilepsy who have IQs of 70 or greater, they found almost 40% repeated a grade at least once prior to the sixth grade; the rate of retention in a comparison sample of children with asthma was only 20.5%.

Within the general population of children with epilepsy, there is variability in learning disability based on seizure variables. Even though one would anticipate that there would be a positive relationship between seizure frequency and cognitive impairment, this relationship is not consistently found (Seidenberg, 1989). Klein (1991) points out, however, that children with seizures resulting from structural brain lesions are most at risk for learning problems, although research with sibling control groups has not been carried out to determine the effect of family history of learning disability in the development of cognitive problems in children with epilepsy (Klein, 1991). Furthermore, research is needed to determine the effect of anticonvulsant medications on both cognitive problems (Bennett, 1992) and mental health problems.

Systematic research also is needed to determine the circumstances and sequence of events that lead to the relationships among learning problems, epilepsy, and mental health problems. Are children with frequent seizures missing important information at school and at home? Are seizures leading to loss of cognitive function and a subsequent decreased ability to cope with stress and therefore increased mental health problems? Do behavior problems result from the child with epilepsy having to adjust to the added stress of also having learning problems? What is the family history for learning problems or poor academic achievement?

SEIZURE VARIABLES

Research that has focused on the relationship between seizure variables and behavior problems in children with epilepsy indicates that age at onset of seizures, duration of epilepsy, seizure control, seizure type, and being on more than one antiepilepsy medication (i.e., polytherapy) are associated with some types of behavior problems in children with epilepsy (Hermann & Whitman, 1986).

Early age of onset has long been reported to be associated with an increased risk of behavior problems (Pond & Bidwell, 1960). More recent research, however, has not supported this relationship. Past research supporting the relationship has included in the sample infantile epileptic syndromes that are associated with mental retardation, such as Lennox-Gastaut syndrome (Steinhausen & Rauss-Mason, 1991). Therefore, the relationship might be a result of the children with earlier age of onset also being the ones who are having more mental health problems. When children with mental retardation were not included in a study of child behavior problems (Austin et al., 1992), no relationship between age of onset and behavior problems was found. Another problem is that age of onset is related to duration of treatment. Research that separates age of onset from duration of treatment indicates that duration of treatment rather than age of onset is related to behavior problems in children with epilepsy (Hoare, 1984a).

The most consistent finding among the seizure variables is that seizure frequency is associated with behavior problems, even though seizure frequency has been measured differently across different studies. Hartlage and Green (1972) found seizure frequency to be negatively related to social maturity. Other authors (Austin, 1988; Austin et al., 1992; Hermann, Whitman, & Dell, 1989; Hoare, 1984a) found seizure frequency to be positively associated with behavioral problems. Austin, Patterson, and Huberty (1991) found seizure frequency to be positively related to the coping behavior of social withdrawal. However, because seizure frequency is often confounded with other variables, especially increased brain damage and higher levels of antiepilepsy medication, it is difficult to determine how much seizure frequency alone contributes to behavior problems (Steinhausen & Rauss-Mason, 1991).

Several researchers have studied the relationship between seizure type and behavior problems. Again, findings are difficult to interpret because a consistent framework has not been used to classify seizures, making it difficult to compare findings from one study to another. Indeed, while much research has been carried out, especially in regard to complex partial seizure type, results are inconsistent. For example, Hoare (1984a) found focal EEG abnormalities and complex partial seizures to be associated with increased psychiatric disturbances. In contrast, Austin et al. (1992) found no differences in behavior problems for children with focal EEG abnormalities and complex partial seizures when compared with other seizure types, and no evidence of focal EEG abnormalities. Furthermore, Whitman, Hermann, Black, and Chhabria (1982) found no relationship between seizures originating from the temporal lobe and psychopathology in children with epilepsy.

MEDICATION VARIABLES

In the past two decades there has been increased interest in the effects of antiepilepsy medication on the cognitive and behavioral functioning of children with epilepsy. Most of the research on effects of antiepilepsy medication has focused on cognitive functioning, and support was found for decreased memory, psychomotor performance, attention, and motor speed, especially with barbiturates and phenytoin (Dodrill, 1990). There is also substantial evidence that antiepilepsy medications can lead to mental health problems in persons with epilepsy. Antiepilepsy medications have been associated with depression, increased irritability, conduct disorder, and hyperactivity (Trimble & Cull, 1989). In general, research indicates that phenobarbital and clonazepam are most frequently associated with behavior problems, while valproate and carbamazepine are least frequently associated with behavior problems (Ferrari, Barabas, & Matthews, 1983; Miles, Tennison, & Greenwood, 1988; Trimble & Cull, 1988, 1989).

Polytherapy is also more likely to be associated with behavior problems than monotherapy (Steinhausen & Rauss-Mason, 1991; Trimble & Cull, 1989). Further supporting the relationship between antiepilepsy medication and behavior problems in children are changes in behavior when medication is decreased. Cull, Trimble, and Wilson (1992) compared changes in behavior for children who were undergoing either a decrease or increase in medication, children who had no change in medication, and a general population control group. Children whose medication was decreased showed significant improvement in areas of conduct problems, anxiety, hyperactivity, and learning problems. Interestingly, children whose medication was increased showed significant improvement in psychosomatic complaints.

One possible mechanism that links antiepilepsy medication with mental changes is decreased folic acid levels, which can be caused by long-term therapy with some antiepilepsy medications. There is substantial evidence that long-term barbiturate or phenytoin therapy can lead to decreased folic acid levels in serum or cerebral spinal fluid (Reynolds, 1986). Furthermore, several studies have demonstrated a link between low folic acid levels and depression in both adults with epilepsy and normal controls (Reynolds, 1986, 1991; Trimble, 1990); decreased folic acid levels have also been found to be associated with depression in children who do not have epilepsy (Trimble, Corbett, & Donaldson, 1980). These findings raised hope that depression could subsequently be reduced through the addition of folic acid to the medication regime. Results of clinical trials where folic acid has been administered, however, have been disappointing. For example, not only has mental status not improved but seizure frequency was also found to increase (Reynolds, 1968) and negative effects on learning were found (Houben, Hommes, & Knaven, 1971).

In conclusion, much of the research linking biological variables and behavior problems in children with epilepsy has been limited by small heterogeneous samples, a lack of a common system for classification of seizures and the measurement of seizure frequency, and a lack of multiple measurements of behavior from both subjective and objective sources. In addition, seizure severity has typically not been considered in the measurement of seizure variables (Baker et al., 1991). Furthermore, even though behavior problems have been found to be related to biological variables, very little variance in behavior problems is accounted for by these variables (Hermann & Whitman, 1986). Finally, in most of the research on biological variables, psychological variables are not included in the design of the research, so interactions between these variables are not known.

PSYCHOLOGICAL FACTORS

In contrast to the large number of studies on biological variables, much less research has been carried out on the relationship between psychological variables and behavior problems in children with epilepsy. Nevertheless, the research that has been conducted indicates strongly that psychological factors are associated with mental health problems in these children. Psychological variables that have been identified in the literature as potential causes of mental health problems include: negative family environment, negative parent and child attitudes, and maladaptive coping strategies on the part of the child.

FAMILY ENVIRONMENT

Because a large percentage of cases of epilepsy begin before age 18 (Hauser & Hesdorffer, 1990), the whole family must make an adjustment to the disorder. It is hypothesized that some families make a poor adaptation to the epilepsy, which leads to a dysfunctional environment for the child with epilepsy and the subsequent development of behavior problems. Because parenting can be difficult even with physically healthy children, it is to be expected that parenting the child with a chronic brain condition would be stressful. Parents are confronted with coping with the epilepsy themselves, helping the child with the epilepsy to deal with the experience, and helping other children in the family and extended family to cope. Dealing with grandparents can also contribute to stress in the family. In open-ended interviews with parents of children with epilepsy, more than two thirds of the families identified the children's grandparents as being sources of stress and impediments to family adjustment (Romeis, 1980).

There is a large amount of clinical impression literature that indicates just living with an unpredictable disorder—one that may entail sudden loss of control over bodily functioning in sometimes frightening displays—can lead to strong emotions in the family. To deal with chronic episodic illnesses, families require flexibility in coping strategies so they can be prepared for both seizures and absence of seizures. The uncertainty of when seizures will occur is one of the difficult aspects for families to deal with in a chronic epilepsy. Rolland (1988) classified epilepsy as a relapsing or episodic illness where there are periods of absence of illness symptoms followed by periods of flare-up. He pointed out that episodic illnesses present unique stressors for the family because even in periods of good seizure control, the possibility of a period of seizures hangs over the families' heads.

Voeller and Rothenberg (1973) found that parents react to epilepsy with fear, anger, guilt, and sadness. Ward and Bower (1978) found that the majority of parents of children with epilepsy had fear surrounding the seizures and were concerned about the physical safety of their children. Mittan (1986) found that family members had several fears about epilepsy, especially of brain damage and death.

There is also indirect support from research that continuing stress from epilepsy in a child can have a negative impact on the mental health of family members. For example, Hoare (1984b) compared the prevalence of psychological disturbance among mothers and siblings of two groups of children with epilepsy, one group newly diagnosed and one with chronic epilepsy. The rate of psychological disturbance was significantly higher in both the mothers and the siblings of the chronic group than in the newly diagnosed group, which suggests that over the long term, epilepsy can adversely affect the psychological health of other family members.

Empirical studies exploring the relationship between aspects of family environment and mental health in children with epilepsy have been limited by small samples and failure to consider seizure and demographic variables in the same analysis with family variables, but family factors have been associated with behavior problems in these children. For example, in a descriptive study of 12 families, Mulder and Suurmeijer (1977) found a positive relationship between parental control and dependency in the child. Hoare and Kerley (1991) found an association between family stress and child behavioral disturbance in 108 families. Austin (1988) found families of children with behavioral problems to have significantly lower levels of family adaptation, less esteem and communication among family members, less social support from extended family, and less financial efficacy than children without behavior problems. Austin et al. (1992) found increased family stress, decreased extended family social support, and decreased family mastery to be the strongest psychological predictors of child behavior problems.

There is also evidence in the literature that parents may have different expectations for children with epilepsy and consequently discipline them differently from their siblings. One study that addressed differences in parent perceptions found that parents expected their children with epilepsy to have more emotional problems and to be more unpredictable and more unstable than their healthy siblings (Long &

Moore, 1979). Unfortunately, however, most of the research focusing on family environment has been cross-sectional, so it is not possible to determine the causal relationship between the family environment and the child's behavioral problems. For example, it is not known if family stress and changes in parental expectations precede or follow child behavior problems.

Nevertheless, the relative importance of family environment variables compared to neurological variables (Austin et al., 1992) is consistent with the broader literature indicating that family variables have a stronger influence on child adjustment than illness severity (Drotar & Bush, 1985). In addition, findings that family adaptive resources are positively related to child adaptation are consistent with models based on family stress theory (McCubbin & Patterson, 1983; Wallander, Varni, Babani, Banis, & Wilcox; 1989), which proposes that increased family resources serve as protective factors for the chronically ill child.

ATTITUDES

Another psychological factor that has consistently been identified as a potential cause of mental health problems in children with epilepsy is the attitudes toward the epilepsy held by the child and family. Because there is a stigma associated with epilepsy in our society, children with epilepsy and their families are confronted with adapting to a stigmatized condition. Bagley (1972) proposed that parental attitudes toward their children's epilepsy are negative as a result of the social stigma; these parental attitudes are believed to lead to behavior problems.

Even though there is a large amount of clinical impression literature indicating that parental attitudes are important, there is a lack of research in the area. Austin, McBride, and Davis (1984) found positive correlations between parental attitudes toward epilepsy and parental adjustment to epilepsy; Austin and McDermott (1988) found positive correlations between parental attitudes and parental coping behaviors of maintaining family integration and use of social support. But only three studies have investigated relationships between parental attitudes and aspects of child mental health. Parental attitudes have, however, been related to social maturity (Hartlage & Green, 1972), although not to dependency in children with epilepsy (Hartlage, Green, & Offutt, 1972), and Bagley (1971), too, found adverse parental attitudes to be correlated with behavior problems in children with epilepsy.

Empirical evidence on the relationship between children's attitudes toward having epilepsy and their mental health outcomes also indicated that attitudes are important. Austin et al. (1991) found children's attitudes toward epilepsy to be positively correlated with adaptive child coping behaviors (e.g., competence) and negatively correlated with maladaptive child coping behaviors (e.g., withdrawal and irritability). Other results from this research (Austin, 1990a; Austin & Huberty, 1993) indicated that children's attitudes toward epilepsy were especially linked to self-concept. This positive association between attitudes and self-concept supports Massie's (1985) contention that negative attitudes toward having a chronic health condition in childhood can become melded into the self-concept and lead to poor self-esteem.

COPING

Coping is another psychological variable that has been identified as important in understanding mental health problems in children with epilepsy. However, the relationship between children's coping with epilepsy and mental health outcomes is probably the least studied area. One approach explaining how child coping leads to mental health problems has focused on children's perceptions of control. It is hypothesized that children with epilepsy have a condition that cannot be predicted or controlled like other physical conditions such as asthma or diabetes because there is not a close link between taking the medication and a seizure occurring. Therefore, children may perceive that the occurrence of a seizure is not dependent on their actions. As a result, they begin to feel helpless and experience a loss of control over their environment. Subsequently, it is proposed, this helplessness may lead to poor self-concept and increased anxiety (DeVellis & DeVellis, 1986; Matthews & Barabas, 1986). Research by Matthews and Barabas found support for the above hypotheses in a comparison of children who had either epilepsy or diabetes with healthy controls. Relative to other children, children with epilepsy were found to have poorer self-concepts, higher anxiety, and greater perceptions of external sources of control.

Austin et al. (1991) also investigated the relationship between coping and mental health outcomes in children with epilepsy and asthma. Based on the theoretical work of McCubbin and Patterson (1983) and Patterson (1988), they took the perspective that children with a chronic illness are faced with both illness-related demands and the other normative demands related to their developmental stage. Austin et al. (1991) then developed a coping scale to measure both adaptive and maladaptive coping behaviors. Results indicated that children with epilepsy adopt two distinct styles of coping: (1) an adaptive style characterized by competence, optimism, compliance, and seeking support from others; and (2) a maladaptive style characterized by irritability, feeling different, and withdrawal from others. The adaptive coping style was found to be positively correlated with self-concept and negatively correlated with behavior problems. The reverse was true of the maladaptive coping style.

In summary, while the clinical anecdotal literature is replete with references to the importance of psychological variables in the development of mental health problems in children with epilepsy, relatively little systematic research has been carried out in this area. In addition, most of the psychological studies have used small samples and have not included biological variables in the study design. Furthermore, samples have often been heterogeneous and included children with a wide range in IQ and degree of neurological deficit. Research in epilepsy has not considered the influence of the child's temperament on child and family adaptation to epilepsy. Even with these methodological limitations, results indicate that psychological variables—such as family environment, attitudes, and coping—influence mental health outcomes in children with epilepsy.

NURSING MANAGEMENT

Even though more than 15 years have passed since the Commission for the Control of Epilepsy and Its Consequences (1979) found that the psychosocial problems surrounding epilepsy were poorly understood, the statement remains true today. The situation regarding cause of behavior problems is complicated by the difficulty in determining if biological and psychological factors are operating independently, additively, or multiplicatively in the development of problems in individual children. This complexity surrounding cause is a most compelling reason for an interdisciplinary approach to the treatment of children with epilepsy and their families.

KEY NURSING PROBLEMS

Within this population of children there is great diversity both in the type of mental health problems found and in how the epilepsy is manifested. Thus, it is essential that a comprehensive assessment be carried out by all members of the inter-disciplinary team and that individualized plans of care be developed that meet the diverse needs of these children and their families.

Similar to findings with other chronic illnesses, Austin (1988) found a wide range of behavior problems in children with epilepsy. Depression, social withdrawal, anxiety, poor self-esteem, hyperactivity, delinquency, and aggressiveness are the most commonly reported. Some behavior problems are context specific. For example, some children experience behavior problems only at school. Likewise, family members of the affected child may exhibit signs of lack of adaptation to the epilepsy, for example, social withdrawal, failure to give antiepilepsy medication as ordered, intrafamily conflict focusing on the epilepsy, excessive fear surrounding epilepsy, and embarrassment about the disorder.

One of the characteristics of epilepsy that makes it challenging for professionals helping these families is the broad spectrum of disability associated with childhood epilepsy. Some children appear to have no or only mild temporary disability, while others are severely disabled. For 80% of the children with epilepsy, seizures can be sufficiently controlled to allow them to lead normal, active lives (Santilli, Dodson, & Walton, 1991). It is the remaining 20% of children who have poor seizure control that experience the most disability. Children who have epilepsy as a result of brain disease are most likely to have early onset of epilepsy, poor seizure control, and intellectual impairment. Furthermore, these children are most likely to be receiving higher doses of antiepilepsy medication in an effort to increase seizure control (Santilli et al., 1991).

Indeed, the fact that epilepsy is sometimes difficult to diagnose can itself be stressful. Some families report that a period of months passed from the time of the first seizure to a definite diagnosis of epilepsy, and even after epilepsy is diagnosed, there is still a great deal of unpredictability surrounding the disorder. For example, some children might become seizure-free rather quickly and be taken off medication after a few years. Other children might be treated with surgery and become seizure-free. School problems might be paramount for some children and not for others. In addition, for a few children the seizures might be caused by a progressive brain disease, which causes them to have both increased mental impairment and seizures over time.

Adolescence, which brings dramatic changes in physical development, can also bring changes in epilepsy. Many children outgrow seizures with the maturing of the central nervous system (Hauser & Hesdorffer, 1990). One particular seizure type, benign rolandic epilepsy, ends in adolescence at about age 16 (Holmes, 1987). In some children, however, seizure type changes or additional seizure types are manifested as the child matures, and adolescents with epilepsy have to deal with these changes in the epilepsy at the same time they are experiencing physical development and changes in relationships with peers and family. It is also during early adolescence that the child begins to assume responsibility for taking the antiepilepsy medication.

Because increased seizure frequency is found to be associated with behavior problems, it might be anticipated that the children with the poorest seizure control would experience the most mental health problems. This is not always the case. Children with well-controlled seizures, as well as those who have been seizure-free for a year or more, can have serious mental health problems.

In summary, epilepsy can be vastly different both within the child over time and across children. In addition, severity of epilepsy is not necessarily strongly associated with mental health problems in the child or adaptation problems in the family. And, finally, the full range of mental health problems is seen in children with epilepsy.

NURSING ASSESSMENT

Nurses need to have a sufficient knowledge of epilepsy, treatment, and all the factors that can influence behavior so they can be full partners in interdisciplinary treatment teams. Regardless of the cause of behavior problems, they generally lead to stress on the whole family. Consequently, both the child and the family should be the target of nursing assessment.

It is important for the nurse to carry out a comprehensive assessment that includes the following: description of seizures; seizure severity; medication effects; presence of other neurological problems; the child's progress in school, perceptions and feelings about having epilepsy, coping strategies, and behavior; the family environment; and other family members' perceptions and feelings about the epilepsy. Resources and instruments that might be helpful for nurses in assessing these areas are presented in Table 6–2. They range from questionnaires that can only be used in the clinical setting to facilitate assessment (e.g., parent description of seizures and common side effects of medications) to well-developed, normed instruments that can be used both for assessment and in research (e.g., Child Behavior Checklist, Pier-Harris Self-Concept Scale, and Child Depression Inventory).

TABLE 6–2. RESOURCES OR INSTRUMENTS FOR ASSESSMENT OF RISK FACTORS

FACTORS	RESOURCES OR SCALES
Seizure severity	Seizure Severity Scale (Baker, Smith, Dewey, Morrow, Crawford, & Chadwick, 1991)
Seizure description	Questionnaire for Parents of Child with Epilepsy (Santilli, Dodson, & Walton, 1991)
Fear of seizures	Sepulveda Epilepsy Battery (Mittan, 1986)
Side effects of medications	Santilli, Dodson, & Walton (1991)
Assessment of development	Quinn (1988)
Behavior problems	Child Behavior Checklist (Achenbach, 1991)
Self-concept	Piers-Harris Self-Concept Scale (Piers, 1984)
	Perceived Competence Scale for Children (Harter, 1982; Harter & Pike, 1984)
	Rosenberg Self-Esteem Scale (Rosenberg, 1965)
Child depression	Child Depression Inventory (Kovacs, 1980/81)
Child attitude	Child Attitude Toward Illness Scale (Austin & Huberty, 1993)
Child coping	Coping Health Inventory for Children (Austin, Patterson, & Huberty, 1991)
Parent attitudes	Parental Attitude Toward Epilepsy (Austin, McBride, & Davis, 1984)
Parent coping	Coping Health Inventory for Parents (McCubbin & Thompson, 1991)
Family environment	Family APGAR—older child and adult (Smilkstein, 1978)
	Family APGAR—young child (Austin & Huberty, 1989)
	Family Inventory for Resources for Management (McCubbin & Thompson, 1991)
	Family Hardiness Index (McCubbin & Thompson, 1991)
	Family Support Scale (Dunst, Trivette, & Deal, 1988)
	Hassles and Uplifts Scale (Lazarus & Folkman, 1989)
	Family Inventory of Life Events and Changes (McCubbin & Thompson, 1991)

NURSING INTERVENTIONS

An examination of the biological risk factors in Table 6–1 indicates that some of the risk factors are not potentially changeable (e.g., age of onset, the number of different seizure types, and the occurrence of neurological deficits). Therefore, interventions for these factors will need to focus on helping the family utilize resources to minimize effects. For example, when a child has learning problems, families can be taught how to work effectively with the school system to obtain the best school situation for the child. Behavioral side effects from medication can sometimes be reduced when antiepilepsy medication is changed, but for some children changing medications is not possible, so it is necessary for the child and family to structure the environment to minimize the negative side effects. On the other hand, the risk factor of seizure frequency is potentially changeable in some children. Indeed, most of the interventions in the literature have focused on reducing seizures. Some of these studies are briefly reviewed here and followed by strategies for reducing psychological risk factors.

INTERVENTIONS FOR REDUCING SEIZURES

Most interventions to reduce seizures have focused on making sure that the child receives a therapeutic dosage of antiepilepsy medication. Behavioral strategies have also been developed to either prevent seizures or stop the progression of seizures once they have occurred. There is also beginning support for the importance of self-monitoring of events surrounding seizure activity to identify interventions that might reduce seizures. Descriptions of the research studies that have been carried out in each of the areas follow.

MAINTAINING A THERAPEUTIC LEVEL OF ANTIEPILEPSY MEDICATION. One of the likeliest causes of poor seizure control is a subtherapeutic level of antiepilepsy medication (Spunt & Black, 1982). Reasons for a subtherapeutic level include drug interaction, the dose being too low for the size of the growing child, altered drug metabolism, and noncompliance (Santilli et al., 1991; Spunt & Black, 1982). Each of these potential causes needs to be assessed to determine the most appropriate intervention. Included in the assessment should be information on other medications the child is taking and recent changes in the child's weight.

Spunt and Black (1982) have found that the most common reason for noncompliance with the antiepilepsy medication regimen is lack of knowledge about how antiepilepsy medications work and how they should be taken for optimal seizure control. Other reasons for failure to take medication as prescribed include confusion regarding the instructions, forgetfulness, and lack of supervision of the child in taking the medication (Santilli et al., 1991). Interventions to address these causes generally include the provision of information about need for consistency in taking medication and strategies to help parents and children remember when the medication should be taken.

Research also indicates that compliance might be influenced by parents' attitudes about giving medication to the child and the parents' perceptions about the treatment team members (Austin, 1989b). If parents hold negative attitudes about their children taking antiepilepsy medication, then interventions could focus on making parents' beliefs and feelings about medicine-giving behavior more positive. For example, Austin (1990b) suggests that correcting parents' erroneous negative beliefs about antiepilepsy medication (e.g., disputing that antiepilepsy medication causes later drug addiction) can lead to more positive attitudes toward giving required doses. Austin's (1989b) research also indicated that parental medicine-giving behavior was influenced by parents' confidence in the physician. She recommended that nurses' interventions could be aimed at strengthening the parents' perceptions of competence in the treatment team.

A final but important consideration with noncompliance is poor psychosocial adjustment to the epilepsy. For example, Friedman et al. (1986) found lack of harmonious family relations and low self-esteem in adolescents were related to noncompliance with antiepilepsy medication. Nursing interventions for these adolescents and their families could be directed at improving family relationships, enhancing self-esteem in the child, and helping the parents and adolescent understand the importance of therapeutic levels of medication. These strategies are covered in more detail in the section on interventions for psychological risk factors.

Behavioral Interventions. The most commonly used behavioral interventions to decrease seizure frequency are biofeedback, relaxation training, and behavior modification. With biofeedback, patients are taught either to increase specifically those cerebral rhythms which have an anticonvulsant effect or to decrease epileptic activity in a nonspecific manner (Fenwick, 1991). Research with adults has indicated that biofeedback can lead to changes in sensory-motor rhythms (SMR) that can have an anticonvulsive effect (Fenwick, 1991). However, Schotte and DuBois (1989) point out that it is not clear if the changes in SMR are a result of the biofeedback per se or result from decreases in afferent thalamic activation brought about by the accompanying muscular relaxation. If the latter, it would mean that relaxation exercises should be as effective as biofeedback.

With relaxation and behavior modification there are also two basic approaches, interventions focused on behavior in general and those focused specifically on seizures; both have been successful in reducing seizures. The most common approach aimed at general behavior is the use of daily progressive relaxation techniques, for which there are five reports of successful seizure reduction (Puskarich et al., 1991). The exact mechanism for this seizure reduction is not known, but it is hypothesized that the relaxation leads to stress reduction, which, in turn, leads to fewer seizures.

There is support for the link between increased stress and seizure frequency in some patients (Legion, 1991; Neugebauer, Paik, Nadel, Hauser, & Susser, 1991; Temkin & Davis, 1984). One link might be hyperventilation, which is present in some people when they are under stress (Legion, 1991). Hyperventilation also affects electrical activity in the brain and is an activator of absence seizures (Holmes, 1987). However, there is also the possibility that the relaxation activity, which includes both cognitive and behavioral actions, might reduce seizures by indirectly affecting electrical activity in the brain.

In general, three main strategies are used for the behavioral approaches targeted specifically to seizures: elimination of stimuli that lead to seizures, counteraction of the first signs of the seizure, and elimination of positive consequences of having seizures. A study by Dahl, Melin, Brorson, and Schollin (1985) combined all three of these approaches. First, a behavioral analysis was carried out to examine the relationship between seizure behavior and the environment in regard to antecedents of the seizures, responses during the seizures, and consequences of the seizures. In the study, children were taught (1) to self-monitor for stimuli that elicited the seizures, (2) to recognize the early signs of the seizure, and (3) to use a seizure-control technique in the form of progressive relaxation. In addition, parents and teachers were encouraged to reinforce the children's use of seizure-control techniques and seizure-free periods. To prevent the further progression of the seizure, children were taught to use relaxation techniques when they were in situations that were likely to stimulate seizures and when they recognized the earliest body signals of a seizure. Children were also observed for environmental reinforcers for having a seizure; the consequences were then changed so that positive reinforcement followed seizure-free periods and use of antiseizure techniques. A trial using all three approaches significantly reduced seizures in 18 children (Dahl et al., 1985).

SELF-MONITORING. Many findings indicate that it might be helpful to teach children to monitor events surrounding seizures, including some research that indicates seizure susceptibility may be related to circadian stage-dependent processes (Poirel & Ennaji, 1991). For example, nocturnal seizures have been frequently found in children with rolandic spikes (Poirel & Ennaji, 1991). Other factors—such as increased fluid intake, fever, consumption of alcohol, sensory stimuli (e.g., certain sounds or lights), and premenstrual changes—have also been identified as having the potential to increase seizures (Johnson, 1982). See Table 6–3 for some examples of interventions that highlight the interface between seizures and behavior.

To determine whether any of these factors is operating in individual children, parents and children should be encouraged to keep seizure diaries that include systematic information on time of seizure, events surrounding seizures, antecedents that might trigger seizures, and consequent events that might reinforce seizures. Younger children could be presented with the notion that they are detectives who are learning more about their bodies. Education about seizures and encouragement of parents to keep a seizure diary might also provide important information that can be used for both the diagnosis and treatment of the seizures. For example, some children have focal seizures that go unnoticed by family members until systematic monitoring leads to the recognition of subtle seizures.

Self-monitoring has also been used in research to reduce seizures. In a study of psychological management of seizures, Gillham (1990) instructed adults in diary-keeping of times of seizures, types of seizures, and events preceding them. Factors that were possible precipitants were identified, and patients were taught seizure-avoidant strategies, such as relaxation. A second treatment included the teaching of effective coping strategies. As a part of the larger study, two groups of patients who had both poorly controlled seizures and psychological disorders received both treatments. The order of the treatment was counterbalanced so that one group received the seizure-avoidant instruction first and one group received the instruction on coping strategies first. Results indicated a significant decrease in seizures and anxiety over a 42-week period. A most intriguing finding was that seizure frequency was reduced in both groups following the first treatment condition. In other words, just the teaching of effective coping strategies led to decreased seizures. These results suggest that interventions that focus on enhancing adaptive coping can both reduce anxiety and improve seizure control.

There is also limited support for thoughts or ideas to influence seizure activity. Research on seizures that are evoked by a specific stimulus, such as a flashing light or reading, indicates that thinking about the stimulus can evoke a seizure (Epstein, 1990). For example, in one patient who had seizures in response to rubbing the right side of his face, the focal EEG abnormality appeared even when the patient was asked only to think about rubbing his face. Epstein concluded that the "idea itself must then have a neural configuration that has physiological power" (p. 70). The use of biofeedback also suggests that thoughts and ideas affect electrical discharges on the brain; if so, it should be possible to use thought to reduce the magnitude of spike waves and consequently reduce seizures through interventions aimed at controlling thoughts.

INTERVENTIONS FOR PSYCHOLOGICAL RISK FACTORS

The major lacuna in the literature is research on the reduction of psychological risk factors. Of the two studies that were found, only one was for children. Lewis

TABLE 6–3. Nursing Intervention Strategies

NURSING INTERVENTION	RATIONALE
Seizure Self-monitoring Teach the parents of young children and older youth to keep a diary of all seizure-related activities including events preceding seizures, times of seizures (e.g., during sleep), types of seizures, factors that were possible precipitants (e.g., lack of sleep, increased fluid intake, and flashing lights), and events following seizures.	In some children there are precipitants for seizures and common patterns that seizures follow. The more that is known about each child's seizure pattern, the better the chance of recognizing if a pattern exists and developing strategies to prevent or reduce seizures. Accurate information on seizures is also helpful in monitoring treatment and in recognizing seizures that might have gone unnoticed.
Teach children to recognize the early signals of an oncoming seizure. Teach children to use relaxation techniques (e.g., progressive muscular relaxation) to control the earliest symptoms of oncoming seizures.	Some children can effectively use relaxation techniques to control seizures through interrupting the beginning stages of the seizure.
Encourage parents to deal with seizures in a neutral manner, not to be attentive only when the child has seizures, and to feel positive about seizure-free periods.	Help the parents avoid any increase in seizures through inadvertent excessive attention to seizures that only reinforce that there can be positive consequences to seizures.
Stress-Management Strategies Teach children to recognize emotional and bodily symptoms of increased stress and anxiety or negative emotion. It is especially important that they learn to recognize anxiety symptoms (e.g., hyperventilation and increased heart rate), behaviors associated with depression, and cues that signal the beginning of depressive moods.	Recognition of early symptoms of stress, particularly with respect to anxiety and depression, is necessary before strategies to manage stress can be effectively used.
Teach children adaptive coping strategies for dealing with increased stress such as perceiving themselves as competent, using friends and family for support, and being optimistic about their ability to deal with whatever happens in life.	Adaptive coping, increased self-esteem, and enhanced ability to deal with stress have been linked to decreased seizures. In addition, problems with poor self-concept, depression, and social withdrawal have been found to remain even after epilepsy is no longer present.
Encourage children to learn methods to manage stress such as increasing physical exercise, frequency of pleasurable activities, positive self-talk, and positive perceptions of self; teach them to stop negative self-talk.	

and colleagues (Lewis, Salas, de la Sota, Chiofalo, & Leake, 1990; Lewis, Hatton, Salas, Leake, & Chiofalo, 1991) evaluated an intervention program for children with epilepsy and their parents. They found that an educational program increased parents' knowledge about epilepsy, decreased parents' anxiety, and increased children's perceived social competence. In the second study, Davis, Armstrong, Donovan, and

TABLE 6–3. NURSING INTERVENTION STRATEGIES *Continued*

NURSING INTERVENTION	RATIONALE
Stress-Management Strategies *(cont)* Help children plan in advance how they will handle stressful situations. Encourage them to keep track of the success of responses so they can improve on their ability to cope effectively. Encourage parents to enhance the child's self-esteem through listening to and valuing their feelings and opinions, accepting their negative feelings, and fostering independence in the child. Teach families stress-management strategies to deal with strain from the seizures and other stressors. For example, they could be taught about the need for an environ-ment that encourages the expression of feelings, identification of resources (e.g., use of extended family social support), and the use of active problem solving to reduce stressors.	Increased family strain has been found to be strongly associated with increased behavior problems in children with epilepsy. Children can also learn positive coping strategies from observing them in their families.
Developing Positive Attitudes Encourage both children and parents to have positive attitudes toward the epilepsy. Encourage parents and children to express their fears, concerns, and worries about the epilepsy so those which are based on inaccurate information can be corrected. Provide new positive informa-tion to help them have more positive beliefs about the epilepsy and conse-quently more positive attitudes. Encour-age interactions with families who hold positive attitudes toward their children's epilepsy. Help families to use reframing and downward comparison to enhance their attitudes toward the epilepsy.	Children's attitudes toward epilepsy have been found to be strongly linked with self-concept. Positive child attitudes toward the epilepsy have been linked to positive coping strategies. Adaptive coping strategies have been linked to reduced seizure activity. Positive parental attitudes toward their children's epilepsy have been found to be associated with their use of adaptive coping strategies.

Temkin (1984) evaluated a skills training program designed to reduce depression in adults with epilepsy. In that intervention, subjects were taught to self-monitor for cues that indicated onset of depression or an increase in negative mood. They were then taught techniques to manage depression, including increasing the frequency of pleasurable activities, increasing physical exercise, being assertive in interpersonal relationships, monitoring self-talk, stopping thoughts, engaging in positive coping behavior, and increasing positive thoughts about self. Results indicated the 6-week intervention significantly decreased depression in the treatment group 6 weeks fol-lowing the intervention.

Even though there is limited empirical testing of interventions designed to en-hance the psychological adaptation of children with epilepsy and their families, there is a large body of literature based on clinical observation that can guide nurs-ing interventions. For example, Leahey and Wright (1985) recommend that interventions be directed at the cognitive, affective, and behavioral levels. At each of these levels, knowledge of both the biological and psychological risk factors can guide interventions.

Cognitive Level. Interventions aimed at the cognitive level provide new information about the illness or the management of the illness (Leahey & Wright, 1985). Parents need information about risk and protective factors that can influence psychosocial adaptation to epilepsy. In addition, parents need information about common fears and concerns of other parents who are in the same situation. Families also can benefit from information about healthy family coping, such as helping the child to be as independent as possible, using good communication strategies, and using social support. Timing of the information for parents also needs to be considered. Parents often report that they were given information during the first visit when they were still trying to come to terms with the idea that their child had epilepsy. Later, when they were ready for specific information, they felt uncomfortable asking nurses to repeat themselves. These parent reports highlight the need for the availability of written materials for parents and the importance of nurses' letting families know that parents should feel free to ask questions as they arise and ask for clarification when things are unclear.

Children with epilepsy also need information. For example, many have unfounded fears about brain damage and death, and children who come to clinics that also provide services to severely disabled children have been found to worry that they will become like those children. Some children may even worry that epilepsy is punishment for bad behavior. Furthermore, the need for education evolves over time as the child grows, is able to understand more, and is confronted with new challenges. It is also important that written materials and/or relevant videotapes be given to children so they incorporate these messages at their own pace at home.

Educational interventions that stress the importance of medicine-taking behavior and self-monitoring for events preceding and following seizures should be taught to children as soon as they are old enough to understand. The stated goal for the self-monitoring should be learning about the body rather than seizure control per se, so that a child does not necessarily feel that he or she failed if/when a seizure occurs.

Affective Level. Legion (1991) reports that people with epilepsy commonly state that emotional upset serves as a precipitant for seizures, which suggests that stress management is important. In addition, the effectiveness of progressive relaxation techniques and effective coping in reducing seizures also supports that children with epilepsy can benefit from strategies that deal with emotion management. Therefore, interventions that lead to effective coping strategies should be aimed at the affective level.

All family members need to be helped to deal with the intense feelings, such as anger and guilt, that can increase strain in the family. For example, helping families to meet other families who are also dealing with childhood epilepsy can be very validating for the family (Brookman, 1988). The Epilepsy Foundation of America has recently developed parent-to-parent networks that use computers to match parents in similar circumstances. Parents report that it is most helpful to talk to another parent who really understands the strong feelings they are experiencing and to learn about strategies that have worked for other families. It also appears that children could benefit from similar networks, especially because social isolation is often a problem. Other examples include encouraging family members' use of downward comparison, so they will realize that there are worse illnesses than epilepsy. Children can also be helped to reframe epilepsy by focusing on positive outcomes of having learned to live comfortably with the epilepsy. For example, children can be reminded how they have learned about feelings and how they have become more understanding of other children with problems.

Based on findings by Dahl et al. (1985), where deemphasizing seizures led to reduced seizures, parents should be taught to deal with seizures in a neutral manner with minimal emotional expression. Davis et al. (1984) suggest that nurses should encourage youth with seizures to self-monitor for cues that signal the onset of depression or negative mood and to use strategies developed by Davis and colleagues (e.g., increasing positive thoughts) for coping with anxiety.

Behavioral Level. Interventions directed at the behavior of the family include encouraging family members to change communication and interaction patterns. For example, strategies could include assigning homework tasks, encouraging participation in more leisure activities, and encouraging the use of respite care to get time away from the demanding care of the severely disabled child. To enhance feelings of control even though seizures may not be controlled, families can be helped to develop plans on how to handle future seizures in different environments, such as school and camp. Because many families are worried that their child will develop poor self-esteem, they are particularly receptive to suggestions aimed at enhancing self-esteem. For example, parents can be taught to listen to and value the child's ideas, help the child focus on positive qualities, accept the child's negative feelings, and involve the child in problem solving. Parents need to be encouraged to make the home environment conducive for the development of independence, initiative, and competence.

Based on research by Davis et al. (1984) and Dahl et al. (1985), children should also be taught to use behavioral strategies that reduce seizures. For example, they should be taught how to keep a diary of events surrounding seizures or negative moods. They could then be encouraged to practice behaviors such as progressive relaxation techniques and thought stopping to prevent and/or reduce seizures and ruminating.

Nursing Curriculum Changes

Currently there is very little information on epilepsy and associated mental health problems in nursing curricula at the undergraduate level, and it is generally not covered in graduate programs in psychiatric nursing because epilepsy is considered a neurological condition. Therefore, content on epilepsy and its treatment needs to be added at both undergraduate and graduate levels if it is to serve as a paradigmatic disorder for the interface of biological and behavioral theoretical frameworks.

Nurses need knowledge about the structure and function of the brain, classification of the different seizure types and epilepsy syndromes, how epilepsy is diagnosed, common causes of epilepsy, actions and side effects of antiepilepsy medications, the effects of antiepilepsy medication on behavior, and assessment of seizures. They also need information on mental health problems in children with epilepsy, including the signs and symptoms of most common mental health problems associated with epilepsy, as well as the biological variables and psychological variables that are risk or protective factors. Information on strategies for self-monitoring of events surrounding seizures and periods of mental health problems also should be included. Graduate program content should also include teaching children the use of cognitive and behavioral strategies such as progressive relaxation therapy. Psychological knowledge should include theories of self-concept development, individual and family stress theory, theories of depression, and social support theory.

The characteristics of epilepsy make it an important disorder to be included in both graduate and undergraduate curricula. It is an excellent disorder to use as an example for studying the interface between the brain and behavior. The unpredictability and chronicity of epilepsy also make it an especially fruitful area for studying adjustment as it relates to dealing with continual uncertainty over time, an area identified as understudied by Mishel (1990). Furthermore, the early age of onset in epilepsy provides an opportunity to learn about the interface between a chronic disorder and the developmental needs of both the individual and the family.

RESEARCH AGENDA

In general, adaptation to epilepsy is an underresearched area, so research is needed in all areas, including the etiology of the behavior problems and the development of interventions to enhance the quality of life for both children and their families. A multietiologic approach is especially needed to understand how the many biological and psychological risk factors interact.

ETIOLOGY

Basic research on etiology needs to be carried out. For example, it is not known when behavior problems begin. No research has been carried out to systematically study the natural history of adaptation to epilepsy beginning with the first seizure. To establish a baseline of mental health functioning, research is also needed that systematically assesses behavior in children and adolescents before the diagnosis of epilepsy and the initiation of antiepilepsy medication. Longitudinal studies are then needed to identify both risk and protective factors.

Another key area is research on the role that family variables play in both the development and the sustainment of behavior problems in children with epilepsy. One consistent observation is that these children experience mental health problems and that family stress is associated with mental health problems. Patterson (1983) proposes that behavior in the child can lead to irritable responses from parents that can set up a cycle of increased family strain and decreased problem-solving ability, but much more needs to be known about the relationship between stress in the family and the child's response. Research on understanding better family responses to irritability and depressed mood is especially germane because antiepilepsy medication has been found to increase irritability and depression (Trimble & Cull, 1989). For example, does teaching families how to respond with less emotion help to reduce irritability in the child? Is there a relationship between parents who are depressed and children who are depressed? What is the relationship between parental anxiety about seizures and the child's anxiety?

Even though most research has focused on the role of seizure variables in the development of psychopathology, more is still needed. Furthermore, whereas past research has tended to focus on adaptation problems or mental health problems globally (e.g., behavior problems), findings by Hermann et al. (1991) that dysphoric mood is associated with frontal lobe dysfunction suggest that more research should focus on specific problems (e.g., dysphoric mood). For example, preliminary findings by Austin indicate that in children with epilepsy, factors leading to poor self-esteem are different from those which lead to externalizing behavior problems; however, research that identifies which factors lead to different types of mental health problems is needed before interventions can be planned to alleviate these problems.

Research is also needed to identify the role that gender plays in the development of mental health problems, especially depression. Main effects for gender were found in self-concept and behavior in both epilepsy and asthma samples by Austin (1989a). Specifically, she found that girls have more negative perceptions about their physical appearance, are more depressed, have more somatic complaints, are more socially withdrawn, and tend to be more hyperactive than boys. Based on these findings, further research questions could address the influence of hormones and parenting as they are related to the differences found in adjustment between boys and girls.

Research on the factors that maintain problems could be another focus area. Recent findings by Post (cited in Holden, 1991) indicate that the kindling response model for the development of epilepsy (where repeated electrical stimulation to the amygdala lowers the threshold for seizures until they occur spontaneously) has relevance for depression. Likewise, once a person has a severe episode of depression, the threshold is lowered for future episodes of depression. Research is especially important in this area because of the implications for prevention of depression. Identifying whether children who have had previous dysphoric mood are at risk for depression when they develop epilepsy and determining if children who develop depression are in families where there is a history of depression are other areas where research is needed.

INTERVENTIONS TO ENHANCE QUALITY OF LIFE

Intervention research is needed to prevent and reduce mental health problems. Because of the great diversity in both epilepsy and the mental health problems manifested, interventions would need to be quite comprehensive and address both biological and behavioral risk and protective factors. This diversity also suggests that interventions will need to be individualized. Research is needed to test whether one-to-one interventions are more effective than group interventions, and research that links specific intervention strategies with specific outcomes is also needed. For example, do interventions that teach positive coping strategies and positive attitudes toward epilepsy lead to lower rates of depression? Does hyperventilation mediate the relationship between stress and seizures?

The presence of poor self-concept is a consistent finding in children with epilepsy. Because poor self-concept can make children vulnerable to depression, research on interventions for families and children that leads to the development of positive self-concepts needs to be developed and tested. For example, does enhancement of social skills increase social competence and self-esteem? Do interventions to help children deal effectively with stigma (i.e., make attitudes toward epilepsy more positive) lead to enhanced self-esteem?

More nursing research is also needed on the whole area of self-management of epilepsy. For example, what roles do sound nutrition, exercise, and regular sleeping habits play in the reduction of seizures or in the prevention of mental health problems? Does teaching self-monitoring lead to reduced fear surrounding seizures? Can children be taught to identify behaviors and thoughts that affect the progression of seizures? Does self-monitoring of events surrounding seizures increase children's perceptions of control over the disorder? Does anxiety mediate the relationship between coping and seizures?

These ideas for research are just a few of the many areas that need attention if nursing practice is to become more research-based. Nurses are in unique positions to contribute to the development of knowledge in the area and play a major role in the development of new and exciting information on the brain-behavior interface.

REFERENCES

Achenbach, T. M. (1991). *Manual for the child behavior checklist 4-18 and 1991 profile.* Burlington, VT: University of Vermont Department of Psychiatry.

Austin, J. K. (1988). Childhood epilepsy: Child adaptation and family resources. *Journal of Child and Adolescent Psychiatric and Mental Health Nursing, 1,* 18–24.

Austin, J. K. (1989a). Comparison of child adaptation to epilepsy and asthma. *Journal of Child and Adolescent Psychiatric and Mental Health Nursing, 2*, 139–144.

Austin, J. K. (1989b). Predicting parental anticonvulsant medication compliance using the theory of reasoned action. *Journal of Pediatric Nursing, 4*, 88–95.

Austin, J. K. (1990a). Childhood epilepsy and asthma: A test of an extension of the Double ABCX Model. ERIC Document Reproduction Service (ED 331 249, EC 300 232).

Austin, J. K. (1990b). Assessment of coping mechanisms used by parents and children with chronic illness. *The American Journal of Maternal/Child Nursing, 15*, 98–102.

Austin, J. K., & Huberty, T. J. (1989). Revision of the family APGAR for use by 8-year-olds. *Family Systems Medicine, 7*, 323–327.

Austin, J. K., & Huberty, T. J. (1993). Development of the child attitude toward illness scale. *Journal of Pediatric Psychology, 18*(4), 467–480.

Austin, J. K., McBride, A. B., & Davis, H. W. (1984). Parental attitude and adjustment to childhood epilepsy. *Nursing Research, 33*, 92–96.

Austin, J. K., & McDermott, N. (1988). Parental attitude and coping behaviors in families of children with epilepsy. *Journal of Neuroscience Nursing, 20*, 174–179.

Austin, J. K., Patterson, J. M., & Huberty, T. J. (1991). Development of the coping health inventory for children. *Journal of Pediatric Nursing, 6*, 166–174.

Austin, J. K., Risinger, M. W., & Beckett, L. (1992). Correlates of behavior problems in children with epilepsy. *Epilepsia, 33*(6), 115–1122.

Austin, J. K., Smith, M. S., Risinger, M. W., & McNelis, A. M. (1994). Childhood epilepsy and asthma: Comparison of quality of life. *Epilepsia, 35*, 608–615.

Bagley, C. (1971). *The social psychology of the child with epilepsy.* London: Routledge & Kegan Paul.

Bagley, C. (1972). Social prejudice and the adjustment of people with epilepsy. *Epilepsia, 13*, 33–45.

Baker, G. A., Smith, D. F., Dewey, M., Morrow, J., Crawford, P. M., & Chadwick, D. W. (1991). The development of a seizure severity scale as an outcome measure in epilepsy. *Epilepsy Research, 8*, 245–251.

Bear, D. M., & Fedio, P. (1977). Quantitative analysis of interictal behavior in temporal lobe epilepsy. *Archives of Neurology, 34*, 454–467.

Bennett, T. L. (1992). Cognitive effects of epilepsy and anticonvulsant medications. In T. L. Bennett (Ed.), *The neuropsychology of epilepsy* (pp. 73–95). New York: Plenum.

Binnie, C. D., & Marston, D. (1992). Cognitive correlates of interictal discharges. *Epilepsia, 33*(Suppl. 6), S11–S17.

Blummer, D. (1984). *Psychiatric aspects of epilepsy.* Washington, DC: American Psychiatric Press.

Breslau, N. (1985). Psychiatric disorder in children with physical disabilities. *Journal of the American Academy of Child Psychiatry, 24*, 87–94.

Brookman, B. A. (1988). Parent to parent support: A model for parent support and information. *Topics in Early Childhood Special Education, 8*, 88–92.

Commission for the Control of Epilepsy and Its Consequences. (1979). *Plan for nationwide action on epilepsy* (Vol. 1). Washington, DC: US Department of Health, Education, and Welfare (Publication Code: NIH 78–276).

Cull, C. A., Trimble, M. R., & Wilson, J. (1992). Changes in antiepilepsy drug regimen and behavior in children with epilepsy. *Journal of Epilepsy, 5*, 1–9.

Dahl, J., Melin, L., Brorson, L., & Schollin, J. (1985). Effects of a broad-spectrum behavior modification treatment program on children with refractory epileptic seizures. *Epilepsia, 26*, 303–309.

Davis, G. R., Armstrong, H. E., Donovan, D. M., & Temkin, N.R. (1984). Cognitive-behavioral treatment of depressed affect among epileptics: Preliminary findings. *Journal of Clinical Psychology, 40*, 930–935.

DeVellis, R. F., & DeVellis, B. M. (1986). An evolving psychosocial model of epilepsy. In S. Whitman & B. P. Hermann (Eds.), *Psychopathology in epilepsy: Social dimensions* (pp. 122–142). New York: Oxford University Press.

Devinsky, O. (1991). Interictal behavior changes in epilepsy. In O. Devinsky & W. H. Theodore (Eds.), *Epilepsy and behavior* (pp. 1–21). New York: Wiley.

Dodrill, C. B. (1990). Neuropsychology. In M. Dam & L. Gram (Eds.), *Comprehensive epileptology* (pp. 473–484). New York: Raven.

Dodrill, C. B. (1992). Interictal cognitive aspects of epilepsy. *Epilepsia, 33*(Suppl. 6), S7–S10.

Drotar, D., & Bush, M. (1985). Mental health issues and services. In N. Hobbs & J. M. Perrin (Eds.), *Issues in the care of children with chronic illness* (pp. 514–550). San Francisco: Jossey-Bass.

Dunst, C., Trivette, C., & Deal, A. (1988). *Enabling and empowering families.* Cambridge, MA: Brookline Books.

Epstein, A. W. (1990). What the reflex epilepsies reveal about physiology of ideation. *Journal of Neuropsychiatry, 2,* 69–71.

Fenwick, P. (1991). The influence of mind on seizure activity. In O. Devinsky & W. H. Theodore (Eds.), *Epilepsy and behavior* (pp. 405–419). New York: Wiley.

Ferrari, M., Barabas, G., & Matthews, W. S. (1983). Psychological and behavioral disturbance among epileptic children treated with barbiturate anticonvulsants. *American Journal of Psychiatry, 21,* 208–212.

Friedman, I. M., Litt, I. F., King, D. R., Henson, R., Holtzman, D., Halverson, D., & Kraemer, H. C. (1986). Compliance with anticonvulsant therapy by epileptic youth. *Journal of Adolescent Health Care, 7,* 12–17.

Gillham, R. A. (1990). Refractory epilepsy: An evaluation of psychological methods in outpatient management. *Epilepsia, 31,* 427–432.

Gross-Tsur, V., & Shinnar, S. (1993). Convulsive status epilepticus in children. *Epilepsia, 34*(Suppl. 1), S12–S20.

Harter, S. (1982). The perceived competence scale for children. *Child Development, 53,* 87–97.

Harter, S., & Pike, R. (1984). The pictorial scale of perceived competence and social acceptance for young children. *Child Development, 55,* 1969–1982.

Hartlage, L. C., & Green, J. B. (1972). The relation of parental attitudes to academic and social achievement in epileptic children. *Epilepsia, 13,* 21–26.

Hartlage, L. C., Green, J. B., & Offutt, L. (1972). Dependency in epileptic children. *Epilepsia, 13,* 27–30.

Hauser, W. A., & Hesdorffer, D. C. (1990). *Epilepsy: Frequency, causes and consequences.* New York: Demos.

Hermann, B. P. (1981). Deficits in neuropsychological functioning and psychopathology in persons with epilepsy: A rejected hypothesis revisited. *Epilepsia, 22,* 161–167.

Hermann, B. P., Seidenberg, M., Haltiner, A., & Wyler, A. R. (1991). Mood state in unilateral temporal lobe epilepsy. *Biological Psychiatry, 30,* 1205–1218.

Hermann, B. P., & Whitman, S. (1984). Behavioral and personality correlates of epilepsy: A review, methodological critique, and conceptual model. *Psychological Bulletin, 95*(3), 451–497.

Hermann, B. P., & Whitman, S. (1986). Psychopathology in epilepsy: A multietiologic model. In B. P. Hermann & S. Whitman (Eds.), *Psychopathology in epilepsy: Social dimensions* (pp. 5–37) New York: Oxford University Press.

Hermann, B. P., & Whitman, S. (1991). Neurobiological, psychosocial, and pharmacological factors underlying interictal psychopathology in epilepsy. In D. Smith, D. Treiman, & M. Trimble (Eds.), *Advances in neurology (Vol. 55): Neurobehavioral problems in epilepsy* (pp. 439–452). New York: Raven.

Hermann, B. P., Whitman, S., & Dell, J. (1989). Correlates of behavior problems and social competence in children with epilepsy, aged 6-11. In B. P. Hermann & M. Seidenberg (Eds.), *Childhood epilepsies: Neurological, psychological and intervention aspects* (pp. 143–157). New York: Wiley.

Hoare, P. (1984a). The development of psychiatric disorder among school children with epilepsy. *Developmental Medicine and Child Neurology, 26,* 3-13.

Hoare, P. (1984b). Psychiatric disturbance in the families of epileptic children. *Developmental Medicine and Child Neurology, 26,* 14–19.

Hoare, P., & Kerley, S. (1991). Psychosocial adjustment of children with chronic epilepsy and their families. *Developmental Medicine and Child Neurology, 33,* 201–215.

Holden, C. (1991). Depression: The news isn't depressing. *Science, 254,* 1450–1452.

Holdsworth, L., & Whitmore, K. (1974). A study of children with epilepsy attending ordinary schools. I: Their seizure patterns, progress and behaviour in school. *Developmental Medicine and Child Neurology, 16,* 746–758.

Holmes, G. L. (1987). *Diagnosis and management of seizures in children.* Philadelphia: Saunders.

Holmes, G. L. (1991). Do seizures cause brain damage? *Epilepsia, 32*(Suppl. 5), 14–28.

Houben, P., Hommes, O., & Knaven, P. (1971). Anticonvulsant drugs and folic acid in young mentally retarded epileptic patients: A study of serum folate, fit frequency and IQ. *Epilepsia, 12,* 2325–2347.

Huberty, T. J., Austin, J. K., Risinger, M. W., & McNelis, A. M. (1992). Relationship of selected variables in children with epilepsy to performance on school-administered achievement tests. *Journal of Epilepsy, 5,* 10–16.

Johnson, B. M. (1982). Nursing priorities in the management of epilepsy. In R. B. Black, B. P. Hermann, & J. T. Shope (Eds.), *Nursing management of epilepsy* (pp. 63–72). Rockville, MD: Aspen.

Klein, S. K. (1991). Cognitive factors and learning disabilities in children with epilepsy. In O. Devinsky & W. H. Theodore (Eds.), *Epilepsy and behavior* (pp. 171–179). New York: Wiley.

Kovacs, M. (1980/81). Rating scales to assess depression in school-aged children. *Acta Paedopsychiatrica, 46,* 305–315.

Lazarus, R. S., & Folkman, S. (1989). *Manual for the Hassles and Uplifts Scales: Research edition.* Palo Alto: Consulting Psychologists.

Leahey, M., & Wright, L. M. (1985). Intervening with families with chronic illness. *Family Systems Medicine, 3,* 60–69.

Legion, V. (1991). Health education for self-management by people with epilepsy. *Journal of Neuroscience Nursing, 23,* 300–305.

Leiderman, D. B., Csernansky, J. G., & Moses, J. A. (1990). Neuroendocrinology and limbic epilepsy: Relationships to psychopathology, seizure variables, and neuropsychosocial function. *Epilepsia, 31*(3), 270–274.

Lewis, M. A., Hatton, C. L., Salas, I., Leake, B., & Chiofalo, N. (1991). Impact of the children's epilepsy program on parents. *Epilepsia, 32,* 365–374.

Lewis, M. A., Salas, I., de la Sota, A., Chiofalo, N., & Leake, B. (1990). Randomized trial of a program to enhance the competencies of children with epilepsy. *Epilepsia, 31,* 101–109.

Long, C. G., & Moore, J. R. (1979). Parental perceptions for their epileptic children. *Journal of Child Psychology and Psychiatry, 20,* 299–312.

Margalit, M., & Heiman, T. (1983). Anxiety and self-dissatisfaction in epileptic children. *International Journal of Social Psychiatry, 29,* 220–224.

Massie, R. K. (1985). The constant shadow: Reflections on the life of a chronically ill child. In N. Hobbs & J. M. Perrin (Eds.), *Issues in the care of children with chronic illness* (pp. 13–23). San Francisco: Jossey-Bass.

Matthews, W. S., & Barabas, G. (1986). Perceptions of control among children with epilepsy. In S. Whitman & B. P. Hermann (Eds.), *Psychopathology in epilepsy: Social dimensions* (pp. 162–184). New York: Oxford University Press.

Matthews, W. S., Barabas, G., & Ferrari, M. (1982). Emotional concomitants of childhood epilepsy. *Epilepsia, 23,* 671–681.

McCubbin, H. I., & Patterson, J. M. (1983). The family stress process: The Double ABCX Model of Adjustment and Adaptation. *Marriage and Family Review, 6,* 7–37.

McCubbin, H. I., & Thompson, A. I. (1991). *Family assessment inventories for research and practice.* Family Stress Coping and Health Project, University of Wisconsin—Madison.

Miles, M. V., Tennison, M. B., & Greenwood, R. S. (1988). Assessment of antiepilepsy drug effects on child behavior using the Child Behavior Checklist. *Journal of Epilepsy, 1,* 209–213.

Mishel, M. H. (1990). Reconceptualization of the uncertainty in illness theory. *IMAGE: Journal of Nursing Scholarship, 22*(4), 256–262.

Mittan, R. J. (1986). Fear of seizures. In S. Whitman & B. P. Hermann (Eds.), *Psychopathology in epilepsy: Social dimensions* (pp. 90–121). New York: Oxford University Press.

Mulder, H. C., & Suurmeijer, T. P. (1977). Families with a child with epilepsy: A sociological contribution. *Journal of Biosocial Science, 9*(1), 13–24.

Neugebauer, R., Paik, M., Nadel, E., Hauser, W. A., & Susser, M. (1991). Association of stressful life events with seizure occurrence in patients with epilepsy. (Abstract). *Epilepsia, 32*(Suppl.), 31.

Patterson, G. R. (1983). Stress: A change agent for family process. In N. Garmezy & M. Rutter (Eds.). *Stress, coping, & development in children* (pp. 235–264). New York: McGraw-Hill.

Patterson, J. M. (1988). Chronic illness in children and the impact on families. In C. S. Chilman, F. M. Cox, & E. W. Nunnally (Eds.), *Chronic illness and disability* (pp. 69–107). Newbury Park, CA: Sage.

Perrine, K. R. (1991). Psychopathology in epilepsy. *Seminars in Neurology, 11,* 175–181.

Piers, E. V. (1984). *Piers-Harris Children's Self-Concept Scale. Revised manual.* Los Angeles, CA: Western Psychological Services.

Poirel, C., & Ennaji, M. (1991). Circadian aspects of epileptic behavior in comparative psychophysiology. *Psychological Reports, 68,* 783–801.

Pond, D. A., & Bidwell, B. H. (1960). A survey of epilepsy in 14 general practices. *Epilepsia, 1,* 285–299.

Puskarich, C. A., Whitman, S., Dell, J., Hughes, J. R., Rosen, A. J., & Hermann, B. P. (1992). Controlled examination of effects of progressive relaxation training on seizure reduction. *Epilepsia, 33,* 675–680.

Quinn, P. (1988). When epilepsy is not the only problem . . . assessing special needs. In H. Reisner (Ed.), *Children with epilepsy: A parents' guide* (pp. 113–146). Kensington, MD: Woodbine House.

Rausch, R., & Victoroff, J. I. (1991). Neuropsychological factors related to behavior disorders in epilepsy. In O. Devinsky & W. H. Theodore (Eds.), *Epilepsy and behavior* (pp. 213–221). New York: Wiley.

Reynolds, E. H. (1968). Mental effects of anticonvulsants and folic acid metabolism. *Brain, 91,* 197–214.

Reynolds, E. H. (1986). Antiepileptic drugs and personality. In M. R. Trimble & T. G. Bolwig (Eds.), *Aspects of epilepsy and psychiatry* (pp. 89–99). New York: Wiley.

Reynolds, E. H. (1991). Interictal psychiatric disorders: Neurochemical aspects. In D. B. Smith, D. M. Treiman, & M. R. Trimble (Eds.), *Advances in neurology* (Vol. 55, pp. 47–58). New York: Raven.

Robertson, M. M., & Trimble, M. R. (1983). Depressive illness in patients with epilepsy: A review. *Epilepsia, 24*(Suppl. 2), 109–116.

Rolland, J. S. (1988). A conceptual model of chronic and life-threatening illness and its impact on families. In C. S. Chilman, E. W. Nunnally, & F. M. Cox (Eds.), *Chronic illness and disability* (pp. 1–68). Newbury Park, CA: Sage.

Romeis, J. C. (1980). The role of grandparents in adjustment to epilepsy. *Social Work in Health Care, 6,* 37–43.

Rosenberg, M. (1965). *Society and the adolescent self-image.* Princeton, NJ: Princeton University Press.

Rutter, M. (1981). Psychological sequelae of brain damage in children. *The American Journal of Psychiatry, 138,* 1533–1544.

Rutter, M. (1993). An overview of developmental neuropsychiatry. *Educational and Child Psychology, 10*(1), 4–16.

Rutter, M., Graham, P., & Yule, W. (1970). A neuropsychiatric study in childhood. *Clinics in Developmental Medicine, 35/36,* 175–185.

Rutter, M., Tizard, J., & Whitmore, K. (1970). *Education, health and behavior.* Huntington, NY: Krieber.

Santilli, N., Dodson, W. E., & Walton, A. V. (1991). *Students with seizures.* Cedar Grove, NJ: HealthScan Inc.

Schotte, D. E., & Dubois, M. A. (1989). Behavioral medicine approaches to enhancing seizure control in children with epilepsy. In B. P. Hermann & M. Seidenberg (Eds.), *Childhood epilepsies: Neurological, psychological and intervention aspects* (pp. 189–200). New York: Wiley.

Scott, D. J. (1978). Psychiatric aspects of epilepsy. *British Journal of Psychiatry, 132,* 417–430.

Seidenberg, M. (1989). Neuropsychological functioning of children with epilepsy. In B. P. Hermann & M. Seidenberg (Eds.), *Childhood epilepsies: Neuropsychological, psychosocial, and intervention aspects* (pp. 71–81). New York: Wiley.

Smilkstein, G. (1978). The family APGAR: A proposal for a family function test and its use by physicians. *Journal of Family Practice, 6,* 1231–1239.

Spunt, A. L., & Black, R. B. (1982). Drug treatment of seizure disorders. In R. B. Black, B. P. Hermann, & J. T. Shope (Eds.), *Nursing management of epilepsy* (pp. 25–41). Rockville, MD: Aspen.

Steinhausen, H. C., & Rauss-Mason, C. (1991). Epilepsy and anticonvulsant drugs. In M. Rutter & P. Casaer (Eds.), *Biological risk factors for psychosocial disorders* (pp. 311–339). Cambridge: Cambridge University Press.

Stores, G. (1978). School-children with epilepsy at risk for learning and behavior problems. *Developmental Medicine and Child Neurology, 20,* 502–508.

Temkin, N. R., & Davis, G. R. (1984). Stress as a risk factor for seizures among adults with epilepsy. *Epilepsia, 25,* 450–456.

Trimble, M. R. (1990). Neuropsychiatry. In M. Dam & L. Gram (Eds.), *Comprehensive epileptology* (pp. 485–494). New York: Raven.

Trimble, M. R., Corbett, J. A., & Donaldson, D. (1980). Folic acid and mental symptoms in children with epilepsy. *Journal of Neurology, Neurosurgery, and Psychiatry, 43,* 1030–1034.

Trimble, M. R., & Cull, C. A. (1988). Children of school age: The influence of antiepileptic drugs. *Epilepsia, 29*(Suppl. 3), 15–19.

Trimble, M. R., & Cull, C. A. (1989). Antiepileptic drugs, cognitive function, and behavior in children. *Cleveland Clinic Journal of Medicine, 56*(Suppl. 1), 140–146.

Voeller, K. K., & Rothenberg, M. B. (1973). Psychosocial aspects of the management of seizures in children. *Pediatrics, 51,* 1072–1082.

Wallander, J. L., Varni, J. W., Babani, L., Banis, T., & Wilcox, K. (1989). Family resources as resistance factors for psychological maladjustment in chronically ill children. *Journal of Pediatric Psychology, 14,* 157–173.

Ward, F., & Bower, B. D. (1978). A study of certain social aspects of epilepsy in childhood. *Developmental Medicine and Child Neurology, 20*(Suppl. 39), 1–63.

Wasterlain, C. G., Fujikawa, D. G., Penix, L., & Sankar, R. (1993). Pathophysiological mechanisms of brain damage from status epilepticus. *Epilepsia, 34*(Suppl. 1), S37–S53.

Whitman, S., Hermann, B. P., Black, R. B., & Chhabria, S. (1982). Psychopathology and seizure type in children with epilepsy. *Psychological Medicine, 12,* 843–853.

Ziegler, R. G. (1985). Risk factors in childhood epilepsy. *Psychotherapeutic Psychosomatics, 44,* 185–190.

CHAPTER

7

Drugs, Children, and Families

Mary R. Haack, PhD, RN, FAAN

ABSTRACT

The chapter explains the magnitude and nature of the problem of drug-exposed infants and their families, describing the physiological and behavioral effects of various commonly used drugs, both illegal (cocaine, heroin) and legal (alcohol, nicotine). It challenges the notion, perpetuated by the popular media, that drug-exposed infants are throwaway kids, pointing out that environmental impact—for example, less effective mothering and unstable home environment—needs to be considered in addition to actual exposure to drugs and concluding that children have a tremendous capacity to recuperate and accommodate to the negative effects of drug exposure if they grow up in an organized, nurturing environment. Therefore, it is important for nurses to expand nursing education in this area and work with others toward changes in health policy that will promote adequate drug abuse treatment programs for addicted pregnant women, rather than prosecution, and provide health and developmental services for children and their families. The chapter then reviews various strategies to ameliorate adverse effects of prenatal drug use, including recommended schedules for detoxification and the need for treatment plans that address the psychiatric and behavioral problems often associated with drug use. For drug-exposed children and their mothers, the chapter recommends adopting a family preservation model of treatment similar to the one developed by the Center for Health Policy Research and the University of Pennsylvania's Transitional Care project. Finally, changes in nursing education and a research agenda in this area are presented.

The growing incidence of substance abuse has gained national prominence, as the problems that attend it continue to devastate all aspects of our nation's social fabric. Substance abusers and their victims have inundated our cities' hospitals (many of them already overburdened and financially distressed), drug treatment centers, child protective services, and prisons. Substance abuse problems of all types have become even more acute among women of childbearing ages, particularly poor and minority women, and have been accompanied by an increasing number of infants born exposed to alcohol, nicotine, and illegal drugs. Psychiatric nursing can play an important role in addressing this national health care issue.

Preparation of this chapter was supported in part by a grant (No. 21920) from The Robert Wood Johnson Foundation.

Although nurses are confronted by the many health and social problems accompanying prenatal drug exposure, barriers such as lack of funding for specialized nursing education programs and lack of adequate treatment systems and reimbursement policies prevent nurses from providing the necessary comprehensive care to this vulnerable and underserved population. Many advanced practice nurses (APNs)—including midwives, neonatal intensive care, pediatric, and psychiatric nurses—have skills and knowledge to improve the care of these families, but their training and practice are not coordinated in such a way that they can work together to deliver a seamless package of services. This chapter will lay the groundwork for a proposed model of advanced practice nursing that promotes the delivery of comprehensive care. What follows is a description of the problem, the biomedical principles underlying the problem, barriers to addressing the problem, and the approaches that are relevant to psychiatric nursing practice.

BACKGROUND

Mother-to-baby drug exposure is rising in the United States, with some estimates showing as many as 375,000 children affected annually. The phenomenon comes at great economic and social cost to the nation. The national price tag for treating drug-exposed infants is estimated at up to $3 billion annually. Short-term human costs are evidenced by premature and low-birth-weight infants, while long-term costs include chronic illness and learning disabilities.

From an international perspective, the U.S. infant mortality and infant low-birth-weight rates rank poorly among other Western countries. Maternal use of alcohol, tobacco, and other drugs is thought to be a contributing factor.

- The United States ranks twentieth in infant mortality and thirty-first in infant low birth weight. Even in Romania, Iran, and the former Soviet Union average birth weights are higher than in the United States. Prenatal use of cocaine and cigarettes and lack of access to prenatal care contribute to the U.S. rankings (Racine, Joyce, & Anderson, 1993).
- Each year 22,000 babies are abandoned at birth; 8 out of 10 of these infants test positive for drugs.
- Between October 1992 and September 1993, reportedly 814 children had AIDS as a result of prenatal exposure from an infected mother. Most maternal AIDS is the result of IV drug use by the mother or her partner (Centers for Disease Control, 1993).
- Median hospital costs for drug-exposed babies range from $1100 to $8450 more than for normal babies (USGAO 1990).
- Inpatient care for one child with AIDS is estimated to cost $34,713 per year.

PROFILE OF ADDICTED PREGNANT WOMAN

Unpublished data indicate that addicted pregnant women access drug treatment late in their drug-taking careers. This is no surprise to nurses who have unsuccessfully tried to refer such clients to treatment. Typically, child protective services and the court system provide the gateway to drug treatment for most pregnant women in most communities. A mother must be seriously impaired to qualify.

Characteristically, the addicted pregnant woman who is a patient in the scarce number of treatment slots available across the country is a 27- to 31-year-old high school dropout with three or four children, either homeless or living in a drug-abusing environment. She has typically been using illegal substances for at least 10 years and has grown up in a home with violence, sexual abuse, and substance-abusing relatives. Her referral to treatment came through child protective services or at the time of delivery if her baby tested positive for drugs. This profile suggests the need for nursing interventions that are augmented by clinical case management, child care, transportation, housing, and education (National Institute on Drug Abuse, 1994).

Although statistics characterize perinatal addiction as primarily affecting poor minorities, recent studies show it affects all social classes. Researchers report minority women are more likely to be identified as drug users because they are more apt to be tested at public clinics and hospitals. Health professionals are, however, reluctant to identify problems they have no way to treat.

U.S. HEALTH CARE POLICIES VERSUS POLICIES OF OTHER WESTERN COUNTRIES

In countries where primary health care services are available to all citizens, it is more likely that addicted women will be treated earlier in their drug-taking careers. The United States is the only Western country that prosecutes addicted pregnant women for using drugs while pregnant. In most of Western Europe, pregnant addicted women have access not only to basic primary care for themselves and their children but also to drug treatment.

For example, under the National Health Service (NHS) in England, addicted pregnant women have priority in access to substance abuse treatment slots. Because heroin is more prevalent in the United Kingdom and the NHS has a policy against treating pregnant women with methadone, women are admitted to the hospital and withdrawn from heroin over a 4-week period. The primary health care services and drug treatment services are coordinated by an interdisciplinary team that includes a psychiatrist and an obstetrician. In addition, the family with a substance-abusing mother is followed indefinitely by a home visitor nurse, social worker, and midwife—all of whom are trained in developmental assessment and case management. The prosecution of women for drug use during pregnancy is unheard of in England.

MAGNITUDE OF THE PROBLEM

Estimates of substance abuse among pregnant women or women of childbearing age in the United States vary, but all indicate a serious and growing problem. It is estimated that approximately 250,362 pregnant women need drug treatment annually; however, in the absence of scientific data the actual numbers are not known (National Association of State Alcohol and Drug Abuse Directors, 1993).

EPIDEMIOLOGY

Of the 59.2 million women of childbearing age (15 to 44) in the United States, over 4.5 million are current users of illegal drugs; 5.6% use marijuana and 1% use cocaine, but estimates of use during pregnancy are not known (National Institute on Drug Abuse, 1991). Approximately 59% to 73% of women between the ages of 12 and 34 drink alcohol during pregnancy (Frank et al., 1988; National Institute on Drug Abuse, 1991). At least 30% of all women in the United States smoke at the time they conceive, and 25% continue to smoke during pregnancy (USDHHS, 1990).

A number of studies illustrate the scope of the problem. For instance, a 1988 study of 36 hospitals across the country conducted by the National Association for Perinatal Addictions Research and Education (NAPARE) found that on average,

11% of pregnant women used heroin, methadone, amphetamines, PCP, marijuana, or cocaine. Another study reported that 17% of pregnant teenagers test positive for alcohol and other drugs by questionnaire, provider report, or urine screen (Kokotailo, Adger, Duggan, Repke, & Jaffe, 1992).

Based on an analysis of the 1988 National Hospital Discharge Survey, the U.S. General Accounting Office (GAO) identified approximately 14,000 infants with indications of maternal drug use during pregnancy. The report, however, states that this figure substantially minimizes the problem because physicians and hospitals do not screen and test all women and their infants for drugs (Chasnoff, Landress, & Barrett, 1990; USGAO, 1990).

Bias toward Poor Women

Studies indicate that poor minority women are more likely to be identified than other pregnant women who are cocaine users. A clinical investigation conducted within Pinellas County, Florida, anonymously tested women entering private obstetric care and women entering public health clinics for prenatal care and found the overall incidence of drug use was similar in both groups (Chasnoff et al., 1990). A 1990 USGAO report found that private hospitals serving primarily non-Medicaid patients screened infants for drug exposure less often than public hospitals. While some researchers have found a prevalence of substance abuse as low as 2%, other studies from inner-city hospitals report that as many as half of all pregnant women test positive for illegal drugs.

A 1992 Rand study found obstetricians in private institutions chose not to screen their patients for presence of illicit drugs because of limited treatment options and significant costs associated with screening. Private physicians also feared losing patients if it became known that they drug screen their patients. The report concluded that private health care providers are reluctant to participate in detecting and reporting maternal drug abuse.

According to public health experts, we lack complete information on the prevalence of addicted pregnant women and drug-exposed children because no studies have attempted to review drug histories over the course of pregnancy in a representative sample of women at delivery and because of somewhat limited methods for acquiring the information through interview or biological assessment (Robins & Mills, 1993).

Pharmacology of Addictive Drugs

To understand why drugs can be so harmful to a pregnant woman and her child, it is important to understand the pharmacological properties of the substance. For example, cocaine produces striking effects on the central nervous system by augmenting the biochemical action of dopamine and by interfering with the normal communication of the catecholamine neurotransmitter in the limbic system, the part of the brain known as the pleasure pathway. Cocaine acts by blocking reuptake of dopamine at the neuronal synaptic junction. Reuptake is the primary mechanism by which dopamine is deactivated in the central nervous system; therefore, by blocking this action, cocaine extends dopaminergic neurotransmission. Many of the behavioral, physiological, and psychological effects of cocaine can be explained by this pharmacological property (Kaplan & Sadock, 1991).

The same catecholamine neurotransmitter mechanism by which cocaine causes a high is thought to be the reason for the crash. Though the exact reason for the crash has not been determined, it is currently thought to be either a result of exhaustion caused by the perpetual excitation of the nerve that occurs in the presence of cocaine or a response to the user's inability to fulfill the greater dosage needed to restore the high. Another possible explanation is that the heightened level of dopamine transmission depletes the dopamine in the system and eventually leads to depression, withdrawal, or crash (Kaplan & Sadock, 1991).

Physiological Effects on the Pregnant Mother

The physiological effects produced by cocaine include flushing, sweating, dilated pupils, increased blood pressure, and slightly increased pulse. Because of the nature of the limbic system, the region of the brain acted on by this drug, excessive energy and physical strength, a decreased need for sleep, decreased appetite, and an increased sexual drive are also caused by the drug. General vasoconstriction and increased muscle activity are responsible for the increased risk for premature labor and abruptio placentae in pregnant cocaine users (Khalsa, 1989). Problems associated with premature birth account for many complications experienced by drug-exposed infants.

Behavioral Effects on the Pregnant Mother

Some of the immediate effects of substance abuse on the behavior of expectant mothers and their infants are known. Cocaine produces mental and physical activation, which leads to a state of euphoria. Self-confidence increases and cognitive, social, or physical tasks seem easier to perform. It is these positive reinforcing properties that make cocaine abusers susceptible to cocaine dependence (Kaplan & Sadock, 1991). However, with prolonged use of cocaine, irritability and aggressiveness may replace euphoria.

These behaviors may drastically interfere with the ability to parent. Users on binges can spend days without eating or sleeping, leading to eventual emotional and physical exhaustion. Paranoid thought processes, delusions, and hallucinations can also result from binges. Then the aftermath of a binge can produce profound depression, characterized by excessive sleep, fatigue, apathy, anhedonia, and psychomotor retardation (Blum, 1984).

Effects of Specific Drug on the Developing Child

Effects of specific drugs have been identified largely through animal studies, but the findings of animal studies cannot always be extrapolated to human beings. There are many interspecies differences for many of the phenomena thought to be drug related (Robins & Mills, 1993).

In any given child, it is also difficult to delineate a single drug effect, since most addicts use several drugs. One drug is usually preferred, but other drugs are used to enhance it, substitute for it, or counteract undesirable effects. Furthermore, almost all addicts use legal drugs such as alcohol and nicotine in conjunction with illegal drugs.

COCAINE

The adverse effects of cocaine use on the developing fetus and the mechanisms by which they work are multiple, inconclusive, and interrelated. Table 7–1 shows the signs and symptoms of prenatal drug exposure related to specific domains of child development. The exact effects of drugs on pregnancy have not been definitely determined, but one problem, premature labor, has been identified and at least partly explained. Because of the increased uterine contractility associated with the increase in catecholamines, the use of cocaine increases risk for premature delivery. Abruptio

TABLE 7–1. DEVELOPMENTAL PROBLEMS ATTRIBUTED TO DRUG EXPOSURE

DOMAIN OF DEVELOPMENT	SIGNS AND SYMPTOMS
Motor and neurological	Tremulousness, irregular sleep patterns, irritability, hypersensitivity to environmental stimuli, muscle rigidity
Affective and behavioral	Lability of emotion, explosive and impulsive behaviors, depressed affect, decreased laughter, difficulty with transitions and changes, difficulty in comforting self and being comforted, increased testing of limits, inability to self-regulate or modulate own behavior
Social and attachment	Decreased use of eye contact, decreased use of gestures, difficulty with attachment and separation, aggressiveness with peers, decreased response to verbal direction or praise, decreased use of adults for solace or comfort
Problem solving	Increased distractibility to extraneous sounds and movements, lack of tolerance for frustration, difficulty organizing behavior
Language	Fewer spontaneous vocalizations from early infancy, delayed acquisition of words, prolonged infantile articulation at the preschool level, difficulty in "word finding" at the preschool level
Play	Decreased spontaneous play, increased aimless wandering, more constricted and impulsive play, difficulty organizing play, difficulty with peer relationships

placentae (the premature detachment of a normally placed placenta) may also result from the same or a similar mechanism. In addition, the increase in metabolism, also resulting from a rise in catecholamines, may contribute to undernutrition of the fetus. Other secondary effects of cocaine use, decreased placental blood flow and maternal malnutrition, may also be responsible for low birth weight.

Further, drug-exposed infants can suffer a wide array of both temporary and enduring consequences, which include not only prematurity and low birth weight but also growth retardation, small head size, cerebral hemorrhage, hyperactivity, sleep disturbance, eating problems, learning difficulties, and withdrawal symptoms (Mitchell, 1993). These conditions can also be associated with other prenatal and environmental conditions.

HEROIN

While there is no identified abstinence syndrome in cocaine-exposed babies, the prenatal use of opiates, such as heroin or methadone, does produce withdrawal symptoms in 60% to 80% of exposed newborns. The neonatal abstinence syndrome involves the central and autonomic nervous systems, gastrointestinal system, and pulmonary system. Central nervous system (CNS) signs include irritability, hypertonia, hyperreflexia, abnormal sucking, and poor feeding. Seizures are seen in 1% to 3%. Gastrointestinal signs include diarrhea and vomiting. Respiratory signs include tachypnea, hyperpnea, and respiratory alkalosis. Autonomic signs include sneezing, yawning, lacrimation, sweating, and hyperpyrexia. If the infant is hypermetabolic, the postnatal weight loss may be excessive and subsequent weight gain less than optimal. Restlessness, agitation, irritability, and poor socialization can persist for 4 to 6 months. Withdrawal from methadone is similar to heroin, with the added complication of an increased incidence of sudden infant death syndrome (SIDS) (Mitchell, 1993). Children whose mothers use both heroin and cocaine have less severe withdrawal symptoms. Cocaine seems to counteract the withdrawal syndrome in newborns.

ALCOHOL

While the problems associated with perinatal substance abuse and addiction have been most visible among users of crack cocaine and heroin, perinatal exposure to alcohol and tobacco smoke can also have devastating effects. Alcoholic drinking can cause a cluster of birth outcomes, known as fetal alcohol syndrome (FAS), including growth deficiencies, facial abnormalities, and mental retardation. Alcohol is the only drug known to have the direct effect of mental retardation and is the third leading cause of birth defects associated with mental retardation. The basic features of FAS are prenatal and postnatal growth retardation; CNS deficits, including developmental delays and neurological/intellectual impairment; and facial feature anomalies, including microcephaly. Many more children are born with milder forms of FAS known as fetal alcohol effect (FAE), conditions that often go undetected. They include cardiac abnormalities, neonatal irritability and hypotonia, hyperactivity, genitourinary abnormalities and skeletal and muscular abnormalities, ocular problems, and hemangiomas.

CIGARETTE SMOKING

Children living within the drug culture are also susceptible to the toxic effects of cigarette smoke and secondary smoke within the environment. The fetal effects of maternal cigarette smoking—premature labor, low birth weight, and SIDS—are very similar to cocaine (Volpe, 1992a; Schoendorf & Kiely, 1992). The National Commission to Prevent Infant Mortality (1992) estimates that a 10% reduction in infant mortality and a 25% reduction in low-birth-weight babies would occur if women stopped smoking cigarettes during pregnancy.

A recent review of nine U.S. studies in *The Lancet* showed fathers who smoked cigarettes also produced smaller babies and babies with higher rates of perinatal mortality. Babies of nonsmoking mothers whose fathers smoked more than 10 cigarettes a day had a greater frequency of severe malformations, independent of parental age and social class (Davis, 1991). Children have also developed neurologic symptoms such as seizures following passive inhalation of vaporized crack (Schwartz, 1989).

INTERACTION BETWEEN LEGAL AND ILLEGAL DRUGS

The interaction of legal drugs with illegal street drugs and the combined effect on pregnancy complications and outcomes has not been adequately studied. It is possible that the reduction of the use of legal drugs during pregnancy would be sufficient to remove the illegal drugs' threat to the pregnancy and developing fetus even when illegal drug use continues (Robins & Mills, 1993).

PROGNOSIS OF DRUG-EXPOSED INFANTS

The presumption is that drug-exposed infants are more likely to have prolonged and chronic health problems and are perhaps more likely to require public assistance as a result of being permanently disabled in some way. This assumption, perpetuated by the media, has led the public to believe that these infants are throwaway kids. It is, however, largely unfounded. Most birth outcomes of substance-abusing mothers are unremarkable. One New York project involving 200 pregnant women reported no complications for two thirds of their deliveries, only 3% congenital anomalies, and five infant deaths (Suffett & Brotman, 1984).

Nevertheless, the long-term impact of drug exposure on a child's physical, mental, and social well-being are as yet unknown. We do, however, know that all children are not physically damaged as a result of maternal drug use. In fact, most effects of prenatal drug exposure are transient and responsive to treatment. A recent meta-analysis of follow-up studies on drug-exposed children found fewer statistically significant differences between children with and without in utero drug exposure later in life than there are at birth (Robins & Mills, 1993). Children have a tremendous capacity to recuperate and accommodate if they grow up in an organized, nurturing environment (Volpe, 1992b; Olegard, 1992; Werner, 1989).

IMPACT OF THE ENVIRONMENT

In general, follow-up studies show that most of the differences observed at birth seem to disappear over time. Many of the behaviors attributed to drug-exposed children are extremely common, especially in small or premature babies. A few adverse outcomes can be attributed to less effective mothering or to an unstable home environment rather than to a woman's use of drugs during pregnancy. The high rate of placement of these children away from the mother also suggests early childhood trauma and separation (Robins & Mills, 1993). It should be noted, however, that some disabling effects of parental substance abuse are the consequence of broader social problems, such as destitution, homelessness, and hunger. Many addicted mothers live with poverty, violence, abuse, neglect, prostitution, mental illness, and psychological and physical abandonment. Physical maltreatment by a chemically involved mother and/or father also has detrimental effects.

Response to any one prenatal or postnatal environmental insult varies. However, cumulative multiple traumas—such as drugs, poor nutrition, inadequate prenatal care, violence, and neglect—are predictive of poorer outcomes (Zuckerman, 1991; Kronstadt, 1991; Werner, 1989). In Werner's study, prenatal complications were consistently related to impairment of physical or psychological development *only* when they were combined with negative environmental factors such as family discord, parental mental illness, chronic poverty, or other consistently poor rearing conditions (Werner, 1989).

WHAT IS NEEDED?

To address the problem of drug-exposed children two broad service needs must be met. The first is drug abuse treatment programs for biological parents of these children. The second is health and developmental services for the children. Presently, neither of these needs is being met.

WHAT ARE THE BARRIERS TO THESE GOALS?

National antidrug efforts are fragmented and lack an overall strategy to combat the problem of perinatal addiction. The complexity and lack of coordinated government funding for health services hinder families from obtaining the comprehensive care they need. While the United States conducts some of the most sophisticated drug research in the world, that research does not always translate into service delivery systems. Indeed, pregnant addicted women and their children have historically been a vulnerable population residing mostly in underserved areas (Aday, 1993). Some policymakers and service providers in the United States have made attempts to respond to the problem of perinatal addiction and drug-exposed children, but little progress has been made in reaching consensus on a national policy.

Prosecution versus Treatment

Eight states now require drug exposure found in newborns to be reported as child abuse, a measure that can lead to termination of parental rights. At least 167 women in 24 states have been prosecuted for exposing a newborn child to drugs. Of the 21 cases that have been appealed, all have been dismissed or overturned (Hansen, 1992).

According to an Intergovernmental Health Policy Project (IHPP) report, 72 bills relating to substance abuse and maternal and child health issues were introduced in 23 states during 1993 (Wilford & Morgan, 1993). Specific substance abuse areas addressed included FAS; mandating health professionals, educators, and community outreach workers to counsel pregnant women about the dangers of using drugs, alcohol, and tobacco; screening newborns and pregnant women for the presence of substances; point-of-purchase warning sign requirements; and the formation of committees to study the extent of the problem of addicted women and their babies and how best to help them.

Although the National Association for Perinatal Addictions Research and Education interprets these actions as a trend away from legislation that is punitive and toward laws that encourage treatment and appropriate intervention (Hansen, 1992), efforts to punish these mothers persist. In 1993, two bills were introduced to the Indiana legislature that would allow addicted pregnant women to be charged with a second-degree felony or subjected to civil commitment. In a state that has only 16 treatment beds for addicted pregnant women, one must ask where these women would be committed. They could be sent to prison.

Punitive approaches have contributed to a tripling of the female prison population since 1980. The most common reason for women being in state prisons is drug convictions (about one third of the female convicts as compared to one fifth of the males). Women are also more likely to be under the influence of drugs when they commit crimes of violence or crimes against property.

Two thirds of the women in prison have children under the age of 18 (Krauss, 1994), and punishment often compounds the problems of these families. Laws that punish addicted mothers are designed to deter drug use, but they also dissuade addicted women from seeking essential prenatal care for fear of losing custody of their children. In prison, addicted pregnant women receive limited health care that often fails to address their needs for prenatal care and drug treatment. The vast majority of addicted inmates lack access to drug treatment programs, and studies show women continue to obtain drugs behind bars. In Washington, DC, 10 Department of Corrections officers were recently charged with taking bribes (often consisting of sexual activity) from inmates at the city jail in return for providing them with cocaine (*The Washington Post*, 1994). Again, the wisdom of incarcerating pregnant and drug-addicted women is questionable.

To date, no national standards have been set in place for addressing the medical and drug treatment needs of female offenders, pregnant or otherwise, with or without HIV infection. Nor has there been any federal program targeting drug abuse research or treatment for women inmates, although there have been some initiatives in this direction. For example, the women's prison facility at Rikers Island, NY, has programs to address the comprehensive needs of their inmates. Of the 14,000 women in this facility, 25% have syphilis, 25% have mental illness, 75% are drug abusers, 27% are HIV-positive, and 10% are pregnant. To address these health problems, the Rikers Health Service has expanded to provide health education and prevention programs as well as treatment. Although Rikers tries to connect the women with community services when they are discharged, the referral often fails because inmates lose eligibility for Medicaid benefits while in prison and have no way to pay for continued treatment (Ragghianti, 1994).

CHILDREN OF ADDICTED MOTHERS

The children in families with addicted parents have been seriously affected by the policies that punish mothers:

- Today, half a million children live in foster homes—more than at any time in history. Neglect and caretaker absence account for the increase in these placements; 8 out of 10 involve parental drug problems (USGAO, 1994).
- Six out of ten foster care children have serious health problems—mostly due to prenatal drug exposure. They include drug withdrawal; FAS; low birth weight; cardiac defects; AIDS; behavioral problems; and the psychological effects of physical, sexual, and emotional abuse (USGAO, 1994).
- Children placed in foster care experience serious disruptions in relationships and home environments. Children cared for in kinship arrangements with a grandmother or great-grandmother may also experience a strained and chaotic home environment (Howard, Beckwith, Rodning, & Kropenske, 1989).

STRATEGIES TO AMELIORATE ADVERSE EFFECTS OF PRENATAL DRUG USE

The lack of appropriate treatment for these families is particularly troublesome because research makes a compelling case for the resilience of drug-exposed children. Many such children have an excellent chance at full and productive lives if they and their mothers receive treatment. Research shows drug treatment for a pregnant woman will benefit the child by decreasing or eliminating the risk of drug exposure before birth and by improving the mother's ability to care for the child after birth.

According to the National Institute of Child Health and Human Development report to Congress, the only scientific information now available concerning the prevention of adverse drug effect during pregnancy is the repeated observation that more prenatal care is associated with fewer adverse pregnancy and birth outcomes. In addition, the practice of transferring heroin users to methadone to improve fetal growth and outcome is the subject of debate (Robins & Mills, 1993).

The advantage of prenatal care may be explained by the differences between women who avail themselves of prenatal care and those who do not. Alternatively, it may be that prenatal care provides access to services that the woman needs to reduce or cease legal and illegal drug use, or to obtain treatment for infections, such as hepatitis or sexually transmitted diseases. Pregnancy offers a critical opportunity when addicted women may be more receptive to treatment that will benefit their babies. With rare exception, mothers want to do what is best for their child.

TREATING BIOMEDICAL PROBLEMS ASSOCIATED WITH DRUG USE

Although cocaine does not produce a classic withdrawal syndrome, a pronounced craving for the substance does occur upon cessation. The crash or postintoxication period gradually progresses from intense craving to symptoms of clinical depression. This period often produces increased risk for suicide. After the depressive phase of the crash, craving may return and be present for weeks or months (Mitchell, 1993).

To withdraw a pregnant woman dependent on cocaine, the Office of Treatment Improvement has drafted possible guidelines for pharmacological intervention (Mitchell, 1993). There are basically four options: (1) no medication; (2) anxiolytics, such as low doses of diazepam or chloridiaze, four times a day for 5 or 6 days; (3) antidepressants, such as doxepin or desipramine, twice a day for 5 days; or (4) barbiturates every 4 to 6 hours for 4 days. Table 7–2 delineates the treatment options for cocaine withdrawal.

The use of psychotropics to withdraw a pregnant mother must be considered on a case-by-case basis, taking into consideration their effects on the mother and fetus, particularly with respect to the potential for teratogenic effects and possible interactions with other drugs, such as methadone.

Behavioral management techniques should be used to minimize the need for medication whenever possible. They include (1) quiet reassurance in a peaceful environment; (2) accepting attitude and avoidance of critical attitudes; (3) friends and relatives to provide support throughout the withdrawal period; (4) accurate drug history to predict possible withdrawal complications; (5) monitoring of vital signs and symptoms of withdrawal; and (6) opportunities for exercise.

Although it is clear that cessation of the use of cocaine during pregnancy is best, the timing of withdrawal is important to the well-being of the mother and her child. Most experts believe withdrawal treatment in the second trimester is the most desirable, since the fetus can be monitored more effectively at that time. Although withdrawal treatment in the first or third trimester has been reported to cause the fetus to abort, motivated women have been withdrawn throughout pregnancy without complications (Robins & Mills, 1993).

TABLE 7–2. TREATMENT OPTIONS FOR WITHDRAWAL FROM COCAINE

No medications	Pregnant patients who are withdrawing from cocaine should not be medicated except in cases of extreme agitation and by an individual order of the health care provider.
Anxiolytics	If medication is needed, low doses of diazepam (Valium) or chlordiazepoxide (Librium) (25 mg by mouth, 4 times a day, x 6 doses) may be used.
Antidepressants	A typical withdrawal guideline for cocaine addicts uses doxepin (Sinequan) or desipramine (Norpramin). For example: Days 1–5: Doxepin 25 mg by mouth 2 times a day. No drug therapy is usually indicated after the first 5 days.
Barbiturates	Days 1–2: Phenobarbital 30–60 mg every 4 hours as needed. Days 3–4: Phenobarbital 30–60 mg every 6 hours as needed.
Bromocriptine	This drug, used to treat menstrual abnormalities and infertility in women, has been shown to provide striking and consistent relief from cocaine craving among inpatients. However, use of this drug in pregnancy is not recommended because of the lack of efficacy and unknown effects on the fetus.

Cocaine Intoxication

The pharmacological understanding of cocaine guides the treatment for intoxication and chronic abuse. The actions of neurotransmitters, for example, dopamine and norepinephrine, are directly affected by stimulant drugs. The immediate intoxication and subsequent potential for psychotic or depressive responses can, in part, be explained by a dysregulation of these neurotransmitters in the brain. This understanding provides the underlying rationale for several pharmacological treatments.

Antipsychotics, such as haloperidol (Haldol) and chlorpromazine (Thorazine), block dopamine receptors in the brain and therefore treat acute, stimulant-induced psychosis. Marked hypotension, however, can be an undesirable side effect of such drugs. Bromocriptine (Parlodel), a dopamine agonist, has also shown promise as a means of decreasing long-term cocaine craving. Other drugs that have been useful are desipramine (Norpramin), amantadine (Symmetrel), and carbamazepine (Tegretol). Unfortunately, however, these agents must be taken for at least 2 weeks to produce an effect. Therefore, the potential for relapse and need for behavioral intervention are great during this period. Acupuncture, an intervention that can be provided by a specially trained nurse, has also been useful for the amelioration of craving and other symptoms associated with cocaine use. Acupuncture is also safe as an adjunctive treatment for pregnant women.

Alcohol Detoxification

Early symptoms of alcohol withdrawal usually appear 6 to 48 hours after cessation of alcohol intake but can occur up to 10 days after the last drink. Mild symptoms include restlessness, irritability, anorexia, nausea, vomiting, sweating, tremor, tachycardia, hypertension, insomnia, nightmares, impaired concentration, impaired memory, and elevated vital signs. More severe symptoms include increased tremulousness, agitation, and sweating; delirium, confusion, disorientation, and impaired memory and judgment; auditory, visual, or tactile hallucinations; delusions with paranoia; and grand mal seizures, which occur within the first 24 hours of withdrawal.

Drugs used to withdraw a pregnant mother include chlordiazepoxide, phenobarbital, and diazepam. Typical withdrawal schedules for each of these are:

- Chlordiazepoxide—25 to 50 mg four times a day for the first 2 days, decreasing gradually to 10 mg four times a day for days 8 through 10;
- Phenobarbital—15 to 60 mg by mouth every 4 to 6 hours as needed for the first 2 days, decreasing gradually to 15 mg by the fourth day;
- Diazepam—10 mg four times a day; or 10 mg every 2 hours as needed for withdrawal symptoms, with a maximum of 150 mg for 24 hours, then decreasing gradually at a rate of 20% to 25% over approximately 5 days (loading dose protocol with diazepam is accomplished with doses given according to withdrawal symptomatology; when withdrawal symptoms are stabilized, the long half-life of diazepam alleviates the need for further medication in most cases) (Mitchell, 1993).

Opiate Withdrawal

Detoxification of pregnant, opiate-dependent women is not recommended by U.S. guidelines. Methadone maintenance is, however, thought to prevent HIV infection if relapse should occur. High-dose methadone ranges between 50 and 150 mg per day. Low-dose methadone ranges between 20 and 25 mg per day. If detoxification is desired, it is recommended that methadone be decreased by 2 to 2.5 mg every

7 to 10 days and that a nonstress test or biophysical profile be done when feasible and indicated (Mitchell, 1993).

Pain during Labor and Delivery

Substance-abusing women often confuse the early signs of labor with signs of withdrawal and medicate themselves with their drug of choice. Therefore, it is important to ascertain an accurate recent drug history so that possible drug interactions during labor and delivery can be avoided. If self-medication has not occurred, analgesia and anesthesia administration during labor may include the same range of options available to all patients, with the following considerations: (1) regional anesthesia may be the drug of choice; (2) a higher dose of short-acting intramuscular narcotics may be required to compensate for tolerance to the drug; and (3) methadone does not provide anesthesia (Mitchell, 1993).

Comorbid Psychiatric Problems

Although psychopharmacological treatment is generally contraindicated during pregnancy, it can be safely used to treat craving, depression, and anxiety after the baby is born. Many providers in the substance abuse treatment community, including members of the self-help community, object to the use of pharmacological treatment to assist in recovery. This conflict is reflective of the lack of coordination between the substance abuse treatment system and the mental health treatment system. Table 7–3 displays the nursing interventions appropriate for women with comorbid psychiatric disorders.

Treating Behavioral Problems Associated with Drug Use

Although crack babies have been erroneously described in the media as hopelessly addicted and suffering from withdrawal, experts believe it is inaccurate to use these terms (Zuckerman, 1991). The neurobehavioral functioning of the prenatally cocaine-exposed infant is not completely understood because research findings are inconsistent.

Cocaine-exposed infants can be poorly responsive and sleepy, or they can be irritable and hypersensitive to stimuli. However, it is not known whether these behaviors are due to a direct effect of cocaine, to changes in the brain's neurotransmitters, or to withdrawal. Nevertheless, these behaviors make the mother-child interaction problematic.

Parent education can begin as soon as possible after the birth to promote effective caregiving and to prevent compounding the problems of the already at-risk infant. It is important for nurses to point out these infants' strengths as well as their weaknesses. Mothers or caregivers can be taught to help the infants relax by avoiding excessive handling and by protecting them from bright lights and noise.

In addition, nurses can design interventions to promote the attachment relationship, establish interactive reciprocity, and develop a communicative dialogue. After the infant is stable at home, care continues through the high-risk follow-up clinic, parent support groups, community liaison, and case management.

The Preschool and School-age Child

Labeling a 3- or 4-year-old child drug-exposed is the most detrimental thing a nurse can do. Even if the child was prenatally exposed to drugs, the current physi-

TABLE 7–3. INTERVENTIONS FOR ADDICTED PREGNANT WOMEN

NURSING INTERVENTION	RATIONALE
Distinguish between drug-induced psychiatric symptoms and a major mental disorder.	Symptoms—such as anxiety, agitation, and paranoia—can be manifestations of a state of drug intoxication or of withdrawal.
Establish any previous history of psychiatric illness before developing the medical withdrawal treatment plan.	Confirmed mental illness may necessitate the continuation of medications such as antidepressants or antipsychotics that have been previously effective in treating the underlying disorder.
Set up consultation to involve psychiatrists where appropriate.	Establish diagnoses and develop treatment plan.
Continue prescribed medications and provide appropriate follow-up for patients who enter alcohol and other drug treatment programs with well-documented, diagnosed psychiatric illnesses that require psychopharmacologic medication.	Comorbid psychiatric disorders can precipitate relapse.
Consider issues of deep trauma from childhood, such as incest, sexual abuse, and family violence.	Treatment plans should include adjunctive therapy specific to the individual.
Use well-validated assessment scales in the diagnosis and follow-up of individual patients.	This will provide a data base to help address the needs of the population.
Individualize medical withdrawal plan for each patient.	Carefully review standard guidelines for withdrawal and amend them if there are significant psychiatric problems to be treated.

cal or emotional problems may be due to other causes. It is more effective to focus on behaviors that signal risk for problems and school failure. Indications of motor and neurological problems include tremulousness, tremors when reaching, increased startling, poor quality of visual following, blanking out, staring spells, bizarre eye movement, and clumsiness in fine motor dexterity. Affective and behavioral development problems are signaled by lability of emotion, rapid shift from apathy to aggressiveness, irritability, hypersensitivity, explosive and impulsive behaviors, depressed affect, decreased laughter, difficulty with transitions and changes, difficulty in comforting self and being comforted, increased testing of limits, and inability to self-regulate or modulate own behavior (easily excited, cannot calm down). Indications of social and attachment problems are decreased use of eye contact to initiate social interaction; decreased use of gestures to initiate social interaction; decreased/absent stranger and separation anxiety; indiscriminate attachment to new people; aggressiveness with peers; decreased compliance to verbal direction; decreased response to verbal praise; decreased use of adults for solace, comfort, and object attainment; and decreased use of adults to gain recognition for accomplishments.

Difficulties with problem solving, attention, and concentration are signaled by poor task orientation, increased distractibility to extraneous sounds and movements, inability to accommodate in problem-solving situations, impulsivity, and persistent use of ineffective problem-solving strategies. Evidence of language development problems is indicated by fewer spontaneous vocalizations from early infancy, delayed acquisition of words, prolonged infantile articulation at the preschool level, and difficulty in work finding at the preschool level. Other problems with play are signaled by decreased spontaneous play with increased aimless wandering, inability to organize play, tendency to be easily overstimulated, and difficulty with peer relationships in unsupervised play (Rodning, Beckwith, & Howard, 1992).

As primary health care becomes increasingly more available in school settings, psychiatric APNs can become an important resource for teachers who must deal with the behavior of drug-exposed children. Because many of these children come from poorly organized environments that lack nurturance and structure, it is important to view the child's behaviors as a deficit in learning that requires special education, rather than as misconduct.

The traditional way to deal with children who appear to be disruptive is to isolate them from the group or give them time-out. The real danger of this practice is the negative self-image that it fosters within young children who have not learned to separate the deed from their own self-worth. Many of these children have experienced such inconsistent punishment that they do not know which behaviors are acceptable and which are not. Early childhood programs such as Head Start, however, are an excellent place to begin teaching organizational skills.

The following are needs of the drug-exposed child at home and in school: (1) an environment with equipment that can be removed to reduce stimuli or added to enrich the activity, when appropriate; (2) assistance in self-organization, facilitated by an orderly, child-appropriate environment; and (3) structure and clarification. In addition, successful programs that intervene with drug-exposed children and other vulnerable populations emphasize a strong relationship between program staff and each child and family. These programs provide a low adult-child ratio to promote the child's attachment and learning. They also establish a partnership with the mother or caregiver both to role model respect and nurturance in interactions with the child and to provide support for the family (Delapena, 1992).

FAMILY PRESERVATION

Like so many interventions designed for intact, middle-class families, traditional family therapy does not lend itself to the needs of addicted mothers and their children. Likewise common drug treatment modalities are generally not appropriate. Table 7–4 delineates the usual treatment approaches. In contrast to these, a more practical approach is the family preservation model. The essential features of the family preservation model are: (1) 24-hour, 7-day-a-week availability for families; (2) small caseloads, usually not more than two families; (3) services provided in the home; (4) intervention that focuses on family needs and strengths; (5) short-term intensive services; and (6) referral to support services and additional counseling.

From a policy perspective, family preservation interventions are timely. Congress has recently enacted the Family Preservation and Family Support Act of 1993, which requires every state's highest court to examine why the family preservation tenets of the Adoption Assistance and Welfare Act of 1980 have not been fulfilled. The act directs courts to work with communities to develop strategies and programs that will serve families more comprehensively while relieving overburdened court systems. Interdisciplinary teams of nurses must help develop practice models to accomplish the federal goals at the community level as communities everywhere search for reform strategies to conform to the law.

TABLE 7–4. TRADITIONAL SUBSTANCE ABUSE TREATMENT MODALITIES

Residential therapeutic community	Best suited for individuals with major impairments, including problems with the criminal justice system. This provides long-term, intensive treatment for 18 to 24 months; structured to provide resocialization, milieu therapy, behavior modification, occupational training and responsibility, and community re-entry.
Methadone maintenance	Designed for heroin addicts; a legal, long-acting narcotic analgesic, methadone is administered in clinically adjusted oral doses to maintain a steady metabolic level that produces little if any behavioral intoxication. Infants who are born to a mother on methadone will experience withdrawal symptoms.
Chemical dependency (CD) treatment	Designed for alcoholics and now has been expanded to include other substances; sometimes referred to as 28-day, 12-step, or Minnesota model, the predominant therapeutic approach is privately financed inpatient and residential programs. CD is an intensive, highly structured inpatient modality utilizing an education-oriented program of lectures and group therapy. Recovery is patterned on step-work as defined by Alcoholic, Cocaine, or Narcotics Anonymous.
Brief intervention	Secondary prevention strategy, designed for use in community-based primary health care settings, to assist individuals to reduce or eliminate their use of alcohol; protocol may be adapted for other drugs.

HEALTH CARE DELIVERY TO FAMILIES WITH SUBSTANCE ABUSE

BARRIERS TO PRIMARY AND SECONDARY PREVENTION

While much is known about the prevention of the effects of perinatal drug use, many barriers exist to the provision of care for these families. The most effective way to prevent prenatal drug exposure is to help the mother to be drug free. As basic as this premise may seem, very few communities have adequate services to accomplish this end. A number of reasons help account for this situation, including fear of legal liability, inadequate insurance coverage, complexity of treatment needs, and community resistance to drug treatment programs.

FEAR OF LEGAL LIABILITY

A survey of 78 drug treatment programs in New York City found that 54% denied treatment to pregnant women (USGAO, 1990). One of the primary reasons cited for refusing treatment to pregnant women is the issue of legal liability.

INSURANCE COVERAGE

Medicaid will cover almost all hospital-based services. In the case of drug treatment, however, Medicaid usually only covers detoxification up to 5 days, which is not adequate for detoxification of most drugs during pregnancy. Follow-up care in a residential treatment program is also difficult. Furthermore, most substance abuse treatment services are provided within nonhospital (freestanding) residential treatment institutions that cannot be covered under Medicaid because of the institution for mental disease (IMD) exclusion (USGAO, 1991). The IMD exclusion is a provision of the Medicaid statute that prohibits coverage for anyone under 65 who is an inpatient in an institution for mental diseases. By finding a residential substance abuse treatment center to be an IMD, any person under the age of 65 residing in that program is excluded from Medicaid coverage, not just for substance abuse treatment but for any Medicaid-covered service, including prenatal care, regardless of where it is provided (USGAO, 1991). The IMD exclusion was not designed by the government to exclude pregnant women from receiving substance abuse treatment. It was designed to exclude the chronically mentally ill from utilizing Medicaid to pay for their psychiatric care because Medicare already covered these services. Nevertheless, the IMD exclusion prevents women from accessing substance abuse treatment even when they are motivated to do so.

COMPLEXITY OF TREATMENT NEEDS

Treatment needs for pregnant and parenting women are more complex than for men. Many pregnant and parenting women with substance abuse problems have multiple diagnoses and require treatment for hepatitis, tuberculosis, and sexually transmitted diseases, which are difficult to accommodate within existing treatment programs. Providing ancillary services such as dental care is also problematic because of the high risk of AIDS among drug populations. The delay in obtaining Medicaid benefits also interferes with the procurement of family planning interventions such as Norplant and tubal ligations.

Addressing the mental health needs of addicted pregnant women also requires specialized staff and services. Women using alcohol and other drugs during pregnancy often face the simultaneous stresses of poverty, addiction, and new motherhood without adequate support and social resources to assist them. Further, part of the problem leading to and resulting from substance abuse is that many of these women suffer from low self-esteem, anxiety, and depression. The lack of appropriate mental health treatment leads to relapse and treatment failure.

COMMUNITY RESISTANCE TO DRUG TREATMENT PROGRAMS

Establishing treatment centers for addicted pregnant women inevitably confronts the NIMBY (not in my backyard) phenomenon. While the need for substance abuse treatment centers is great, people needing treatment are often seen as undesirable and dangerous. Moreover, communities are often fearful that the presence of substance abuse treatment centers will encourage and foster increased drug use or present dangers for children and other adults. This fear contributes to the maintenance of substance abuse treatment programs as satellites of mainstream medical and mental health services and ultimately encourages a climate of mistrust and lack of coordination between substance abuse treatment and mental health services.

DEMONSTRATION PROJECTS

Since a war on drugs was launched in 1986, the federal government's policy has been based on the premise that illegal drug use is morally wrong and unacceptable, and users must be punished. However, within the past 5 years, federal and state governments have also begun to encourage substance abuse treatment programs for pregnant women through federally funded demonstration projects and federal block grant money. These grant programs, subject to congressional appropriations on a time-limited basis, usually award funds that are nonrenewable and extend for 3 to 5 years. Their intent is to provide limited support for innovation and research for projects that will eventually be assimilated into the service delivery system and financed through a stable source. However, with addicted mothers-to-be, the sources for continuation funding are very limited. While a fraction of the women who need treatment have been able to take advantage of these programs, the majority still go untreated.

The reason for the lack of resources resides in the way the government funds services. Federal funding for antidrug activities is controlled by 75 committees and subcommittees within Congress. None of the activities is coordinated. The Center for Health Policy Research (CHPR) reviewed more than 250 federal and private sources of funding and concluded that most funding is targeted toward either the condition of pregnancy or the infant, rather than the mother and her family. Only three federal programs are aimed at comprehensive care for drug-exposed children and their families (Haack, Budetti, & Darnell, 1993).

COMPREHENSIVE MODEL OF CARE FOR FAMILIES WITH AN ADDICTED MOTHER

It is useful to look at a comprehensive model of care to analyze how services can be improved and to identify the potential role of the psychiatric nurse in delivering those services. The model developed by the CHPR is based on information from key state and federal agencies concerned with substance abuse prevention and treatment. The sources included published research, conference proceedings, and special analyses. The contributing agencies included four agencies within the Department of Health and Human Services, the New York State Division of Substance Abuse Service, and the National Association for Perinatal Addiction Research and Education.

The CHPR comprehensive model is built on the assumption that infants have a sequence of developmental tasks to accomplish, each dependent on successful mastery of the earlier task, and that the mother has an indispensable role in this process. Drugs can disturb either side of this relationship by impairing the mother's ability to care for her child or by making the child irritable and difficult to care for. Prenatal drug abuse interferes with the normal regulation of the infant's prenatal physiologic processes, and postnatal drug abuse impairs the mother's ability to communicate with and respond to the infant.

Children need a nurturing mother and a safe environment in which to grow. Services that improve an addicted mother's chances to live a drug-free existence enhance the child's chances to grow and develop normally. Services that prevent or treat a child's developmental delays strengthen the potential for a healthy relationship between mother and child (USDHHS, 1992).

A typical addicted pregnant woman will be identified through child protective services if the existing children in the family are thought to be neglected or if the baby tests positive for drugs at the time of delivery. If the family is homeless or without food, they will need services to address hunger and safety before they will need substance abuse treatment. Once the mother is detoxified and treated for substance abuse, she will need skills to help her live a drug-free life. She may need language and literacy skills and communication assistance with providers or services. She may need education in parenting, life skills, and employment skills as well as support and information concerning how to negotiate the numerous public and private systems that can provide assistance. She may even need access to a telephone to call for appointments or to notify agencies of where the family is living.

When the community services were organized in a time sequence or according to when the family might be ready for services, categories emerged as building blocks. In reality, the services within the model build on each other, and the strength or weakness of one service has the ability to weaken the effectiveness of other services. Interagency linkages and coordination and case management were added to maximize the synergistic potential of the services. Transportation and child care are integrated throughout the model to improve access and compliance to treatment.

THEORETICAL FRAMEWORK

The guiding principles of Maslow's work (1954) were used as the theoretical framework for the model. Maslow's hierarchy is built on two fundamental premises. First, people's needs depend on what they have, and they are motivated only by needs not yet satisfied; and second, people's needs are arranged in a hierarchy of importance. Figure 7–1 demonstrates the application of Maslow's hierarchy of needs to the CHPR comprehensive model of care for drug-exposed infants and their families. As shown in Figure 7–1, there are five need categories: (1) physiological, (2) safety and security, (3) affection and social activity, (4) esteem and status, and (5) self-realization. Figure 7–2 displays the model components, arranged according to Maslow's

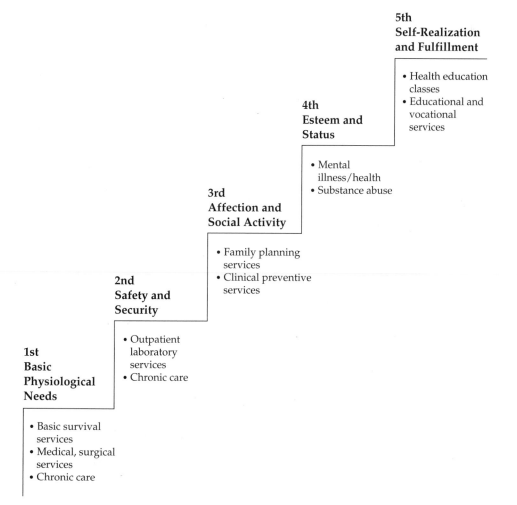

FIGURE 7–1. Maslow's hierarchy of needs applied to the comprehensive service delivery model.

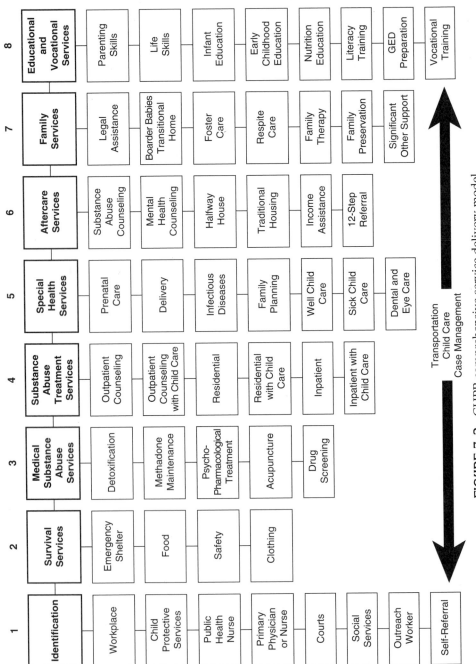

FIGURE 7-2. CHPR comprehensive service delivery model.

152

hierarchy of needs. Basic physiological needs begin at the left side of the page and progress to higher needs, such as esteem and self-fulfillment, on the right; the effectiveness of the services on the right side of the model are dependent on the strength of the services on the left. Furthermore, the critical components of transportation, case management, and child care are integrated throughout the service delivery model to enhance the ability of families with an addicted mother to make the transition from one stage to the next.

NEED FOR SPECIALIZED TRAINING

Most psychiatric nurses are ill-prepared to manage the complex needs of an addicted pregnant woman and her children. Until recently, medical and nursing school curricula were lacking in substance abuse content. For the most part, clinical training in substance abuse treatment is regarded as an unnecessary or optional component of nursing education.

In addition, the psychiatric treatment system and the substance abuse treatment system have different philosophies, clinical training programs, staffing patterns, and service delivery. Kalb and Propper (1976) have compared training in the substance abuse treatment system—built upon the ideology of self-help groups such as AA—to a craft model and training in the psychiatric treatment system to a scientific model. These approaches can be distinguished by differences in acquisition of knowledge, implementation of knowledge, and the nature of loyalty among its members. A craftsman gains knowledge through direct observation and experience under the tutelage of a master craftsman. Research and critical analysis of traditional practice is discouraged. Mutual agreement is the basis for loyalty among its members. On the other hand, the scientifically trained professional obtains knowledge through a mentorship relationship and the teaching of others. Independent thinking and critical analysis are encouraged. Scientific research provides the basis for practice.

There are also theoretical and practice differences between traditional prenatal, mental health, and substance abuse services that impede the ability of APNs to work collaboratively for the patient. Most psychiatric and other specialty nurses with expertise in substance abuse treatment obtain their skills through apprenticeship, inservice, and continuing education in substance abuse treatment programs. The work of reconciling the domains of conflict has been left to the individual nurse.

The complex needs of addicted pregnant women and their families require assistance from many agencies within the health care and social service delivery systems. Often nurses in the mental health treatment, substance abuse treatment, and obstetrical and pediatric systems of care lack skills in interdisciplinary and interagency referral and cooperation. Therefore, coordination of the many required services is rare. The result is deficient care for pregnant women with drug abuse problems.

MODELS OF NURSING CARE

Psychiatric nurses are uniquely qualified to supervise a family preservation team and case manage the complex medical and mental health needs of families with substance abuse problems. A prototype of care that is appropriate for the addicted woman and her child is the graduate training project, Transitional Care, at the University of Pennsylvania School of Nursing. Transitional Care has been used effectively to treat low-birth-weight babies, HIV-positive infants, and pregnant women with other high-risk conditions such as diabetes and hypertension (Brooten et al., 1986; Finkler, Brooten, & Brown, 1988). Skills in assessing the comprehensive needs of families and in teaching families to care for their illness are the key factors that contribute to the success of the model (Brooten et al., 1991; Cohen, Arnold, Brown, & Brooten, 1991).

Although the Transitional Care prototype was not designed for families with substance abuse problems, the problems of high-risk infants addressed by this model are similar to those of addicted pregnant women and their children. Indeed, the model has already been adapted to HIV-positive infants, who are often drug-exposed; perinatal transmission accounts for 84% of reported childhood AIDS cases, and prenatal exposure to HIV infection is strongly linked to maternal drug use. In these cases, the source of the mother's HIV infection was almost always her intravenous drug use or that of a sexual partner (Centers for Disease Control, 1993).

The transitional care for HIV-positive infants was developed by a University of Pennsylvania team of nurse researchers and clinicians who work in collaboration with an interdisciplinary team of the Special Immunology Clinic at The Children's Hospital of Philadelphia. The structure of the clinical interventions parallels the family preservation model.

The Transitional Care protocol is compatible with the CHPR Comprehensive Model of Care in that the APN is trained to assess a wide range of health and social problems of the HIV-positive child and family and to case manage and facilitate the amelioration of those problems through education and referral to professional and community agencies and services. The APN assists the family by teaching members how to care for their own needs when possible and how to access appropriate agencies when necessary.

The Transitional Care APN functions as a primary care professional who assists the child and family through a five-step process:

1. Assessment of the physical and psychological problems of the mother and child, including developmental screening of the child (Table 7–5 lists the instruments that can assist the nurse in this process);
2. Diagnosis of the problems;
3. Identification of a plan of care for each problem, including a prioritization of which problems should be addressed immediately and which should be addressed at a later time;
4. Designation of a therapeutic intervention appropriate for each problem, to be delivered directly by the APN or indirectly by referral to another professional or agency;
5. Evaluation of the effectiveness of the interventions, including an appraisal of the child's or family's ability to follow through on referrals and to access the needed services.

The five steps of the nursing process are repeated for each level of services in the CHPR model of comprehensive care and are followed sequentially by the nurse practitioner in treating the affected family. For example, the family may suffer from poor nutrition due to lack of money and knowledge about diet. The nurse practitioner would first address this survival need by assisting the family in obtaining an emergency grant to pay for food. Assistance with the application for food stamps and WIC would follow.

At the same time, the nurse will assess the child for symptoms associated with HIV such as diarrhea and other gastrointestinal disturbances, as well as for symp-

TABLE 7–5. NURSING ASSESSMENT TOOLS

Addiction Severity Index	Clinical research instrument to assess seven problem areas: medical condition, employment, drug use, alcohol use, illegal activity, family relations, and psychiatric condition. The tool has been adapted for addicted pregnant women through the NIDA Perinatal 20 Program (McClellan et al., 1985)
SCL-90-R	Self-report measure of psychological symptom patterns; appropriate for use with addicted pregnant women (Derogatis, Rickels, & Rock, 1976)
Brazelton Neonatal Behavioral Assessment Scale	Assessment of reflexes and behaviors of the newborn; has been adapted for use with drug-exposed infants (Eisen et al., 1991)
Moos Family Environment Scale (FES)	Measurement of cohesion, expressiveness, conflict, independence, achievement orientation, intellectual-cultural orientation, active-recreational orientation, moral-religious emphasis, organization, and control within the family (Moos & Moos, 1984)
Clinical Withdrawal Assessment for Alcohol (CIWA)	Rating scale for the assessment of the severity of withdrawal; has been adapted for cocaine, narcotic, and alcohol withdrawal; available from the Addiction Research Foundation, Toronto, Canada (Devenyi & Saunders, 1986)
Drug screening	Testing of urine, hair, and meconium provides information about the types of drugs that have been used and the subsequent potential for withdrawal symptoms. Drugs can be detected in urine over varying amounts of time, ranging from 12 hours for alcohol to 30 days for barbiturates and marijuana. Radioimmunoassay of maternal and infant hair and infant meconium are also used to screen for perinatal drug use.

toms associated with drug exposure, such as central nervous system hypersensitivity, tremors, high-pitched cry, hyperactive moro reflex, increased muscle tone, sleep disturbance, and seizure activity. If the child is severely dehydrated or running a high fever, the child may be referred to the Special Immunology Clinic at the University Hospital. If not, the nurse will teach the mother how to control the diarrhea symptoms through diet. Concurrently, the nurse will assess the mother's ability to understand the instructions and the willingness to provide the diet. Good nutrition is critical to the maintenance of the compromised immune system of the HIV-positive child.

If the child is having seizures or experiencing other serious signs of drug effects, the child will be transferred to an acute care setting. If not, the nurse will teach the mother comforting techniques such as swaddling, vertically rocking the child, and protecting the child from bright lights and noise. The mother will also be encouraged to soothe the child with frequent warm baths and gentle handling. If the mother is under the influence of mood-altering drugs, the APN will assess the physiologic need for detoxification and substance abuse treatment.

Although the Transitional Care program at the University of Pennsylvania has not yet developed a protocol that allows the pediatric nurse practitioner to collaborate with a psychiatric APN to address the psychiatric needs of the mother, such a protocol would be ideal. Addicted women require an extended period of support and counseling because their addiction is often complicated by other comorbid problems. In addition to a substance abuse disorder, many suffer from posttraumatic stress that is related to physical and sexual abuse. They also suffer from low self-esteem and poor interpersonal relationships.

Pediatric and Psychiatric Advanced Nursing Practice Team

If the nurse successfully links the mother with a community substance abuse treatment program, the psychiatric APN can continue to work with the treatment staff to establish a comprehensive plan of care during treatment and after discharge. For instance, a mother's agitation and oppositional or impulsive behavior can be manifestations of cognitive impairments, such as attention deficit disorder, limited intelligence, mild retardation, or psychotic illness. Patients with these behaviors can appear to have difficulty comprehending or complying with treatment expectations. Psychiatric nurses can assess for cognitive problems and recommend appropriate educational programs. Awareness of these deficits can help the substance abuse staff manage these problems and adapt treatment methods to minimize or avoid unnecessary confrontations.

The economic status and eligibility for Medicaid will always be a concern to APNs who care for these families. For instance, the mother may have difficulty obtaining work because of literacy problems. The nursing team can help the mother improve not only her self-esteem but also her chances of securing a job both by discussing the feelings of shame and working with the substance abuse treatment staff to include literacy training in the mother's aftercare program.

Factors such as the mother's own upbringing and the chaotic environment of the drug culture may contribute to her inappropriate response to her children. The nurse may role model good parenting by playing with the mother and child. The nurse may also teach the mother how to be consistent in handling the inevitable frustrations that arise with parenthood.

As shown in Figure 7–3, the University of Pennsylvania nurse practitioner directly facilitates access to treatment for HIV-related problems as well as to the limited number of substance abuse services in the Philadelphia area. The nurse practitioner helps the family to combat additional problems by linking them with other professionals and agencies. Interventions are aimed not only at the HIV-affected child but also at other members of the family. The Transitional Care model emphasizes the importance of addressing the health of the entire family as a means of improving the environment in which the infant grows.

Rather than taking care of the family's needs, the APN team works together to empower the family to take care of their own needs wherever the infant and family are, across a continuum of situations and settings—the home, community, outpatient clinic, or hospital. Rather than provide expensive direct care that cannot be sustained over a long period, the APN team helps the family by teaching them how to access appropriate health and social services and by instructing them to carry out certain procedures to care for themselves and other members of the families. Direct care is provided, of course, in emergency situations.

The missing piece of the University of Pennsylvania model is long-term mental health counseling to treat posttraumatic stress, clinical depression, and anxiety. It also lacks psychopharmacological treatment and monitoring. Clearly, these services could be provided by a psychiatric APN if barriers were removed. Figure 7–4 depicts the services provided by the psychiatric APN.

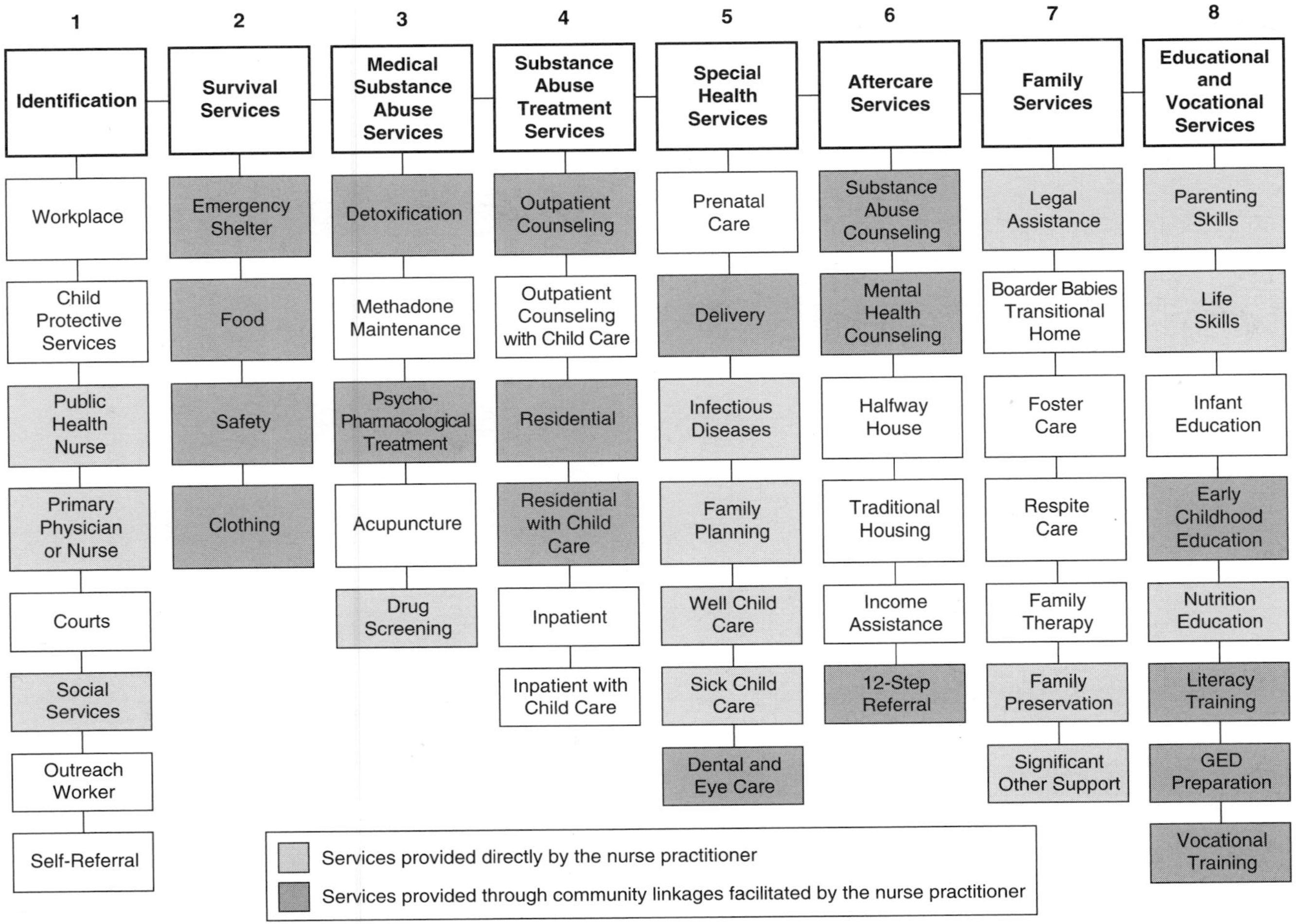
1
Identification
Workplace
Child Protective Services
Public Health Nurse
Primary Physician or Nurse
Courts
Social Services
Outreach Worker
Self-Referral
2
Survival Services
Emergency Shelter
Food
Safety
Clothing
3
Medical Substance Abuse Services
Detoxification
Methadone Maintenance
Psycho-Pharmacological Treatment
Acupuncture
Drug Screening
4
Substance Abuse Treatment Services
Outpatient Counseling
Outpatient Counseling with Child Care
Residential
Residential with Child Care
Inpatient
Inpatient with Child Care
5
Special Health Services
Prenatal Care
Delivery
Infectious Diseases
Family Planning
Well Child Care
Sick Child Care
Dental and Eye Care
6
Aftercare Services
Substance Abuse Counseling
Mental Health Counseling
Halfway House
Traditional Housing
Income Assistance
12-Step Referral
7
Family Services
Legal Assistance
Boarder Babies Transitional Home
Foster Care
Respite Care
Family Therapy
Family Preservation
Significant Other Support
8
Educational and Vocational Services
Parenting Skills
Life Skills
Infant Education
Early Childhood Education
Nutrition Education
Literacy Training
GED Preparation
Vocational Training
Services provided directly by the nurse practitioner
Services provided through community linkages facilitated by the nurse practitioner

FIGURE 7–3. University of Pennsylvania School of Nursing HIV transitional care project.

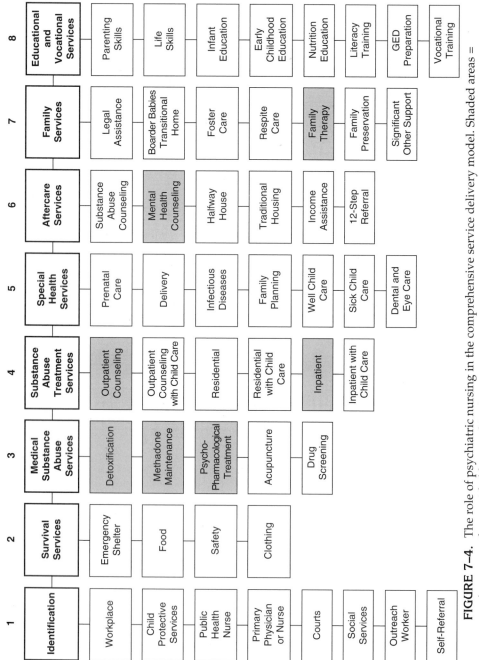

FIGURE 7–4. The role of psychiatric nursing in the comprehensive service delivery model. Shaded areas = services currently provided by psychiatric nurses.

NURSING EDUCATION
UNDERGRADUATE CURRICULUM

It is no longer reasonable to reserve course content on drug addiction to the senior year. Drug addiction is such a critical health care problem that course content should be integrated throughout the curriculum. The most important learning task for the undergraduate nursing student is to experience drug-addicted women and their children as sick people who deserve treatment. This can best be accomplished by clinical placements in health care systems that exemplify effective comprehensive treatment for addicted women and their children. Undergraduate substance abuse curriculum guides are available from the Ohio State University School of Nursing and the University of Connecticut School of Nursing.

The ability to utilize information about the interaction between the biochemical and behavioral aspects of drug addiction among pregnant women can be greatly hampered by punitive and moralistic attitudes on the part of the nurse. The urge to punish these women is often motivated by the belief that punishment of the mother will somehow protect the child. Drug treatment is also thought to be easy when, in fact, it usually is a long and painful process. The American Nurses Association and the American College of Obstetricians and Gynecologists are among the 13 professional groups who oppose criminal prosecution of addicted mothers. Students should be knowledgeable about these important policy positions.

In the junior year, pediatric and obstetric nursing courses should contain accurate information on the consequences of prenatal drug exposure and other environmental factors that can influence the health of a child. Pediatric clinical rotations should include time in Head Start programs that educate children who have been exposed to maternal drug abuse. It should also include experience with support groups or parenting classes for parents of high-risk babies. Medical-surgical courses should contain information on assessment for drug withdrawal and protocols to treat drug withdrawal.

In the senior year, psychiatric nursing courses should contain information on different modalities of treatment that are appropriate for addicted pregnant women. Community health courses should contain content on how to refer clients to appropriate services that meet the comprehensive needs of addicted pregnant women and their children. They should also provide some understanding of how state mandatory reporting laws impact nurses' ability to practice and provide services.

GRADUATE NURSING EDUCATION

It is no longer appropriate to teach students isolated pieces of the health delivery system. Students need to know how to work with several disciplines in multiple agencies. Graduate programs need to be exposed to models of interdisciplinary collaboration and interagency cooperation in the treatment of families with an addiction problem. Perhaps this is best accomplished by a faculty who can role model such behaviors.

Graduate programs need to provide clinical experiences that allow pediatric APN students to work with graduate psychiatric students to treat the same addicted mother and her child. This will provide opportunities to gain a greater understanding of how to work together.

As research on treatment progresses, it will become easier to identify critical characteristics of addicted individuals that can be matched to specific treatments.

Graduate programs in psychiatric nursing need to include didactic material on a broad range of treatment modalities, including both behavioral and pharmacological interventions. This process will enable psychiatric nurses to create with greater accuracy a comprehensive treatment plan individualized to the patient.

While family therapy is theoretically significant, students should be taught other family treatments that are more appropriate for indigent families. Clinical experiences should include the opportunity to work with a family preservation team.

Graduate programs should also teach about government policy and how it influences the provision of health care services. Students need to understand how policy affects funding and access to health care. They also need to understand that politicians control policy.

NURSING RESEARCH

CLINICAL AND BASIC RESEARCH

Because we know that prenatal exposure to drugs can create biological changes in the developing fetus, there needs to be more research on how to decrease the negative impact of that exposure. For example, Robins and Mills (1993) suggest studies on interventions that help women to stop or reduce their use of legal as well as illegal drugs. So much attention is focused on the illegal drugs, we have no way of knowing if the reduction of legal drugs can reduce the harm of the illegal substance. To study such interventions successfully, patients and investigators need to be protected from adverse legal consequences. Researchers should vigorously pursue federal confidentiality certificates (42 USC § 242a[a]). Because a history of depression may well interfere with stopping illegal drug use, just as it does with stopping smoking, we also need studies on the use of antidepressants in helping women in recovery (Robins & Mills, 1993).

Other areas to explore include the efficacy of nontraditional treatments such as acupuncture and brief intervention with addicted pregnant women. Such studies have been carried out with alcohol but never with illicit drugs. If such services could be effectively integrated with the service of a midwife, the prevention of prenatal drug exposure could be enhanced.

We also need to know more about the vulnerability of some children to drug exposure, for example, why some children are seriously affected, while others sustain no effect; and the unique biological characteristics of resilient children. Ideally, these studies should include pregnancy data on type and timing of in utero drug exposure, adequacy of prenatal care, and the presence of infections during the prenatal period; IQ neuropsychological testing of the mother and father; data on adequacy of parenting and child care; and exposure to drugs at home, in school, and in the neighborhood (Robins & Mills, 1993).

SERVICE RESEARCH

We need demonstration projects to study how pediatric and psychiatric APNs can work collaboratively with each other to improve access to comprehensive health care services for vulnerable populations such as drug-exposed children and their families. We also need studies that demonstrate the cost effectiveness of such a service delivery model. European models of interdisciplinary care may provide some guidance on developing models that are appropriate for APNs in managed care environments.

POLICY RESEARCH

Policy research is needed to determine how psychiatric nurses are prevented from providing services to drug-exposed children and their families because of regulatory or reimbursement policies. Studies that show how APNs have overcome those barriers in specific states can be used to demonstrate lessons learned.

CONCLUSION

As states, cities, and communities grapple with the immediate financial, medical, and social needs of substance-abusing women, policymakers have struggled with the problem by developing an array of programs for treatment as well as prevention. The prospect of health care reform provides an opportunity to create new models of care and new roles for the psychiatric APNs. Psychiatric nursing can contribute at every level to the amelioration of this complex problem. The traditions of the specialty and the history within the community mental health movement have provided the foundation on which to build.

It is clear that no one institution, agency, or discipline can provide a comprehensive model of care for addicted mothers and their children. The problem is bigger than the eradication of a drug within a pregnant woman or the jailing of an addicted pregnant woman. It reflects the weakest links of our social, medical, and mental health service delivery system.

The ability to address the complex problems of addicted mothers and their families requires contributions from many sources. It demands the coordination and collaboration of institutions as well as disciplines. It requires that we learn to work together. It necessitates an understanding of biological, social, and political sciences and knowledge about how groups and systems work. The challenge is to carve out a role for psychiatric nursing within the context of a reformed health care delivery system that allows APNs to work together to provide comprehensive care.

ACKNOWLEDGMENTS. I gratefully acknowledge Julie Darnell and Laura Barta for their assistance in the development of this manuscript.

REFERENCES

Aday, L. (1993). *At risk in America: The health and health care needs of vulnerable populations in the United States.* San Francisco: Jossey-Bass.

Blum, K. (1984). *Handbook of abusable drugs.* New York and London: Gardner.

Brooten, D., Gennaro, S., Knapp, H., Jovene, N., Brown, L., & York, R. (1991). Functions in early discharge of very low birthweight infants. *Clinical Nurse Specialist, 5*(4), 196–201.

Brooten, D., Kumar, S., Brown, L., Butts, P., Finkler, S., Bakewell-Sachs, S., Gibbons, A., & Delivoria-Papadoupoulos, M. (1986). A randomized clinical trial of early hospital discharge and home follow-up of very-low-birth-weight infants. *New England Journal of Medicine, 315,* 834–939.

Centers for Disease Control. (1993, April). US AIDS cases reported through March, 1993. *HIV/AIDS Surveillance Report, 5.*

Chasnoff, I. J., Landress, H. J., & Barrett, M. E. (1990). The prevalence of illicit-drug or alcohol use during pregnancy and discrepancies in mandatory reporting in Pinellas County, Florida. *The New England Journal of Medicine, 322,* 1202–1206.

Cohen, S., Arnold, L., Brown, L., & Brooten, D. (1991). Taxonomic classification of transitional follow-up care nursing interventions of low birthweight infants. *Clinical Nurse Specialist, 5*(1), 31–36.

Davis, D. L. (1991). Parental smoking and fetal health. *The Lancet, 337*(12), 123.

Delapena, L. B. (1992). Strategies for teaching young children at risk and/or prenatally exposed to drugs. Unpublished manuscript, Hillsborough County Public Schools, Tampa, Florida.

Devenyi, P., & Saunders, S. J. (1986). *Physicians' handbook.* Toronto, Canada: Addiction Research Foundation and the Ontario Medical Association.

Derogatis, L. R., Rickels, K., & Rock, A. F. (1976). The SCL-90 and the MMPI: A step in the validation of a new self-report scale. *British Journal of Psychiatry, 128,* 280–289.

Eisen, L. N., Field, T. M., Bandstra, E. S., Robert, J. P., Morrow, C., Larson, S. K., & Steele, B. M. (1991). Perinatal cocaine effects on neonatal stress behavior and performance on the Brazelton scale. *Pediatrics, 88*(3), 477–480.

Finkler, S., Brooten, D., & Brown, L. (1988). Utilization of inpatient services under shortened lengths of stay: A neonatal care example. *Inquiry, 25*(2), 271–280.

Frank, D., Zuckerman, B., Aboagye, K., Bauchmer, H., Cabrel, H., Fried, L., Hingfon, S., Kayne, H., Levinson, S., Parker, S., Reece, H., & Vinci, R. (1988). Cocaine use during pregnancy: Prevalence and correlates. *Pediatrics, 82,* 888–895.

Haack, M. R., Budetti, P. P., & Darnell, J. (1993). *Analysis of resources to AID drug-exposed children and their families.* Washington, DC: The George Washington University Center for Health Policy Research (ERIC Document Reproduction Service No. ED 359 734).

Hansen, M. (1992). Courts side with mom in drug case. *American Bar Association Journal, 78,* 18.

Howard, J., Beckwith, L., Rodning, C., & Kropenske, V. (1989). The development of young children of substance-abusing parents: Insights from seven years of intervention and research. *Zero to Three, 9,* 8–12.

Kalb, M., & Propper, M. S. (1976). The future of alcohology: Craft or science? *American Journal of Psychiatry, 133*(6), 641–645.

Kaplan, H. I., & Sadock, B. J. (1991). *Synopsis of psychiatry, behavioral sciences, clinical psychiatry* (6th ed.). Baltimore: Williams & Wilkins.

Khalsa, J. H. (1989). *Epidemiology of maternal drug abuse and its health consequences: Recent findings.* Rockville, MD: National Institute on Drug Abuse.

Kokotailo, P. K., Adger, H., Duggan, A. K., Repke, J., & Jaffe, A. (1992). Cigarette, alcohol, and other drug use by school-age, pregnant adolescents: Prevalence, detection, and associated risk factors. *Pediatrics, 90*(3), 328–334.

Krauss, C. (1994, July 3). Women doing crime. Women doing time. *The New York Times,* E3.

Kronstadt, D. (1991). Complex developmental issues of prenatal drug exposure. In C. S. Larson (Ed.), *The future of children: Drug-exposed infants* (pp. 36–49). Los Altos, CA: The David and Lucile Packard Foundation.

Kumpfer, P. (1991). Treatment programs for drug-abusing women. In C. S. Larson (Ed.), *The future of children: Drug-exposed infants* (Vol. 1, pp. 50–60). Los Altos, CA: The David and Lucile Packard Foundation.

Maslow, A. H. (1954). *Motivation and personality.* New York: Harper & Row.

McLellan, T. A., Luborsky, L., Cacciola, M. A., Griffith, J., Evans, F., Barr, H. L., & O'Brien, C. P. (1985). New data from the addiction severity index: Reliability and validity in three centers. *The Journal of Nervous and Mental Disease, 173*(7), 412–422.

Mitchell, J. L. (1993). *Treatment improvement protocols (TIPS): Pregnant, substance abusing women.* Rockville, MD: Office of Treatment Improvement.

Moos, R., & Moos, B. (1984). The process of recovery from alcoholism: Comparing functioning in families of alcoholic and matched control families. *Journal of Alcohol Studies, 45,* 111–118.

National Association of State Alcohol and Drug Abuse Directors. (1993). *Highlights of results from recent NASADAD survey on state and alcohol and drug agency use of FY 1989 federal and state funds.* Washington, DC: Author.

The National Commission to Prevent Infant Mortality. (1992). *Troubling trends persist: The shortchanging of America's next generation.* Washington, DC: Author.

National Institute on Drug Abuse (NIDA). (1991). *Household survey on drug abuse 1990.* Rockville, MD: Author.

National Institute on Drug Abuse. (1994). *Technical review: The Perinatal-20: A program of treatment research on drug-exposed women and their children.* West Palm Beach, FL: The Breakers.

Olegard, R. (1992). Effects of cocaine use on the fetus. *The New England Journal of Medicine, 327*(6), 399–407.

Racine, A., Joyce, T., & Anderson, R. (1993). The association between prenatal care and birth weight among women exposed to cocaine in New York City. *JAMA, 270,* 1581–1586.

Ragghianti, M. (1994, February 6). Save the innocent victims of prison. *The Washington Post Parade Magazine,* 14–15.

Robins, L. N., & Mills, J. L. (1993). Effects of in utero exposure to street drugs. *American Journal of Public Health, 83*(Suppl.), 3–32.

Rodning, C., Beckwith, L., & Howard, J. (1992) Spontaneous play and development of young children. In S. Quinton & S. A. Johnson (Eds.), *OSAP prevention monograph 11: Identifying the needs of drug-affected children: Public policy issues* (pp. 87–91). (DHHS No. (ADM) 92-1814). Washington, DC: U.S. Department of Health and Human Services.

Schoendorf, K. C., & Kiely, J. L. (1992). Relationship of Sudden Infant Death Syndrome to maternal smoking during and after pregnancy. *Pediatrics, 90*(6), 905–938.

Schwartz, R. H. (1989). Passive inhalation of marijuana, phencyclidine, and freebase cocaine ("crack") by infants. *American Journal of Diseases of Children, 143*(6), 644.

Suffet, F., & Brotman, R. A. (1984). A comprehensive care program for pregnant addicts: Obstetrical, neonatal and child development outcomes. *International Journal of Addictions, 19,* 199–219.

U.S. Department of Health and Human Services. (1990). *Healthy people 2000: National health promotion and disease prevention objectives.* Washington, DC: Author.

U.S. Department of Health and Human Services. (1992). OSAP monograph: Identifying the needs of drug-affected children: Public policy issues (DHHS No. (ADM) 92-1814). Washington, DC: U.S. Department of Health and Human Services.

U.S. General Accounting Office. (1990). *Drug-exposed infants: A generation at risk.* Report to the Chairman, Committee on Finance, U.S. Senate (GAO/HDR 90-138). Washington, DC: Author.

U.S. General Accounting Office. (1991). *Substance abuse treatment: Medicaid allows some services but generally limits coverage.* Report to Congressional requesters (GAO/HRD-91-92). Washington, DC: Author.

U.S. General Accounting Office. (1994). Foster care: Parental drug abuse has alarming impact on young children (Report 4/4/94, GAO/HEHS-94-89). Washington, DC: Author.

Volpe, J. J. (1992a). Mechanisms of disease: Effect of cocaine use on the fetus. *The New England Journal of Medicine, 327*(6), 399–407.

Volpe, J. J. (1992b). Alcohol and narcotics: Epidemiology and pregnancy risks. *International Journal of Technology Assessment in Health Care, 8*(Suppl. 1), 101–105.

The Washington Post (1994, April 4). Editorial: Will corrections escape again?, A20.

Weitzman, M., Gortmaker, S., & Sobol, A. (1992). Maternal smoking and behavior problems of children. *Pediatrics, 90*(3), 342–349.

Werner, E. E. (1989, April). Children of the garden island. *Scientific American, 260,* 106–111.

Wilford, B. B., & Morgan, J. (1993). *Substance abuse and maternal and child health. 1993 legislative activity. State ADM reports* (Intergovernmental Health Policy Project). Washington, DC: George Washington University.

Zuckerman, B. (1991). Drug-exposed infants: Understanding the medical risk. In C. S. Larson (Ed.), *The future of children: Drug-exposed infants* (Vol. 1, pp. 26–35). Los Altos, CA: The David and Lucile Packard Foundation.

CHAPTER

8

BULIMIA NERVOSA

Jane Howarth White, DNSc, RN, CS

ABSTRACT

The chapter reviews research studies that propose various theories, hypotheses, and/or critiques on the biological, psychological, sociocultural, and comorbidity factors that influence the development of bulimia nervosa. The literature suggests that none of these four main categories alone can explain the etiology and maintenance of this disorder; rather, a model based on the interrelationship of the risk factors should prove most useful in addressing key nursing issues. The chapter then explains what is necessary for a thorough assessment in which biological and behavioral components are considered, noting the complexity of the disorder and the need for multimodal treatment approaches. Various clinical instruments and nursing interventions are discussed, including the role of self-monitoring, cognitive-behavioral therapy, insight-oriented individual and family therapy, psychopharmacology, and medical follow-up, as well as the timing of various interventions. Also noted is the advocacy role of nurses, who are called to treat society as well as individuals. In keeping with the latter, the chapter suggests curricular changes in nursing education and a proposed research agenda.

Bulimia nervosa refers to a pattern of binge eating followed by compensatory behaviors to prevent weight gain, for example, laxative use, vomiting, or overexercising (American Psychiatric Association, 1994). Other clinical features of this disorder are food, weight, and shape preoccupation; fluctuations in weight; a morbid fear of becoming obese; and a feeling of lack of control over eating (Mitchell & Pyle, 1985). Palmer (1979) coined the term *dietary chaos syndrome* to describe these bulimic characteristics.

The prevalence of bulimia nervosa is difficult to determine because of the secrecy surrounding the bingeing and purging. Additionally, prevalence rates differ when self-report questionnaires, as opposed to clinical interviews, are used to determine prevalence. Prevalence has been estimated in self-report studies at 3% to 19%, while those investigations using an interview report a substantially lower prevalence of 1% to 3% (Fairburn & Beglin, 1990). One study on population-based estimates reported a weighted estimate of bulimia among American adolescents of 4% for girls and 0.2% for boys (Whitaker et al., 1990). Their study did not rely exclusively on self-report questionnaires.

Bulimic behavior has been estimated to occur 8 to 10 times more often in female than in male college students (Hsu, 1989). In studies that used questionnaire data alone, the mean prevalence of bulimia in males was 0.8%. In studies on men using an interview-based design, the mean prevalence was 0.2% (Carlatt & Carmargo, 1991). The age of onset for bulimia nervosa is usually midadolescence to the early twenties.

Bulimia nervosa is a relatively new psychiatric disorder. At present it is viewed as primarily a psychological illness with a strong cognitive-behavioral focus—that is, the behaviors of bingeing and purging are understood as a response to a particular way of thinking about one's weight, size, or shape. There is also some support for the idea that mood or emotional factors, such as fears, play a role in the development of the disorder and result in the behaviors of bingeing and purging.

At present there is only beginning support for biological theories of etiology. In fact, it is more appropriate to label this knowledge as hypothetical formulations. Such issues as the role of neurotransmitters and stringent dieting are, to date, two of the biological issues that are only in an infancy stage of research. Additionally, more so than any other disorder today, bulimia nervosa is viewed as a disorder whose development is clearly influenced by sociocultural factors—that is, the environment (in this case Western societies) is a significant etiological factor.

As with most psychiatric disorders, there has been a recent shift away from environment and toward biological research. However, this shift has been slow because first it is important to refine the conceptualization and definition of this relatively new disorder.

A great deal of the current literature supports a need for etiological theory, but to date only *factors* (biological, psychological, and sociocultural) that influence the development of bulimia nervosa have been identified. In addition, comorbidity is a significant issue in its development. A discussion of these factors will allow for a presentation of key nursing problems with strategies for assessment and intervention. Following this, the development of nursing curricula and an agenda for nursing research are proposed.

THE DEVELOPMENT OF BULIMIA NERVOSA
PSYCHOLOGICAL FACTORS
DEVELOPMENTAL THEORIES

Among the important issues facing clinicians and researchers today is the role that the psychological development of the female adolescent plays in the development of bulimia nervosa. Identity has been one factor cited as influencing eating, dieting, and bulimia nervosa. Identity for the female adolescent has both role and body-image aspects.

According to Lidz (1968), achieving a firm identity has become increasingly more difficult for many girls because they are caught up in a historical crisis—they are "brought up on the planned limitation of childbearing, women's increased education, the altered structure of the family, etc., that has been changing women's place in society and thereby the adolescent girl's image of herself and her future self" (p. 232).

In today's society and in the changing American family, the adolescent female may experience conflict over what the group's ideals are—that is, which ideals are to be incorporated. Food obsessions and a preoccupation with shape, body, and weight are ways to hesitate or to cease one's development because of this unresolved conflict. Taking on the lean, male-looking body, now increasingly muscular, might represent a hope to be able to move forward without choosing the new feminine image over mother (Chernin, 1985).

Another key psychological theory is the issue of separation-individuation. Ritvo (1984) claimed that for most bulimic women, the eating disturbance began with their leaving home for the first time. During puberty and adolescence the pre-oedipal struggle is revived in an intense way. Beattie (1988) described the relationship of separation-individuation to eating disorders as most typically beginning when the teenage girl experiences a physical or psychological separation from her mother, such as going away to camp or dating. The initial response is often to overeat and gain weight because this is a common way of dealing with loss or with depression of a transient nature. Overeating is followed by dieting as a way of overcoming passive-dependent feelings and restoring perfection. Then, the dieting itself can get out of hand and impulses to eat can break through, leading in turn to binge eating and purging.

Body image has long been considered a contributing factor to eating disorders. In fact, the overevaluation of one's size, shape, and weight has been considered a key criterion for an eating disorder (Garfinkel, 1992). Physical attractiveness, a part of body image, has been considered important to the female in this society (Brumberg, 1988), and female adolescence depends a great deal on self-evaluation of body image. Because the current ideal is a slender, toned physique, the developing adolescent is placed in conflict. Curves and breasts begin to develop and fat increases in the female at puberty just when she desires to seek out and conform to the "controlled tight body" image. At this time, adolescents need more than ever to be accepted, to be attractive, to be liked (all considered by them the same accomplishment). It is understandable how the female would be concerned with and unhappy about her new fat. Diet and exercise become ways to master this "self-fat."

COGNITIVE-BEHAVIORAL THEORIES

Important to both the development and maintenance of bulimia nervosa are cognitive and behavioral patterns. Numerous research and clinical articles have indicated that these patterns are extremely influential in this disorder (Agras, 1991; Cooper & Fairburn, 1987).

Behaviors such as binge eating and purging are maintained, according to behaviorists, through cues or stimuli. For example, visual cues often stimulate eating for most individuals. For the bulimic woman, a refrigerator filled with food or a cupboard containing easily eaten carbohydrates (crackers and cereal) are cues. Behaviors can often occur in chains, and several behaviors (one leading to the other) can set up an unwanted consequence (response) such as bingeing. Such a chain might be (1) entering the kitchen, (2) opening the refrigerator, (3) choosing a food, and so on. Cue elimination, breaking behavioral chains, and learning alternate responses to the cues (rather than eating) are interventions that are often *taught* and will be discussed later.

Few clinicians consider behaviors without cognitions in the maintenance of this disorder. Thought patterns perpetuating the behaviors of bingeing and purging are distortions about body size, shape, weight, and eating. The specific thought patterns often noted are (1) overgeneralization (the tendency to draw a general conclusion on the basis of a single incident); (2) personalization (the tendency to relate external events to oneself without any justification); (3) catastrophizing (the tendency to interpret an event as being a disaster without justification); (4) selective abstraction (the tendency to concentrate on a detail taken out of context and ignore other salient features of the situation); and (5) dichotomizing (the tendency to see the world, including foods, as black or white, good or bad) (Dritchel, Williams, & Cooper, 1991).

While a great deal of research on body size and shape distortion has concluded that these patterns are present in normal-weight women in this society, it must be emphasized that this factor must be clustered with other symptoms for a diagnosis

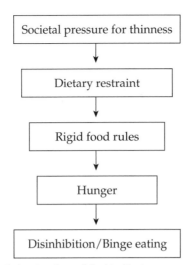

FIGURE 8–1. A cognitive-behavioral model of bulimia nervosa. (From Agras, W. S. [1991]. Nonpharmacologic treatments of bulimia nervosa. *The Journal of Clinical Psychiatry, 52*[Suppl. 10], 30. Copyright 1991 by Physicians Postgraduate Press, Inc. Reprinted by permission.)

of bulimia nervosa. In other words, how one reacts to these distortions is important in determining abnormal from normal distinctions.

Agras (1991) has related cognitions and behaviors in a simple figure in which rigid rules (dietary "dos" and don'ts") mediate thinking and behaving (see Fig. 8–1). One can see that biological status (hunger) is also part of this maintenance equation.

These psychological factors, interacting with both the sociocultural factors and with the family and biological predispositions, put a young female at risk for developing bulimia nervosa.

THE FAMILY

Many researchers have concluded that eating disorders are a symptom of a dysfunctional family and that certain characteristics contribute to the development of an eating disorder. Some research has focused on particular characteristics of the families of "bulimic females" that seem to put the daughter at risk. Achievement, success, control, and overprotectiveness have been themes in these studies.

Pole, Waller, Stewart, and Parkin-Feigenbaum (1988) studied overprotectiveness and parental caring of bulimic individuals. The women were compared to controls, and these researchers concluded that bulimics perceived their mothers as significantly less caring than the control subjects perceived theirs. This finding approached significance for fathers as well. While mothers were perceived as less caring, there was also a trend to view them as high in protection.

Other researchers have found achievement and success to be emphasized by mothers of bulimics when compared to mothers of controls (Sights & Richards, 1984). In a recent study, Steiger, Liquornik, Chapman, and Hussain (1991) noted family disturbance on self-report by bulimic women—in the form of poor communication, affective unresponsiveness, and general family functioning—when compared to normal subjects. In contrast to many other studies, these researchers found no differences between bulimic women who restrict and bulimic women who purge as ways to control weight.

In summary, the family of the bulimic woman presents a profile of dysfunction in the form of a focus on success and achievement, overprotectiveness on the part of the mother, poor communication, and a lack of affective responsiveness, often interpreted as noncaring.

Sociocultural Risk Factors

The role of environment in the development of bulimia nervosa is significant. Sociocultural factors are norms, standards, or values of a society or culture. Among the factors that put women at risk for bulimia nervosa are (1) the value placed on a thin and toned physique and search for perfectionism; (2) the expectations of certain occupations; and (3) the influence of the media on these values. Each of these factors will be presented. It should be noted that a great deal of literature exists on the feminist analysis that can be made of eating disorders.

The current preference in Western societies for a thin body has, for women, become associated with a preoccupation with weight and shape. The shift, historically, from a more rounded body preference to the Twiggy model of the 1970s is well-documented (Brumberg, 1988; Silverstein, Perdue, Peterson, Vogel, & Fantini, 1986). In a recent study, girls as young as nine preferred a body type that was thinner than the one they had, even though being overweight was not a characteristic of these young girls (Collins, 1991). Today, the emphasis on a toned body, as well as a thin one, has not changed the value of this ideal; rather, even more stringent criteria have been added for the ideal look. Exercising and dieting are used and overused to reach and maintain this ideal. Additionally, the pursuit of perfection is a sociocultural phenomenon today, and women are more at risk for eating disorders in a society that stresses perfection because, as a gender class, women are expected to be more concerned with their body image and appearance. Historically, their perfection has been defined in terms of the perfect body, shape, and weight. As a result of this societal pressure, perfecting the body may have symbolic meaning, such as control, power, and improving the state of the soul (White, 1991).

Without a doubt, certain careers promote personal appearance and weight standards that put young women at risk for developing abnormal eating and exercise patterns. Dancers, flight attendants, athletes, and fashion models are expected to have particular appearances (McKenna, 1989). It might be debated that certain women, who are preoccupied with weight and shape and are already bulimic, choose certain professions and life-styles to perpetuate the disorder, but no data are available to support this. What is known is that there is a greater incidence of eating pathology in those individuals when compared to individuals whose professions are unrelated to personal appearance; further, it appears that the pathology begins after the woman has entered the profession (Crago, Yates, Beutler, & Arizmendi, 1985).

A significant amount of research has been undertaken to demonstrate the relationship between media influence and eating disorders. Garner, Garfinkel, Schwartz, and Thompson (1980), after reviewing weight and height data for both *Playboy* magazine centerfolds and Miss America contestants between 1959 and 1978, concluded that there was a 10% decrease in weight over a 20-year period. Concomitantly, they discovered a sixfold increase in the number of diet articles in six popular women's magazines during the same 20-year period.

Recently, Wiseman, Gray, Mosimann, and Ahrens (1992) investigated body measurements of *Playboy* magazine centerfolds and Miss America contestants from 1979 to 1988 and concluded that body weight was 13% to 19% below expected weight for women in that age group. Additionally, when tabulating diet-for-weight-loss and exercise articles in six women's magazines for the years 1959 to 1988, these researchers found a significant increase in both types of articles during this period. These findings suggest that the overvaluation of thinness in the media continues, and this ideal is now sought through both dieting and exercise.

A discussion of the risk factors associated with bulimia nervosa would be lacking without mention of the feminist viewpoint. The literature abounds with this sociocultural, political perspective. Four important critiques have been developed by feminist theorists: (1) the effect of the diet and fashion industries on women; (2) the conflict between traditional and contemporary roles available for women today; (3) the sick role as a response to patriarchal power; and (4) the body as symbol representing oppression.

Orbach (1979), Bordo (1990), Chernin (1981, 1985), and Woodman (1980, 1982) have advanced the thesis that the changing role of women in the last half of this century has contributed to the development of eating disorders. Chernin, in particular, argues that the changing awareness of women in this society has divided itself into two divergent movements: one, a movement toward feminist power; the other, a retreat from it, supported by the fashion and diet industries, which fear that women's power will repel their products and hurt them financially.

A second hypothesis offered by these writers suggests that today's adolescent female is faced with social changes that converge with the usual anxieties confronted in the transition to adult womanhood. Today's young women face open-ended possibilities, unlike their mothers. In this conflict, young women of today are unsure what parts of tradition they want to keep or leave behind. Today's woman, it is claimed, wants it all; thus, seeking this Superwoman ideal becomes a striving for the perfect self and body (since self is often interpreted as physical self).

Third, feminist critiques have contributed to our understanding of eating disorders as a form of protest for women in this society. Some writers have noted that, historically, the sick role could be viewed as a means for women to sabotage their traditional roles. In particular, anorexia nervosa has been viewed as a disorder in which women are, at early adolescence, actually rejecting the female role (body) and regressing into childhood (Bruch, 1985).

Last, feminist writings on society and culture have viewed the female body as a symbol of women's attempts to equalize their position with respect to males. It has been frequently noted that in times of gender change in society, the consuming-woman theme proliferates in art and literature, and the dominant construction of the female body becomes more sylphlike (Bartky, 1988; Michie, 1987). MacKenzie (1985) also argues that gender issues in society are interpreted through the body. He contends that women may be more vulnerable to the importance of the size of the body because, traditionally, achievements accessible to them have been those concerned with controlling their size.

While feminism underscores the sociocultural factors that are important in the development of eating disorders, many hypotheses about the psychological, biological, and family risk factors also continue to be advanced.

BIOLOGICAL RISK FACTORS

Among the cited biological hypotheses in the development of bulimia nervosa are dieting; neurotransmitter disturbances, such as hyposerotonergic function; and issues related to genetic transmission. As research continues, numerous other factors are, of course, likely to surface as biological risk factors. However, for this disorder the three areas represented here are the most commonly discussed.

DIETING

Many studies have demonstrated that there are genetic and developmental determinants of adult obesity (Crisp, 1988). There is a substantial amount of evidence that obesity occurs in generations of families. Because obesity is linked to dieting, and dieting is linked to the development of eating disorders, a discussion of these relationships is important (Bruch, 1978; Boskind-White & White, 1983).

Normally, fat is accumulated in the body during infancy, prepubescence, and pregnancy. Thus, the risk of developing an eating disorder for those who are genetically predisposed to overweight may be greater especially at these times. The fact that eating disorders have their origins in puberty cannot be overlooked.

When the fat-to-lean ratio is determined, women are more fat than men. The prepubescent female, who may be heavier than her peers during childhood, is confronted with a society that prefers a slender, and now toned, body type. Dieting ensues and can be an important link in this relationship of obesity to the development of an eating disorder (Wooley & Wooley, 1982).

Dieting is a culturally accepted norm (Polivy & Herman, 1985). However, it is now well established that biologically, dieting can contribute to a subsequent weight gain rather than a loss because of the lowering of metabolic rate (Garrow, 1978; Steen, Oppliger, & Brownell, 1988; Wooley, Wooley, & Dryenforth, 1979). This may apply especially to women, who already have a lower metabolic rate than men (determined by lean-to-fat body composition). Yet women diet to control added fat and weight, a tendency that is particularly important during prepubescence. One study demonstrated that 80% of girls, compared to 10% of boys, reported being on a weight-loss diet (Hawkins, Turrell, & Jackson, 1983). Also, Polivy and Herman (1985) have reported that dieting can actually increase eating because it is associated with feelings of deprivation. Their research on *dietary restraint,* the process by which amounts or specific types of foods are restricted, is also important. Women tend to binge on the very foods that were restricted.

It is easy to conclude that dieting can relate biologically to eating disorders: With each restrictive diet, basal metabolic rate further decreases, and it becomes more and more difficult to lose fat; starving and/or bingeing and purging may then take over.

NEUROTRANSMITTER DISTURBANCES

Although specific neurotransmitter disturbances have been found in patients with bulimia nervosa, the cause of these disturbances is thus far not known. Serotonin and norepinephrine are among the neurotransmitter systems known to modulate feeding, mood, and neuroendocrine function, but the reason that mood, feeding, weight, and neuroendocrine function are linked is not well understood. It has been hypothesized, for instance, that such disturbances could be secondary to some state-related factor such as malnutrition (Kaye & Weltzin, 1991), since much of the hypothetical information regarding the role of neurotransmitters in bulimia nervosa is based on the long-recognized fact that disturbances of mood, appetite, weight regulation, and neuroendocrine function coexist in certain disorders. According to Kaye and Weltzin (1991), one hypothesis is "that these functions are linked because each of these systems is modulated by the same neurotransmitter(s)" (p. 22).

Support is limited for the hypothesis that disturbances in norepinephrine (e.g., hypothalamic norepinephrine systems are activated) or serotonin (systems are inhibited) are a cause of bulimia nervosa in women. What is known is that when bulimic patients binge, they have an increased rate of eating and an increase in duration of eating (Kaye, Gwirtsman, George, Weiss, & Jimerson, 1986), and certain neurotransmitters regulate different aspects of eating, such as rate, duration, and size of meals. Further, Leibowitz and Shor-Posner (1986) and Leibowitz (1990) found that bingeing behavior is consistent with overactivity of the hypothalamic noradrenergic system and underactivity of the hypothalamic serotonergic system, or a combination of both.

Kaye and Weltzin (1991) also noted that interventions that *diminish* serotonergic neurotransmissions or serotonin receptor activation reportedly increase food consumption and promote weight gain. Serotonin administration to rats has been reported to *decrease* size and duration of meals and rate of eating, and the fact that serotonin may also decrease carbohydrate consumption (foods usually consumed by bulimics during a binge episode) and spare protein selection has led to hypotheses about the role of antidepressants or serotonin agonists in bulimia. Kaye and Weltzin (1991) explain this mechanism further, stating that *hypo*serotonergic function in bulimia nervosa patients could contribute to reduced satiety; increased meal size, meal duration, and rates of eating; and increased ingestion of grams of carbohydrate.

Norepinephrine disturbances in bulimia nervosa have also been studied, but whether or not these disturbances are secondary to alterations in nutritional status, mood, hormonal status, physical activity, or neuroendocrine systems is questioned. While studies have consistently found alterations in noradrenergic activity in bulimia nervosa patients, it is again uncertain whether there is an upregulation of hypothalamic receptors, or whether noradrenergic disturbances contribute to pathologic eating behaviors.

Many other neurochemical studies regarding bulimia nervosa are being undertaken. For example, the function of cholecystokinin (CCK), which promotes satiety, might be impaired in bulimia nervosa. Also, disturbances in opioids and peptides, which regulate appetite, may contribute to the abnormal patterns of food intake in bulimic women (Kaye & Weltzin, 1991). Findings on these neurochemicals remain inconclusive, however (Blundell & Hill, 1993; Kaye & Weltzin, 1991).

GENETIC TRANSMISSION

While a number of hypotheses exist concerning the genetic factors predisposing young women to bulimia, none has conclusively determined that it is genetically transmitted. However, it is important to address these hypotheses and the conflicting findings thus far.

Hudson, Pope, Jonas, Yurgelun-Todd, and Frankenburg (1987) employed the family history method to determine genetic underpinnings of bulimia nervosa. In diagnosing 283 first-degree relatives of 69 bulimic probands, 149 relatives of community controls, and 104 relatives of 24 probands with major affective disorder (a disorder known to be genetically transmitted), they found bulimia nervosa in only 1.7% of relatives of bulimics. This rate does not differ from the prevalence in the general population, estimated to be between 1 and 3%.

On the other hand, when Kassett et al. (1989) used the family study method, they found a threefold increase in morbid risk of bulimia nervosa (9.6%) when they compared first-degree relatives of 40 bulimic probands to normal controls. Therefore, some evidence exists that bulimia nervosa aggregates in families, but the exact nature of this intergenerational transmission is, to date, undetermined.

Twin studies have also demonstrated a genetic link to some degree. However, as Strober (1991) has suggested, twin studies thus far, although showing a higher percentage of bulimia nervosa than in the general population and a higher percentage in monozygotic versus dizygotic twins, are fraught with confounding influences, such as recruitment (volunteers) that might overselect for monozygotic twins. Small sample sizes also contribute to questionable findings.

Studies associating affective disorders with eating disorders have attempted to demonstrate a unitary model to explain the transmission of eating disorders. Because many women who have bulimia nervosa also have a mood disorder, it was hypothesized that the eating disorder could also be genetic. These studies do, in fact, report increased rates of unipolar depression among first- and second-degree relatives of bulimia probands. However, Strober, Lampert, Morrell, Burroughs, and Jacobs (1990) found that familial risks for anorexia nervosa and bulimia nervosa were no greater than those in the general population when they investigated the cross-transmission of eating disorders among relatives of probands with both unipolar and bipolar affective illness. Thus the evidence is conflicting, but it seems to argue against a unitary model of familial etiology (Strober, 1991)—that is, the association of mood and eating disorders appears to be constructed along independent although possibly interacting pathways.

COMORBIDITY

A number of research articles have concluded that bulimia nervosa is associated with other forms of psychopathology, such as affective disorders, substance abuse, anxiety disorders, and personality disorders (Mitchell, Specker, & de Zwaan, 1991). It is possible that these other disorders might help to contribute to the development and maintenance of this eating disorder.

The presence of depression in women with eating disorders is well documented, and one hypothesis is that depression develops because of the social and psychological consequences of bulimia. In one study, for example, Laessle, Kittl, Fichter, Wittchen, and Pirke (1987) noted that improvement in depression paralleled improvement in the eating disorder symptoms. One issue in the maintenance of bulimia nervosa is that depressive symptoms can often mask an eating disorder; for example, the patient in treatment finds it easier to seek help for a mood disorder or stress than for eating pathology. Conversely, many individuals treated by this author in dynamic psychotherapy appear to use their eating pathology (e.g., preoccupation with weight and size, bingeing and purging followed by self-deprecating thoughts) as a "defense" against depression. In this way, they maintain their eating disorder to avoid a painful, or more painful, experience of dealing with their psychopathology.

The association between alcohol and drug problems and eating disorders (substance use/abuse disorder) is another area being studied. For example, Mitchell, Hatsukami, Eckert, and Pyle (1985) reported that of 275 outpatient women with bulimia nervosa, 34% had a history of problems with alcohol and drugs, and 17.7% had prior chemical dependency treatment. The high prevalence of eating disorders in substance abuse populations also adds support for this association. However, the literature does not support viewing bulimia nervosa, on the whole, as an "addiction" (Scott, 1983; Vandereycken, 1990). While there are some similarities—for example, secrecy, denial, loss of control, and craving—there are also many differences—for example, lack of "tolerance" and withdrawal symptoms—that cannot be ignored when considering an addiction explanation. It is, however, possible that, just as with the affective disorders, substance abuse and eating pathologies are used to cope with negative affect. When those suffering from both bulimia nervosa and substance abuse seek treatment from self-help groups for substance abuse, an accompanying eating disorder may go untreated, thus perpetuating the latter.

The research literature has also frequently suggested an association of bulimia nervosa with the Cluster "B" personality disorders, such as borderline, histrionic, narcissistic, and antisocial disorders (Mitchell et al., 1991). Additionally, of the cluster "C" personality disorders, avoidant disorder has been diagnosed in 30 to 35% of both anorexic and bulimic patients (Mitchell et al., 1991). Several hypotheses for this association have been formulated. With respect to the maintenance of bulimia nervosa, one probable explanation is that personality disorders may predispose individuals to develop clinical syndromes such as eating disorders; further, the personality disorder and eating disorder might each interact to alter the features of the other. When a personality disorder is not diagnosed, it can contribute to the maintenance of bulimic symptoms. One such example is the feature of impulsivity in individuals with borderline personality disorder. Treatment of food impulses may be ineffective through usual cognitive-behavioral procedures when the impulse issue is a *personality* feature that responds to dynamic, rather than cognitive-behavioral, treatment.

High rates of anxiety disorders, such as phobias and obsessive compulsive disorder, have also been found in groups of women with bulimia nervosa. One might hypothesize that when these disorders are untreated, they can lead to eating pathology as a way to control anxiety and panic. However, according to Mitchell and his colleagues (1991), these associations have only been studied recently. More research on the exact mechanism of this group of disorders and its relationship to the maintenance of eating pathology is warranted.

SUMMARY OF ETIOLOGIC FACTORS

In summary, many factors have been identified as contributing to the development of bulimia nervosa. Some of these are theories, some are hypotheses, and some are critiques of existing explanations or paradigms, such as the feminist analysis. Table 8–1 summarizes the four main categories of factors and significant issues within each category. It is important, however, to stress that a single factor, or cause-effect model, is *not* considered plausible in the development of bulimia nervosa. It is most useful to approach the etiology of this disorder using an interrelationship model. A discussion of how this model would work is presented below.

THE INTERRELATIONSHIP OF ETIOLOGIC FACTORS

The relationship of the major categories of factors—sociocultural, psychological (including developmental), biological, and comorbidity—is best described by example. White's (1992a; 1992b) summary of how this may be viewed is based on Katz's (1985) work on this disorder (see Figure 8–2). Although the comorbidity issue is not discussed by Katz, it must be considered in both the development and the maintenance of bulimia nervosa.

TABLE 8–1. FACTORS IN THE DEVELOPMENT OF BULIMIA NERVOSA

Psychological	*Biological*
Identity and role conflict	Obesity
Separation-individuation issues	Dieting
Body image	Neurotransmitter disturbances
Dysfunctional family patterns	Genetic predisposition
Cognitive dysfunction	
Ineffective behavioral styles	*Comorbidity*
	Affective disorders
Sociocultural	Substance abuse disorders
Valuing thinness/perfectionism	Personality disorders
Occupational choice	Anxiety disorders
The media	
Oppression of women	

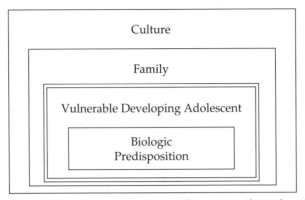

FIGURE 8–2. Relationships among biological predisposition; the vulnerable, developing adolescent; his or her family; and the sociocultural context in the development of an eating disorder. (Adapted from Katz, J. L. [1985]. Some reflections on the nature of the eating disorders: On the need for humility. *The International Journal of Eating Disorders, 4,* 618. Copyright © 1985 by John Wiley & Sons, Inc. Adapted by permission John Wiley & Sons, Inc.)

With the young female, the developmental issue is separation-individuation. An older adolescent or young adult female may confront this emotional issue when faced with a physical separation, such as going away to college. In this case, the separation would be from a particular type of family. For example, the family might be one that is chaotic, oriented toward achievement and success, and influenced by a mother who is overprotective but experienced as uncaring or unresponsive in affect. Biologically, this young woman might have been predisposed to an overweight state, a serotonin or norepinephrine disturbance may be present, and she has begun practicing dietary restraint (the restricting of particular foods), leading to binge eating.

Fearful of becoming fat in a society with so much pressure to be thin, she cannot allow the binged food to remain in her body. She begins purging by vomiting, laxative use, or overexercising. This binge eating might also be the result of psychosocial problems. For example, anxiety can often occur from feelings of inadequacy related to a lack of independence or individuation, and from emotional separation issues. Although she wants to achieve and be successful—family traits with which she is familiar—this woman is ill-equipped to do so. Therefore, the binge-purge cycle ensues. Once this cycle begins, however, many factors and systems function to maintain this disorder, such as depression, isolation, and more dieting or dietary restraint.

KEY NURSING PROBLEMS

Patients with bulimia nervosa present a challenge to the professional because of both the biological and psychological issues facing this population. Some individuals present with more cognitive dysfunction (distorted thinking about weight, shape, and size); some with more interpersonal difficulties (e.g., anxiety, difficult relationships); some with comorbidity (depression); and some with a significant physiologic component (omitting foods, as in dietary restraint). Each individual may be different in the underlying causes of the bingeing and purging. Therefore, an accurate assessment—using a variety of clinical instruments on eating disorders along with the clinical interview—will help define interventions that are specific and individualized. Table 8–2 outlines the key assessment categories to be addressed.

Several methods are available for the assessment of bulimia nervosa. The clinical interview and the DSM-IV (American Psychiatric Association, 1994) criteria are

TABLE 8–2. BULIMIA NERVOSA: ASSESSMENT CATEGORIES

Behavioral	Cognitions
Developmental	Knowledge deficits
Family	Interpersonal
Biological/dietary	Intrapersonal
Physiologic symptoms/	Comorbidity
medical complications	Weight history
DSM-IV criteria	Exercise

most often used. Instruments developed by clinicians and researchers in the field of eating disorders are also available. The major goal of assessment is to outline for the clinician the specific interventions necessary to relieve the symptoms of bingeing and purging, as well as any accompanying comorbidity, such as depression.

CRITERIA FOR ASSESSMENT

Using the DSM-IV (American Psychiatric Association, 1994) criteria for bulimia nervosa and the literature on risk factors and maintenance factors presented earlier, a systematic assessment is possible. However, in addition to criteria already discussed, medical or physical symptoms must also be considered during assessment. Table 8–3 lists the DSM-IV criteria and Table 8–4 lists the common medical complications and symptoms associated with bulimia that also need to be assessed in the initial interview.

CLINICAL INSTRUMENTS

Two important and useful tools are the Eating Disorder Examination (EDE) developed by Cooper and Fairburn (1987) and the well-known Eating Disorder Inventory (EDI) developed by Garner, Olmstead, and Polivy (1983). Both can be used for clinical or research purposes. Validating a clinical interview with instruments may often be necessary to differentiate the eating disorders from each other and/or

TABLE 8–3. DSM-IV CRITERIA FOR BULIMIA NERVOSA

A. Recurrent episodes of binge eating. An episode of binge eating is characterized by both of the following:
   (1) eating, in a discrete period of time (e.g., within any 2-hour period), an amount of food that is definitely larger than most people would eat during a similar period of time and under similar circumstances
   (2) a sense of lack of control over eating during the episode (e.g., a feeling that one cannot stop eating or control what or how much one is eating)
B. Recurrent inappropriate compensatory behavior in order to prevent weight gain, such as self-induced vomiting; misuse of laxatives, diuretics, enemas, or other medications; fasting; or excessive exercise.
C. The binge eating and inappropriate compensatory behaviors both occur, on average, at least twice a week for 3 months.
D. Self-evaluation is unduly influenced by body shape and weight.
E. The disturbance does not occur exclusively during episodes of anorexia nervosa.

From American Psychiatric Association (1994). *Diagnostic and statistical manual of mental disorders* (4th ed.). Washington, DC: Author.

TABLE 8–4. PHYSIOLOGICAL SYMPTOMS AND MEDICAL COMPLICATIONS IN BULIMIA NERVOSA

Symptoms

Lethargy	Swelling or fluid retention
Constipation	Heart fluttering
Abdominal pain or discomfort	Heart skipping beats
Absent menstrual periods	Feeling bloated
Irregular menstrual periods	Nausea
Feeling cold often	Puffy cheeks
Slow heart rate	Excessive dental problems
Dry skin	Finger callouses from inducing vomiting
Brittle nails	Leg pains or cramps
Hair thinning or loss	Blood or blood streaks when vomiting
Chest pain or burning	

Possible Medical Complications

Electrolyte imbalance	Cardiac arrythmia
Hypotension	Dental enamel erosion
Liver damage	Kidney damage or malfunction

Adapted from J. White & G. Litovitz (1994). A comparison of inpatient vs. outpatient women with eating disorders on selected variables. [Study in progress]. The table uses language for patient understanding. Some symptoms are associated with anorexia nervosa, and this disorder must be ruled out.

for identifying *specific* symptoms that are measurably more problematic to a *specific* patient. In some patients, for example, preoccupation with weight, shape, and size is more of a problem than loss of control over eating. Instruments such as the EDI, the EDE, and the Bulimia Test (BULIT) are useful in this way. Additionally, an initial interview would include questions about physiological as well as psychological issues.

THE EATING DISORDERS EXAMINATION

This semistructured interview, which takes approximately 45 minutes, was designed to assess specific core psychopathology of patients with eating disorders. The interviewer questions the patient's behaviors, beliefs, and values about eating, shape, weight, and size. The 62-item interview guide uses the framework of the past 4 weeks for each question to elicit present pathology. The strength of this instrument rests on the premise that beliefs and values about eating, size, and shape are difficult to obtain through self-report measures and lend themselves best to an interview. Structuring the interview in the form of subscales also provides the clinician with an objective measure. The five subscales are (1) restraint, (2) overeating, (3) eating concern, (4) shape concern, and (5) weight concern. The higher the score, the more pathology. However, the independent subscales can also be used to determine areas of pathology most significant in individual patients. These data can then be used to individualize interventions. Test-retest reliability and a variety of validity measures have been established for the EDE (Cooper & Fairburn, 1987; Wilson & Smith, 1989).

THE EATING DISORDER INVENTORY

The original version of the EDI (Garner et al., 1983) and the newer EDE-2 (Garner, 1991) both use a self-report format. The original version contained 64 items on eight subscales to assess eating pathology. The eight subscales measure (1) drive for thinness, (2) bulimia, (3) body dissatisfaction, (4) ineffectiveness, (5) perfectionism, (6) interpersonal distrust, (7) interoceptive awareness, and (8) maturity fears. The subscale scores aid in differentiating individuals with anorexia nervosa and bulimia from those who are normal or have an overall eating pathology. This version has been widely used and has excellent reliability and validity (Garner et al., 1983; Wear & Pratz, 1987).

The EDI-2 is similar to the original version except for the addition of three subscales: (9) asceticism; (10) impulse regulation; and (11) social insecurity. These scales have been added to assess other important pathologies associated with eating disorders. To date, these subscales are labeled provisional because further work is needed in testing for reliability and validity, but they have excellent concurrent validity so far (Garner, 1991).

The EDI is useful in assessing an eating disorder and is frequently used with a screening interview for diagnostic purposes. The authors suggest administering the EDI, then following up those individuals with scores about the cutoff point with a clinical interview to determine a diagnosis of bulimia nervosa or anorexia nervosa.

THE BULIT

The Bulimia Test (BULIT) (Smith & Thelen, 1984) is a 36-item inventory designed to assess the symptoms of bulimia in the DSM-III (American Psychiatric Association, 1980). It discriminates between patients with bulimia and normal controls and has adequate reliability and validity. It includes items on purging and weight change as well as those on eating habits.

THE CLINICAL INTERVIEW

In addition to assessing if the patient meets the DSM-IV criteria (American Psychiatric Association, 1994), it will also be necessary to form a list of questions about the physical manifestations of bulimia because many of these, such as dental erosion, may need intervention. Table 8–4 lists some common physiological symptoms that occur with bulimia. Questions about eating and dietary restraint will also need to be included. The nurse may, for instance, want to request a week of food records to assess the specific amount of abnormal eating (dietary restraint, bingeing) and purging that occurs. This technique is called self-monitoring.

SELF-MONITORING

A variety of methods can be used for self-monitoring. Some programs have developed food diaries that are used by each individual. Whatever the form, the diary should include the type of food, the amount of food, the location where food was eaten, and the social or emotional context of the eating. Clients should indicate whether eating episodes were actual or perceived binges and record each purge as well. Some clients consider any *unplanned* eating episode a binge, and self-monitoring helps define client distortions about food amounts that later will benefit from a cognitive intervention.

The disadvantages of self-monitoring are compliance and accuracy. Individuals should be instructed to write down intake of food within 15 minutes of consumption to minimize inaccuracies. Compliance is a problem because of the increased anxiety evoked around actually realizing the amount of food consumed. Compliance is best when self-monitoring is embedded into an actively collaborative relationship between the assessor and the patient (Meichenbaum & Turk, 1989), although this may be difficult to achieve at a first session.

NURSING INTERVENTIONS

The most significant interventions for the client with bulimia nervosa address (1) the resolution of the binge-purge cycles; (2) the development of insight into the underlying issues (family, developmental, and interpersonal-intrapersonal dynamics); (3) the treatment of neurotransmitter disturbances; and (4) the correction of knowledge and nutritional deficits. The overall result is physical and emotional health for the client. Table 8–5 presents key interventions and their rationale. In addition, the psychiatric nurse in advanced practice should become an advocate with respect to society's role in this disorder, contribute to curriculum development, and support developing a research agenda to address this disorder.

COGNITIVE-BEHAVIORAL THERAPY

One of the most successful treatments for bulimia nervosa has been cognitive-behavioral therapy (Agras, 1991; Fairburn, 1985). The goal of this time-limited program is to change behavior and restructure thinking through a systematic, step-by-step intervention that addresses behaviors such as binge eating, restraint, and purging. The behavioral techniques used are self-monitoring (record keeping), cue elimination (controlling one's environment), reinforcement, successive approximation, and alternate-response adoption. Successive approximation refers to the achievement of smaller goals that, in succession, get closer and closer to the final goal. Alternate-response adoption means choosing a different response and adopting it to be used when the stimulus is presented. The premise is that behaviors are learned and can be unlearned, and that cues can be eliminated to prevent the response (e.g., removing visual food cues prevents binge eating).

Along with this behavioral component is the cognitive restructuring aspect. Individuals are helped to restructure, or change, their thinking by challenging distortions and presenting more realistic thinking patterns. The well-known work of Beck, Rush, Shaw, and Emery (1979) is an example of using cognitive therapy with depressed patients.

White (1990) developed a 12-week cognitive-behavioral program for bulimic women and piloted it on a university campus with 10 women who met the DSM-III-R (American Psychiatric Association, 1987) criteria for bulimia nervosa. This program was designed to test the effects of a time-limited cognitive-behavioral program on the symptoms of bingeing and purging and on the specific core psychopathology of bulimia nervosa. The preoccupation with body shape and size, depressive symptoms and negative thinking, perfectionism, dietary restraint, and frequency of bingeing and purging were measured in a pretest-posttest format. The program was adapted from Fairburn (1985), Lacey (1985), and Agras (1989). Agras's (1989) manual is available to clinicians.

The format for this program was a mixture of individual (30-minute) and group (90-minute) sessions. Individual cognitive sessions challenged dysfunctional thinking patterns; they were conducted individually because many of the subjects had different patterns of thinking that were dysfunctional. In the group format, topics included changing behavior, learning about bulimia, and learning about nutrition. Group sessions—didactic presentations followed by discussion—were also used to reinforce the new thinking patterns being developed through individual sessions.

The posttest data revealed that these college students had decreased their bingeing and purging, increased their knowledge about bulimia and eating and nutrition, decreased their practice of dietary restraint, and decreased their dissatisfaction with

TABLE 8–5. NURSING INTERVENTION STRATEGIES

NURSING INTERVENTION	RATIONALE
Behavioral Techniques Self-monitoring Cue elimination Successive approximation Alternate-response adoption	The more that is known about the particular eating style and binges, the more specific the nurse can be in helping each individual eliminate the stimuli or cues, plan small goals to approximate an end goal, or present alternatives to stimuli that cannot be removed. Self-report also helps clients to self-manage at a later point. Behavioral intervention has significantly decreased binge/purge behaviors.
Cognitive Techniques Restructuring of thinking that is dysfunctional, such as dichotomous thinking, catastrophizing, and/or overgeneralizing	Clients often respond to dysfunctional cognitive patterns by bingeing and purging. Restructuring thinking to be more realistic decreases the probability of binges and has been demonstrated to effect a more realistic (less ideal or perfectionistic) view of size, shape, and weight.
Insight Development Developing insight into ineffective relationships, coping, emotions, and roles	Underlying problems such as role conflict, relationship difficulties, and ineffective coping often lead to emotional states such as anxiety and depression, which may, in turn, lead to bingeing. Uncovering and correcting the causes of these has effectively decreased binge and purge behaviors. Although the exact mechanism is unknown, the nurse clinician should encourage the client to reflect on current conflicts, emotions, and coping, and assist in the process of identifying causes for the development of these difficulties. Facilitating awareness about their development is a first step. Clients then need to be helped to develop healthier ways of relating, coping, or responding that are a combination of support, teaching, suggesting, and role modeling on the part of the therapist.
Psychopharmacology Referral for antidepressant medication Monitoring of medications for effectiveness and side effects	A significant treatment for bulimia nervosa is the administration of antidepressant medication for the treatment of both depression and binge-purge behavior. Nurse clinicians are in a position to determine effects and side effects because of the frequency with which they are in contact with their clients for other treatment.
Nutritional Education Education about the role of dietary restraint in bingeing Referral to a dietitian (as necessary)	Clients with bulimia nervosa are often bingeing on high-carbohydrate, high-fat foods, and alternately restricting these foods. Structured eating plans that also provide flexibility have been shown to alleviate this type of behavior. Therefore, the value of a diet that is structured, flexible, and includes all food groups should be discussed.

Table continued on following page.

TABLE 8–5. NURSING INTERVENTION STRATEGIES *Continued*

NURSING INTERVENTION	RATIONALE
Family Work	
Family therapy, education, and support (especially for families of young bulimic patients)	Bulimia is often described as a "family disorder," especially when separation-individuation is an issue. Helping the family know more about the disorder and work through their own issues has facilitated recovery for the bulimic individual. Therefore, they should be involved in learning about the signs and symptoms, the causes, and the changes that all will need to make, especially if family dynamics are counterproductive to recovery.
Support Groups	
Conducting a support group (especially for recovered bulimic clients)	Relapse is a significant problem with bulimia nervosa. Continuing to involve the client on a long-term basis in a group will help with relapse prevention or early intervention in relapse.

their bodies after the 12 weeks. After this 12-week intervention, an 8-month support phase was instituted to reinforce behavior change, healthy cognitive patterns, and obtained knowledge. These were discussion sessions lasting one and one-half hours weekly. The findings after the 12 weeks remained the same—that is, the change made during the intervention phase remained stable when measured after the support phase.

As expected, however, in some cases interpersonal problems—like maturity fears (measured by the EDI) and interpersonal distrust—were not changed through this cognitive-behavioral program. Still, it is important to remember that the goal of this type of treatment modality is symptom relief, and underlying interpersonal issues need to be addressed in another mode of therapy.

INSIGHT-ORIENTED INDIVIDUAL THERAPY

A great number of clinicians who work with women who have bulimia nervosa report that insight-oriented therapy is effective in addressing and resolving underlying issues such as role conflict, low self-esteem, guilt, ineffective coping, and separation-individuation (White, 1984, 1986). Nevertheless, while some also report the cessation of the bingeing-and-purging cycle with this type of dynamic work, it is unclear what mechanism might be involved here (Agras, 1991). How the eating behavior changes as a result of insight is an unknown process.

Weekly or twice-weekly sessions are necessary, and the orientation of the nurse will dictate the way the sessions are conducted. Each clinician depends on her or his own training and experience to conduct these sessions, and it is not within the scope of this chapter to present the many different types of or orientations to dynamic therapy, such as analytic, object-relations, self-psychology, and interpersonal. Regardless of orientation, however, the role of the clinician focuses on uncovering the causes of problematic relating, coping, or responding because facilitating this awareness can assist clients in changing current behavior. An exploration of the causes often results in understanding ineffective behaviors or relating, as well as a need and hope for change. This realization is then followed by adoption of new behaviors or emotions.

It is difficult to engage the patient in insight-oriented work when her eating is out of control or concentration is a problem. It is best to manage the eating, possibly with cognitive-behavioral work, before introducing psychotherapy with such clients.

FAMILY THERAPY

Many authors believe that an eating disorder is a disorder of the family, so the entire family needs to be treated. Whether to include the family as the focus of the entire treatment or as just one part of the management of a particular client's care will depend on the philosophical orientation of the nurse. This chapter has, however, already pointed out the interrelationship of family dysfunctioning and the developing young woman, and it seems imperative that the family be included in some way. As previously discussed, most families of the woman with bulimia nervosa need help with boundaries, communication, conflict resolution, and separation from the daughter (White, 1984, 1986). If the family lives in another town, suggestions can be made for treatment there. While some nurse specialists do both the individual and family work, it is common to collaborate with another therapist around the family work.

PSYCHOPHARMACOLOGY

Many research studies have concluded that antidepressants are useful in bulimia nervosa to help with the cessation of the bingeing-and-purging cycle. Two hypotheses (a neurotransmitter disturbance and/or an accompanying affective disorder) have been advanced as the explanation for these positive results with antidepressants (Walsh, 1991). The most often recommended and prescribed medications are the selective serotonin reuptake inhibitors, such as sertraline (Zoloft) or fluoxetine (Prozac), although the older tricyclic antidepressants and monamine oxidase inhibitors also have demonstrated utility in treating bulimia.

Psychiatrists who specialize in neuropharmacology are helpful in assessing the need for such medication and the treatment of the client with medication, so collaboration is again essential. It is also important to clarify monitoring responsibilities.

MEDICAL TREATMENT AND CONSULTATION

Many serious complications can result from repeated bingeing and purging (Pomeroy & Mitchell, 1989), as indicated in Table 8–4; therefore, referral to a physician for monitoring and collaboration is essential in managing care for a bulimic client. Further, it is important to refer to physicians who are familiar with the disease because there is much shame associated with this diagnosis, and women might be reluctant to discuss symptoms with a physician who does not seem knowledgeable.

NUTRITIONAL COUNSELING

Many cognitive-behavioral programs include nutritional-dietary information because it is so closely related to the behaviors and cognitions of women with bulimia nervosa. Indeed, key nursing interventions include providing basic information about dietary restraint and its role in binge eating, as well as an assessment of diet and food intake with suggestions for change. In some instances, however, referral to and collaboration with a dietitian may also be necessary. Many dietitians are familiar with eating disorders, but it is helpful to discuss the overall goals of treatment with this clinician, especially the problem of dietary restraint. In this way, the dietitian will not be working in a counterproductive way by prescribing a diet that might reinforce dietary restraint.

HOSPITALIZATION

Referral for inpatient treatment is another option for the psychiatric nurse specialist. Decisions to seek hospitalization are based on (1) the presence of medical complications; (2) a danger on the part of the client to herself or others (as in severe depression and suicidal ideation); and/or (3) an inability to make progress in the outpatient setting. An inpatient stay on a unit or in a program specifically designed for patients with eating disorders is optimum. The nurse will, of course, collaborate with the inpatient team around the care of her client and continue work with her, as permitted, while she is hospitalized. For example, ongoing individual psychotherapy can be continued by the nurse during an inpatient stay.

OPERATIONALIZING BIOLOGICAL-BEHAVIORAL-COGNITIVE INTERVENTIONS

Sessions with clients who have bulimia nervosa must include many types of interventions, which are summarized in Table 8–5. The timing of these interventions is important because the biological, behavioral, and cognitive aspects of the disorder are linked.

It is important to educate the client first with respect to the biological basis of the disorder. This paves the way for the referral for psychopharmacology treatment, suggestions about diet, exercise, and overall symptom management. Clients are often relieved to know there is a biological component for their binge eating that is related to serotonergic function. Obsessive thoughts about food are also a typical complaint and are improved by medication.

Following psychopharmacology interventions and dietary prescriptions, monitoring for medication effects and side effects is important. Through the monitoring procedures the therapist uses, clients can learn a great deal about the link between serotonergic dysfunction and eating and thought patterns. In this way, the client can later learn to self-monitor. For example, when asked specifically about food obsessions, clients note the decrease after the start of medication. This enables them to assess their own progress in this area, noting changes that may suggest medication-dosage adjustment.

Almost immediately and throughout the work with the client, direct cognitive interventions are important. This requires systematically challenging distorted thought patterns and then replacing them with more realistic thinking.

Insight-oriented therapy is best introduced following some progress with the disturbed eating patterns because most clients feel too out-of-control when first in treatment to work on anything but their eating and purging—that is, their anxiety is directly related to an inability to control eating. Early biological interventions (diet, exercise, education, and psychopharmacology) help decrease these dysfunctional behaviors, however, and can also lead to a decrease in anxiety. Once anxiety is reduced, the client can better focus on the intra- or interpersonal issues underlying the disorder.

This author presents treatment goals to the client early on so that the client is aware of the multifaceted, research-based approach necessary for effective treatment. Evaluation of the various interventions is, of course, ongoing and individualized. Not all clients, for example, need diet interventions.

CLIENT ADVOCACY

While most of this chapter focused on the individual client, it is necessary before leaving treatment to discuss the need for society to be treated as well. In considering advocacy for the client with an eating disorder, the nurse must consider women and society in general, as discussed thoroughly by White (1991, 1992a, 1992b). One avenue for advocacy is involvement in organizations that advocate for the healthy, equal treatment of women and the defocus on women's appearances as paramount in their evaluation. Recently, for example, eating disorder advocacy groups have lobbied heavily for the removal of advertising in magazines that reach adolescent girls and feature fad dieting, the need to be thin, and so on (Too Rich or Too Thin, 1989). Additionally, more information written by clinicians needs to reach the lay literature on topics such as the danger of bulimia nervosa and its need for professional treatment. Psychiatric nurses can make an impact in these areas.

CURRICULUM DEVELOPMENT AND BULIMIA NERVOSA

As nurses begin to address the interface between the biological and behavioral components of psychiatric problems, eating disorders must be included. While it is probably not feasible to include an entire course on eating disorders, a graduate curriculum in psychiatric nursing should contain some essential content, including such areas as risk factors, the types of effective treatment modes, and the biological basis for these disorders. Since the literature abounds with research that supports cognitive-behavioral therapy as an effective strategy for bulimia nervosa, a program could also include training in this modality. Furthermore, the research to date has demonstrated that this disorder is prevalent in college-aged women, so a curriculum that focuses on adolescent health *across* specialty programs should also include the risk factors for and treatment of this problem.

Because this disorder is often a "closet" one and can often accompany another disorder or be masked by another psychiatric problem, assessment criteria such as those included in this chapter are other important content areas for psychiatric nurses. Thorough assessments in differentiating eating disorders from each other (anorexia, bulimia) are important at the graduate level and necessary in independent practice and primary care settings. Several assessment instruments, developed for research and clinical work in bulimia nervosa, have been widely used and could be incorporated into graduate course work. Such tools—objective measures and clinical interview schedules—are efficient and provide reliable, valid data; they also support the traditional history-taking methods of nursing.

Finally, graduate curricula must begin to address neuroscience—neuroanatomy, neurophysiology, and neurochemistry—for the psychiatric nurse of today to manage and care for clients with eating disorders. An understanding of both the biological and behavioral bases for this disorder advances client health and prevents further dysfunction. To date, however, few curricula require such courses.

Undergraduate curricula generally include eating disorders as a nutritional problem and as a psychiatric inpatient problem. They tend to focus on the nursing interventions of support, education, and monitoring, but as more knowledge, particularly biological, becomes available, the content must be expanded to include early detection and assessment criteria.

BULIMIA NERVOSA: A RESEARCH AGENDA

Without question, nurses can make a significant contribution in research on eating disorders. Four important areas are necessary for the future: (a) studies that investigate treatment outcomes so that the exact mechanism of the effect is known; (b) feminist studies that take society and culture into account; (c) qualitative studies that address the problem from the perspective of the client with bulimia nervosa; and (d) risk-factor studies.

Thus far, the literature supports cognitive-behavioral therapy, psychopharmacology, and insight-oriented therapy as effective treatments, but it is unclear which treatment is effective for which patients. The disorder is often discussed in the literature by such subtypes as restricters and bingers, or exercisers and purgers, but little information is available on the most effective treatment for these subtypes, or even for clients with specific characteristics. Such studies are, however, warranted.

Much of the research in the literature is presented from a biomedical, individual client perspective. Yet it is well known that society and culture play an important role in the development of this disorder. Streigel-Moore (1990), for example, outlined the following emergent criteria for feminist research: (1) it takes a contextual approach that examines units of analysis that are larger than the individual; (2) it affirms a positive view of women; (3) it utilizes a broad spectrum of research methods, exploring experiences and establishing a collaborative relationship with the research participant; and (4) it considers the findings for social rather than individual-based change.

No studies have been found in the extant literature that address this disorder from the perspective of the patient or client. Phenomenological studies would, however, be helpful in addressing the meaning bulimia has for the client. For example, much of the literature presents role conflicts and a changing society as precipitants, but little is known, except in clinical vignettes, about these difficulties. By systematically examining these areas from an insider's view, however, researchers might gain insights about bingeing as a coping mechanism or lend support for previously mentioned notions about role conflict.

Last, there are few *prospective* studies on the risk factors for eating disorders. Yet prevention must be a part of the psychiatric nurse's research agenda. Prospective studies on families who present with dysfunctions like those described earlier are therefore warranted. Subsequently, early family and parent treatment could be developed based on these types of research findings. Prospective studies on young girls prior to prepubescence must also be included to determine preventable risk factors.

SUMMARY

This chapter has presented the disorder of bulimia nervosa, the risk factors in its development, how they contribute to the etiology and maintenance of this disorder, and what is necessary for a thorough assessment in which biological and behavioral components are considered. Because bulimia nervosa is a complex disorder, management of it must include multimodal treatment approaches. Cognitive-behavioral therapy, insight-oriented individual and family therapy, psychopharmacology, and medical follow-up are all parts of the treatment. Additionally, collaboration skills are an important aspect for the psychiatric nurse managing the bulimic client's care. As a result, both nursing curricula and nursing's research agenda need reformulating in light of the extensive body of knowledge on this biological-behavioral phenomenon.

ACKNOWLEDGEMENTS. The author wishes to thank Christopher Brush and Dody Breen for their technical assistance with this chapter.

REFERENCES

Agras, W. S. (1989). *Cognitive behavioral treatment therapist manual: Stanford bulimia nervosa treatment studies* (rev. ed.). Stanford: Stanford University.

Agras, W. S. (1991). Nonpharmacologic treatments of bulimia nervosa. *The Journal of Clinical Psychiatry, 52*(Suppl. 10), 29–32.

American Psychiatric Association. (1980). *Diagnostic and statistical manual of mental disorders* (3rd ed.). Washington, DC: Author.

American Psychiatric Association. (1987). *Diagnostic and statistical manual of mental disorders* (3rd ed. rev.). Washington, DC: Author.

American Psychiatric Association. (1994). *Diagnostic and statistical manual of mental disorders* (4th ed.). Washington, DC: Author.

Bartky, S. (1988). Foucault, femininity, and the modernization of patriarchal power. In J. Diamond & L. Quinby (Eds.), *Feminism and Foucault: Reflections on resistance* (pp. 61–86). Boston: Northeastern University Press.

Beattie, H. J. (1988). Eating disorders and the mother-daughter relationship. *International Journal of Eating Disorders, 7*(4), 453–457.

Beck, A. T., Rush, A. J., Shaw, B. F., & Emery, G. (1979). *Cognitive therapy of depression.* New York: Guilford.

Blundell, J., & Hill, A. (1993). Binge eating: Psychological mechanisms. In C. Fairburn & G. T. (Eds.), *Binge eating: Nature assessment and treatment* (pp. 206-223). New York: Guilford.

Boskind-White, M., & White, W. C. (1983). *Bulimarexia: The binge-purge cycle.* New York: Norton.

Bordo, S. (1990). Reading the slender body. In M. Jacobus, E. F. Keller, & S. Shuttleworth (Eds.), *Body/politics, women, and the discourses of science* (pp. 83–112). New York: Routledge, Chapman and Hall.

Bruch, H. (1978). *The golden cage: The enigma of anorexia nervosa.* New York: Random House.

Bruch, H. (1985). Four decades of eating disorder. In D. M. Garner & P. E. Garfinkel (Eds.), *Handbook of psychotherapy for anorexia nervosa and bulimia* (pp. 7–18). New York: Garfield.

Brumberg, J. J. (1988). *Fasting girls: The emergence of anorexia nervosa as a modern disease.* Cambridge: Harvard University Press.

Carlatt, M. S., & Carmargo, C. (1991). Review of bulimia nervosa in males. *American Journal of Psychiatry, 148*(7), 831–843.

Chernin, K. (1981). *The obsession: Reflections on the tyranny of slenderness.* New York: Harper & Row.

Chernin, K. (1985). *The hungry self: Women, eating and identity.* New York: Harper & Row.

Collins, M. E. (1991). Body figure perceptions and preferences among preadolescent children. *International Journal of Eating Disorders, 10*(2), 199–208.

Cooper, L., & Fairburn, C. (1987). The eating disorder examination: A semi-structured interview for the assessment of the specific pathology of eating disorders. *International Journal of Eating Disorders, 6*(1), 1–8.

Crago, M., Yates, A., Beutler, L. E., & Arizmendi, T. A. (1985). Height/weight ratios among female athletes: Are collegiate athletics the precursors to anorexic syndrome? *International Journal of Eating Disorders, 4,* 79–82.

Crisp, A. H. (1988). Some possible approaches to prevention of eating and body weight/shape disorders, with particular reference to anorexia nervosa. *International Journal of Eating Disorders, 7*(1), 1–17.

Dritchel, B. H., Williams, K., & Cooper, P. (1991). Cognitive distortions amongst women experiencing bulimic episodes. *International Journal of Eating Disorders, 10,* 539–547.

Fairburn, C. G. (1985). A cognitive-behavioral treatment for bulimia. In D. M. Garner & P. E. Garfinkel (Eds.), *Handbook of psychotherapy for anorexia nervosa and bulimia* (pp. 160–192). New York: Guilford.

Fairburn, C. G., & Beglin, S. J. (1990). Studies of the epidemiology of bulimia nervosa. *The American Journal of Psychiatry, 147,* 401–408.

Garfinkel, P. E. (1992). Evidence in support of attitudes to shape and weight as a diagnostic criterion of bulimia nervosa. *International Journal of Eating Disorders, 4,* 321-325.

Garner, D. M. (1991). The EDE-2. Odessa, FL: Psychological Assessment Resources.

Garner, D. M., Garfinkel, P. E., Schwartz, D., & Thompson, M. (1980). Cultural expectations of thinness in women. *Psychological Reports, 47,* 483–491.

Garner, D. M., Olmstead, M., & Polivy, J. (1983). Development and validation of a multidimensional eating disorder inventory for anorexia nervosa and bulimia. *International Journal of Eating Disorders, 2*(1), 15–34.

Garrow, J. (1978). The regulation of energy expenditure. In A. Bray (Ed.), *Recent advances in obesity research* (pp. 200–210). London: Newman.

Hawkins, R., Turrell, S., & Jackson, L. (1983). Desirable and undesirable masculine and feminine traits in relation to students' dieting tendencies and body image. *Sex Roles, 6,* 765–781.

Hudson, J. I., Pope, H. G., Jonas, J. M., Yurgelun-Todd, D., & Frankenburg, F. R. (1987). A controlled family history study of bulimia. *Psychological Medicine, 17,* 883-890.

Hsu, L. K. G. (1989). The gender gap in eating disorders: Why are the eating disorders more common among women? *Clinical Psychology Review, 9,* 393-407.

Kassett, J. A., Gershon, E. S., Maxwell, M. E., Guroff, J. J., Kazuba, D. M., Smith, A. L., Brandt, H. A., & Jimerson, D. C. (1989). Psychiatric disorders in the first-degree relatives of probands with bulimia nervosa. *American Journal of Psychiatry, 146,* 1468–1471.

Katz, J. L. (1985). Some reflections on the nature of the eating disorders: On the need for humility. *International Journal of Eating Disorders, 4*(4A), 617–626.

Kaye, W., & Weltzin, T. (1991). Neurochemistry of bulimia nervosa. *The Journal of Clinical Psychiatry, 52*(Suppl. 10), 21–28.

Kaye, W. H., Gwirtsman, H. E., George, D. T., Weiss, S. R., & Jimerson, D. C. (1986). Relationship of mood alterations to bingeing behavior in bulimia. *British Journal of Psychiatry, 149,* 479–485.

Lacey, J. H. (1985). Time-limited individual and group treatment for bulimia. In D. M. Garner & P. E. Garfinkel (Eds.), *Handbook of psychotherapy for anorexia nervosa and bulimia* (pp. 431–457). New York: Guilford.

Laessle, R. G., Kittl, S., Fichter, M., Wittchen, H. U., & Pirke, R. M. (1987). Major affective disorder in anorexia nervosa and bulimia: A descriptive diagnostic study. *British Journal of Psychiatry, 151,* 785–789.

Leibowitz, S. F. (1990). The role of serotonin in eating disorders. *Drugs, 39,* 33–48.

Leibowitz, S. F., & Shor-Posner, G. (1986). Brain serotonin and eating behavior. *Appetite, 7,* 1–13.

Lidz, T. (1968). *The person.* New York: Basics.

MacKenzie, M. (1985). The pursuit of slenderness and addiction to self-control: An anthropological interpretation of eating disorders. *Nutrition Update, 5,* 174–194.

McKenna, M. (1989). Assessment of the eating disordered patient. *Psychiatric Annals, 19*(9), 467–472.

Meichenbaum, D., & Turk, D.C. (1989). *Facilitating treatment adherence.* New York: Plenum.

Michie, H. (1987). *The flesh made word: Female figures and women's bodies.* Oxford: Oxford University Press.

Mitchell, J., & Pyle, R. (1985). Characteristics of bulimia. In J. Mitchell (Ed.), *Anorexia nervosa and bulimia: Diagnosis and treatment* (pp. 29–47). Minneapolis: University of Minnesota Press.

Mitchell, J., Specker, S., & de Zwaan, M. (1991). Comorbidity and medical complications in bulimia nervosa. *The Journal of Clinical Psychiatry, 52*(Suppl. 10), 13–21.

Mitchell, J. E., Hatsukami, D., Eckert, E. D., & Pyle, R. L. (1985). Characteristics of 275 patients with bulimia. *American Journal of Psychiatry, 142,* 482–485.

Orbach, S. (1979). *Fat is a feminist issue.* Berkley, CA: Berkley Press.

Palmer, R. L. (1979). The dietary chaos syndrome: A useful new term? *British Journal of Medical Psychology, 52,* 187–190.

Pole, R., Waller, D., Stewart, S., & Parkin-Feigenbaum, L. (1988). Parental caring versus over-protection in bulimia. *International Journal of Eating Disorders, 7*(5), 601–606.

Polivy, J., & Herman, C. P. (1985). Dieting and bingeing: A causal analysis. *American Psychologist, 40,* 193–201.

Pomeroy, C., & Mitchell, J. E. (1989). Medical complications and management of eating disorders in adolescence. *Psychiatric Annals, 19*(9), 488-493.

Ritvo, S. (1984). The image and uses of the body in psychic conflict with special reference to eating disorders in adolescence. *Psychoanalytic Study of the Child, 39,* 449–469.

Scott, D. W. (1983). Alcohol and food abuse: Some comparisons. *British Journal of Addictions, 78,* 339–349.

Sights, J., & Richards, H. (1984). Parents of bulimic women. *International Journal of Eating Disorders, 3*(4), 3–24.

Silverstein, B., Perdue, L., Peterson, B., Vogel, L., & Fantini, D. (1986). Possible causes of the thin standard of bodily attractiveness for women. *International Journal of Eating Disorders, 5,* 907–916.

Smith, M. C., & Thelen, M. H. (1984). Development and validation of a test for bulimia nervosa. *Journal of Consulting and Clinical Psychology, 52,* 863–872.

Steen, N., Oppliger, R., & Brownell, K. (1988). Metabolic effects of repeated weight loss and gain in adolescent wrestlers. *Journal of the American Medical Association, 260*(1), 47–50.

Steiger, H., Liquornik, K., Chapman, J., & Hussain, N. (1991). Personality and family disturbances in eating disorder patients. *International Journal of Eating Disorders, 10*(5), 501–512.

Streigel-Moore, R. (1990, April 28). *Emergent criteria for feminist research.* Paper presented at the Fourth International Conference on Eating Disorders, New York, NY.

Strober, M. (1991). Family-genetic studies of eating disorders. *The Journal of Clinical Psychiatry, 52*(Suppl. 10), 9–12.

Strober, M., Lampert, C., Morrell, W., Burroughs, J., & Jacobs, C. (1990). A controlled family study of anorexia nervosa: Evidence of familial aggregation and lack of shared transmission with affective disorders. *International Journal of Eating Disorders, 9*(3), 239–253.

Too rich or too thin (Advertisement) [sic]. (1989). *Obesity and Health, 3*(11), 8.

Vandereycken, W. (1990). The addiction model in eating disorders: Some critical remarks and a selective bibliography. *International Journal of Eating Disorders, 9*(1), 95–101.

Walsh, T. (1991). Psychopharmacologic treatment of bulimia nervosa. *The Journal of Clinical Psychiatry, 52*(Suppl. 10), 34–38.

Wear, R., & Pratz, O. (1987). Test-retest reliability for the eating disorder inventory. *International Journal of Eating Disorders, 6*(6), 767–769.

Whitaker, A., Johnson, J., Shaffer, D., Rapaport, J. L., Kalikow, K., Walsh, B. T., Davies, M., Braiman, S., & Dolinsky, A. (1990). Uncommon troubles in young people: Prevalence in a non-referred adolescent population. *Archives of General Psychiatry, 47,* 487–496.

White, J. H. (1984). Bulimia: Utilizing individual and family therapy. *Journal of Psychosocial Nursing, 22*(4), 22–28.

White, J. H. (1986). The patient with an eating disorder. In J. Durham & S. Hardin (Eds.), *The nurse psychotherapist in private practice* (pp. 157–172). New York: Springer.

White, J. H. (1990). Pilot study: The effects of a time-limited cognitive-behavioral program on bulimia in women. Unpublished research.

White, J. H. (1991). Feminism, eating and mental health. *Advances in Nursing Science, 13*(3), 68–80.

White, J. H. (1992a). Women and eating disorders: Significance and sociocultural risk factors. *Health Care for Women International, 13*(4), 351–362.

White, J. H. (1992b). Women and eating disorders: Developmental, family and biologic risk factors. *Health Care for Women International, 13*(4), 363–373.

White, J. H., & Litovitz, G. (1994). Eating disorders symptom checklist. Unpublished research in progress.

Wilson, G., & Smith, D. (1989). Assessment of bulimia nervosa: An evaluation of the eating disorders examination. *International Journal of Eating Disorders, 8*(2), 173–179.

Wiseman, C. V., Gray, J. J., Mosimann, J. E., & Ahrens, A. H. (1992). Cultural expectations of thinness in women: An update. *International Journal of Eating Disorders, 11*(1), 85–91.

Woodman, M. (1980). *The owl was a baker's daughter: Anorexia nervosa and the repressed feminine.* Toronto: Inner City Books.

Woodman, M. (1982). *Addiction to perfection: The still unravished bride.* Toronto: Inner City Books.

Wooley, O. W., Wooley, S. C., & Dryenforth, S. R. (1979). Obesity and women II: A neglected feminist topic. *Women's Studies International Quarterly, 2,* 81-92.

Wooley, S., & Wooley, O. W. (1982). The Beverly Hills eating disorders: The mass marketing of anorexia nervosa. *International Journal of Eating Disorders, 1*(3), 57–69.

CHAPTER

9

CARING FOR DEPRESSED CHILDREN AND ADOLESCENTS

Maureen Reed Killeen, PhD, RN, FAAN, and Cynthia Frame Bongarten, PhD

ABSTRACT

While it is now widely recognized that depression does occur during childhood and adolescence, three overlapping issues must be addressed: the validity of specific diagnoses, developmental aspects of the psychopathology, and the relative influences of nature and nurture on the etiology and treatment of childhood depression. This chapter reviews existing research on the biology and psychology of depression and problems associated with the diagnosis, treatment, and nursing care of depressed children and adolescents. Despite the tendency to adapt adult-focused interventions to children, research indicates that major differences exist between children and adults in the biological correlates of depression, symptoms, and responses to treatments. Research issues related to assessment and diagnosis are explored, curricular changes are proposed, and the need for programmatic research in nursing care of childhood depression is noted. The chapter asserts that psychiatric nursing must integrate the biological and psychosocial approaches and utilize transactional models, which take into account the characteristics of both parents and children and their mutual influences on each other.

It is now widely recognized that depression occurs during childhood and adolescence. Among child psychiatric clinic attendees, approximately 15% meet criteria for depressive disorders defined by the American Psychiatric Association in its *Diagnostic and Statistical Manual of Mental Disorders* (DSM-IV) (American Psychiatric Association, 1994; Angold & Rutter, 1992). In addition, childhood depression is often chronic, treatment resistant, and associated with poor outcomes (Geller, 1993). Thus, depressive disorders in children represent a serious mental health problem, often requiring psychiatric nursing interventions for both the children and their families. Because depressive symptoms include changes in physical, psychological, and social functioning, depression presents an excellent vehicle for examining issues related to the integration of biomedical and psychological research in child and adolescent psychiatric nursing.

Whenever psychopathology is studied in children and adolescents, three issues must be addressed. The first concerns the existence of mental disorders in children and the validity of specific diagnoses for them. Some researchers have questioned whether depression exists during childhood and, if it does, whether it exists as merely a symptom of negative mood or affect, or as a disease or disorder (Rutter 1988; Seifer, Nurcombe, Scioli, & Grapentine, 1989).

The second issue concerns the developmental aspects of psychopathology, including the developmental trajectory of specific disorders and continuities and discontinuities in mental disorders over time. Developmental psychopathology focuses on whether childhood depression predicts adult depression and on age-related changes in depressive symptoms and in treatment efficacy.

The third issue concerns the relative influences of nature and nurture on the etiology and treatment of mental disorders in children. Questions focus on whether childhood depression is best predicted by biological variables, environmental influences, or both, and whether childhood depression is best treated biologically, psychosocially, or with combined treatments.

In reality, these questions overlap, so that both the validity and the developmental psychopathology issues can be examined from both biological and psychological perspectives, and in terms of the contributions of nature and nurture. Throughout this chapter, questions related to these three issues will be addressed by examining the existing empirical information on childhood depression and exploring the implications of findings from both biomedical and psychological research for the nursing care of children with depression.

PHENOMENOLOGY OF DEPRESSION IN CHILDHOOD
VALIDITY OF THE DIAGNOSIS

Prior to the 1980s, many theorists disputed the validity of depression as a diagnosis for children. Psychoanalysts asserted that depression stemmed from guilt or from an unrealized ideal self (Rie, 1966) and that it required a well-developed superego. Because it was assumed that children's superegos remained immature until adolescence, it was thought that children could not experience depression. As a result, childhood depression was neither studied nor treated.

During the 1970s, others asserted that depression could be experienced during childhood, but that the symptoms were unlike those experienced by adults. However, "masked depression" was said to be the underlying problem of children who expressed their psychopathology by temper tantrums, hyperactivity, noncompliance, somatic complaints, underachievement, and numerous other symptoms of distress (Cytryn & McKnew, 1974). Masked depression is no longer regarded as a useful construct (Cytryn, McKnew, & Bunney, 1980; Kovacs & Beck, 1977). A more fruitful approach to the issues of symptom expression and diagnosis has been advanced by those who suggest that childhood depression exists but might be difficult to diagnose because it is sometimes manifested by symptoms that differ from those of adult depression, or is accompanied by symptoms of other childhood disorders (Carlson & Cantwell, 1980; Sroufe & Rutter, 1984). Such thinking has led to many studies on the correlates of depression, comorbidity, and age-related changes in symptoms of depression.

A third theoretical position proposed that depressive symptoms that emerged during childhood were normal developmental phenomena, were quite prevalent, and would dissipate over time (Lefkowitz & Burton, 1978). Proponents of this position, which has also fallen into disrepute, claimed that mental health professionals need not diagnose or treat depression in children. The more widely accepted view is that although specific symptoms of depression (such as poor appetite or crying) may be quite prevalent during particular age periods, this does not preclude the existence of a depressive disorder (Kazdin, 1988).

DEFINITIONS AND DESCRIPTIONS

Despite some disagreement (Seifer et al., 1989), the generally accepted view is that childhood depression exists, and the essential features of the disorder are very similar to depression in adults (American Psychiatric Association, 1994). Although depression can be diagnosed in children and adolescents using the same criteria as for adults (Kazdin, 1990), this does not mean that the manifestations of the disorder are necessarily identical. Rather, the prevalence rates, specific symptoms, and clinical course can vary with age.

PREVALENCE

Estimates of the prevalence of depression in children vary with the type of assessment instrument, diagnostic criteria, and type of sample. The most widely cited prevalence estimate for all childhood psychiatric disorders is 11.8% (Gould, Wunsch-Hitzig, & Dohrenwend, 1981). More recent studies have estimated that between 14% and 20% of children and adolescents suffer from moderate to severe psychopathology, with the prevalence of severe disorder at about 7% (Brandenburg, Friedman, & Silva, 1990). Epidemiological studies of major depression (Anderson, Williams, McGee, & Silva, 1987; Fleming & Offord, 1990; Kashani et al., 1987; Kazdin, 1990) have found that pure depression is rare in children and adolescents; that the prevalence of major depression is lower in children than in adults (2% to 3% of general populations and 10% to 20% of clinical populations) and increases in adolescence; that high comorbidity of depressive and nondepressive disorders exists; and that comorbidity increases as the severity of the depression increases. Further, depressive symptoms and disorders are persistent, recur, and are associated with poor academic and psychosocial outcomes (Kovacs & Goldston, 1991; McCauley et al., 1993).

Sex differences in the prevalence of depression either have not been found in clinic and nonclinic samples of 5- to 12-year-olds or have shown higher rates among prepubertal boys. Among adolescents, however, both the prevalence and the severity of depression have been higher among females. Rates of depression in adolescent girls are twice as high as for younger girls or adolescent boys (Angold & Rutter, 1992).

SYMPTOMS

The essential features of major depressive disorders (MDD) include

- *Melancholic symptoms,* such as dysphoria or negative mood (or irritability in children), a loss of interest or pleasure, and a lack of responsiveness to ongoing activities
- *Cognitive symptoms,* including feelings of unworthiness or guilt, or helplessness and hopelessness
- *Vegetative symptoms,* such as changes in sleep patterns, appetite, and energy, and often
- *Suicidal ideas*

In addition, there is some degree of social impairment, and the condition persists for weeks or months (Rutter, 1988). Table 9–1 displays the DSM-IV (American Psychiatric Association, 1994) criteria for major depression and dysthymia.

TABLE 9-1. DSM-IV Diagnostic Criteria for Major Depressive Episode and Dysthymic Disorder

DSM-IV Diagnostic Criteria for Major Depressive Episode

A. Five or more of the following symptoms have been present during the same two-week period and represent a change from previous functioning; at least one of the symptoms is either (1) depressed mood, or (2) loss of interest or pleasure.

    Note: Do not include symptoms that are clearly due to a general medical condition, or mood-incongruent delusions or hallucinations

    (1) depressed mood most of the day, nearly every day, as indicated by either subjective report (e.g., feels sad or empty) or observation made by others (e.g., appears tearful) **Note:** In children and adolescents, can be irritable mood

    (2) markedly diminished interest or pleasure in all, or almost all, activities most of the day, nearly every day (as indicated either by subjective account or observation made by others)

    (3) significant weight loss when not dieting or weight gain (e.g., a change of more than 5% of body weight in a month), or decrease or increase in appetite nearly every day. **Note:** In children, consider failure to make expected weight gains

    (4) insomnia or hypersomnia nearly every day

    (5) psychomotor agitation or retardation nearly every day (observable by others, not merely subjective feelings of restlessness or being slowed down)

    (6) fatigue or loss of energy nearly every day

    (7) feelings of worthlessness, or excessive or inappropriate guilt (which may be delusional) nearly every day (not merely self-reproach or guilt about being sick)

    (8) diminished ability to think or concentrate, or indecisiveness, nearly every day (either by subjective account or as observed by others)

    (9) recurrent thoughts of death (not just fear of dying), recurrent suicidal ideation without a specific plan, or a suicide attempt or a specific plan for committing suicide

B. The symptoms do not meet criteria for a Mixed Episode.

C. The symptoms cause clinically significant distress or impairment in social, occupational, or other important areas of functioning.

D. The symptoms are not due to the direct physiological effects of a substance (e.g., a drug of abuse, a medication) or a general medical condition (e.g., hypothyroidism).

E. The symptoms are not better accounted for by Bereavement, i.e., after the loss of a loved one, the symptoms persist for longer than 2 months or are characterized by marked functional impairment, morbid preoccupation with worthlessness, suicidal ideation, psychotic symptoms, or psychomotor retardation.

There is little controversy concerning symptoms of major depression in adults. Melancholic symptoms, cognitive symptoms, vegetative symptoms, and suicidal ideas are all included in both DSM-IV (American Psychiatric Association, 1994) and Research Diagnostic Criteria (RDC) (Spitzer, Endicott, & Robbins, 1978). Developmental research, however, shows mixed results on whether specific symptoms of depression vary with age and gender. Although some investigators have failed to find developmental differences in symptoms (Mitchell, McCauley, Burke, & Moss, 1988), studies have generally found that while the severity and frequency of symptoms does not vary between children and adolescents diagnosed with depression, the pattern of symptoms does differ (Ryan, Puig-Antich, Ambrosini, et al., 1987). Table 9-2 displays symptoms typical of children and adolescents diagnosed with major depression. Dysphoric mood, somatic complaints, and social withdrawal are the most common symptoms experienced by prepubertal children, while adolescents' symptoms are similar to those of depressed adults, including suicidal ideas and attempts (Puig-Antich, 1982).

TABLE 9–1. DSM-IV DIAGNOSTIC CRITERIA FOR MAJOR DEPRESSIVE EPISODE AND DYSTHYMIC DISORDER *Continued*

DSM-IV Diagnostic Criteria for Dysthymic Disorder

A. Depressed mood for most of the day, for more days than not, as indicated either by subjective account or observation by others, for at least two years. **Note:** In children and adolescents, mood can be irritable and duration must be at least 1 year.

B. Presence, while depressed, of two (or more) of the following:
   (1) poor appetite or overeating
   (2) insomnia or hypersomnia
   (3) low energy or fatigue
   (4) low self-esteem
   (5) poor concentration or difficulty making decisions
   (6) feelings of hopelessness

C. During a two-year period (1 year for children and adolescents) of the disturbance, the person has never been without the symptoms in Criteria A and B for more than 2 months at a time.

D. No Major Depressive Episode has been present during the first 2 years of the disturbance (1 year for children and adolescents); i.e., the disturbance is not better accounted for by chronic Major Depressive Disorder, or Major Depressive Disorder, In Partial Remission.

   Note: There may have been a previous Major Depressive Episode provided there was a full remission (no significant signs or symptoms for 2 months) before development of the Dysthymic Disorder. In addition, after the initial 2 years (1 year in children or adolescents) of Dysthymic Disorder, there may be superimposed episodes of Major Depressive Disorder, in which case both diagnoses may be given when the criteria are met for a major Depressive Episode.

E. There has never been a Manic Episode, a Mixed Episode, or a Hypomanic Episode, and criteria have never been met for Cyclothymic Disorder.

F. The disturbance does not occur exclusively during the course of a chronic Psychotic Disorder, such as Schizophrenia or Delusional Disorder.

G. The symptoms are not due to the direct physiological effects of a substance (e.g., a drug of abuse, a medication) or a general medical condition (e.g., hypothyroidism).

H. The symptoms cause clinically significant distress or impairment in social, occupational, or other important areas of functioning.

From American Psychiatric Association (1994). *Diagnostic and statistical manual of mental disorders* (4th ed.). Washington, DC: Author.

CLINICAL COURSE

How childhood depression fits into the larger picture of developmental psychopathology is unclear at present. Most adults diagnosed with depressive disorder do not appear to have suffered from depression during childhood (Rutter, 1986). Yet recent research demonstrates that depressive disorder in childhood is not transient. A single episode lasts for 9 to 10 months on average, and about two thirds of depressed youngsters experience recurrence of the disorder prior to adulthood (Kovacs, 1989; Kovacs & Goldston, 1991; McCauley et al., 1993; McGee & Williams, 1988). Preliminary findings suggest that prepubertal onset of depression may be associated with a higher loading of familial depression (Fleming & Offord, 1990; Orvaschel, 1990).

The outcome and clinical course for children suffering from depression also might depend on whether they have other psychiatric disorders. Comorbidity of depression and anxiety disorders is well documented (Ryan, Puig-Antich, Ambrosini, et al., 1987; Weissman et al., 1987) and is associated with increased severity of symp-

TABLE 9–2. Symptoms of Major Depression Most Often Exhibited by Adults, Children, and Adolescents

ADULTS	CHILDREN	ADOLESCENTS
Melancholic Symptoms		
Depressed mood	Irritable mood	Depressed or irritable mood
	Sadness	
Anhedonia	Boredom	Anhedonia
	Decreased pleasure	
	Social withdrawal	
Vegetative Symptoms		
Significant weight loss or gain	Decreased appetite	Weight change
	Somatic complaints	Failure to gain expected weight
Insomnia or hypersomnia	Hyposomnia	Hypersomnia
Psychomotor agitation or retardation	Agitation	
	Listlessness	
Cognitive Symptoms		
Excessive guilt		Guilt
Feelings of worthlessness		Low self-esteem
Diminished concentration	Academic difficulties	Difficulty concentrating
Indecisiveness		
Thoughts of death	Morbid thoughts	Hopelessness
Suicidal ideas		Suicidal ideas
Suicide attempts		Suicide attempts
Mood-congruent delusions and hallucinations	Possible hallucinations	Possible delusions or hallucinations

toms (Bernstein, 1991). Comorbidity of depression and conduct disorder also leads to less positive outcomes than depression alone. One longitudinal study, which followed depressed child and adolescent patients and nondepressed controls into adulthood, found 21% of the depressed group also had conduct disorder (CD) (Harrington et al., 1991). Although the depressed children with comorbid CD did not differ from depressed children without CD in demographics or depressive symptoms, they had a worse short-term outcome, a higher risk of adult criminality, and a trend toward lower risk of depression in adulthood. In a similar study (Fleming, Boyle, & Offord, 1993), adolescents with either depressive syndrome or CD had significant psychosocial morbidity 4 years later.

The major developmental psychopathology question regarding depression is whether there are links among depressive phenomena in childhood, adolescence, and adulthood. Few studies address this question, primarily because of the difficulty in designing and implementing life-span studies of any psychiatric disorder. Despite limitations, the existing empirical literature suggests that depression in youth is associated with increased risk of depression later in life (Cantwell, 1990; Kovacs et al., 1984; Poznanski, Krahenbuhl, & Zrull, 1976) and with substantial risk of suicidal behavior during later recurrences of depression (Kovacs, Goldston, & Gatsonis, 1993; Rao, Weissman, Martin, & Hammond, 1993).

RELIABILITY OF THE DIAGNOSIS

There are two types of assessment of depression in children: diagnostic assessment and target symptom assessment. The goal of diagnostic assessment is to determine the presence and type of disorder. The purpose of target symptom assessment is often to establish the extent of one or more features of the disorder, so that the degree of change resulting from therapy can be measured and analyzed. Research reports authored by psychiatrists most often use diagnostic assessments, while reports by psychologists and psychiatric nurses tend to use assessments of target symptoms and behaviors, within a context of diagnostic assessment. The reliability of the diagnosis is a major issue for both types of assessment and for research on treatment and nursing care.

SOURCES OF INFORMATION

Much of the controversy over whether depression exists in children is due to differences in assessment results, depending on who is questioned, the content of the questions, and the methods used to collect information. In the classic Isle of Wight studies, Rutter and his colleagues (Rutter, 1989; Rutter, Tizard, & Whitmore, 1970, cited in Cantwell, 1988) found that a parental interview was distinctly the best instrument when used alone, and that a child interview was the least useful for detecting a disorder that had been missed by other measures. Child interviews were useful in detecting mild depressive episodes that others missed, however, and in distinguishing types of disorders.

Since then, numerous studies have examined the reliability and convergence of assessments of childhood depression by various informants and have found very complex results. In general, agreement among children, parents, teachers, and peers is low to moderate (Angold et al., 1987). Edelbrock, Costello, Dulcan, Kalas, and Conover (1985) found that the reliability of the child interview was substantially lower than that of the parent, but that there was an inverse relationship with age. Children became better informants as they became older, with adolescents being as reliable as their parents. Children below age 10, however, usually were not reliable in reporting on their own symptoms. Conversely, parents became less reliable informants as their children became older. Children appear to be better informants about their internal experiences, while parents and teachers are better informants about observable behaviors. Parental reports of children's depression frequently contain false negatives, but few false positives (Angold et al., 1987).

Despite the lack of agreement, it is important to obtain reports from multiple sources because each informant's reports have been correlated with other indices. Children's self-reports of depression correlate with suicidal attempts and ideas, hopelessness, and low self-esteem, while parental reports of their children's depression correlate with the children's decreased social interactions and with expressive affects. Teacher and peer reports are associated with academic performance and popularity, respectively (Kazdin, 1990). These studies clearly suggest that the use of multiple informants provides a more comprehensive view of children's symptoms and disorders.

ASSESSMENT METHODS

A second issue in reliability of diagnosis concerns the form in which information is collected about children. Table 9–3 displays a list of assessment instruments used with children and adolescents. A detailed review of these instruments is beyond the scope of this chapter, but an overview will be provided. Excellent reviews of depression instruments and of more general instruments having depression subscales are included in Kazdin (1988) and Rehm, Gordon-Leventon, and Ivens (1987).

TABLE 9–3. SELECTED DEPRESSION INSTRUMENTS FOR CHILDREN AND ADOLESCENTS

INSTRUMENT	AUTHOR	TYPE	INFORMANT
Schedule for Affective Disorders and Schizophrenia (SADS)	Puig-Antich & Chambers (1978)	Semi-structured/ structured interview	Parent Child
Diagnostic Interview Schedule for Children	Costello, Edelbrock, & Costello (1985)	Structured interview	Parent Child
Diagnostic Interview for Children and Adolescents	Herjanic, Herjanic, Brown, & Wheatt (1975)	Structured interview	Parent Child
Children's Depression Rating Scale (CDRS)	Poznanski, Cook, & Carroll (1979)	Interview rating scale	Clinician
Children's Depression Inventory (CDI)	Kovacs & Beck (1977)	Self-report Forced choice	Child Adolescent
Scale for Suicide Ideation (SSI)	Beck, Kovacs, & Weissman (1979)	Semi-structured interview Self-report Rating scale	Trained interviewer Child Adolescent
Suicidal Ideation Questionnaire (SIQ)	Lewinsohn et al. (1989)	Self-report Rating scale	Child Adolescent

Diagnostic assessment is most often conducted by means of standardized questionnaires and/or a structured or unstructured clinical interview. Parents and children are the most frequent respondents. Most psychiatric nurses are very familiar with *unstructured clinical interviews*. Typically, the interview begins with conversations and activities that are designed to put children at ease and get them to talk about themselves. Drawing and talking about favorite activities, pets, or school often are helpful in getting started. Depressive symptoms and other difficulties can be assessed through questions about the present and recent past. Because children often have difficulty relating events in time, tying symptoms to a specific event is often helpful in assessing the duration of symptoms. For example, a child may be asked, "Have you been feeling sad since your birthday?" or "Have you felt sick at school?" The clinical unstructured interview has the advantage of flexibility, allowing the interviewer to follow the child's lead and link questions naturally within the flow of conversation. A potential disadvantage is that diagnostic assessment using this approach requires a skilled interviewer who is knowledgeable about cognitive and social development as well as diagnostic criteria. It is also difficult to assess the reliability and validity of diagnoses based on unstructured clinical interviews.

A number of *structured interviews* are available for diagnosing childhood psychopathology (Edelstein & Berler, 1987). The Diagnostic Interview Schedule for Children (DISC) (Costello, Edelbrock, & Costello, 1985) is a highly structured interview that can be conducted with the child or parent as respondent. The interviewer reads aloud the questions about a wide variety of psychiatric symptoms and indicates whether each item was endorsed. All questions are asked of each respondent in the same order, and no areas of inquiry are skipped. The scoring indicates whether the child qualifies for each DSM diagnosis. Although one advantage of structured interviews lies in their ability to reduce interviewer bias or error, thereby enhancing the reliability and validity of the diagnoses, the reliability and validity of the DISC and its revisions are only now being established (Fisher et al., 1993; Schwab-Stone et al., 1993; Shaffer et al., 1993). The primary weakness of structured interviews is their inflexibility. Children and adults may have difficulty with the wording of questions or with attending to questions in lengthy interviews.

Semistructured interviews are more flexible, allowing interviewers some latitude in using clinical judgment in the conduct of the interview and coding of responses. One that is widely used is the Kiddie-SADS (Puig-Antich & Chambers, 1978), adapted from the adult version of the Schedule of Affective Disorders and Schizophrenia (SADS) (Endicott & Spitzer, 1978). This diagnostic interview initially is semistructured, allowing the interviewer to establish rapport and gain information about the presenting problem and history. The second part of the interview is a more structured assessment of the child's symptoms. Yet detailed questions can be skipped if a symptom is denied on an initial screening question. Reliability and validity information on the Kiddie-SADS is also limited (Edelstein & Berler, 1987).

Interviews are frequently supplemented with *standardized questionnaires.* The Children's Depression Inventory (CDI) (Kovacs, 1981), a widely used children's self-report instrument, is used to indicate the severity of depressive symptoms in children aged 7 to 17. The CDI has been shown to have high internal consistency and moderate test-retest reliability, to distinguish clinic from nonclinic children, and to correlate positively with measures of related constructs; however, it does not necessarily predict depression scores from other instruments and is weak in discriminating depression from other diagnoses (Kazdin, 1988). Reliability estimates vary markedly among studies. For example, Kazdin (1989) found little overlap in the children identified as depressed by parents' CDI ratings of their children, children's CDI self-reports, and DSM-III-R diagnoses (American Psychiatric Association, 1987). Although the CDI is one of the most researched measures of childhood depression, it needs further psychometric evaluation.

SUMMARY

In general, diagnostic assessment of depression in children and adolescents is fraught with difficulty. Different informants and different assessment methods identify different children as depressed, prompting the recommendation that multiple informants and multiple methods of assessment be utilized. This is not a trivial problem. The evaluation of the role of both physiological and psychological measures and treatments in childhood depression depends on accurate identification and diagnosis.

MODELS OF DEPRESSION

The controversy surrounding the phenomenology of depression is not the only theoretical dispute in this area. Until recently, two separate models of depression guided research on the etiology, correlates, and treatment of depression in both children and adults. Biological models of depression focused on within-person pathology, with the goal of identifying the biological sources of symptoms and discovering medical interventions to treat the disorder. Psychosocial models focused on environmental causes of psychopathology, with the goal of identifying psychological treatments for alleviating target symptoms. Increasingly, these two research traditions are being blended in contemporary research projects (Abraham, Fox, & Cohen, 1992). McBride (1990) has argued that psychiatric nursing has devalued biological knowledge and favored a focus on psychosocial theories and psychotherapy in caring for the mentally ill. She suggests that there is a tremendous need to integrate knowledge from the biological and behavioral sciences in the practice of psychiatric nursing. By examining research findings from both the biological and psychological models of childhood depression, some important insights can be gained about etiology, treatment, and appropriate nursing interventions for children with depression.

BIOLOGICAL MODELS OF DEPRESSION

As with other areas of research, studies of the biological correlates of childhood depression have resulted from efforts to generalize findings from adults to children. Biological research has generally focused on two broad areas of inquiry: heritability of depression and neurophysiological abnormalities.

GENETIC MODELS

Depressive disorders are much more common among close relatives of persons with major depression than in the general population (Burke & Puig-Antich, 1990). Among monozygotic twins, the concordance rate is 65%, while only 14% of dizygotic twins are concordant for depression. The genetic data also show some specificity for type of disorder, with relatives of adult patients with unipolar depression having an increased risk only for unipolar illness and relatives of bipolar patients having increased risk for both bipolar and unipolar depressions (Gold, Goodwin, & Chrousos, 1988a).

Age of onset is also related to family risk for MDD. The highest rates of depression in families are found in relatives of probands with early onset of depression. Weissman et al., (1988) found a 14-fold increase in risk of early onset (before age 13) of MDD in children whose parents were less than 20 years old at the time of their first depressive episode. These findings have been replicated for adolescent-onset bipolar and unipolar depression (Kutcher & Marton, 1991).

In addition, families of both unipolar and bipolar adolescent probands had significantly higher rates of other psychiatric disorders, such as alcoholism and anxiety disorders, than the relatives of normal controls. Over half of the relatives of adolescents with either unipolar or bipolar disorder had some psychiatric illness, compared to less than 11% of the relatives of normal controls. For children of adults with depression, the morbidity risk increases as a function of parental depression, family history of psychiatric disorders, and associated diagnoses of panic disorder or agoraphobia (Burke & Puig-Antich, 1990; Kutcher & Marton, 1991).

Despite this clear evidence of increased risk of psychiatric disorder among relatives of depressed adolescents, concordance evidence alone does not implicate genetics. Rather, familial concordance may be due to shared environmental influences. For example, Cadoret, Gorman, Heywood, and Troughton (1985) found that depression was not correlated with affective illness in the biological relatives of adoptees. Rather, factors in the adoptive families such as alcoholism, family members' behavior problems, or death of an adoptive parent were also important (Burke & Puig-Antich, 1990). Other studies have reported findings that indicate genetic heterogeneity among persons vulnerable to major affective disorders (Gershon, 1988).

Nongenetic risk factors for depression may also have biological implications, providing an illustration of environmental effects on biological factors. An example comes from Gershon's (1988) analysis of cohort differences in depression and suicide. The cohort of persons born since 1940 has higher lifetime prevalence of affective disorders and a higher age-specific suicide rate than do cohorts born earlier. Gershon interprets this finding as reflecting cultural influences on the rate of affective illness, possibly related to the increased incidence of substance abuse among those from younger cohorts who commit suicide. The combination of a cohort difference in substance abuse with genetic risk for depression may lead to the observed cohort differences in suicidality.

NEUROPHYSIOLOGICAL ABNORMALITIES

NEUROTRANSMITTERS

Several biological models of affective disorders in adults have been proposed (Gold et al., 1988a; 1988b). Initially, studies of the biological basis of MDDs examined the role of neurotransmitters. The original catecholamine hypothesis, the first biological theory of depression, asserted that depression results from a functional *deficit* of norepinephrine at critical sites in the central nervous system. However, more recent studies of noradrenergic functioning have found *increased* levels of norepinephrine in cerebrospinal fluid and plasma and increased levels of 3-methoxy-4-hydroxyphenylglycol (MHPG), a metabolite of norepinephrine, in cerebrospinal fluid and urine of adults with MDD. In addition, antidepressant medications decrease the levels of norepinephrine metabolites in the brain and the firing rate of the locus coeruleus, a site for synthesis of norepinephrine. These studies support a conclusion that is the opposite of the original catecholamine hypothesis: that in adults with major depression, the locus-coeruleus-norepinephrine system is *activated* (Gold et al., 1988a).

The locus coeruleus is also involved in responses to threatening situations. Stimulation of the locus coeruleus produces intense anxiety, hypervigilance, and inhibition of exploratory behavior in primates. Abnormally high activation of the locus coeruleus has been associated with effects on areas of the brain that are activated by fear, while low levels of activation were characterized by inattention, impulsivity, carelessness, recklessness, and fearlessness. Furthermore, measures of noradrenergic function tend to be higher in adults with anxiety disorders and in children with behavioral inhibition (Kagan, Reznick, & Snidman, 1987; Rogeness, Javors, Maas, & Macedo, 1990).

Because separation anxiety disorder and MDD in children are related to adult disorders that have shown increased noradrenergic function, it might be expected that children with MDD would show increased levels of norepinephrine or its metabolites. However, a recent review (Yaylayan, Weller, & Weller, 1990/1991) found no clear support for increased levels of norepinephrine metabolites in children with MDD. Nevertheless, in a study of children with a variety of diagnoses, anxiety and depressive disorders were associated with increased noradrenergic function, while undersocialized conduct disorder was associated with decreased noradrenergic function (Rogeness et al., 1990).

NEUROENDOCRINE ABNORMALITIES

Because many symptoms of depression reflect alterations in the hypothalamic centers governing food intake, libido, circadian rhythms, and the release of neurohormones, the hypothalamic-pituitary-adrenal (HPA) axis has been studied (Weller & Weller, 1988). Animal research has shown that neurohormones influence adaptive behaviors during threatening situations. For example, the administration of corticotropin-releasing hormone (CRH) in rats leads to arousal, anorexia, decreased libido, enhancement of conditioned fear responses, and reduction in exploration of unfamiliar surroundings (Gold et al., 1988b).

In adults, MDD has also been associated with neuroendocrine abnormalities, including increased secretion of cortisol, and with an earlier-than-expected rise in cortisol secretion during sleep, with a return to normal cortisol secretion upon recovery of the depressive syndrome (Sachar, 1975). Similar abnormalities in cortisol have been reported in some studies of children with MDD (Puig-Antich, Blau, Marx, Greenhill, & Chambers, 1978) but not all (Doherty et al., 1986; Puig-Antich et al., 1989). Recent studies with depressed adolescents have also failed to find consistent abnormalities in cortisol secretion (Dahl et al., cited in Burke & Puig-Antich, 1990). The inconsistent findings may be due to an age effect on cortisol hypersecretion, or they may be due to the difficulties inherent in studying the neuroendocrine system. Hormones are sensitive to stress and can be affected by nutritional variables, age, circadian rhythms, psychotropic medications, and estrogen. In addition, there is marked variation in basal cortisol levels, and there is no specific level of cortisol that separates depressed from nondepressed adults (Weller & Weller, 1988). As a result, a number of other potential biological markers for depression have been used. These markers include *state* markers, which are abnormal only through the depressive episode and return to normal during recovery, and *trait* markers, which persist through recovery and are presumably abnormal throughout life (Yaylayan et al., 1990/1991).

Biological Assessment Methods

Dexamethasone Suppression Test (DST)

The DST has been extensively studied as a potential state marker in both adult and childhood depression. Typically, a 1 mg PO dose of dexamethasone is given to adults and adolescents, while a 0.5 mg dose is given to prepubertal children, usually around 11 PM; then cortisol is measured at 8 AM and 4 PM. Dexamethasone usually suppresses the blood levels of cortisol for at least 24 hours; however, over 40% of adults with endogenous depression have been found to be nonsuppressors. Nonsuppressors are those whose plasma cortisol levels return to 5 µg/dl, or above, within 24 hours after administration of the dexamethasone.

The many differences in the methods used in various studies make it difficult to generalize across studies. However, three reviews of the literature on DST as a biological marker for depression in children and adolescents have found age differences (Casat, Arana, & Powell, 1989; Weller & Weller, 1988; Yaylayan et al., 1990/1991). These reviews also found markedly different ranges in the following:

1. DST *sensitivities* (proportion of depressed subjects with positive tests)
2. DST *specificities* (proportion of nondepressed subjects with a negative test)
3. *Predictive values* (the likelihood that a subject with a positive DST is depressed)

Birmaher, Ryan, et al. (1992) also failed to find evidence that the DST discriminated among depressed children, nonaffective psychiatric controls, and normal controls, despite a well-controlled study. Yaylayan et al. (1990/1991) conclude that the DST does not clearly identify prepubertal children with major depression. Furthermore, abnormal DST results also are found in children with separation anxiety disorder, autism, and eating disorders.

In addition to examining the relationship of DST to diagnosis, studies have focused on its utility in assessing suicidal risk, evaluating treatment response, and following the status of depressed patients. As in other reports, the findings have been mixed. A positive DST has been associated with lethality of suicide attempts among adolescents and with response to antidepressant treatment in a small study of children. In recent studies, however, the DST has not distinguished between children or adolescents with MDD and controls; suppressors and nonsuppressors have also not differed on suicidality, endogenous features, or psychotic symptoms (Birmaher, Dahl, et al., 1992; Birmaher, Ryan, et al., 1992; Dahl et al., 1993). Follow-up studies of adults and children have found that continued positive DST may be associated with poorer outcomes, although the treatment response rate is not different between adults with positive and negative DST results (Weller & Weller, 1988; Yaylayan et al., 1990/1991).

In summary, despite its promise as a biological marker for depression in adults, the DST has not been found to be consistently related to any aspects of depression in children. The small number of studies and the contradictory results preclude generalization about the potential usefulness of DST with children in clinical settings. At present, its usefulness as a state marker for depression in childhood is limited.

GROWTH HORMONE SECRETION

Growth hormone secretion has been studied as another potential marker for childhood depression. Changes in secretion of growth hormone—in response to clonidine challenge, insulin challenge, and sleep patterns—have been reported in depressed adults (Jarrett, Miewald, & Kupfer, 1990). Among depressed children, however, a small number of studies have reported a different pattern of results.

Although basal levels of growth hormone are not affected in adults with depression, Myer et al. (cited in Yaylayan et al., 1990/1991) found significantly *lower* concentrations of growth hormone during the day, at night, and during sleep in a small sample of depressed boys. Further studies have found that depressed children *hypersecrete* growth hormone during sleep (Puig-Antich, Goetz, Davies, Fein, et al., 1984), and this hypersecretion persists into recovery and remission (Puig-Antich, Goetz, Davies, Tabrizi, et al., 1984). Thus growth hormone hypersecretion during sleep may be a trait marker for major depression in children. In depressed adolescents, however, no differences have been found in growth hormone secretion during sleep. Yaylayan et al. (1990/1991) interpret these findings as suggesting an age effect, wherein growth hormone secretion during sleep decreases with age in depressed persons.

In response to challenge tests using insulin and clonidine, depressed children have had significant hyposecretion compared to controls, while adolescents have not. In general, the findings point to similarities in the growth hormone response to challenge among prepubertal children and postmenopausal women, and differences with adolescents and premenopausal adults (Burke & Puig-Antich, 1990).

POLYSOMNOGRAPHIC FINDINGS

There is considerable evidence that there are abnormalities in the sleep architecture (the length and timing of sleep stages) of depressed adults (Gold et al., 1988a). Changes in the stages of non-rapid-eye-movement (non-REM) sleep include increased sleep latency, decreased arousal threshold, and early morning awakening.

The first REM sleep period usually begins after 70 to 100 minutes of sleep, with three or five additional REM periods typically occurring during the latter part of the night. Among depressed adults, there is a short REM latency. REM sleep periods, which typically increase in length as the night progresses, are redistributed to the first half of the night. Antidepressants either restore a normal pattern of REM sleep in depression or decrease the frequency and intensity of REM sleep. Wehr, Wirz-Justice, and Goodwin (1979) attributed these changes to phase advances in the circadian rhythms during depression. They found that advancing the sleep phase by having patients sleep from 5 PM to 2 AM produced remission in depression in some adults.

In contrast, studies of EEG sleep in childhood depression have failed to find consistent sleep abnormalities before puberty (Burke & Puig-Antich, 1990; Yaylayan et al., 1990/1991). Among prepubertal children, two studies (Puig-Antich et al., 1982; Young, Knowles, MacLean, Boag, & McConville, 1982) have found no abnormalities in slow wave sleep, in sleep efficiency, in REM latency, or in the temporal distribution of REM sleep during the night, while others did find abnormalities in both REM sleep and sleep latencies (Emslie, Rush, Weinberg, Rintelmann, & Roffwarg, 1990). Some studies of depressed adolescents have found that changes in REM sleep latency occur only in late adolescence, but others suggest that abnormalities in sleep latency and continuity occur earlier in adolescence. Finally, the sleep changes that typify depressed adults have also been found in prepubertal children who are recovering from depression. Yaylayan et al. (1990/1991) suggest that these contradictory findings may be the result of developmental changes in sleep itself. Although there appear to be age-related sleep abnormalities during and following depressive episodes, the data for children and adolescents require further study.

SUMMARY

Studies of changes in the neuroendocrine system, neurotransmitters, and sleep architecture, which typify depression in adults, have found conflicting results in children and adolescents. Additional well-controlled research is needed.

BIOLOGICAL TREATMENT OF DEPRESSION: MEDICATIONS

Adults with major depressive disorders are often treated with antidepressant medications (Table 9–4) (Johnson, Hannah, & Zerr, 1992; Ryan, 1990). *Heterocyclic antidepressants* consist of the tricyclics (TCAs), such as imipramine, desipramine, amitriptyline, and nortriptyline, and pharmacologically similar compounds, such as maprotilene and trazadone. *Selective serotonin reuptake inhibitors* (SRIs) include fluoxetine and sertraline. *Monoamine oxidase inhibitors* (MAOIs) include phenelzine and tranylcypromine. Because of the danger of serious drug and diet interactions, MAOIs are rarely used for treatment of depression in children and adolescents.

The exact mechanisms by which the TCAs and other drugs produce their antidepressant effects are not known; however, it is assumed that by blocking uptake of serotonin or norepinephrine in the nerve ending (Johnson et al., 1992; Keltner & Folks, 1993; Ryan, 1990), these drugs correct an imbalance or deficiency in neurotransmitters such as norepinephrine or serotonin. The TCAs are most effective in adults suffering from severe depression who exhibit greater vegetative symptoms and melancholia. Because TCAs have both antihistaminic and anticholinergic effects, however, they often sedate patients and cause annoying side effects, such as dry mouth, blurred vision, constipation, and urinary retention. Weight gain also often accompanies treatment with TCAs. Furthermore, although it takes at least 2 weeks for the antidepressant effects of these drugs to become evident, the sedating and anticholinergic effects are noticeable very early in treatment. Other adverse effects of TCAs are manifested in the cardiovascular system, including orthostatic hypotension, and at high doses, TCAs may increase the risk of tachycardia and other cardiac arrhythmias. In addition to the adverse effects at therapeutic doses, acute heterocyclic antidepressant poisoning from overdose can be fatal. Symptoms of overdose include coma, seizures, cardiac arrhythmias, and conduction abnormalities.

Fluoxetine and sertraline produce their effects by inhibiting reuptake of serotonin. In contrast to the TCAs, fluoxetine may cause weight loss, anxiety, insomnia

TABLE 9–4. SELECTED ANTIDEPRESSANT MEDICATIONS USED WITH CHILDREN AND ADOLESCENTS

NAME	FDA GUIDELINES AGE LIMIT	INDICATIONS
Tricyclics		
Imipramine	6 years old	Enuresis in children
Desipramine	Not recommended for children	Depression in adolescents
		Attention deficit disorder
Amitriptyline	12 years old	Depression in adolescents
Nortriptyline	Not recommended for children	Depression in adolescents
Other Heterocyclics		
Maprotilene	18 years old	Major depression
Trazodone	18 years old	Major depression
Fluoxetine	No FDA limit provided	Major depression

General Precautions
ECG monitoring at each dose increase and at frequent intervals. PR interval less than 0.21 seconds; QRS interval widening less than 30% over baseline. Heart rate less than 130 beats/min. Systolic pressure less than 130 mm Hg; diastolic pressure less than 85 mm Hg.

Common Side Effects
Cardiac conduction slowing (increase in PR and QRS interval)
Tachycardia
Anticholinergic effects, especially dry mouth and constipation

Serious Adverse Effects
Heart block or arrhythmia
Psychosis
Confusion
Seizures
Withdrawal effects
Occasional adverse effects
Toxicity
Drug interactions

Occasional Adverse Effects
Rash
Tics
Photosensitivity
Gynecomastia
Galactorrhea and breast enlargement

U.S. Food and Drug Administration.

or drowsiness, tremors, dizziness, excessive sweating, and gastrointestinal symptoms such as nausea, diarrhea, and anorexia.

The mechanism for MAOIs is thought to be the inhibition of monoamine oxidase enzymes, which inactivate norepinephrine, dopamine, and serotonin. Thus, MAOIs increase the levels of neurotransmitters by inhibiting neurotransmitter breakdown; they stimulate rather than sedate, and they supress REM sleep. The MAOIs are more difficult to use than heterocyclics, however, because drug-diet interactions and drug interactions can lead to hypertensive crises during treatment and for several weeks after the discontinuation of the MAOI. Patients taking MAOIs must be placed on diets free from tyramine and tryptophan (e.g., no aged cheese, chianti wine, preserved and fermented foods, chocolate, yogurt), and patients must refrain from all over-the-counter and prescription sympathomimetic drugs (e.g., those containing amphetamines, norepinephrine, dopamine), tricyclics, and serotonin reuptake inhibitors (Townsend, 1990).

ANTIDEPRESSANT MEDICATION USE IN CHILDREN AND ADOLESCENTS

With the prevailing view that MDD exists among prepubertal children and that it has the essential features reported by adults, one would expect childhood depression to be treated with antidepressant medications; however, neither heterocyclic antidepressants nor MAOIs are recommended for treatment of depression in prepubertal children (Keltner, 1991). Nevertheless, clinicians do prescribe antidepressants for MDD in children and adolescents (Ryan, 1990).

Riddle, Nelson, et al. (1991) described the process by which psychotropic medications may become recognized as effective treatments for children. Typically, they are initially studied in adults and specifically marketed for adults. Despite the fact that few studies of effectiveness in children are included in the preliminary clinical trials, reports of efficacy in small, short-term studies of children are disseminated at scientific meetings and later published. Thus, medications may become widely prescribed for treating clinical disorders, such as depression, in children without the support of the systematic studies that typically precede their use in adults.

TRICYCLICS

The TCAs are used to treat a variety of psychiatric disorders of childhood, including enuresis, attention deficit hyperactivity disorder, anxiety disorders, and separation anxiety disorder, as well as MDD (Ambrosini, Bianchi, Rabinovich, & Elia, 1993a; Ryan, 1990). They are most consistently effective for treating enuresis and attention deficit hyperactivity disorder (Ambrosini, Bianchi, Rabinovich, & Elia, 1993b). Results of antidepressant treatment for affective disorders in children and adolescents have been more disappointing (Ambrosini et al., 1993a).

In several reviews of the use of antidepressants for MDDs in prepubertal children, fewer than 10 studies were cited (Burke & Puig-Antich, 1990; Ryan, 1990), and these studies produced little evidence that antidepressant medication was superior to placebo. More recently, Ambrosini et al. (1993a) reviewed 15 published reports—seven on studies of antidepressant treatment of prepubertal children and eight on adolescents. Only four of the studies on prepubertal children were double-blind and placebo-controlled, and only a total of 153 subjects were studied. The adolescent studies included four open trials and four placebo-controlled, double-blind studies of antidepressant treatment. They reported findings for 162 depressed adolescents who were given antidepressants and 66 who were given placebos. Concurring with the earlier reviews, Ambrosini et al. (1993a) concluded that the data do not support the efficacy of antidepressant medications for child and adolescent MDD. Following is a review of the major findings and the issues that were raised by the existing studies of the efficacy and safety of antidepressant medications in the treatment of childhood depression.

Several small preliminary studies found that imipramine was superior to placebo in the treatment of depression in prepubertal children (Petti & Law, 1982; Preskorn, Weller, & Weller, 1982), while another study (Kashani, Shekim, & Reid, 1984) failed to find significant differences between treatment with amitriptyline and placebo. Puig-Antich et al. (1987) conducted the first double-blind, placebo-controlled study of TCAs with children that used an adequate sample size, RDC diagnostic criteria for depression, adequate assessment procedures, and adequate doses of imipramine. They found only 56% of the medication group responded to treatment, while 68% of the placebo group did.

One potential explanation for this finding concerns the age-related metabolism rates of TCAs. Children metabolize TCAs more rapidly than adolescents, who metabolize them more rapidly than adults. In addition, there are wide individual variations in the ranges of plasma levels of the drugs. Thus, it was thought that children might respond to some optimum plasma level of the antidepressant. When the relation between plasma levels of imipramine and clinical response were examined, Preskorn et al. (1982) found that all the responding children in their study had plasma levels between 125 and 225 ng/ml. They concluded that there is a curvilinear relationship between plasma level of imipramine and clinical response. Although similar findings have been demonstrated in a small study using nortriptyline (Geller, Perel, Knitter, Lycak, & Farook, 1983), Puig-Antich et al. (1987) failed to find a curvilinear relationship between plasma levels of imipramine and clinical response.

Finally, the first double-blind, placebo-controlled study of nortriptyline in children with MDD recently has been reported (Geller et al., 1992). This study randomly assigned 50 prepubertal 6- to 12-year-olds with Research Diagnostic Criteria and DSM-III-R MDD to a placebo washout period of 2 weeks. This was followed by a double-blind, placebo-controlled phase with weekly plasma-level monitoring. Treatment group subjects had their doses adjusted to maintain a plasma level of nortriptyline at 60 to 100 ng/ml. Outcome measures revealed a poor response rate in both the treated and placebo groups. Only 30.8% of the actively treated subjects and 16.7% of the placebo-treated group reached criteria for response to medication. There were no significant differences between groups on any of the categorical or continuous outcome measures. All subjects receiving active treatment reached steady-state plasma levels in the desired fixed range of the study, and there were no significant differences between responders and nonresponders in plasma levels or in total doses of nortriptyline. Contrary to typical findings with adults treated with TCAs, none of the subjects experienced anticholinergic side effects, such as dry mouth, constipation, or difficulty with urination, and on average they gained less weight than did the controls.

Despite the use of standard diagnostic criteria, careful monitoring of treatment levels, and assessment or control of potential confounds, no clear benefits of treatment with nortriptyline were found. The authors discussed a number of issues that may be relevant to studies of the effectiveness of treatment of childhood depression with TCA. They noted that previous reports of successful treatment with tricyclics involved studies that were case reports or uncontrolled studies, in which parents and children knew they were receiving a medication that the investigators expected to work. Thus, parental expectations may have constituted a placebo effect that influenced the results.

Two other issues require exploration. First, children and adults may respond very differently to TCAs. Children in the Geller et al. (1992) study did not experience the anticholinergic symptoms that usually accompany tricyclic use in adults. The authors suggest that this finding may indicate age-specific differences in drug-tissue interaction. Similarly, the decrement in weight gain observed in this sample is the opposite of the usual problems with weight gain observed in adults treated with tricyclics.

The most important differences between studies of tricyclics reported in the adult literature and the studies with children (Puig-Antich et al., 1987; Geller et al., 1992) are the characteristics of the samples. The children in these studies had a severe degree of depression and many suffered from comorbid conditions such as separation anxiety or conduct disorder. Geller et al. (1992) suggest that severity and comorbidity may predict poor response in children. In addition, these children had an unremitting, chronic course of MDD, rather than the episodic course that typifies adults. Thus, their resistance to treatment with tricyclics may be a function of the comorbid conditions, the severity and chronicity of their depression, or age-related differences in response to medications. Ambrosini et al. (1993a) suggest that MDD in youth may be a more severe illness or may represent a distinct biological subtype that is resistant to pharmacotherapy. They further suggest efficacy studies with specific serotonin reuptake inhibitors to clarify whether early-onset MDD is more serotonergically based. Whatever the reason for the poor response to TCAs in well-controlled studies, it is clear that further research is needed before consistent guidelines for prescribing TCAs for prepubertal children with MDD can be developed.

Similar problems plague the literature on drug treatment of MDD in adolescents. Of the few studies reported, several have found disappointing results. One found that placebo was as effective as amitriptyline (Kramer & Feiguine, 1983), while another (Ryan et al., 1986) found that only 33% of endogenously depressed, and 44% of all depressed, subjects responded to imipramine. No relationship between plasma level of the drug and clinical response was found. Ryan (1990) concludes that the lack of established efficacy makes it impossible to offer recommendations regarding the use of tricyclics in adolescent depression.

Another difficulty is that when TCAs are used for treatment of childhood depression, there is a risk of switching to mania or rapid cycling for a subset of patients (Ambrosini et al., 1993b). Switching refers to the development of mania during treatment with TCAs for a depressive episode, while rapid cycling refers to four or more episodes of mood disorder per year (Geller, Fox, & Fletcher, 1993). Recent studies have found evidence of development of manic symptoms and rapid cycling in prepubertal children treated with TCAs (Geller et al., 1993; Strober, Lampert, Schmidt, & Morrell, 1993); therefore, the authors recommend caution in using TCAs for children with a psychotic depressive episode or a family history of bipolar disorder, and they urge hypervigilance concerning symptoms of hypomania.

A final caveat concerning the use of TCAs for children with MDD stems from recent reports of deaths of children who were being treated with desipramine (Popper & Elliott, 1990; Riddle, Nelson, et al., 1991). These reports have led to the recommendation that increased caution be used in treating prepubertal children with TCAs. Reanalysis of these cases (Riddle, Geller, & Ryan, 1993) and findings of naturalistic studies of desipramine effects on cardiovascular function (Biederman et al., 1993; Wilens et al., 1993) have led researchers to conclude, however, that it is safe to administer TCAs to children with normal cardiovascular functioning. Children appear to be at no greater risk for ECG changes than adults taking desipramine. Neither Biederman et al. nor Wilens et al. found significant correlations between serum desipramine levels and heart rate or conduction problems. Although desipramine was associated with tachycardia, the cardiovascular effects were considered benign. Nevertheless, the following guidelines have been recommended concerning the use of TCAs in children (Ambrosini et al., 1993b; Ryan, 1990):

1. A baseline ECG should be obtained prior to initiation of medication treatment, at each dose increase, and at frequent intervals during the period of dose elevation. Serum TCA concentrations and ECGs should be monitored especially when daily doses are above 3 mg/kg.
2. Heart rate should be no more than 130 beats per minute.

3. Blood pressure readings should be less than 130 to 140 mm Hg systolic and 85 to 90 mm Hg diastolic.
4. ECG should maintain PR intervals below 0.21 msec, QRS less than 130% of baseline.
5. TCAs may be contraindicated in children with prolonged QT intervals on baseline ECGs, and in children whose QT_c exceeds 0.425 to 0.450 seconds while on medication.
6. History should include review of the patient's cardiovascular system and family history of cardiac illnesses, unexplained syncope, or sudden death.

OTHER MEDICATIONS

Few studies have examined the efficacy of the nontricyclic antidepressants. No double-blind, placebo-controlled studies of fluoxetine treatment of childhood or adolescent depression were found. However, in a recent study of children and adolescents treated with fluoxetine for a variety of diagnoses, half the subjects experienced two or more of the following side effects: motor restlessness, sleep disturbances, social disinhibition, or a subjective sense of excitation (Riddle, King, et al., 1991). In all 12 of the children, these side effects were resolved within 2 weeks of discontinuation or decrease in drug dosage. More serious is the report of the emergence of intense self-injurious ideation or behavior among a group of 10- to 17-year-old boys and girls receiving fluoxetine for treatment of obsessive-compulsive disorder (King et al., 1991). One study also reported fluoxetine-induced mania in five adolescents being treated for depression (Venkataraman, Naylor, & King, 1992). As with TCAs, the risk factors for mania or hypomania included comorbid attention deficit hyperactivity disorder, affective instability, major depression with psychotic features, and self or family history of bipolar disorder.

SUMMARY

In summary, the research literature on drug treatment of major depression in children and adolescents is quite limited. Despite reports of successful open trials of antidepressant treatment for child and adolescent depression, those well-controlled studies that do exist have found little evidence of medication efficacy. In addition, there exist sporadic reports of serious adverse consequences of antidepressant treatment for children. Yet clinicians continue to prescribe these medications for children and adolescents with depression because there are serious sequelae of unremitting depression, and antidepressants do appear to help some children. It is therefore imperative that nurses be aware of the need for close monitoring of side effects, especially cardiovascular changes, hypomania, motor restlessness, sleep difficulties, and suicidal ideation.

ELECTROCONVULSIVE THERAPY

Although electroconvulsive therapy (ECT) has been used to treat depression in children as young as 5 years of age, few studies have been conducted, and no carefully controlled studies exist (Black, Wilcox, & Stewart, 1985). After reviewing case reports involving 10 youth with depression and 22 children and adolescents with bipolar disorders, Bertagnoli and Borchardt (1990) concluded that ECT is beneficial to children and adolescents with bipolar disorder and depression. They noted, however, that each of the reports based treatment response on the observer's clinical impression and that none of the reports included control groups, rigid diagnostic criteria, or outcome measures. Furthermore, a number of complications of ECT were reported, including a brief period of organic impairment (with mild impairment and disinhibition possibly persisting for a few months), anxiety reactions, and alteration of seizure thresholds. The authors suggest that much more research needs to be done, including studies of long-term follow-up, neuropsychological functioning following ECT, and controlled studies of medication nonresponders.

PHOTOTHERAPY

Recent recognition of the existence of seasonal affective disorder (SAD) has led to studies of the use of phototherapy for treatment of depression that fits the criteria for this diagnosis, namely, a seasonal pattern of recurrent major depression or bipolar disorder (Betrus & Elmore, 1991; Elmore, 1991). SAD has been reported in children (Mghir & Vincent, 1991; Rosenthal et al., 1986). The seven children and adolescents in these studies, aged 6 to 17, reported symptoms of sadness, irritability, and anxiety during the winter months and remission of symptoms during the summer. Additional symptoms included fatigue, sleep changes, appetite changes, carbohydrate cravings, headaches, and difficulties in school or in social relations. Both studies reported reversal of these symptoms during trials of phototherapy. Mghir and Vincent reported full relapse of symptoms during discontinuation of phototherapy and reversal of symptoms following resumption of treatment.

SLEEP DEPRIVATION

Because of the disruptions in circadian rhythms experienced by depressed adults, a number of studies have examined the utility of sleep deprivation as a treatment for depression (Wu & Bunney, 1990). Sleep deprivation has been used in a variety of ways: as an adjunct or alternative to antidepressant treatment, for example, to hasten the onset of action of antidepressant medications or to prevent recurrent mood cycles; as a diagnostic probe; and as a predictor of response to antidepressant medications or ECT (Liebenluft & Wehr, 1992). As with many studies of treatment for depression, there are inconsistent results and a number of methodological difficulties. In general, the adult studies show that partial late sleep deprivation (awake from 2 AM to 10 PM) is as effective as total sleep deprivation (awake for 36 hours) and more effective than early sleep deprivation (awake until 2 AM). Several controlled studies that examined the effect of sleep deprivation in hastening the onset of action of antidepressant medication and in preventing recurrent mood cycles were quite promising.

Only one study included a child (King, Baxter, Stuber, & Fish, 1987). An 11-year-old receiving imipramine improved following an initial night of partial sleep deprivation, but these gains were not consistently replicated in subsequent trials. Several methodological complications in this case study hinder clear interpretation of the findings.

Naylor et al. (1993) conducted the first standardized assessment of the effects of total sleep deprivation on depressed adolescents. The participants were kept awake for 36 hours, from 8 AM on day 1 to 8 PM on day 2. Severity of depression was assessed at 8 AM and 8 PM on days 1 and 2, and on day 3 following recovery sleep. Severely depressed adolescents showed significant decrease in depressive symptoms following sleep deprivation, while mildly depressed patients did not. Those with depression in remission and the nondepressed psychiatric controls increased in severity of depression following sleep deprivation. In contrast to adult studies in which the antidepressant effects were immediately reversible with any amount of sleep, the adolescents showed benefits for 3 to 5 days. The authors suggest that sleep deprivation may be an effective intervention for suicidal adolescents for whom a quick antidepressant response is necessary to minimize risk of suicide during treatment.

SUMMARY

Biological therapies, such as phototherapy for SAD and sleep deprivation, have been studied with adults, but only one or two small studies have been completed with children. Each of these studies indicated that children and adolescents responded positively to the treatments. Further research with children is needed before any recommendations can be drawn.

PSYCHOSOCIAL MODELS OF DEPRESSION

A number of psychosocial etiologic theories have been postulated for depressive disorders in adults. These models describe intrapsychic, interpersonal, behavioral, and/or cognitive contributions to the onset of depression. Although many of them have been used as both explanations of depressive phenomena in children and as rationales for treatment, few authors have clearly delineated the specific theoretical underpinnings for depression during childhood and adolescence. Each of these models has been described elsewhere (Brantly & Takacs, 1991; Kazdin, 1990) and will be only briefly reviewed.

PSYCHOANALYTIC MODELS

Psychoanalytic models of depression emphasize unsatisfied libidinal strivings and identification with harsh parental values as the precursors to the emergence of a punitive superego. The self-rejection and criticism that describe many persons with depression are viewed as a reflection of this punitive superego. Psychoanalysts further maintain that depression cannot occur in childhood because of the immaturity of the superego. In fact, Freud (cited in Kazdin, 1990) viewed self-criticism as stemming from anger and hostility toward the parent. Alternative psychoanalytic views suggested, however, that depression in adulthood was due to aggression turned toward the self, fixation at the oral stage, craving for narcissistic gratification, unsatisfied needs for affection, and repeated disappointments with parents during childhood (Kazdin, 1990).

Among the psychoanalysts most known for their work with children are Anna Freud, Melanie Klein, Margaret Mahler, and John Bowlby. Each of these theorists focused on developmental aspects of parent-child relations—specifically, *object loss*—as important contributors to childhood psychopathology (see Brantly & Takacs, 1991). With the exception of the vast research literature initially based on Bowlby's views of attachment, psychoanalytic theory has not generated much research; however, the notion that the experience of an early loss is a significant factor in depression has been empirically studied.

DEPRESSION AND LOSS

The experience of early loss of a significant person, specifically the mother, has been suggested as an important contributor to depression in adults (Bowlby, 1980); yet a relationship between loss and depression has been found in only some studies. Brown and his colleagues (Brown & Harris, 1978; Brown, Harris, & Bifulco, 1986) suggest that the inconsistencies in the research findings on loss and depression are due to faulty specification of the important variables for individuals experiencing a depressive episode that is precipitated by a current severe event involving loss. These include whether the individual is vulnerable to depression because of early experiences with loss or a current lack of social support. They view early loss and lack of social support as contextual variables that increase the risk of depression only in the presence of a severe precipitating event.

Gold et al. (1988b) suggest that this predisposition to become depressed as a result of early stressful experiences may be due to long-term changes in the responsivity of the central nervous system. They suggest that kindled limbic seizures or the sensitization of limbic substrates may account for many features of affective illness, such as gradual worsening of episodes over time and progressively shorter time lags between episodes. They describe a process of behavioral sensitization in which experimentally induced stress lowers the threshold for stimulation and can produce an increase in behavioral and neurochemical abnormalities in laboratory animals. Furthermore, lithium, which can block behavioral sensitization, is known to be effective in preventing depression in bipolar disorder. Others (Post et al., cited in Gold et al., 1988b) have suggested that sensitization to repeated stresses, such as painful separations, could have a role in the progression of recurrent affective disorders. Thus, what began as a psychoanalytic explanation for the relationship between early loss and later depression has found preliminary support in the neuroscience literature.

BEHAVIORAL MODELS

Behavioral models focus on problems in interacting with the environment. Different theorists have described these problems as stemming from inadequate levels of reinforcement, a lack of skill in gaining rewards, and faulty cognitions.

REINFORCEMENT

Several theorists have proposed that depression is due to reduced levels of positive reinforcement for an individual (Lewinsohn, 1974; Rehm, 1977). Reinforcement may be diminished by a lack of contact with previously rewarding persons or situations (i.e., a loss). Lewinsohn suggests that this reduction in reinforcement leads to passivity and diminished social interaction, which subsequently leads to more reduced levels of reinforcement and depression. Accordingly, the level of pleasant events must be increased to relieve the depression. It is assumed that the other symptoms of depression will remit when the level of positive reinforcement is sufficiently high.

Rehm's theory posits that the depressed individual's ability to self-monitor, evaluate performance, and reward the self for accomplishments is deficient. Depressed persons are viewed as having overly strict evaluation criteria that focus on negative performances and provide little reinforcement to themselves. For Rehm, the key to successful intervention for depression is in teaching individuals to monitor, recognize, and reward their own positive behaviors.

SOCIAL SKILLS

Other behaviorists posit poor or unpleasant interpersonal interactions as playing a central role in depression. In some cases, aversive interpersonal interactions and subsequent social withdrawal are assumed to be the result of poor social skills. Social skills deficits in the amount of interaction and in making friends, initiating conversation, and expressing affect have been demonstrated in depressed children (Kazdin, 1990). The treatment of choice for these difficulties is social skills training, consisting of instruction, modeling, behavioral rehearsal, feedback, and generalization training. When aversive interactions are due to parental inconsistency or marital conflict, training in parenting skills or family therapy are the treatments of choice. Parents may be taught a variety of approaches, including the use of reinforcers, negotiation with adolescents, and problem-solving techniques (Patterson, 1975; 1982).

COGNITIVE-BEHAVIORAL MODELS

Several theorists have proposed cognitive models of depression. A revision of the learned helplessness model of depression (Abramson, Seligman, & Teasdale, 1978) proposes that depression results from the person's expectations that behavior will not influence life events. The individual feels helpless, and thus depressed, as a result of faulty cognitive attributions about causal events. The depressed person attributes uncontrollable negative events to causes that are personal, stable, and global and attributes positive events to causes that are external, unstable, and specific. As a result, the depressed person is more likely to feel responsible for bad things that happen and not responsible for good things that happen. Further, self-blame arises from the belief that negative events are due to a lack of ability rather than to bad luck or lack of effort, while positive events are seen as being due to luck. The learned helplessness model has been supported in studies of children (Curry & Craighead, 1990; Seligman et al., 1984).

Beck's (1976) cognitive theory of depression focuses on cognitive distortions that reflect errors in judgment in interpreting the world. He emphasizes a *cognitive triad of depression*—negative views of oneself, the world, and the future—as the basis for affective, motivational, and behavioral symptoms of depression. Studies based on this model have shown that depressed children also have a negative view of themselves, the world, and the future (Worchel, Little, & Alcala, 1990). These negative cognitions have been found to mediate the relations between stressful life events and depression in youth (Hammen, 1988).

PSYCHOSOCIAL ASSESSMENTS

Although many clinical investigators utilize the DSM-IV diagnosis of major depression as the focus of treatment, others target specific behaviors or symptoms for intervention. For example, prior to the initiation of behavioral treatment, behavior therapists usually conduct a diagnostic assessment, followed by a baseline assessment of selected target symptoms. The target symptoms are reassessed frequently to determine change. Treatment is considered successful when the target symptom reaches a normal, or at least acceptable, level. Often, however, the diagnostic assessment is not repeated following intervention, thus preventing an assessment of whether the disorder has remitted, or whether treatment gains are limited to target behaviors.

Psychosocial assessments include observations, participant-observations, interviewing, and ratings by informants such as parents, teachers, and peers (Ollendick & Hersen, 1984; Schaefer & O'Connor, 1983). The specific assessment methods utilized depend on the specific psychosocial model guiding assessment and the age of the child or adolescent. Therapists oriented toward psychoanalysis and psychodynamic models are more likely to use play therapy assessments for young children and projective tests for adolescents. Behaviorists are more likely to observe parent-child and parent-adolescent interactions, focusing on contingencies in social interactions. Cognitive-behaviorists are more likely to assess attributions and negative cognitions.

TARGET SYMPTOM ASSESSMENT: SUICIDAL RISK

Of all the consequences of MDD in youth, suicide and suicide attempts are clearly the most serious. Suicide is the second leading cause of death for 15- to 24-year-olds (Rosenberg, Smith, Davidson, & Conn, 1987). The demographic picture of suicidality in youth is complex. For example, *suicide completers* are predominantly male, and their death rates increase into young adulthood (Earls, 1989), while *suicide attempters* are predominantly female, and the frequency of suicide attempts decreases with age. Female suicide attempters often later complete a suicidal act, however, so accurate assessment of risk is extremely important. Also, some accidental suicides may occur among youth who make a suicidal gesture but who misjudge the lethality of the act or are not discovered in time for intervention (Hawton, 1986).

Among the risk factors for suicidality identified in studies of heterogeneous diagnostic groups of adolescents are age, impulsive and aggressive behaviors, feelings of hopelessness and worthlessness, negative self-perceptions, recent stressful life events, inflexible parenting styles, family conflict, parental depression, and parental suicide (Myers et al., 1991; Valente, 1989). In addition, lack of social support, loss of a boyfriend, recent school changes, and recent sexual abuse have been associated with suicidal behavior among adolescent females (Pfeffer, Newcorn, Kaplan, Mizruchi, & Plutchik, 1988).

Although adolescent suicide is not specific to any particular diagnosis, it is clear that depression is an important risk factor (Kovacs et al., 1993; Myers et al., 1991; Rao et al., 1993). Ryan (Ryan, Puig-Antich, Ambrosini, et al., 1987) found that 26% of a sample of adolescents with MDD had attempted suicide within the current episode and that only 39% had no suicidal ideation. Several studies have examined the correlates of suicidal thoughts, attempts, and completions among adolescents with MDD. Myers et al. found that among 7- to 17-year-olds from both inpatient and outpatient mental health settings, conduct problems and extent of depressive thinking emerged as the most powerful predictors of suicidality among both the depressed and nondepressed groups. In a study of factors that may increase suicidal risk for hospitalized adolescents in addition to depressive illness (Brent, Kolko, Allan, & Brown, 1990), earlier onset, longer duration of affective illness, and greater self-rated depression characterized the suicidal group. In addition, suicidal depressed youth had more cognitive distortion, less assertiveness, more life stresses within the past year, and greater exposure to family suicidality. Among the patients who were admitted for an actual suicide attempt, severity of suicidal intent was related to having MDD superimposed on a pre-existing dysthymia, comorbid substance abuse or conduct disorder, family conflict, nonassertiveness, and family history of suicidality.

Impulsivity has often been identified as a risk factor for youth suicide and suicide attempts (Brown, Overholser, Spirito, & Fritz, 1991). Brown et al. examined the importance of planning in 12- to 17-year-old suicide attempters seen in a general hospital. They found that premeditative suicide attempters displayed higher levels of depression, hopelessness, and suicidal ideation than impulsive suicide attempters. Impulsive attempters were more likely to come from impoverished circumstances, while the premeditated group were from diverse economic backgrounds.

INSTRUMENTS

A number of instruments for the assessment of adolescent suicidal risk exist (Lewinsohn, Garrison, Langhinrichsen, & Marsteller, 1989). Most of these instruments measure suicidal ideas, while others are general diagnostic assessments that include items tapping suicidality. Two examples of specific scales are the *Scale for*

Suicide Ideation (SSI) (Beck, Kovacs, & Weissman, 1979) and the *Suicidal Ideation Questionnaire* (SIQ) (Reynolds, 1987). The SSI consists of 19 items designed to measure the intensity, pervasiveness, and characteristics of an individual's thoughts, plans, and wishes about suicide. Ratings are made by a trained interviewer on the basis of a semistructured interview. Two additional forms of the scale exist: a self-report form and a more structured interview form for use by paraprofessionals. All forms yield similar results and discriminate between suicide attempters and nonattempters (Lewinsohn et al., 1989).

The SIQ was designed as a screening instrument for assessing severity and frequency of suicidal ideation among middle and high school students. Respondents are asked to indicate on a seven-point scale "how often this thought was on my mind." Each version provides a single score for severity of suicidal ideation and critical items related to specific plans. Adequate reliability and validity have been reported. Lewinsohn et al. (1989) suggest that it is among the best screening instruments available but requires further information on sensitivity and specificity before recommending general use for nonresearch purposes.

PSYCHOSOCIAL INTERVENTIONS

There are few controlled studies of psychosocial interventions for children with depression. Psychosocial interventions for individual children encompass traditional verbal psychotherapies, play therapies, and behavioral and cognitive-behavioral treatments.

In a review of published reports of nonbehavioral child and adolescent psychotherapy, including play therapy, none of the studies focused on treatment of children or adolescents with MDD (Barnett, Docherty, & Frommelt, 1991). In addition, none met the need for rigorous research delineating which treatment procedures are effective with which types of patients, with what kinds of problems, and with what kind of therapist. Barnett et al. conclude that this body of literature cannot be summarized because of the magnitude of the flaws in basic psychotherapy research methodology.

BEHAVIORAL TREATMENT

Although reviews of behavioral and cognitive-behavioral therapies generally attest to their effectiveness in treating specific behavioral disorders in children (Barnett et al., 1991), there are even fewer studies of the psychological treatment of childhood depression than there are medication studies (Kazdin, 1989). In addition, the behavioral literature is marred by a preponderance of single-subject studies and by outcome criteria that do not specifically address the disorder of depression.

Most behavioral treatments for childhood depression have been modeled after treatments for adults and are derived from models of adult depression. Behavioral treatments include reinforcement models, social skills training models, cognitive-behavioral models, and parent training. There is little empirical evidence to guide clinicians in a choice of treatment methods. Although virtually all the studies comparing psychosocial treatment methods have found that depressive symptoms decreased in treated children compared to waiting list controls, significant differences among treatment methods have not been found (Kazdin, 1990).

Frame and Cooper (1993) suggest that the therapist attend to the apparent deficits in the child's behavioral repertoire and tailor interventions to the specific problem area. For children with several behavioral deficits, a levels-of-treatment approach (Winnett, Bornstein, Cogswell, & Paris, 1987) may be used. In this approach, treatments are categorized into four levels. Lower levels include direct reinforcement of appropriate behaviors and selective ignoring of depressive behaviors by therapist, parents, and other social agents. Higher levels represent greater complexity of treatment and greater degree of voluntary participation by the child, as well as the requirement of more advanced cognitive functioning and more training for generalization to other situations. Higher level treatments include social skills training, problem-solving training, and self-control training. The choice of appropriate strategy depends on the age and other characteristics of the child being treated, as well as on the ability of the parents to assist in the treatment.

BEHAVIORAL TREATMENT STUDIES

About half the existing research on behavioral treatment of childhood depression has utilized single-subject studies, including multiple-baseline designs. Most studies have utilized social skills training to modify depression-related behaviors and have produced promising results (e.g., Calpin & Cinciripini, 1978, cited in Kazdin, 1988). Several have examined social skills training in children who were also being treated with antidepressant medication (Petti, Bornstein, Delameter, & Connors, 1980; Schloss, Schloss, & Harris, 1984). Although specific depressive symptoms decreased, the concurrent use of medication clouds the interpretation of these effects.

Frame, Matson, Sonis, Fialkov, and Kazdin (1982) successfully utilized social skills training to reduce the depressive behaviors of a hospitalized 10-year-old boy. This study is notable in that the child had a DSM-III diagnosis of depression and was not being treated with psychotropic medications. The targets for change were inappropriate body position, lack of eye contact, poor speech quality, and bland affect. The treatment consisted of instruction, modeling, behavioral rehearsal, and performance feedback provided in daily individual therapy sessions over a 5-week period. The study utilized a multiple-baseline design across behaviors. Following an 8-week baseline period, appropriate target behaviors were taught, one at a time. Marked improvement was noted in each behavior after specific training was instituted, and treatment gains were maintained at a 3-month follow-up.

Despite the promising results, there are a number of limitations to these case studies. For example, none evaluated the children's impressions of improvement or their self-reports of depression following treatment, so it is unclear whether behavioral improvement was accompanied by reductions in subjective distress or remission of the depressive disorder.

Several group-outcome intervention studies with depressed youth in school settings have been reported (Butler, Miezitis, Friedman, & Cole, 1980; Kahn, Kehle, Jenson, & Clark, 1990; Reynolds & Coates, 1986; Stark, Reynolds, & Kaslow, 1987). Each compared at least two active treatments with a control condition and utilized children and adolescents with high self-reported depression. Most included random assignment to groups. Treatments examined in the different studies were social skills training, self-control training, relaxation training, behavioral problem-solving therapy, increasing reinforcement levels, cognitive-behavioral therapy, and self-modeling. All studies found that active treatments were superior to control conditions in decreasing the symptoms of depression, but none of the between-treatment comparisons were significantly different. In another study using a similar array of cognitive-behavioral interventions to treat clinically depressed adolescents (Lewinsohn, Clarke, Hops, & Andrews, 1990), there was a strong trend favoring combining a parent intervention with the group intervention for the adolescent. Treated participants improved significantly on the depression measures, and gains were maintained for 2 years.

Although the group treatment studies deal with several of the confounds in the case studies, they are also characterized by a number of problems. First, the participants were recruited from schools rather than from clinical populations. With the exception of Lewinsohn et al. (1990), participants were not assessed for a DSM or RDC diagnosis of depression. Thus, their success may be due to the characteristics of the samples and may not be generalizable to the very distressed children found in clinical populations. Furthermore, problems found in medication treatment studies may also plague behavioral treatment studies with clinical populations. For example, it might be difficult to demonstrate effectiveness of behavioral treatments for depressed children with comorbid conditions. Second, the numbers of subjects in the group treatment studies remain small, and results have not been replicated. Frame and Cooper (1993) suggested that several of the group studies themselves represent case-study methodology because treatments were provided to groups rather than to individuals. Had the statistical requirements for analyzing these data as cases been followed, there would have been an insufficient number of cases for analysis. Finally, the specificity of these treatments for depression, rather than general distress, has not been sufficiently demonstrated. Given the methodological difficulties, Kazdin (1990) concludes that psychological intervention studies of childhood depression lag behind pharmacotherapy trials.

TRANSACTIONAL MODELS AND NURSING

Both biological and psychosocial models of childhood depression are adaptations of models initially derived for adults. They are essentially linear models, which focus on single root causes. The genetic theories postulate that heredity causes depression, while the psychosocial theories essentially suggest that depression is caused either by adverse environments and experiences or by their effects on cognitions. Most contemporary researchers have abandoned this nature-nurture dichotomy in favor of discovering how each influences development and on how adverse outcomes come about and can be prevented. More often, theorists are espousing a transactional view that both children and their parents are shaped by their biological endowments and their social experiences with each other, and with contextual sources of stress and support (Belsky, 1984; Sameroff & Seifer, 1983). Individuals are seen as bringing certain competencies and risks to their interactions, and the outcome is viewed as the culmination of chronic and pervasive influences throughout their lives.

Transactional models often stress the self-righting and integrative tendencies of children as they attempt to adapt to environmental change, indicating that deviant development is the result of *continuous* malfunction in person-environment transactions over time (Sameroff & Chandler, 1975). Continuous malfunctions require a profound insult to the child's integrative capacities, from a serious neurological deficit or from adverse environmental influences present throughout development. Characteristics of children themselves have been found to buffer the effects of adverse environments. For example, studies of resilient children (Garmezy, 1987; Werner & Smith, 1982) have found that the ability to seek and find support from an adult outside the family, to engage in positive peer relations, and to develop a sense of self independent of the functioning of one's parents are characteristics that may protect the child from adverse outcomes associated with dysfunctional parenting.

Nurses have long recognized that how individuals develop depends on both their constitutional vulnerabilities and the risk factors present in their environments (Rose & Killian, 1983). Transactional models, like system models (Whall, 1991), take into account the biological, psychological, and social forces operating on children and families. From a transactional view, interventions that strengthen any of the positive biological or psychosocial influences—and limit any negative influences—will have reverberating, escalating, and continuous effects on children and their environments. Transactional models are beginning to be applied to the study of children of depressed parents, as these children are both genetically vulnerable and at environmental risk for depression.

Some investigators (e.g., Dodge, 1990; Hammen, Burge, & Stansbury, 1990; Miller, Birnbaum, & Durbin, 1990) have studied the etiology of childhood depression by focusing on intergenerational transmission. In general, studies of children of depressed mothers indicate an increased risk for problems in adjustment and psychopathology generally, and for clinical depression specifically (see Downey & Coyne, 1990, for a review). These difficulties are evident as early as infancy, and they emerge in reports of teachers and peers as well as in parent and self-reports. This finding has led researchers to examine environmental influences on children genetically at risk for depression.

Using Brown's (Brown et al, 1986) notions of increased *vulnerability* to depression as a result of early loss and increased *risk* as a function of precipitating negative life events, Miller et al. (1990) examined the impact of parental depression and adverse experiences in the lives of depressed children. They concluded that children of depressed parents experience both early loss (through the impaired family interactions of depressed parents) and direct precipitating negative events. The lives of families with *either* a depressed parent or a depressed child include more negative events and significantly less family support and resources. Family interactions of depressed children were found to be more negative than those of controls. Compared to parents of normal controls, parents of depressed children display less affection, exhibit less positive affect, set more stringent standards, and generally suppress self-expression and autonomy.

The relationship between depression in children and their parents may be the result of genetics, impaired parenting of depressed parents, or difficulties in the broader interpersonal context. In reviewing each of these possibilities, Downey and Coyne (1990) concluded that genetic models alone do not account for the incidence of depression in the offspring of depressed parents. A number of studies have found that depressed mothers' interactions with their children are characterized by lower rates of behavior and affective expression in general, and by the use of childrearing strategies such as coercion or withdrawal rather than negotiation. Depressed mothers respond less positively, less quickly, and less frequently to attention-seeking efforts of their children and are more likely to be hostile, irritable, and negative in their interactions with them.

Yet further review reveals that these parenting difficulties are not unique to clinically depressed parents. Rather, they are common to mothers who experience other stressors such as marital conflict, divorce, poverty, and physical or other psychiatric illnesses (Downey & Coyne, 1990; Goodman & Brumley, 1990; Gordon et al., 1989). There is still insufficient evidence to conclude that the parenting difficulties of depressed parents are a specific consequence of their depression (Downey & Coyne, 1990). In fact, Hammen et al. (1990) found a very complex pattern of causal influences in depressed mother-child relations, in which both children and mothers contributed to each other's unhappiness and distress and to the child's future outcome. Furthermore, Downey and Coyne noted data showing that marital conflict accounts for the relation between parental depression and children's disturbed behavior, and they assert that these data challenge the view that depression is transmitted intergenerationally through the parenting behavior of depressed mothers; instead, the data point to the need to look at the broader interpersonal context of maternal depression and the child's contribution to that context.

The impact of children on their depressed parents has been studied only recently. For example, children of depressed parents have more problems than children of normal parents and may be more difficult to parent. Hammen's (Hammen et al., 1990) findings of bidirectional influences between depressed mothers and their children are consistent with other studies (e.g., Barkley & Cunningham, 1979) that have found changes in mothers' parenting behaviors as a result of treatment of children's disorders. Others have found that mothers' depression declines with improvements in their children's behavior problems (Forehand, Wells, & Griest, 1980).

Finally, virtually all the studies of parent-child relations and depression examine mother-child relations. There is a great need for studies examining father-child relations in families in which a child or parent is depressed.

SUMMARY

A large number of models of the etiology of childhood depression exist, yet most have generated little research. Although the evidence for a genetic basis for depression is strong, the preponderance of the evidence suggests that depression is multidetermined. Adverse environmental influences, in addition to genetic vulnerability to depression, appear to best explain the incidence of major depressive disorder in both adults and children. Transactional models that take into account the characteristics of both parents and children—and their mutual influences on each other—may best fit the data on etiology of depression in childhood and adolescence. For the most part, transactional models have not been tested directly in families in which a child is depressed.

NURSING DIAGNOSES AND BEHAVIORAL TARGETS OF INTERVENTION

In assessing the biopsychosocial needs of depressed children and their families, nurses utilize transactional models. Nursing diagnoses typically represent specific responses to areas of alteration or impairment of functioning in both the child and family. These areas of concern are not unique to depression, however, and therefore may be considered examples of specific target behavior assessments rather than psychiatric diagnostic assessments. The psychiatric nursing literature contains examples of both the North American Nursing Diagnosis Association (NANDA) nursing diagnostic system and the American Nurses Association Psychiatric–Mental Health (PMH) Nursing Classification System of Human Responses (O'Toole & Loomis, 1989) for assessing nursing problems of adults with depressive disorders. West and Pothier (1989) discussed the utility of the PMH human response classification system with a school-age child, while Coler (1989) has suggested combining NANDA and DSM-III-R diagnoses for child psychiatric nursing.

Because nursing diagnoses currently are made independently of DSM-IV diagnoses, there is no specific subset of diagnoses that is uniquely appropriate for children or adolescents with depression. Indeed, because of the variability in manifestations of depression in youth, it is not possible to completely predict nursing diagnoses for depressed children from those of depressed adults. Further, the meaning of specific behaviors, alterations, impairments, or human responses may differ depending upon age, psychiatric diagnosis, and treatment (e.g., whether it includes medication for depression). As a result, psychiatric nurses often utilize nursing diagnoses in the context

Table 9–5. Selected Nursing Diagnoses for Children and Adolescents with Depression

Anxiety	Noncompliance
Communication, impaired verbal	Nutrition, altered
Coping, ineffective individual	Self-esteem disturbance
Family processes, altered	Sleep pattern disturbance
Fatigue	Social interaction, impaired
Grieving, dysfunctional	Social isolation
Growth and development, altered	Thought processes, altered
Hopelessness	Violence, potential for self-directed
Knowledge deficit	

of DSM-IV diagnoses before identifying appropriate nursing interventions. For example, hyperphagia, an alteration in nutrition, has different meanings for adolescents with depression, seasonal affective disorders, or bulimia, and requires different interventions. Table 9–5 includes several of the most common nursing diagnoses for problems emanating from depression (Doenges, Townsend, & Moorhouse, 1988).

There have been no empirical articles addressing the utility of these nursing diagnoses for children and adolescents with major depression. Indeed, Scahill (1991) suggests that nursing diagnoses may not be as efficient and effective in indicating appropriate nursing interventions for child psychiatric inpatients as is multidisciplinary goal-oriented treatment planning.

In summary, the use of nursing diagnoses with children and adolescents leaves much to be desired. Currently, there are at least two systems of nomenclature, and the relation between nursing diagnosis and intervention is unexplored for depressed youth. There is essentially no empirical nursing literature on assessment or treatment of children with depression. Nursing diagnoses that are appropriate for depressed adults might be appropriate for children and should probably be utilized until further information about the prevalence of nursing problems in children with depression is available. The need for studies on nursing assessment and diagnosis of depressed youth is critical.

Nursing Interventions

Nursing interventions focus on treating responses to actual or potential health problems. Thus, nurses utilize knowledge gained from both biological and psychosocial research in planning interventions for depressed youth and their families. The problems that plague the research on assessment and complicate both biomedical and psychosocial treatments for depression in children and adolescents also make recommendations of nursing interventions difficult. First, there are *no* published empirical studies of the efficacy of specific nursing interventions for children with depression. Second, the literature that has been reviewed demonstrates major differences in the responses of adults and children with depression. Findings from studies of biological correlates, patterns of symptoms, and responses to medications indicate that children and adolescents differ from adults in a number of ways that may influence their nursing care. Despite these differences, there are enough commonalities that we can derive some tentative suggestions from the empirical literature and from nursing care of depressed adults (Bradley-Corpuel, 1992; Doenges et al., 1988; Sipple, 1992) for use with children and youth. Table 9–6 summarizes nursing interventions for selected nursing problems of depressed children and youth.

TABLE 9–6. NURSING INTERVENTIONS FOR CHILDREN AND ADOLESCENTS WITH MAJOR DEPRESSION

NURSING INTERVENTION	RATIONALE
Potential for Self-directed Violence	
Arrange therapeutic environment to promote safety. Remove potentially harmful objects, including sharp items, poisons, mirrors, and belts. Explain rationale to patient.	Adolescents with depression or comorbid conduct disorder or who are substance abusers are at high risk for suicide. Suicide is the third leading cause of death among persons 15 to 24 years old.
Observe closely for self-destructive behaviors. Supervise closely according to level of suicide precautions (every 10 to 15 minutes to constant observation).	Suicide by children or adolescents is often impulsive, but may be planned.
Ask about suicidal thoughts, plans, actions, and friends or family who committed suicide.	Youth who have a close friend or relative who attempted or completed suicide are at increased risk for suicide.
Observe for changes in mood, activity level, and statements about leaving.	As energy increases and hypersomnia decreases, the risk of suicide increases.
Observe closely when administering medications.	Children and adolescents may "save up" medications to attempt suicide.
Teach parents to identify signs of depression, risk factors, and stressors that may precipitate a suicide attempt. Teach parents to recognize the seriousness of any suicidal idea, threat, or act.	Parents may dismiss suicidal ideas or gestures because of denial or because of the adolescent's keeping thoughts private. Parents have been found to underestimate the degree of depression of their children. Children's and adolescents' self-reports of depression are correlated with suicide attempts.
Knowledge Deficit Related to Depression and Treatment	
Teach youth and parents about biology of depression.	Explanations centering on biology may interrupt the child's or adolescent's tendency to self-blame. Parents' recognition of early signs of depression may lead to earlier intervention and treatment of recurrence.
Teach youth and parents to observe for therapeutic actions of medications, side effects, and serious adverse effects.	Knowledge encourages child or adolescent and parent to collaborate on a plan for medication use and periodic medication evaluations by a psychiatrist.
Teach parents recommended monitoring guidelines for specific medication. Discuss ECG, blood work, and blood pressure monitoring schedules. Teach about procedures for laboratory tests.	Antidepressant medications have been associated with deaths of several prepubertal children. Frequent monitoring of ECGs and vital signs at increasing doses is recommended.
Teach child or adolescent using principles of learning and child development. Teach parents principles of child or adolescent development and effective parenting strategies.	Ability of children to think abstractly is limited. Compliance and self-esteem may be enhanced by having child participate in the treatment plan.
Administer biological interventions. Observe child's or adolescent's responses to biological therapies.	Children's and adolescents' responses to biological therapies may differ from typical adult responses.

Table continued on following page.

TABLE 9–6. NURSING INTERVENTIONS FOR CHILDREN AND ADOLESCENTS WITH MAJOR DEPRESSION *Continued*

NURSING INTERVENTION	RATIONALE
Sleep Pattern Disturbance	
Observe for changes in hours of sleep and pattern of sleep.	Prepubertal children may sleep less when depressed, while adolescents often sleep more than usual. Circadian rhythms are disturbed in depression, but consistent sleep difficulties have been found only in late adolescence.
Limit caffeine-containing beverages in late afternoon or evening. Teach relaxation exercises. Encourage physical activity (e.g., walking or exercise) during the day.	Difficulty in falling asleep may be due to over stimulation or anxiety, or to inactivity.
Discourage napping during the early part of the day. May utilize altered sleep pattern to readjust circadian rhythms and possibly ameliorate depression. Teach parents and children/adolescents about changes in sleep cycles with depression.	Sleeping from 5 PM to 2 AM has been found to produce remission of depression in some adults. Sleep deprivation from 2 AM to 10 PM has been found to hasten the onset of efficacy of antidepressants in adults.
Altered Nutrition	
Observe for decreased appetite or failure to make expected gains in weight. Observe for cravings for carbohydrates and effects of high carbohydrate meals on mood and energy.	Changes in appetite may lead to reduced growth and weight gain in children and adolescents. Adults with SAD have been shown to respond atypically to high carbohydrate meals (with increased energy and more positive mood).
Provide attractive balanced meals with sufficient protein and vitamins, fiber, and fluid intake.	Fiber and fluids may prevent constipation due to inactivity and antidepressant medications.
Self-Esteem Disturbance	
Assist children and adolescents to identify negative thoughts about the self as they occur.	Negative thoughts and attributions are often "automatic" cognitive symptoms of depression.
Assist youth in distinguishing important and unimportant areas of performance. Assist in setting realistic standards for performance in important areas.	Depressed youth are often realistic about the *quality* of their performance, but unrealistic in the *standards* they set (e.g., extremely high achievement in all areas).
Assist in identifying progress toward goals. Do not use global reassurance.	Depressed youth often discount accomplishments and reassurance and notice only perceived failures.
Assist in reframing and problem-solving approaches for unmet goals.	Cognitive therapy approaches have been successfully used with depressed youth.
Set up positive contingencies for meeting realistic goals.	Depressed youth are prone to punish, but not reward, self.
Teach positive parenting practices to parents, including rewarding children with attention, warmth, and tangible rewards, setting realistic limits, and using nonhostile interactions when negative consequences are used.	Depressed youth often get fewer rewards. Lack of rewarding experiences may underlie depression. Positive parenting practices are associated with higher self-esteem. Hostile interactions are associated with diminished self-esteem.

TABLE 9–6. NURSING INTERVENTIONS FOR CHILDREN AND ADOLESCENTS WITH MAJOR DEPRESSION *Continued*

NURSING INTERVENTION	RATIONALE
Impaired Social Interaction	
Utilize behavioral methods such as instruction, modeling, behavioral rehearsal, and performance feedback to enhance social skills.	Enhanced social skills may lead to more rewarding social interactions.
Utilize group interventions in conjunction with social skills training.	Practicing social skills with peers on a real group task has been found to be more effective in fostering positive peer relations than has social skills training alone.
Utilize activities of daily living to foster positive social interactions (e.g., meals, recreation times, school projects) during hospitalization. Assist parents to set up a behavior modification system for rewarding positive peer and sibling interactions.	Utilizing natural opportunities for using social skills fosters generalization to new settings.

SAFETY

The highest priority is always patient safety. Although suicide is rare among prepubertal children, both children and adolescents should be assessed for suicide potential. Adolescents with comorbid depression and conduct disorder are at increased risk. In most hospital settings, suicide precautions include very close supervision, varying from 15-minute checks to one-to-one observation, depending on the degree of assessed risk. The nurse should routinely check for potentially hazardous objects and ensure that medications are swallowed. Impulse control should also be assessed for all youths who have thoughts of self-injury.

Safety is also an important area of concern for children receiving medications. Vital signs should be checked frequently, and any unusual pulse or blood pressure should be reported immediately—especially after an increase in dosage. It is particularly important to distinguish between the common depressive symptom of somatic complaints and signs of adverse effects of medication. Children taking fluoxetine should be carefully monitored for complaints of restlessness, sleep disturbances, or thoughts of self-injury. Any physical complaints by children taking tricyclics should also be investigated, and children should be observed for evidence of anticholinergic side effects of tricyclics because their presence or absence may provide clues to how children are absorbing and utilizing these drugs. Since researchers have found little evidence that tricyclics are more effective than placebo in the treatment of childhood depression, nurses should be especially vigilant in assessing and reporting signs of medication efficacy. Nursing observations should include specific information on each target behavior, especially eating, sleeping, activities, peer interactions, presence of negative thoughts, and suicidal ideas.

SLEEP

Children and adolescents should be carefully observed for alterations in sleep patterns and subsequent levels of depression. Patterns of sleep alteration with depression in children and adolescents may differ markedly from those in adults. Hypersomnia rather than insomnia is common among adolescents. We could find no data to support either a recommendation that adolescents with hypersomnia be allowed to sleep throughout the day, or that they be awakened at a regular time and provided a regular schedule of activities. Still, supportive measures that promote sleep should be considered, for example, a regular pattern of exercise (as energy level permits) and milk prior to bedtime (because of its tryptophan content) (Nihart, 1993). In addition, for youth receiving therapeutic trials of sleep deprivation, nurses must be available to provide support and distraction during the night. All children and adolescents with depression should also be assessed for diurnal variation in mood. This is an important marker for positive response to therapeutic sleep alteration in adults but does not always accompany childhood depression.

NUTRITION

Nutritional assessment should include not only weight loss but whether the child has gained as much weight as expected for her age. Cravings for carbohydrates and evidence of positive or negative effects on mood and energy should also be noted. Meals should be attractive and balanced, providing sufficient protein, carbohydrates, and sources of vitamins to promote growth and weight gain. In addition, diet should include sufficient fluids and fiber because of the potential for elimination problems as a result of decreased activity and side effects of medications.

COGNITIONS AND SOCIAL SKILLS

Psychosocial interventions for children and adolescents must take into account their negative self-schemas, cognitive distortions, and attribution errors. Helping depressed youths identify misperceptions and negative thoughts may interrupt and decrease their negative views (Bednar, Wells, & Peterson, 1989; Stuart & Sundeen, 1991). For example, such thoughts can be identified as symptoms of depression by using comments like, "It's hard to think that you'll ever feel better, but this is a symptom of clinical depression, and it does get better when the depression lifts." Clinicians should avoid trying to raise the self-esteem of depressed youth through vague reassurance. Rather, they have a better chance of influencing children's and adolescents' self-views if they help the children and adolescents notice real progress and have a positive affective tone in interactions with them (Killeen, 1992). Children and young adolescents have a great deal of difficulty holding both positive and negative views of the self and others. Unlike youth with high self-esteem, those with low self-esteem have difficulty discounting the importance of areas in which they do not perform well (Harter, 1986). Nurses can assist in identifying which areas of competence are important and which are relatively unimportant. Nurses can also help depressed youth increase the level of rewards in their daily lives by helping them to set realistic goals and arrange positive contingencies.

Nurses should attend to promoting cognitive and social development as well as physical growth. For example, children and adolescents should be fully informed about their care, and they should be given the opportunity to make decisions within the rules of the hospital, clinic, or school setting. They should also have opportunities to discuss their perceptions of events and be guided through a problem-solving approach. Discussion of alternatives, potential consequences of events, and opportunities to practice interactions can assist children and adolescents to develop skill in problem solving and can increase their sense of self-efficacy (Bandura, 1977). The fact that negative feelings often occur in a social context provides an opportunity for teaching social skills; they should be accepted and discussed within the framework of problem solving.

FAMILY EDUCATION

Consistent with a transactional model, nurses emphasize the importance of family and patient education. Parents are often the "therapists" for children and adolescents receiving behavioral treatments. They should be taught age-appropriate parenting strategies, especially the use of positive reinforcements, and should be clearly instructed regarding the nature and course of depression, signs of potential relapse, and warning signs of suicidal behavior (Brent, Poling, McKain, & Baugher, 1993). Providing information about etiology of depression can help prevent parents from blaming themselves for their child's illness. Parents also administer medications and must be aware of potential adverse reactions. Most important, parents should be given a number to call if they are concerned about an adverse reaction to medications or their child's or adolescent's potential for self-injurious behavior. Also important are referral to support groups such as the National Alliance for the Mentally Ill and provision of educational materials for parents.

IMPLICATIONS FOR NURSING RESEARCH AND EDUCATION

Despite the fact that there have been hundreds of studies on depression during childhood and adolescence, there remain many unanswered questions. Chief among these are questions related to effective nursing interventions for depressed children and youth. What is needed to address these questions is a cadre of psychiatric nurse researchers with sufficient background in both biomedical and psychosocial research on depression and in developmental psychopathology, as well as expertise in psychiatric nursing interventions. Several authors have discussed ways in which psychiatric nurses with these areas of expertise might be educated (e.g., Killeen, 1990; McBride, 1990; McEnany, 1991).

Efforts should begin at the undergraduate level. First, the role of the nurse in caring for youth with mental illnesses must be emphasized (McBride, 1990). Nursing programs have done an excellent job of emphasizing mental health promotion and prevention of serious mental health problems. However, the typical undergraduate psychiatric nursing course devotes very little time to serious mental disorders in children. There are very few guidelines for nursing care of children with depression, and none are the product of carefully controlled studies of nursing interventions. For example, there is no empirically based guideline for structuring sleep or activity policies for depressed adolescent inpatients. Similarly, there is little guidance for dietary interventions. There must be a dual commitment to teaching what is known about physiological aspects of depression with adults and potential differences with children, and a challenge to students to test nursing interventions for children with diagnosed mental disorders. The connections between research findings on the physiology and psychology of depressive disorders and specific nursing measures in caring for children and adolescents must be made explicit in undergraduate nursing courses.

Much more emphasis must be placed on findings from research in undergraduate psychiatric nursing courses, but the major changes must occur in graduate programs if we are to produce faculty who can teach these principles and a cadre of researchers to test nursing interventions. Both doctoral and master's degree programs must emphasize the need for clinical nursing interventions and clinical nursing research and must provide the foundation for this clinical focus through coursework on biological and psychological correlates of mental disorders. Rather than emphasizing psychotherapy skills, master's programs might focus on graduating clinicians with expert assessment skills and detailed knowledge of applying biological and psychosocial research findings to children with diagnosed mental disorders. Coursework in assessment issues across the life span, pathophysiology of mental disorders, and empirically based psychopathology would help to lay the foundation for nursing assessments and interventions. Strengths and weaknesses of clinical interviews, laboratory findings, and diagnostic instruments should be included at all levels of the curriculum in psychiatric nursing.

Finally, a clear listing of the nursing problems or diagnoses and specific interventions in the context of diagnosed mental disorders is important. Psychiatric nurses can no more ignore the implications of specific psychiatric diagnoses, such as MDD, than medical nurses can ignore the implications of diagnoses such as diabetes mellitus. DSM-IV diagnoses are utilized by all disciplines who care for psychiatric clients. These diagnoses are imperfect, but they can convey substantial information about the clinical course and potentially effective treatments. As nurses develop interventions based on understanding the relationships among behavioral symptoms, pathophysiology, and psychopathology, guidelines for interventions should become more specifically related to the nursing diagnosis and the diagnosed mental disorder. Abraham et al. (1992) have argued that increasing biological knowledge will expand the opportunities for psychiatric nursing. They illustrate the kinds of biopsychosocial interventions that nurses can undertake and argue that true biopsychosocial integration will lead to development of holistic and multidisciplinary care.

The body of research reported here also points to the direction that doctoral education should take to prepare researchers in child psychiatric nursing. There should be a focus on preparing scholars to pursue research on psychiatric nursing interventions, with an emphasis on the biomedical and psychological underpinnings of nursing practice. Gross, Fogg, and Conrad (1993) described four sources of information for developing a strong theoretical and empirical foundation for nursing interventions. These include an explicit theory for the intervention, supporting descriptive data, preliminary evaluation of potential interventions consistent with the theory and descriptive data, and the use of focus groups to examine the feasibility and generality of the intervention.

In addition, developmental research, particularly studies addressing issues derived from transactional models, is needed. Cantwell (1990) has reviewed the existing literature on the developmental course of depression in children and youth and has identified the research issues that must be addressed to assess the links among depressive phenomena across different age ranges. These issues are also relevant for studies of nursing interventions. Researchers must concern themselves with the accuracy of the diagnosis in the index sample. Valid and reliable operational criteria must be used. The characteristics of the index sample (e.g., inpatients, outpatients, or children with comorbid conditions) and the comparison groups (normal or psychiatric controls) must be chosen carefully, so that the findings are generalizable to other populations. The time frame for follow-up assessment is another important consideration. Some studies may follow children or adolescents into adulthood, while others may be interested in shorter-term development and outcomes. Finally, the choice of intervening variables and strategies for measuring them is particularly problematic because many instruments that are useful for assessment of children may be inappropriate for adults.

In addition, because nursing care so often focuses on the family, studies are needed that explore the links between family processes–child outcomes and depression in youth-family outcomes. Although nurses typically focus their interventions on all family members, psychiatric nursing research has not often identified the effects of interventions on specific outcomes for family members. Research similar to Barnard's (Barnard, Snyder, & Spietz, 1991; Bee, Hammond, Eyres, Barnard, & Snyder, 1986) and Austin's (1988), which take into account family transactions, is needed for children with depression.

SUMMARY

This chapter reviewed existing research on the biology and psychology of childhood depression, its treatment, and nursing care. Despite the ubiquitous tendency to adapt adult-focused interventions to children, the research indicates that major differences exist between children and adults in the biological correlates of depression, symptoms, and responses to biological treatments. Research issues related to assessment and diagnosis were explored, and the need for programmatic research in nursing care of childhood depression was emphasized. Implications for nursing education and research were explored.

CASE STUDY

Eleven-year-old Mitch was referred by his family nurse practitioner to the child psychiatry clinic. He was subsequently admitted to the child unit of a private psychiatric hospital for evaluation. Mitch's mother had become concerned about his behavior over the last 6 months. Mitch had increasingly come home directly from school and had stopped going out to play with his friends. He was taking frequent naps in the afternoons and evenings, was eating poorly, and was often irritable. Mitch had complained of headaches and stomachaches and often asked to stay home from school because he "just didn't feel well." On his last report card, his grades had dropped considerably. He explained the poor report by saying he "just wasn't smart enough to do better."

During the admission interview, it was learned that Mitch's parents had divorced over a year ago, and his father had moved to a neighboring city. Mitch and his older brother spent every other weekend with their father. Family history revealed that Mitch's mother had been treated for depression with fluoxetine 2 years ago.

During the first few days on the child unit, Mitch continued to eat little and to sleep 12 hours a night. He often returned to his room during the day "for naps" and had to be continually encouraged to attend the school program and other activities. Neurological examination was normal. Neuropsychological assessment found Mitch to be above average in intelligence and without evidence of learning disability or other neuropsychological impairment. He was diagnosed as having a major depressive episode. The presence of a severe psychosocial stressor (parents' divorce) was noted.

A baseline electrocardiogram (ECG) was normal. Vital signs were: BP 104/70; P 76; R 20. Weight 36 kg, Height 145 cm.

Treatment plan included:

1. Imipramine 25 mg b.i.d. PO for 1 week, gradually increasing to 50 mg b.i.d. Monitor ECG with each dose increase, and monitor plasma level of imipramine at regular intervals.
2. *Coping with Divorce* group attendance for Mitch.
3. Individual cognitive-behavioral therapy for Mitch.
4. Family education program on depression for Mitch, his mother, father, and brother.
5. Social skills group following discharge, if indicated.

Mitch was discharged from the hospital after 3 weeks, following stabilization of his medication dosage and improvement in his ability to attend to schoolwork and engage in activities on the unit. He continued weekly group therapy and biweekly medication checks for 3 months as an outpatient. Over the 3 months there was a gradual decrease in depressive symptoms and increase in activity. Medications were gradually withdrawn after 6 months, with no recurrence of symptoms.

REFERENCES

Abraham, I. L., Fox, J. C., & Cohen, B. T. (1992). Integrating the bio into the biopsychosocial: Understanding and treating biological phenomena in psychiatric–mental health nursing. *Archives of Psychiatric Nursing, 6,* 296–305.

Abramson, L. Y., Seligman, M. E., & Teasdale, J. D. (1978). Learned helplessness in humans: Critique and reformulation. *Journal of Abnormal Psychology, 87,* 49–74.

Ambrosini, P. J., Bianchi, M. D., Rabinovich, H., & Elia, J. (1993a). Antidepressant treatments in children and adolescents: I. Affective disorders. *Journal of the American Academy of Child and Adolescent Psychiatry, 32,* 1–6.

Ambrosini, P. J., Bianchi, M. D., Rabinovich, H., & Elia, J. (1993b). Antidepressant treatments in children and adolescents: II. Anxiety, physical, and behavioral disorders. *Journal of the American Academy of Child and Adolescent Psychiatry, 32,* 483–493.

American Psychiatric Association. (1987). *Diagnostic and statistical manual of mental disorders* (3rd ed. rev.). Washington, DC: Author.

American Psychiatric Association. (1994). *Diagnostic and statistical manual of mental disorders* (4th ed.). Washington, DC: Author.

Anderson, J. C., Williams, S., McGee, R., & Silva, P. A. (1987). DSM-III-R disorders in preadolescent children: Prevalence in a large sample from the general population. *Archives of General Psychiatry, 44,* 69–76.

Angold, A., & Rutter, M. (1992). Effects of age and pubertal status on depression in a large clinical sample. *Development and Psychopathology, 4,* 5–28.

Angold, A., Weissman, M., John, K., Merikangas, K. R., et al. (1987). Parent and child reports of depressive symptoms in children at low and high risk of depression. *Journal of Child Psychology and Psychiatry and Allied Disciplines, 28,* 901–915.

Austin, J. K. (1988). Childhood epilepsy: Child adaptation and family resources. *Journal of Child and Adolescent Psychiatric and Mental Health Nursing, 1,* 18–24.

Bandura, A. (1977). Self-efficacy: Toward a unifying theory of behavioral change. *Psychological Review, 84,* 191–215.

Barkley, R. A., & Cunningham, C. E. (1979). The effects of methylphenidate on the mother-child interactions of hyperactive children. *Archives of General Psychiatry, 36,* 201–208.

Barnard, K., Snyder, C., & Spietz, A. (1991). Supportive measures for high-risk infants and families. In A. L. Whall & J. Fawcett (Eds.), *Family theory development in nursing* (pp. 139–178). Philadelphia: Davis.

Barnett, R. J., Docherty, J. P., & Frommelt, G. M. (1991). A review of child psychotherapy research since 1963. *Journal of the American Academy of Child and Adolescent Psychiatry, 30,* 1–14.

Beck, A. T. (1976). *Cognitive therapy and the emotional disorders.* New York: International Universities Press.

Beck, A. T., Kovacs, M., & Weissman, A. (1979). Assessment of suicidal intention: The Scale for Suicide Ideation. *Journal of Consulting and Clinical Psychology, 47,* 343–352.

Bednar, R. L., Wells, M. G., & Peterson, S. R. (1989). *Self-esteem: Paradoxes and innovations in clinical theory and practice.* Washington, DC: American Psychological Association.

Bee, H. L., Hammond, M. A., Eyres, S. J., Barnard, K. E., & Snyder, C. (1986). The impact of parental life change on the early development of children. *Research in Nursing and Health, 9,* 65–74.

Belsky, J. (1984). The determinants of parenting: A process model. *Child Development, 55,* 83–96.

Bernstein, G. A. (1991). Comorbidity and severity of anxiety and depressive disorders in a clinic sample. *Journal of the American Academy of Child and Adolescent Psychiatry, 30,* 43–50.

Bertagnoli, M. W., & Borchardt, C. M. (1990). Case study: A review of ECT for children and adolescents. *Journal of the American Academy of Child and Adolescent Psychiatry, 29,* 302–307.

Betrus, P. A., & Elmore, S. K. (1991). Seasonal affective disorder: 1. A review of the neural mechanisms for psychosocial nurses. *Archives of Psychiatric Nursing, 5,* 357–364.

Biederman, J., Baldessarini, R. J., Goldblatt, A., Lapey, K. A., Dolye, A., & Hesslein, P. S. (1993). A naturalistic study of 24-hour electrocardiographic recordings and echocardiographic findings in children and adolescents treated with desipramine. *Journal of the American Academy of Child and Adolescent Psychiatry, 32,* 805–813.

Birmaher, B., Dahl, R., Ryan, N. D., Rabinovich, H., Ambrosini, P., Al-Shabbout, M., Novacenko, H., Nelson, B., & Puig-Antich, J. (1992). The dexamethasone suppression test in adolescent outpatients with major depressive disorder. *American Journal of Psychiatry, 149,* 1040–1045.

Birmaher, B., Ryan, N. D., Dahl, R., Rabinovich, H., Ambrosini, P., Williamson, D. E., Novacenko, H., Nelson, B., Lo, E. S., & Puig-Antich, J. (1992). Dexamethasone suppression test in children with major depressive disorder. *Journal of the American Academy of Child and Adolescent Psychiatry, 31,* 291–297.

Black, D., Wilcox, J., & Stewart, M. (1985). The use of ECT in children: Case report. *Journal of Clinical Psychiatry, 46,* 98–99.

Bowlby, J. (1980). *Attachment and loss: Vol. 3. Loss: Sadness and Depression.* New York: Basic.

Bradley-Corpuel, C. (1992). Applying the nursing process with adolescents. In H. S. Wilson & C. R. Kneisl (Eds.), *Psychiatric nursing* (4th ed.) (pp. 839–866). Redwood City, CA: Addison-Wesley.

Brandenburg, N. A., Friedman, R. M., & Silva, S. E. (1990). The epidemiology of childhood psychiatric disorders: Prevalence findings from recent studies. *Journal of the American Academy of Child and Adolescent Psychiatry, 29,* 76–83.

Brantly, D. K., & Takacs, D. J. (1991). Anxiety and depression in preschool and school-aged children. In P. Clunn (Ed.), *Child psychiatric nursing* (pp. 351–365). St. Louis: Mosby.

Brent, D. A., Kolko, D. J., Allan, M. J., & Brown, R. V. (1990). Suicidality in affectively disordered adolescent inpatients. *Journal of the American Academy of Child and Adolescent Psychiatry, 29,* 586–593.

Brent, D. A., Poling, K., McKain, B., & Baugher, M. (1993). A psychoeducational program for families of affectively ill children and adolescents. *Journal of the American Academy of Child and Adolescent Psychiatry, 32,* 770–774.

Brown, G. W., & Harris, T. O. (1978). *Social origins of depression.* New York: Free Press.

Brown, G. W., Harris, T. O., & Bifulco, A. (1986). Long term effects of early loss of parent. In M. Rutter, C. E. Izard, & P. B. Read (Eds.), *Depression in young people: Developmental and clinical perspectives* (pp. 251–296). New York: Guilford.

Brown, L. K., Overholser, J., Spirito, A., & Fritz, G. K. (1991). The correlates of planning in adolescent suicide attempts. *Journal of the American Academy of Child and Adolescent Psychiatry, 30,* 95–99.

Burke, P., & Puig-Antich, J. (1990). Psychobiology of childhood depression. In M. Lewis & S. M. Miller (Eds.), *Handbook of developmental psychopathology* (pp. 327–339). New York: Plenum.

Butler, L., Miezitis, S., Friedman, R., & Cole, E. (1980). The effect of two school-based intervention programs on depressive symptoms in preadolescents. *American Educational Research Journal, 17,* 111–119.

Cadoret, R. J., Gorman, T. W., Heywood, E., & Troughton, E. (1985). Genetic and environmental factors in major depression. *Journal of Affective Disorders, 9,* 155–164.

Cantwell, D. (1988). DSM-III studies. In M. Rutter, A. H. Tuma, & I. S. Lann (Eds.), *Assessment and diagnosis in child psychopathology* (pp. 3–36). New York: Guilford.

Cantwell, D. (1990). Depression across the early life span. In M. Lewis & S. M. Miller (Eds.), *Handbook of developmental psychopathology* (pp. 311–325). New York: Plenum.

Carlson, G. A., & Cantwell, D. P. (1980). Unmasking masked depression in children and adolescents. *American Journal of Psychiatry, 137,* 445–449.

Casat, C. D., Arana, G. W., & Powell, K. (1989). The DST in children and adolescents with major depressive disorders. *American Journal of Psychiatry, 146,* 503–507.

Coler, M. (1989). Diagnoses for child and adolescent psychiatric nursing: Combining NANDA and the DSM III-R. *Journal of Child and Adolescent Psychiatric Mental Health Nursing, 2,* 115–122.

Costello, E. J., Edelbrock, C. A., & Costello, A. J. (1985). Validity of the NIMH Diagnostic Interview Schedule for Children: A comparison between psychiatric and pediatric referrals. *Journal of Abnormal Child Psychology, 13,* 579–595.

Curry, J. F., & Craighead, W. E. (1990). Attributional style in clinically depressed and conduct disordered adolescents. *Journal of Consulting and Clinical Psychology, 58,* 109–115.

Cytryn, L., & McKnew, D. H. (1974). Factors influencing the changing clinical expression of the depressive process in children. *American Journal of Psychiatry, 131,* 879–881.

Cytryn, L., McKnew, D. H., & Bunney, W. E. (1980). Diagnosis of depression in children: A reassessment. *American Journal of Psychiatry, 137,* 22–25.

Dahl, R. E., Kaufman, J., Ryan, N. D., Perel, J. M., Al-Shabbout, M., Birmaher, B., Nelson, B., & Puig-Antich, J. (1993). The dexamethasone suppression test in children and adolescents: A review and a controlled study: Erratum. *Biological Psychiatry, 33,* 64–69.

Dodge, K. A. (1990). Developmental psychopathology in children of depressed mothers. *Developmental Psychology, 26,* 3–6.

Doenges, M. E., Townsend, M. C., & Moorhouse, M. F. (1988). *Psychiatric care plans: Guidelines for client care.* Philadelphia: Davis.

Doherty, M. B., Madansky, D., Kraft, J., Carter-Ake, L. L., Rosenthal, P. A., & Coughlin, B. F. (1986). Cortisol dynamics and test performance of dexamethasone suppression test in 97 psychiatrically hospitalized children aged 3–16 years. *Journal of the American Academy of Child Psychiatry, 25,* 400–408.

Downey, G., & Coyne, J. (1990). Children of depressed parents: An integrative review. *Psychological Bulletin, 108,* 50–76.

Earls, F. (1989). Studying adolescent suicidal ideation and behavior in primary care settings. *Suicide and Life-Threatening Behavior, 19,* 99–107.

Edelbrock, C., Costello, A. J., Dulcan, M. K., Kalas, R., & Conover, N. C. (1985). Age differences in the reliability of the psychiatric interview of the child. *Child Development, 56,* 265–275.

Edelstein, B. A., & Berler, E. S. (1987). Interviewing and report writing. In C. L. Frame & J. L. Matson (Eds.), *Handbook of assessment in childhood psychopathology* (pp. 341–372). New York: Plenum.

Elmore, S. K. (1991). Seasonal affective disorder: 2. Phototherapy, an expanded role of the psychosocial nurse. *Archives of Psychiatric Nursing, 5,* 365–372.

Emslie, G. J., Rush, A. J., Weinberg, W. A., Rintelmann, J. W., & Roffwarg, H. P. (1990). Children with major depression show reduced rapid eye movement latencies. *Archives of General Psychiatry, 47,* 119–124.

Endicott, J., & Spitzer, R. L. (1978). A diagnostic interview: The schedule of affective disorders and schizophrenia. *Archives of General Psychiatry, 35,* 837–844.

Fisher, P. W., Shaffer, D., Piacentini, J., Lapkin, J., Kafantaris, V., Leonard, H., & Herzog, D. B. (1993). Sensitivity of the Diagnostic Interview Schedule for Children, 2nd edition (DISC 2.1) for specific diagnoses of children and adolescents. *Journal of the American Academy of Child and Adolescent Psychiatry, 32,* 666–673.

Fleming, J. E., Boyle, M. H., & Offord, D. R. (1993). The outcome of adolescent depression in the Ontario Child Health Study follow-up. *Journal of the American Academy of Child and Adolescent Psychiatry, 32,* 28–33.

Fleming, J. E., & Offord, D. R. (1990). Epidemiology of childhood depressive disorders: A critical review. *Journal of the American Academy of Child and Adolescent Psychiatry, 29,* 571–580.

Forehand, R., Wells, K., & Griest, D. (1980). An examination of the social validity of a parent training program. *Behavior Therapy, 11,* 488–502.

Frame, C. L., & Cooper, D. K. (1993). Major depression in children. In R. T. Ammerman & M. Hersen (Eds.), *Handbook of behavior therapy with children and adults: A developmental and longitudinal perspective.* Boston: Allyn & Bacon.

Frame, C. L., Matson, J. L., Sonis, W. A., Fialkov, M. J., & Kazdin, A. E. (1982). Behavioral treatment of depression in a prepubertal child. *Journal of Behavior Therapy and Experimental Psychiatry, 13,* 239–243.

Garmezy, N. (1987). Stress, competence, and development: Continuities in the study of schizophrenic adults, children vulnerable to psychopathology, and the search for stress resistant children. *American Journal of Orthopsychiatry, 57,* 159–174.

Geller, B. (1993). Longitudinal studies of depressive disorders in children [Introduction]. *Journal of the American Academy of Child and Adolescent Psychiatry, 32,* 7.

Geller, B., Cooper, T., Graham, D., Fetner, H., Marsteller, F., & Wells, J. (1992). Pharmokinetically designed double-blind, placebo-controlled study of nortriptyline in 6- to 12-year-olds with major depressive disorder. *Journal of the American Academy of Child and Adolescent Psychiatry, 31,* 34–44.

Geller, B., Fox, L. W., & Fletcher, M. (1993). Effect of tricyclic antidepressants on switching to mania and on the onset of bipolarity in depressed 6- to 12-year-olds. *Journal of the American Academy of Child and Adolescent Psychiatry, 32,* 43–50.

Geller, B., Perel, H., Knitter, E., Lycak, H., & Farook, Z. (1983). Nortriptyline in major depressive disorder in children: Response, steady state plasma levels, predictive kinetics, and pharmacokinetics. *Psychopharmacology Bulletin, 19,* 62–65.

Gershon, E. S. (1988). Discovering biologically specific risk factors and genetic linkage markers in affective disorders. In D. L. Dunner, E. S. Gershon, & J. E. Barrett (Eds.), *Relatives at risk for mental disorder* (pp. 127–141). New York: Raven.

Gold, P. W., Goodwin, F. K., & Chrousos, G. P. (1988a). Clinical and biochemical manifestations of depression: Relation to the neurobiology of stress. Part 1. *New England Journal of Medicine, 319,* 348–353.

Gold, P. W., Goodwin, F. K., & Chrousos, G. P. (1988b). Clinical and biochemical manifestations of depression: Relation to the neurobiology of stress. Part 2. *New England Journal of Medicine, 319,* 413–420.

Goodman, S., & Brumley, H. (1990). Schizophrenic and depressed mothers: Relational deficits in parenting. *Developmental Psychology, 26,* 31–39.

Gordon, D., Burge, D., Hammen, C., Adrian, C., Jaenicke, C., & Hirohoto, D. (1989). Observations of interactions of depressed women with their children. *American Journal of Psychiatry, 146,* 50–55.

Gould, M. S., Wunsch-Hitzig, R., & Dohrenwend, B. (1981). Estimating the prevalence of childhood psychopathology: A critical review. *Journal of the American Academy of Child Psychiatry, 20,* 462.

Gross, D., Fogg, L., & Conrad, B. (1993). Designing interventions in psychosocial research. *Archives of Psychiatric Nursing, 7,* 259–264.

Hammen, C. (1988). Self-cognitions, stressful events, and the prediction of depression in children of depressed mothers. *Journal of Abnormal Child Psychology, 16,* 347–360.

Hammen, C., Burge, D., & Stansbury, K. (1990). Relationship of mother and child variables to child outcomes in a high-risk sample: A causal modeling analysis. *Developmental Psychology, 26,* 24–30.

Harrington, R., Fudge, H., Rutter, M., Pickles, A., & Hill, J. (1991). Adult outcomes of childhood and adolescent depression: 2. Links with antisocial disorders. *Journal of the American Academy of Child and Adolescent Psychiatry, 30,* 434–439.

Harter, S. (1986). The determinants and mediational role of global self-worth in children. In N. Eisenberg (Ed.), *Contemporary issues in developmental psychology* (pp. 219–242). New York: Wiley.

Hawton, K. (1986). *Attempted suicide among children and adolescents.* Beverly Hills, CA: Sage.

Herjanic, B., Herjanic, M., Brown, F., & Wheatt, T. (1975). Are children reliable reporters? *Journal of Abnormal Child Psychology, 3,* 21–28.

Jarrett, D. B., Miewald, J. M., & Kupfer, D. J. (1990). Recurrent depression is associated with a persistent reduction in sleep-related growth hormone secretion. *Archives of General Psychiatry, 47,* 113–118.

Johnson, G. E., Hannah, K. J., & Zerr, S. R. (1992). *Pharmacology and the nursing process* (3rd ed.). Philadelphia: Saunders.

Kagan, J., Reznick, J. S., & Snidman, N. (1987). The physiology and psychology of behavioral inhibition in young children. *Child Development, 58,* 1459–1473.

Kahn, J. S., Kehle, T. J., Jenson, W. R., & Clark, E. (1990). Comparison of cognitive-behavioral, relaxation, and self-modeling interventions for depression among middle-school students. *School Psychology Review, 19,* 196–211.

Kashani, J., Shekim, W., & Reid, J. (1984). Amitriptyline in children with major depressive disorder: A double-blind crossover pilot study. *Journal of the American Academy of Child Psychiatry, 23*, 348–351.

Kashani, J. H., Carlson, G. A., Beck, N. C., Hoeper, E. W., Corcoran, C. M., McAllister, J. A., Fallahi, C., Rosenberg, T. K., & Reid, J. C. (1987). Depression, depressive symptoms, and depressed mood among a community sample of adolescents. *American Journal of Psychiatry, 144*, 931–934.

Kazdin, A. E. (1988). Childhood depression. In E. J. Marsh & L. G. Terdal (Eds.), *Behavioral assessment of childhood disorders* (pp. 157–195). New York: Guilford.

Kazdin, A. E. (1989). Identifying depression in children: A comparison of alternative selection criteria. *Journal of Abnormal Child Psychology, 17*, 437–454.

Kazdin, A. E. (1990). Childhood depression. *Journal of Child Psychology and Psychiatry and Allied Disciplines, 31*, 121–160.

Keltner, N. (1991). Psychopharmacology. In P. Clunn (Ed.), *Child psychiatric nursing* (pp. 380–395). St. Louis: Mosby.

Keltner, N., & Folks, D. (1993). *Psychotropic drugs*. St. Louis: Mosby.

Killeen, M. R. (1990). Challenges and choices in child and adolescent mental health–psychiatric nursing. *Journal of Child and Adolescent Psychiatric and Mental Health Nursing, 3*, 113–119.

Killeen, M. R. (1992, February). *A transactional model of self-esteem*. Presented at the Third State of the Art and Science of Psychiatric Nursing Conference, NIMH, Bethesda, MD.

King, B. H., Baxter, L. R., Stuber, M., & Fish, B. (1987). Therapeutic sleep deprivation for depression in children. *Journal of the American Academy of Child and Adolescent Psychiatry, 26*, 928–931.

King, R. A., Riddle, M., Chappell, P. B., Hardin, M. T., Anderson, G. M., Lombroso, P., & Scahill, L. (1991). Emergence of self-destructive phenomena in children and adolescents during fluoxetine treatment. *Journal of the American Academy of Child and Adolescent Psychiatry, 30*, 179–186.

Kovacs, M. (1981). Rating scales to assess depression in school-aged children. *Acta Paedopsychiatrica, 46*, 305–315.

Kovacs, M. (1989). Affective disorders in children and adolescents. *American Psychologist, 44*, 209–215.

Kovacs, M., & Beck, A. T. (1977). An empirical clinical approach towards a definition of childhood depression. In J. G. Schulterbrandt & A. Raskin (Eds.), *Depression in children: Diagnosis, treatment, and conceptual models* (p. 125). New York: Raven.

Kovacs, M. M., Feinberg, T. L., Crouse-Novak, M. A., Paulauskas, S. L., Pollack, M., & Finkelstein, R. (1984). Depressive disorders in childhood: 2. A longitudinal study of the risk for a subsequent major depression. *Archives of General Psychiatry, 41*, 643–649.

Kovacs, M., & Goldston, D. (1991). Cognitive and social cognitive development of depressed children and adolescents. *Journal of the American Academy of Child and Adolescent Psychiatry, 30*, 388–392.

Kovacs, M., Goldston, D., & Gatsonis, C. (1993). Suicidal behaviors and childhood onset depressive disorders: A longitudinal investigation. *Journal of the American Academy of Child and Adolescent Psychiatry, 32*, 8–20.

Kramer, E., & Feiguine, R. (1983). Clinical effects of amitriptyline in adolescent depression. *Journal of the American Academy of Child Psychiatry, 20*, 636–644.

Kutcher, S., & Marton, P. (1991). Affective disorders in first-degree relatives of adolescent onset bipolars, unipolars, and normal controls. *Journal of the American Academy of Child and Adolescent Psychiatry, 30*, 75–78.

Lefkowitz, M. M., & Burton, N. (1978). Childhood depression: A critique of the concept. *Psychological Bulletin, 85*, 716–726.

Leibenluft, E., & Wehr, T. A. (1992). Is sleep deprivation useful in the treatment of depression? *American Journal of Psychiatry, 149*, 159–168.

Lewinsohn, P. M. (1974). A behavioral approach to depression. In R. J. Friedman & M. M. Katz (Eds.), *The psychology of depression: Contemporary theory and research* (pp. 157–184). New York: Wiley.

Lewinsohn, P. M., Clarke, G. N., Hops, H., & Andrews, J. (1990). Cognitive-behavioral treatment for depressed adolescents. *Behavior Therapy, 21,* 385–401.

Lewinsohn, P. M., Garrison, C. Z., Langhinrichsen, J., & Marsteller, F. (1989). The assessment of suicidal behavior in adolescents: A review of scales suitable for epidemiologic and clinical research. Rockville, MD: National Institute of Mental Health.

McBride, A. B. (1990). Psychiatric nursing in the 1990s. *Archives of Psychiatric Nursing, 4,* 21–28.

McCauley, E., Myers, K., Mitchell, J., Calderon, R., Schloredt, K., & Treder, R. (1993). Depression in young people: Initial presentation and clinical course. *Journal of the American Academy of Child and Adolescent Psychiatry, 32,* 714–722.

McEnany, G. W. (1991). Psychobiology and psychiatric nursing: A philosophical matrix. *Archives of Psychiatric Nursing, 5,* 255–261.

McGee, R., & Williams, S. (1988). A longitudinal study of depression in nine-year-old children. *Journal of the American Academy of Child and Adolescent Psychiatry, 27,* 342–348.

Mghir, R., & Vincent, J. (1991). Phototherapy of seasonal affective disorder in an adolescent female. *Journal of the American Academy of Child and Adolescent Psychiatry, 30,* 440–442.

Miller, S., Birnbaum, A., & Durbin, D. (1990). Etiologic perspectives on depression in childhood. In M. Lewis & S. M. Miller (Eds.), *Handbook of developmental psychopathology* (pp. 311–325). New York: Plenum.

Mitchell, J. R., McCauley, E., Burke, P. M., & Moss, S. J. (1988). Phenomenology of depression in children and adolescents. *Journal of the American Academy of Child and Adolescent Psychiatry, 27,* 12–20.

Myers, K., McCauley, E., Calderon, R., Mitchell, J., Burke, P., & Schloredt, K. (1991). Risks for suicidality in major depressive disorder. *Journal of the American Academy of Child and Adolescent Psychiatry, 30,* 86–94.

Naylor, M. W., King, C. A., Lindsay, K. A., Evans, T., Armelagos, J., Shain, B. N., & Greden, J. F. (1993). Sleep deprivation in depressed adolescents and psychiatric controls. *Journal of the American Academy of Child and Adolescent Psychiatry, 32,* 753–759.

Nihart, M. A. (1993). The development of neurotransmitter systems. *Journal of Child and Adolescent Psychiatric and Mental Health Nursing, 6,* 23–24.

Ollendick, T. H., & Hersen, M. (Eds.). (1984). *Child behavioral assessment principles and procedures.* New York: Pergamon.

Orvaschel, H. (1990). Early onset psychiatric disorder in high risk children and increased familial morbidity. *Journal of the American Academy of Child and Adolescent Psychiatry, 29,* 184–188.

O'Toole, A. W., & Loomis, M. E. (1989). Revision of the phenomena of concern for psychiatric mental health nursing. *Archives of Psychiatric Nursing, 3,* 288–299.

Patterson, G. R. (1975). *Families; Applications of social learning to family life* (rev. ed.). Champaign, IL: Research Press.

Patterson, G. R. (1982). *Coercive family processes.* Eugene, OR: Castalia.

Petti, T. A., Bornstein, M., Delameter, A., & Connors, K. (1980). Evaluation of multimodal treatment of a depressed prepubertal girl. *Journal of the American Academy of Child Psychiatry, 19,* 690–702.

Petti, T. A., & Law, W. (1982). Imipramine treatment of depressed children: A double-blind pilot study. *Journal of Clinical Psychopharmacology, 2,* 107–110.

Pfeffer, C. R., Newcorn, J., Kaplan, G., Mizruchi, M. S., & Plutchik, R. (1988). Suicidal behavior in adolescent psychiatric inpatients. *Journal of the American Academy of Child and Adolescent Psychiatry, 27,* 357–361.

Popper, C. W., & Elliott, G. R. (1990). Sudden death and tricyclic antidepressants: Clinical considerations for children. *Journal of Child and Adolescent Psychopharmacology, 1,* 125–132.

Poznanski, E., Cook, S., & Carroll, B. (1979). A depression rating scale for children. *Pediatrics, 64,* 442–450.

Poznanski, E. O., Krahenbuhl, V., & Zrull, J. P. (1976). Childhood depression—a longitudinal perspective. *Journal of the American Academy of Child Psychiatry, 15,* 491–501.

Preskorn, S., Weller, E., & Weller, R. (1982). Depression in children: Relationship between plasma imipramine levels and response. *Journal of Clinical Psychiatry, 43,* 450–453.

Puig-Antich, J. (1982). Major depression and conduct disorder in prepuberty. *Journal of the American Academy of Child Psychiatry, 21,* 118–128.

Puig-Antich, J., Blau, S., Marx, N., Greenhill, L. L., & Chambers, W. (1978). Prepubertal major depressive disorder: A pilot study. *Journal of the American Academy of Child Psychiatry, 17,* 695–707.

Puig-Antich, J., & Chambers, W. (1978). *Schedule for affective disorders and schizophrenia for school-aged children (6-16 years) (Kiddie-SADS).* New York: New York State Psychiatric Institute.

Puig-Antich, J., Dahl, R., Ryan, N., Novacenko, H., Goetz, D., Goetz, R., Twomey, J., & Klepper, T. (1989). Cortisol secretion in prepubertal children with major depressive disorder: Episode and recovery. *Archives of General Psychiatry, 46,* 801–809.

Puig-Antich, J., Goetz, R., Davies, M., Fein, M., Hanlon, C., Chambers, W. J., Tabrizi, M. A., Sachar, E. J., & Weitzman, E. D. (1984). Growth hormone secretion in prepubertal children with major depression: 2. Sleep-related plasma concentrations during a depressive episode. *Archives of General Psychiatry, 41,* 463–466.

Puig-Antich, J., Goetz, R., Davies, M., Tabrizi, M. A., Novacenko, H., Hanlon, C., Sachar, E. J., & Weitzman, E. D. (1984). Growth hormone secretion in prepubertal children with major depression: 4: Sleep related plasma concentrations in a drug-free fully recovered clinical state. *Archives of General Psychiatry, 41,* 479–483.

Puig-Antich, J., Goetz, R., Hanlon, C., Tabrizi, M. A., Davies, M., & Weitzman, E. D. (1982). Sleep architecture and REM sleep measures in prepubertal children with major depression: A controlled study. *Archives of General Psychiatry, 39,* 932–939.

Puig-Antich, J., Perel, J., Lupatkin, W., Chambers, W., Tabrizi, M., King, J., Goetz, R., Davies, M., & Stiller, R. (1987). Imipramine in prepubertal major depressive disorders. *Archives of General Psychiatry, 44,* 81–89.

Rao, U., Weissman, M. M., Martin, J. A., & Hammond, R. W. (1993). Childhood depression and risk of suicide: A preliminary report of a longitudinal study. *Journal of the American Academy of Child and Adolescent Psychiatry, 32,* 21–27.

Rehm, L. P. (1977). A self-control model of depression. *Behavior Therapy, 8,* 787–804.

Rehm, L. P., Gordon-Leventon, B., & Ivens, C. (1987). Depression. In C. L. Frame & J. L. Matson (Eds.), *Handbook of assessment in childhood psychopathology* (pp. 341–372). New York: Plenum.

Reynolds, W. (1987). Major depression. In M. Hersen & C. G. Last (Eds.), *Child behavior therapy casebook* (pp. 85–100). New York: Plenum.

Reynolds, W. M., & Coates, K. I. (1986). A comparison of cognitive-behavioral therapy and relaxation training for treatment of depression in adolescents. *Journal of Consulting and Clinical Psychology, 54,* 653–660.

Riddle, M., Geller, B., & Ryan, N. (1993). Case study: Another sudden death in a child treated with desipramine. *Journal of the American Academy of Child and Adolescent Psychiatry, 32,* 792–797.

Riddle, M., King, R., Hardin, M., Scahill, L., Ort, S., Chappell, P., Rasmussen, A., & Leckman, J. (1991). Behavioral side effects of fluoxetine in children and adolescents. *Journal of Child and Adolescent Psychopharmacology, 1,* 193–198.

Riddle, M. A., Nelson, J. C., Kleinman, C. S., Rasmussen, A., Leckman, J. F., King, R. A., & Cohen, D. J. (1991). Case study: Sudden death in children receiving Norpramin: A review of three reported cases and commentary. *Journal of the American Academy of Child and Adolescent Psychiatry, 30,* 104–108.

Rie, M. (1966). Depression in childhood: A survey of some pertinent contributors. *Journal of the American Academy of Child Psychiatry, 5,* 653–685.

Rogeness, G. A., Javors, M. A., Maas, J. W., & Macedo, C. A. (1990). Catecholamines and diagnoses in children. *Journal of the American Academy of Child and Adolescent Psychiatry, 29,* 234–241.

Rose, M. H., & Killian, M. (1983). Risk and vulnerability: A case for differentiation. *Advances in Nursing Science, 5*(3), 60–73.

Rosenberg, M. L., Smith, J. C., Davidson, L. E., & Conn, J. M. (1987). The emergence of youth suicide: An epidemiological analysis and public health perspective. *Annual Review of Public Health, 8,* 417–427.

Rosenthal, N. E., Carpenter, C. J., James, S. P., Parry, B. L., Rogers, S. L., & Wehr, T. A. (1986). Seasonal affective disorder in children and adolescents. *American Journal of Psychiatry, 143,* 356–358.

Rutter, M. (1986). The developmental psychopathology of depression: Issues and perspectives. In M. Rutter, C. E. Izard, & P. B. Read (Eds.), *Depression in young people* (pp. 491–519). New York: Guilford.

Rutter, M. (1988). Depression. In M. Rutter, A. H. Tuma, & I. S. Lann (Eds.), *Assessment and diagnosis in child psychopathology* (pp. 347–376). New York: Guilford.

Rutter, M. (1989). Isle of Wight revisited: Twenty-five years of child psychiatric epidemiology. *Journal of the American Academy of Child and Adolescent Psychiatry, 32,* 633–653.

Ryan, N. D. (1990). Heterocyclic antidepressants in children and adolescents. *Journal of Child and Adolescent Psychopharmacology, 1,* 21–31.

Ryan, N. D., Puig-Antich, J., Ambrosini, P., Rabinovich, H., Robinson, D., Nelson, B., Iyengar, S., & Twomey, J. (1987). The clinical picture of major depression in children and adolescents. *Archives of General Psychiatry, 44,* 854–861.

Ryan, N. D., Puig-Antich, J., Cooper, T. B., Rabinovich, H., Ambrosini, P., Davies, J., King, J., Torres, D., & Fried, J. (1986). Imipramine in adolescent major depression: Plasma level and clinical response. *Acta Psychiatrica Scandinavia, 73,* 275–288.

Ryan, N. D., Puig-Antich, J., Cooper, T. B., Rabinovich, H., Ambrosini, P., Fried, J., Davies, M., Torres, D., & Suckrow, R. F. (1987). Safety of single versus divided dose imipramine in adolescent major depression. *Journal of the American Academy of Child and Adolescent Psychiatry, 26,* 400–406.

Sachar, E. J. (1975). Neuroendocrine abnormalities in depressive illness. In E. J. Sachar (Ed.), *Topics in psychoneuroimmunology* (pp. 135-156). New York: Grune & Stratton.

Sameroff, A. J. , & Chandler, M. J. (1975). Reproductive risk and the continuum of caretaking casualty. In F. D. Horowitz, M. Hetherington, S. Scarr-Salapatek, & G. Siegel (Eds.), *Review of child development research* (Vol. 4, pp. 187–244). Chicago: University of Chicago Press.

Sameroff, A. J., & Seifer, R. (1983). Familial risk and child competence. *Child Development, 54,* 1254–1268.

Scahill, L. (1991). Nursing diagnosis vs. goal-oriented treatment planning in inpatient child psychiatry. *Image: Journal of Nursing Scholarship, 23,* 95–98.

Schloss, P. J., Schloss, C. N., & Harris, L. (1984). A multiple baseline analysis of an interpersonal skills training program for depressed youth. *Behavioral Disorders, 9,* 182–188.

Schaefer, C. E., & O'Connor, K. J. (Eds.). (1983). *Handbook of play therapy.* New York: Wiley.

Schwab-Stone, M., Fisher, P., Piacentini, J., Shaffer, D., Davies, M., & Briggs, M. (1993). The diagnostic interview schedule for children—revised version (DISC-R): 2. Test-retest reliability. *Journal of the American Academy of Child and Adolescent Psychiatry, 32,* 651–657.

Seifer, R., Nurcombe, B., Scioli, A., & Grapentine, W. L. (1989). Is major depressive disorder in childhood a distinct diagnostic entity? *Journal of the American Academy of Child and Adolescent Psychiatry, 28,* 935–941.

Seligman, M. E., Peterson, C., Kaslow, N., Tanenbaum, R. L., Alloy, L. B., & Abramson, L. Y. (1984). Attributional style and depressive symptoms among children. *Journal of Abnormal Psychology, 93,* 235–238.

Shaffer, D., Schwab-Stone, M., Fisher, P., Cohen, P., Piacentini, J., Davies, M., Conners, C. K., & Regier, D. (1993). The diagnostic interview schedule for children—revised version (DISC-R): 1. Preparation, field testing, interrater reliability, and acceptability. *Journal of the American Academy of Child and Adolescent Psychiatry, 32,* 643–650.

Sipple, B. (1992). Applying the nursing process with children. In H. S. Wilson & C. R. Kneisl (Eds.), *Psychiatric nursing* (4th ed.) (pp. 810–838). Redwood City, CA: Addison-Wesley.

Spitzer, R. L., Endicott, J., & Robins, E. (1978). Research diagnostic criteria: Rationale and reliability. *Archives of General Psychiatry, 35,* 773–782.

Sroufe, L. A., & Rutter, M. (1984). The domain of developmental psychopathology. *Child Development, 55,* 17–29.

Stark, K. D., Reynolds, W. M., & Kaslow, N. J. (1987). A comparison of the relative efficacy of self-control therapy and a behavioral problem-solving therapy for depression. *Journal of Abnormal Child Psychology, 15,* 91–113.

Strober, M., Lampert, C., Schmidt, S., & Morrell, W. (1993). The course of major depressive disorder in adolescents: 1. Recovery and risk of manic switching in a follow-up of psychotic and nonpsychotic subtypes. Special section: Longitudinal studies of depressive disorders in children. *Journal of the American Academy of Child and Adolescent Psychiatry, 32,* 34–42.

Stuart, G. W., & Sundeen, S. J. (Eds.). (1991). Disturbances of mood. In *Principles and practice of psychiatric nursing* (4th ed.) (pp. 413–458). St. Louis: Mosby.

Townsend, M. C. (1990). *Drug guide for psychiatric nursing.* Philadelphia: Davis.

Valente, S. M. (1989). Adolescent suicide: Assessment and intervention. *Journal of Child and Adolescent Psychiatric and Mental Health Nursing, 2,* 34–39.

Venkataraman, S., Naylor, M. W., & King, C. (1992). Case study: Mania associated with fluoxetine treatment in adolescents. *Journal of the American Academy of Child and Adolescent Psychiatry, 31,* 276–281.

Wehr, T. A., Wirz-Justice, A., & Goodwin, F. K. (1979). Phase advance of the circadian sleep-wake cycle as an antidepressant. *Science, 206,* 210–213.

Weissman, M. M., Gammon, G. D., John, K., Merikangas, K. R., Warner, V., Prusoff, B. A., & Sholomskas, D. (1987). Children of depressed parents: Increased psychopathology and early onset of major depression. *Archives of General Psychiatry, 44,* 847–853.

Weissman, M. M., Warner, V., Wickramaratne, P., & Prusoff, B. A. (1988). Early onset major depression in parents and their children. *Journal of Affective Disorders, 15,* 269–277.

Weller, E. B., & Weller, R. A. (1988). Neuroendocrine changes in affectively ill children and adolescents. *Neurologic Clinics, 6,* 41–54.

Werner, E. E., & Smith, R. S. (1982). *Vulnerable but invincible: A longitudinal study of resilient children and youth.* New York: McGraw-Hill.

West, P. P., & Pothier, P. C. (1989). Clinical application of human responses classification system: Child example. *Archives of Psychiatric Nursing, 3,* 300–304.

Whall, A. L. (1991). Family system theory: Relationship to nursing conceptual models. In A. L. Whall & J. Fawcett (Eds.), *Family theory development in nursing* (pp. 317–342). Philadelphia: Davis.

Wilens, T. E., Biederman, J., Baldessarini, R. J., Puopolo, P. R., & Flood, J. (1993). Electrocardiographic effects of desipramine and 2-hydroxydesipramine in children, adolescents, and adults treated with desipramine. *Journal of the American Academy of Child and Adolescent Psychiatry, 32,* 798–804.

Winnett, R. L., Bornstein, P. H., Cogswell, K. A., & Paris, A. E. (1987). Cognitive-behavioral therapy for childhood depression: A levels of treatment approach. *Journal of Child and Adolescent Psychotherapy, 4,* 283–286.

Worchel, F., Little, V., & Alcala, J. (1990). Self-perceptions of depressed children on tasks of cognitive abilities. *Journal of School Psychology, 28,* 97–104.

Wu, J. C., & Bunney, W. E. (1990). The biological basis of an antidepressant response to sleep deprivation and relapse: Review and hypothesis. *American Journal of Psychiatry, 147,* 14–21.

Yaylayan, S. A., Weller, E. B., & Weller, R. A. (1990/1991). Biology of depression in children and adolescents. *Journal of Child and Adolescent Psychopharmacology, 1,* 215–227.

Young, W., Knowles, J. B., MacLean, A. W., Boag, L., & McConville, B. J. (1982). The sleep of childhood depressives. Comparison with age-matched controls. *Biological Psychiatry, 17,* 1163–1168.

CHAPTER

10

DEPRESSION IN WOMEN

Linda S. Beeber, PhD, RN, CS

ABSTRACT

This chapter reviews ways that depression has been categorized and described, then discusses the predispositional, biological, and interpersonal factors that create a dynamic balance of threats and buffers, thereby influencing women's potential to become depressed or to grow through interactions with the environment. Predispositional factors include sex, age, and family history. Studies exploring the biological processes link depression to the limbic system and the hypothalamus, and the dysregulation hypothesis unifies the relationship between stress and depression, given that women predictably experience clustered and chronic stressors in their classic roles as caregivers, for example, during the perinatal period. The role of interpersonal processes is discussed in the context of the need to reformulate the theoretical model of depression from the classical theories—which viewed "unhealthy dependency" as a pathological outgrowth of a failed process of differentiation—to a self-in-relation framework—which recognizes that interpersonal processes are essential to women's sense of self and self-esteem. The chapter then describes interventions within the context of a therapeutic relationship that are intended to (1) restore and protect biological regulatory systems, for example, through pharmacology, sleep deprivation, phototherapy, and aerobic conditioning; (2) modulate mood, thought, and action to help the depressed woman develop self-efficacy and reduce immobilization; (3) restore and strengthen self-worth through activities that enhance self-awareness by using the therapeutic relationship and groups as "learning laboratories"; and (4) restore social integration and enhance meaningful social involvement. The chapter concludes with a discussion of new directions for practice, research, and education.

In her dreams, a depressed young woman visualized herself as a Southern belle, dressed in a long, white gossamer gown and wearing tiny lace shoes with no soles. She carried a parasol and waited under a tree for a man in a black suit, who approached her, swept her into his arms, and placed her into a rowboat. When she picked up the oars in her tiny gloved hands, they were onerously heavy, and as she tried to row, the oars became mired in heavy muck surrounding the boat. When she awoke, she left herself in that dream, suspended in the heat and mire of her momentumless journey.

The dream expressed the fusion of femininity and helplessness, the loss of purpose and soul, the inadequate efficacy, and the romantic rescue and passionate se-duction of depression, represented by the black-suited lover. For this woman, depression had appeared in the midst of a seemingly fully realized life. Only retrospectively would she recognize that the source of her torment was a complex of interrelated factors that worked synergistically to increase stresses in her life while simultaneously eroding her resources. This chapter will present depression as an expression of biological, interpersonal, and social processes that coalesce to create a vulnerability for women. Because nursing practice uses concepts of prevention, multidimensional treatment, and holism, the specialty practice of psychiatric nursing is positioned to develop effective interventions for depression.

DEPRESSION AND WOMEN: THE CONTEXT

Depression is a disorder of mood characterized by a persistent sad mood, lack of pleasure, difficulty in concentration, loss of energy, a profound sense of worthlessness, somatic changes, and suicidal preoccupation and action (American Psychiatric Association, 1994). Additional characteristics include social withdrawal, preoccupation with morbid ideas, diminished motivation for meaningful interpersonal involvement, loss of the will for meaningful achievements, and self-neglecting behaviors. Scientific understanding of depression has led to social, interpersonal, and intrapsychic explanations of these phenomena. Newer biological data confirm alterations of basic brain physiology in depression. Although the explosion of biological data has dominated recent discussions of depression, it is clear that depression, perhaps more clearly than other mental disorders, arises out of the multiple interactions of persons and their environments. Predictably, as knowledge about depression has become more sophisticated, the models depicting its epidemiology and course have become more complex. With its concentration on human biology and behavior in health (Gortner, 1983), nursing science is an ideal discipline in which to develop models that will accurately depict depression as a complex entity.

An intriguing aspect of depression to emerge from more sophisticated epidemiologic study is the overrepresentation of the disorder in women (Weissman & Klerman, 1981). More than a decade of investigation has not yielded a definitive answer to this observation but has raised interesting questions about depression that are instructive in challenging older models of the disorder. In addition to the efforts to demonstrate genetic and sex-hormone bases for depression, researchers have proposed other explanations, such as the selective valuing of one sex over another in society (Miller, 1976; 1983; 1984) and differences in the presentation of disorders between men and women (Egeland & Hostetter, 1983). Depression prevalence fluctuates with periodicities in social change, suggesting that individual propensities for developing the disorder are affected by changes in larger environmental systems. In noting that depression prevalence is highest in periods of relative social calm and prosperity, Paykel (Weissman & Paykel, 1974) observed, "Depression seems to arise not when things are at their worst, but when there is a discrepancy between one's aspirations and the likelihood that reality will fulfill these wishes and hopes" (p. x). Clearly, this factor could also be relevant in the appearance of the disorder in contemporary women, especially those struggling to take advantage of expanded opportunities.

The prevalence of depression in women and the insidious nature of this disorder present a clear and present danger to the personal development of women. Except in its most severe forms, depression masquerades as fatigue, laziness, confusion, lack of organization, and a variety of qualities that are maligned in the contemporary American quest for productivity and efficiency. As these qualities resonate with deeply held attitudes that women are not capable of achieving excellence, the appearance of these behaviors is not viewed with alarm, but rather a perception that the expected has materialized. Qualities associated with depression—such as social withdrawal, blunted reactivity to situations, and diminished ability to act efficaciously—invite those around the depressed woman to back away, ignore the problem, and overlook the gradual decline. These attitudes confirm the depressed woman's perception that her contribution was never intrinsically worth much at all. Consequently, the young woman who is failing a course, the mother who cannot energetically nurture her young children, the career woman whose productivity is faltering, and the older woman who isolates herself after her husband dies are all treated with a shrug, or worse, a moralistic "get yourself moving" approach. The losses are immeasurable because in many ways, traditional forms of women's work do not lend themselves to traditional measures of worth. Although there is reason to be concerned about the potential lethality of depression by virtue of its relationship with suicide, death in more subtle ways must also be of concern to those who care for women.

Another danger that depression presents to women is the progressive nature of the disorder. Far from being a quiescent phenomenon, depression produces unrelenting symptoms that, over time, destroy meaningful human connections to work and love. Depression ideally requires aggressive, sustained interventions within a context of a deep, professional commitment to another person. The episodic, short-term nature of the American mental health care system does not allow for this type of relationship, creating a treatment response that is primarily symptom focused; it aims to restore previous functioning rather than to seek a better-than-previous functional outcome. Treatment systems are restricted, and the options that are offered to a client often reflect an institution's philosophy rather than the treatment options that are best for the person in question.

Within this context, depression as a health problem for women emerges as a challenge for psychiatric nursing that requires a commitment to holism, humanism, and care in the context of the professional relationship. The remainder of this chapter will present selected biological, social, and interpersonal elements of the environment that have an empirically supported relationship with depression. The chapter will demonstrate the use of these relationships in crafting interventions intended to be used within the context of the therapeutic relationship developed by the nurse and the client.

AN INTEGRATED UNDERSTANDING OF THE PHENOMENA ASSOCIATED WITH DEPRESSION

DESCRIPTIVE AND DIAGNOSTIC FRAMEWORKS FOR DEPRESSION

Depression has been described for the purposes of delineating categories (and hence defining treatments), for creating severity scales to stage its development, and for predicting responses to interventions. The *Diagnostic and Statistical Manual of Mental Disorders*, fourth edition (DSM-IV) (American Psychiatric Association, 1994) is the accepted American standard for categorical nomenclature, although much of the available epidemiological and pharmacological outcome data are based on DSM-III and DSM-III-R categories.

The DSM-IV includes three categories of depression:

1. Major depressive disorder
2. Dysthymic disorder
3. Depressive disorder not otherwise specified (American Psychiatric Association, 1994).

An episode of major depression includes the presence of the following symptoms: depressed mood, loss of interest or pleasure in all or almost all activities, appetite and weight loss when not dieting, insomnia or hypersomnia, psychomotor agitation or retardation, fatigue or loss of energy, feelings of worthlessness or excessive guilt, diminished ability to concentrate, recurrent thoughts of death, and suicidal ideation or attempt. At least five of these, including either depressed mood or loss of interest, must be present on a nearly daily basis during a 2-week period and represent a change in previous functioning. Symptoms may include delusions and hallucinations, and the disorder is differentiated from bereavement, organicity, and other related mental disorders.

Dysthymic disorder is characterized by a chronic depressed mood for most of the day more days than not; this depressed mood has persisted for at least a 2-year period without remission for more than 2 months. In addition, two of the following are present: undereating or overeating, insomnia or hypersomnia, low energy, low self-esteem, poor concentration or decisionmaking, or feelings of hopelessness. During this period the symptoms never meet all the criteria for major depressive episode.

Nurses have developed descriptive severity continua that describe clinical phenomena associated with shifts from mild to severe forms of depression (Swanson, 1978; Beeber, 1980; Kerr, 1987). These are useful in managing acutely depressed persons, particularly in predicting suicide attempts and in assessing responses to interventions. The other commonly used nomenclature has been developed by the North American Nursing Diagnosis Association (NANDA). The current list of 98 approved diagnoses does not include depression as a distinct entity, requiring the use of more global diagnoses (e.g., ineffective individual coping) or related problem diagnoses (e.g., social isolation, altered thought processes). Based on work by Loomis and colleagues (1987), additional diagnoses specific to psychiatric nursing have been identified; these provide a rich matrix in which to classify phenomena more specifically associated with depression (e.g., suicidal ideation, psychomotor retardation). MacFarland and Thomas (1991) developed 50 nursing diagnoses, including depression, from the work by Loomis and colleagues. In this context, the defining characteristics of depression include despair, guilt, anger, low self-esteem, hopelessness, anhedonia, suicidal ideation; apathy, decreased interaction, anxiety, withdrawal, frequent crying, poor eye contact; sleep disturbances, changes in activity level, and appetite changes. While in need of further validation and development, as a group these defining characteristics are useful in distinguishing depression from similar phenomena such as grieving. However, several defining characteristics associated with biological alterations are absent (biological rhythm disturbances, nonreactive affect, somatization, psychomotor retardation, weight loss, constipation), and characteristics associated with severe forms of depression are not included (depressive rumination, self-hatred, self-neglect or harm, delusions, hallucinations). In addition, the aspects of depression associating it with a self- and energy-conserving process are not addressed, thus defining depression as only a health alteration. This approach is not consistent with a holistic framework, which examines behaviors in terms of both alteration *and* actualization of health. For example, depression may also be viewed as a health-seeking behavior in which the withdrawal of energy from the environment and the investment of energy in the self is a healing process appropriately mobilized for a complex injury (Gut, 1989).

It is clear that there is congruence across disciplines concerning the phenomena associated with depression. The next section will focus on some of these phenomena and the scientific knowledge related to them.

SELECTED PHENOMENA ASSOCIATED WITH DEPRESSION

As the intent of this chapter is to view depression in a holistic framework, the following three categories of phenomena will be reviewed: (1) predispositional factors, (2) biological processes, and (3) interpersonal processes. Within each category, evidence is focused on women across the life span. Table 10–1 summarizes selected instruments and assessment strategies useful in identifying and monitoring phenomena associated with depression.

TABLE 10–1. RESOURCES OR INSTRUMENTS FOR ASSESSING RISK FACTORS

FACTORS	RESOURCES/SCALES
Depression symptoms or severity	Schedule for Affective Disorders and Schizophrenia (SADS) (Endicott & Spitzer, 1978) Interview Guide
	Hamilton Rating Scale for Depression (Hamilton, 1960; Elkin, Parloff, Hadley, & Autry, 1985) Interview Guide
	Beck Depression Inventory (Beck, Ward, Mendelson, Mock, and Erbaugh, 1961) Self-report
	Zung Self-Rating Depression Scale (Zung, 1965) Self-report
	Center for Epidemiologic Studies Depression Scale (Radloff, 1977) Self-report
Geriatric depression	Geriatric depression scale (Yesavage et al., 1983) Self-report
Previous episodes of depression	Schedule for Affective Disorders and Schizophrenia (Lifetime version)
	Inventory to Diagnose Depression (Zimmerman, Coryell, Corenthal, & Wilson, 1986) (Lifetime version) Self-report
Change in depression severity	Schedule for Affective Disorders and Schizophrenia (Change version)
	Beck Depression Inventory
Biological or rhythm alterations	
Appetite or eating patterns	Personal journal detailing patterns for 1 week
Sleep patterns	Personal journal detailing sleep and wake times for 1 week
Menstrual patterns and mood	Premenstrual Assessment Form (Halbreich, Endicott, & Nee, 1983)
	Moos Menstrual Distress Questionnaire (Moos, 1968)
Suicide	Hopelessness Scale (Beck, Weissman, Lester, & Trexler, 1974)
	Suicide Assessment Scale (Hoff, 1989)
	Assessment of Suicidal Potentiality—Los Angeles Suicide Prevention Center (Stuart & Sundeen, 1995)
Self-worth or self-esteem	Describe Yourself (Stake & Orlofsky, 1981)
	Rosenberg Self-Esteem Scale (Rosenberg, 1965)
Social support or social integration	Interpersonal Relationship Inventory (Tilden & Nelson, 1988)
	Barrett-Lennard Relationship Inventory Empathy Subscale (Barrett-Lennard, 1962)
	Family Environment Scale (Moos & Moos, 1986)
Marital adjustment	Dyadic Adjustment Scale (Spanier, 1976)
	Life Stress Schedule of Recent Life Events/Recent Life Change Questionnaire (Lin, Dean, & Ensel, 1986)

FACTORS PREDISPOSING WOMEN TO DEPRESSION

The following four factors have been shown to predispose women to depression: (1) sex, (2) age, (3) family history of mood disorders, and (4) previous episodes of depression.

SEX. Women are twice as liable to become depressed as men. Data collected in the National Institute of Mental Health Epidemiologic Catchment Area (ECA) program indicates that 2.5% to 4.6% of males and 5.4% to 9.1% of women are liable to suffer a major depression in their lifetime (Regier, 1985). This trend has been demonstrated in multiple studies over several decades in industrialized countries (Weissman & Klerman, 1981). The culturally consistent treatment of women as inherently less valued than men has been implicated as a causal factor by numerous studies (Belle, 1982; Radloff, 1975; Hirschfield & Cross, 1981; Orr, 1984; Pitts, Schuller, Rich, & Pitts, 1979), with the suspected vulnerability being the constriction of self-esteem and worth, both of which are central to depression (Arieti & Bemporad, 1978; Miller, 1976; Beeber, 1987).

A sex-linked vulnerability for depression has been investigated and found to be inconclusive (Simmons-Alling, 1990; Kovacs, Feinberg, Crouse-Novak, Paulauskas, & Finkelstein, 1984). The latter study demonstrated the same 2:1 ratio in prepubertal children as in postpubertal children. These data seriously challenge a sex-hormone basis for the disorder, as the prepubertal ratios would be expected to equal each other in such a disorder. Studies of the Amish indicated nearly equal ratios in the sexes, which was hypothesized to result from men being barred from drinking and antisocial activities (Egeland & Hostetter, 1983). Similar findings in prepubertal children suggested that the ratio may result from a difference in the presentation of distress between sexes (Kovacs et al., 1984). In reviewing earlier data that were similar, Weissman and Klerman (1981) concluded that the disproportionate ratio in men and women could be explained as well by social factors as biological factors. This conclusion was supported by Nolen-Hoeksema (1987) in an extensive review of additional social and biological data on sex differences. These reviews suggest that in contrast to other mental disorders where genetic and biochemical data are clearer, depression is an outgrowth of multiple factors that interact to create the disorder.

AGE. Younger women are at greater risk for depression than any other population group. Across several community studies, women born after 1970 have a greater risk of developing depression, with a median age of onset in the mid- to late twenties (Weissman, 1986; Weissman & Klerman, 1985; Dean, 1985; Weissman et al., 1984). It is unclear, however, whether this finding is an age or a cohort effect. Depression rates in elderly women are decreasing, but because of the demographic shift toward greater numbers of elderly persons, the actual number of depressed elderly women is expected to increase. Because the diagnosis and treatment of depression in the elderly is complex, these women present an especially vulnerable group in need of nursing care.

FAMILY HISTORY. Women who have a parent who was depressed are three times more liable to develop depression, and the risk for cyclothymic, bipolar, and depressive disorder increases if first-degree relatives have bipolar disorder (Gershon, 1983; Rice et al., 1984; Weissman et al., 1984; Winokur, Tsuang, & Crowe, 1982). In addition, women whose parent was depressed are more at risk for anxiety disorders, substance abuse, accidents, health problems, and academic difficulties (Weissman, 1986). There is weak evidence for a genetic linkage in depression (Weissman, 1986) and strong evidence that supports familial patterns of relatedness as causal agents in the histories of depressed persons (Perris et al., 1986). Stuart, Laraia, Ballenger, and Lydiard (1990) identified three characteristics—chronic disease, minimal interactions, and low interpersonal resources—in the histories of depressed women.

These characteristics differentiated depressed women from women who were bulimic or normal (Stuart et al., 1990).

PREVIOUS EPISODES. Women who become depressed have a greater risk for subsequent depression. Two factors, age of onset and initial severity, have been shown to relate to the persistence of depression. Giles, Jarrett, Biggs, Guzick, and Rush (1989) found that the onset of depression before age 20 predicted recurrence of depression. Initial levels of depression have been shown to be the strongest predictor of subsequent depression in adults (Lin & Ensel, 1984) and in elderly persons (Phifer & Murrell, 1986). Once depression is present, its persistence has a devastating association with close relationships. Relationships among persistently depressed persons have been shown to have greater strain and lower functionality (Mitchell, Cronkite, & Moos, 1983), and even when symptoms remit, relationships with significant others never approach the functional level of those of nondepressed persons (Billings & Moos, 1984). In one study, chronically dysthymic persons were more severely compromised in social functioning than persons who experienced episodes of major depression (Klein, Taylor, Dickstein, & Harding, 1988). Although effective treatment is available for depression, as many as 75% of those persons who recover from depression with treatment will relapse within 2 years (Hirshfield, 1982; Agency for Health Care Policy and Research, 1993). These studies illustrate the importance of aggressive intervention in initial episodes of depression, as well as attention to moderate, persistent forms of depression.

BIOLOGICAL PROCESSES IN DEPRESSION

Rapid progress has been made in understanding some of the biological processes involved in depression. This knowledge has brought evidence about feelings (drawn predominantly from personal realms of knowing) closer to evidence about autonomic, cognitive, and behavioral manifestations. These latter elements can be observed empirically. Anatomically, the expression of affect is linked to two areas in the brain, the limbic system and the hypothalamus. The limbic system is sandwiched between the brainstem and the cerebral cortex (Kolb & Whishaw, 1985). Few connections between the limbic system and higher brain centers exist, and as Stephens (1976) pointed out, "although neocortex and limbic systems do interact, it is typical of emotions that they are only slightly under the control of reasoning areas of the brain" (p. 595). Functions influenced by these areas include biological rhythms, motivation, feeding activities, sleep-wakefulness, body temperature, and endocrine and pituitary activity. Norepinephrine, a neurotransmitter, is transported from the locus coeruleus by six noradrenergic tracts projecting to the hypothalamus, thalamus, limbic system, neocortex, cerebellum, and spinal cord. Serotonin originates in nine clusters of cells in the pons and upper brainstem known as the raphe nuclei and is transported widely throughout the brain (Kolb & Whishaw, 1985).

The connection between the brain and depression arose putatively from linking the effect of antidepressant medications to neurotransmitter functioning at synaptic levels throughout the brain. Antidepressants were thought to reverse depressive symptoms by increasing the synaptic availability of two neurotransmitters, norepinephrine and serotonin. This led to an initial hypothesis that depressive phenomena resulted from a deficit of these neurotransmitters (Bunney & Davis, 1965; Schildkraut, 1965). Some data supported this hypothesis, most notably in studies of the primary metabolite of norepinephrine known as 3-methoxy-4-hydroxy-phenylglycol (MHPG) and studies of cortisol secretion patterns. Because norepinephrine cannot be assayed directly in the synapse, MHPG as an end product of norepinephrine breakdown was used as a proxy measure. MHPG studies have demonstrated reduction of MHPG excretion in some, but not all, depressed persons (Kalin, Risch, & Murphy, 1982; Zis & Goodwin, 1982; Thase, Frank, & Kupfer, 1985; Mallet et al., 1987; McEnany, 1990). Furthermore, the 4- to 6-week lag in response to antidepressant therapy raised questions about the deficit hypothesis, as the effect of the antidepressants would theoretically be immediate if a deficit of neurotransmitters were the problem (Noll, Davis, & DeLeon-Jones, 1985).

Further investigation involved acetylcholine (ACTH) by virtue of studies that linked depressive symptoms with cholinergic agonists (chemicals that combine with a synaptic receptor to initiate a reaction) (Janowsky, Risch, Parker, Huey, & Judd, 1980; Risch, Cohen, Janowsky, Kalin, & Murphy, 1980), and abnormalities in REM sleep cycles in depressed persons (Janowsky, Risch, & Gillin, 1983). These studies suggested that it was the role of ACTH in maintaining a balance among norepinephrine, serotonin, and acetylcholine that was critical to depressive symptoms, rather than a deficiency in the neurotransmitter concentration. As serotonin and norepinephrine modulate the secretion of hormones by the hypothalamus, it was predicted that hypothalamic function in depressed persons would be abnormal. Initial studies of depressed persons demonstrated that about 50% secrete excessive amounts of cortisol in the evening and that, unlike nondepressed persons, about 40% of depressed persons do not stop secreting cortisol when given dexamethasone, whereas nondepressed controls do (Carroll, 1982; Holsboer, Steiger, & Maier, 1983; Thase et al., 1985). These studies suggested a more elaborate process involving abnormalities in a dynamic, interactive process in which depressive symptoms would arise from a blunted or inappropriate response to environmental stimuli.

These developments brought regulatory systems under scrutiny. Presynaptic receptors regulate the supply of agonists by inhibiting (alpha2 receptors) and stimulating (beta receptors) the release of neurotransmitters. In this model, depressive symptoms arise from receptor malfunction either in activity or in sensitivity (downregulation). Garcia-Sevilla, Guimon, Garcia-Vallejo, and Fuster's (1986) demonstration of greater alpha2 sensitivity in depressed persons lent support to this hypothesis. Extension of the regulatory hypothesis was proposed by Siever and Davis (1985), who found that multiple factors—such as time and environmental stimuli—interact with regulatory processes, including not only the synaptic structures but also the central regulatory processes. In fact, deficits in neurotransmitters may reflect only one abnormality in a dysregulated system that is poorly modulated in response to environmental stimuli. The dysregulation of neurotransmitters may also extend to alterations in more central oscillators that regulate biological rhythms, such as sleep, temperature regulation, menses, metabolism, appetite, and sex drive, all of which have been observed to be dysregulated in depressed persons.

The dysregulation hypothesis unifies the relationship between stress and depression that has been extensively documented (Lin, Dean, & Ensel, 1986; Brown, 1987; Monroe, Bromet, Connell, & Steiner, 1986). It appears that depressed persons respond poorly to environmental pressures. Thus, stress in any form—physiological or psychological—may present a demand that exposes a vulnerability in responsiveness that becomes most obvious under stressful circumstances. As a result, timing becomes critical in this model. Clustered stressors (many at one time) have been demonstrated to be associated more with depression than single stressors, regardless of potency (Propst, Pardington, Ostrom, & Watkins, 1986; Catalano & Dooley, 1977; Turner & Noh, 1988). This finding suggests a threshold effect by which the vulnerable person may lose the ability to regulate, or may experience more erratic biological regulation, if stressors reach a certain intensity. Similarly, chronic stressors have been shown to have a strong relationship with depression, especially stressors that involve close-tie relationships (Barnett & Gotlib, 1988). By the same reasoning, exposure to a stressor over time without relief may favor extensive dysregulation.

Although men and women both experience stressors of these sorts, women *predictably* experience clustered and chronic stressors in their classic roles as caregivers. Further, points of high vulnerability for depression, such as the perinatal period, present psychosocial and biological challenges unique to women. Seiver and Davis (1985) proposed a "diabetes model" for depression in which predispositional factors (including biological ones) interact with environmental ones to produce the syndrome. The fascinating question that remains is whether the appearance of biological dysregulatory processes signals a permanent change in the biological substrate of the person and predicts a more chronic, recurrent pattern of depressive symptoms.

The importance of hypothalamic involvement in this process must be emphasized. The hypothalamus is the oscillator that integrates energy production with environmental changes by controlling physiological systems that regulate temperature, appetite, and physical activity. In addition, the hypothalamus controls pituitary and thyroid activity, as well as other "pacemakers" that generate ultradian (less than 20- to 24-hour periodicity), circadian (20- to 24-hour periodicity), and infradian (longer than 24-hour periodicity) rhythms. If erratic norepinephrine production miscues the hypothalamus, not one but many systems regulated by the hypothalamus are affected (Rosenthal, Sack, Carpenter, et al., 1985; Rosenthal, Sack, James, et al., 1985; Rosenthal, Sack, & Skwerer, 1988). Because this understanding is relatively new and may be inaccurate, one must restrain the urge to make "therefore" statements, linking specific dysregulatory processes with the phenomena seen in depression. However, understanding these relationships does begin to instruct us to attend to the interrelationships between clinical phenomena and biological processes and to change some of our intervention strategies.

If vulnerability for depression is linked to poorly modulated regulatory processes, then certain sources of stress known to interact with regulatory systems should show an association. Likely candidates would be stressors affecting neurotransmitters, the hypothalamus, the pituitary and adrenal cortex, and rhythm-disrupting stressors. This hypothesis is somewhat supported by clinical data. Certain physical disorders are strongly associated with depression. These include disorders of the thyroid or parathyroids and adrenal glands, central nervous system events (cerebral vascular accident, encephalitis), neurologic disorders (multiple sclerosis, Huntington's chorea), and neoplasms of the central nervous system or the pancreas (see Kathol, 1985, for a fuller discussion; Field, 1989). Associated with depression are the antihypertensive, analgesic, antiparkinsonian, cardiovascular, and psychotropic medications (see Flomenbaum, Freedman, Levy, Simpson, & Talley, 1984, for a more exhaustive listing), each group of which interacts with either neurotransmitters or a central regulatory process.

Some of the rhythm-disrupting events that affect biological periodicities have special implication for women. Pregnancy and childbirth have been associated not only with greater depression but also with greater mental disorders of all types for women (Weissman & Klerman, 1981; Norbeck & Tilden, 1983). Childbirth involves sleep-disrupting infant care and, by virtue of that, may be a particularly potent stressor with a potential triple-punch combination of hormonal, neurochemical, and rhythm-disrupting effects. Frequently, women are in caretaking roles in regard to spouses and parents with age- or Alzheimer's-related dementias. These women suffer as much sleep disruption as do the parents of infants. Other sleep disruptions unique to women are associated with women's multiple roles (McBride, 1988), in that women who are motivated to achieve rob themselves of sleep time to juggle full-time family and social roles in addition to work and educational commitments. Shiftwork that does not follow a forward rotation (days to evenings to nights) with adequate adjustment for each rotation may also present a stressor. Further, these special stressors for women are often combined with other rhythm-disrupting processes, such as seasonal light changes, thereby creating a rhythm-disrupting effect in short and long biological rhythms. Regulation of these rhythm-disrupting factors is a complex process that has excellent potential as an intervention in women who are vulnerable to depression. Some aspects of this will be discussed in depth later.

INTERPERSONAL PROCESSES IN DEPRESSION

Interpersonal processes have been the core dimension of psychiatric nursing, with a particular focus on using the self as a therapeutic medium through which change can be produced (Peplau, 1952; 1988). Because the difference between "therapeutic use of self" and "therapy" has been unclear, many of the principles taught in psychiatric nursing have mimicked the prescriptions of psychoanalytic theorists, in which the data generated interpersonally, especially data originating in the therapist-self, were not actually used for intervention purposes. Rather, interpersonal principles have been integrated in a global way in psychiatric–mental health nursing practice literature. Therefore, the development of interpersonal interventions that are designed to enact focused interpersonal change and use the "self" as a major part of the therapeutic dialogue is the next frontier in psychiatric–mental health nursing (Beeber, 1989a). The unique dimensions of this field of practice identified by Fagin (1967) (e.g., using the 24-hour clock, capitalizing on interactions played out over extended time periods, and caring for the whole person) fit into this agenda and would expand the opportunities for client change. This approach requires liberating our practice from restrictive traditions.

A first step might be to reformulate the theoretical model of depression. Classical theories of depression proposed that women's vulnerability to depression grew out of their unhealthy dependence on relationships for the definition of self and self-esteem maintenance (Jack, 1987a; Arieti & Bemporad, 1978; Beck, Rush, Shaw, & Emery, 1979). Unhealthy dependency was viewed as a pathological outgrowth of a failed process of differentiation, and field-dependency or relativity in the definition of the self and self processes was seen as a less healthy way of organizing experience. It has become clearer, however, that these theories using the experiences of men as the standard for determining healthy development may not hold for women (Jack, 1987a).

The work of feminist scholars and psychotherapists has resulted in a reformulation of developmental theories that allows for different worldviews for men and women. Most notable are the self-in-relation theorists, whose work offers a new direction for treating depression and for integrating interpersonal dimensions in psychiatric nursing practice. Chodorow (1978, 1985) observed that universally, infant care is women's work. As a consequence, male and female babies form their first object relation with a female. In order to adopt the identity of their genetic sex, males and females must accomplish different orientations to this first object. Females fuse the experience of attachment with identity, whereas males reactively differentiate themselves from their first object to become not-like mother. As a result, females emerge into womanhood through a longer, more connected process of identity formation carried out in relation to the mother. This process results in a greater capacity for empathy, an identity predicated on involvement with others, and more anxiety over separation. In contrast, males make a clearer demarcation of the self and reach adulthood with a sense of self formed in differentiation from others. They are more at ease with issues of separation and have more anxiety over closeness and fusion. Traditional theories that describe normal development only in terms of differentiation are therefore inadequate in describing women's world orientation, which is more contextual in the sense of self and self-esteem (Jack, 1987a; Gilligan, 1982). Whereas developmental arrest in males may well be a failure to differentiate, in females, developmental arrest is the failure to connect.

Problems for women arise not out of the process, but out of a preferential valuation of men over women in society (Miller, 1976; 1984). As a consequence, a daughter's identification with her mother is weakened by an inherent difficulty in accepting the mother—and hence the self—as valued. Additional socialization encourages women to develop qualities associated with caretaking (other-focusing, selflessness), which inherently are devalued in comparison to men's work (Bernardez, 1988). Not only does this predispose women to lower self-esteem derived from their appraised contributions (Beeber, 1987); it also "silences the self" (Jack, 1987b) by anesthetizing the woman to her own needs (Beeber, 1989b). Without this information, the woman cannot shape her relationships to meet her needs, and as a consequence her self-definition and self-esteem suffer. As disrupted self-esteem is a core dimension of depression, these factors predispose women to depression.

Self-in-relation theory also provides a conceptual umbrella to explain the finding that social support prevents the development of depression during stressful times (Ensel, 1985; Lin, et al., 1986; Cohen & Wills, 1985); indeed, such support has an even stronger effect for women than for men (Dean & Ensel, 1982). The interpersonal aspects of social support (advising, emotional support, affection, empathy, praise, feedback, reciprocity, physical touch, intimacy) have been demonstrated to protect self-esteem against threatening events (Thoits, 1985; Beeber, 1987) and, in turn, prevent depression (Pearlin, Menaghan, Lieberman, & Mullan, 1981). Those with whom the woman maintains her closest ties are both the greatest resource and the greatest danger to her self-esteem, ultimately influencing whether she becomes and remains depressed. In younger women, these ties may be with her family and friends, whereas in maturing women, the partner or spouse becomes central to this process (Brown, 1987; Brown & Harris, 1978; Barnett & Gotlib, 1988). The New Haven Epidemiologic Catchment Area (ECA) study revealed that women were three times more likely than men to be depressed if their marriages were unhappy (Weissman, 1986). Recovery from depression is also related to the overall quality of close relationships, with the level of intimacy, helpfulness, and critical emotions being influential in whether women recover or relapse from depression (Barnett & Gottlib, 1988; Hooley, Orley, & Teasdale, 1986; Belsher & Costello, 1988).

The residual effect of depression is particularly insidious as it is played out in intimate relationships. In one study, asymptomatic formerly depressed women were compared to nondepressed controls. Eight months after "recovery," the remitted women were inhibited in their communication and had more friction in their intimate relationships (Paykel & Weissman, 1973). Four years later, the same women continued to have greater interpersonal friction and more marital problems than their nondepressed counterparts (Bothwell & Weissman, 1977). If, consistent with self-in-relation theory, women are socialized to "do" the caretaking and connecting functions in a relationship, it would follow that depression in the woman would have devastating effects not only on her own self-esteem but also on the quality of her relationships. In one study, marital conflict returned to normal after depression in a spouse only if the affected spouse was the husband. Depression in the wife led to long-term marital friction after the wife had "recovered" (Gotlib, 1986).

Interpersonal processes are essential to women's sense of self and self-esteem and appear, through well-supported evidence, to be related to whether a woman becomes depressed. The capability of good interpersonal relationships to prevent depression has been demonstrated over a variety of stressful conditions, including those with profound physiologically dysregulating qualities (e.g., pregnancy, cancer, chronic physical disease). Thus, it would appear that relationships are a powerful force in combating the influence of stressors in women, especially in the development of depression. This realization should shape psychiatric nursing practice. The empirically supported protective qualities of interpersonal relationships (availability, feedback, praise, advice) are different from the qualities that therapists are taught to maintain (structured availability, neutrality, nonadvising). If, however, as predicted by self-in-relation theory, women gain their sense of self within the context of the significant relationship, the qualities modeled by therapists working in traditional models are not those most helpful for the woman to reciprocally create in her real relationships. The outcome of a reformulation of the theoretical and empirical basis for women's development and mental health may be changes in clinical approaches within the context of the therapeutic relationship. These will be proposed in a subsequent section.

INTEGRATING PREDISPOSITIONAL, BIOLOGICAL, AND INTERPERSONAL DYNAMICS IN A MODEL OF DEPRESSION

These three factors are linked in a model portraying the human as a complex being with multiple levels of sentience and volition and a capacity to adapt to the environment. Predispositional, biological, and interpersonal elements create a dynamic balance of threats and buffers that create a unique potential for women to become depressed, or to grow through interactions with the environment. In certain combinations, predispositional factors, developmental factors, threats to biological processes, and the climate of significant interpersonal relationships can overwhelm resources and create dysregulatory processes on multiple levels. These same factors can create a moment of opportunity, however. Recognition of the unique combination of these factors, and the collaborative creation of strategies to offer clients becomes the role of the psychiatric nurse.

This model creates fascinating questions. For example, how linked are the biological phenomena (immobilization as a synaptic response from dysregulated norepinephrine) and interpersonal phenomena (interpersonal immobilization)? Which comes first, or is there a reciprocal interaction between biological and behavioral activity? Obviously, neither biological nor interpersonal explanations are sufficient to explain depressive phenomena, because treatment approaches that use only one of these systems are insufficient for most clients. Further research may reveal the critical linkages, as well as the staging of the interconnection between biological and interpersonal phenomena.

Regardless of the scientific connections between body and mind, it is clear that the client who is depressed tries to organize the experience. If biological immobilization occurs under threat, the person may describe the experience through language and feeling as one of "being powerless." If one aspect of the immobilization is interpersonal withdrawal, the woman may feel a weakened sense of social connection and, through that perception, a weakened sense of self-identity and self-esteem. These feelings gain increasing congruence with the biological depletion and immobilization. In response, others in the interpersonal field may interpret the woman's withdrawal as a hostile move and become alienated. Sensing this, the woman may withdraw further as an energy-conserving move to prevent further loss of self, interpersonal "failures," and negative evaluations from her significant others. These behavioral shifts may synergize biological changes, and a cycle of reciprocal interactions may continue. These are hypothetical relationships, as the essential connections between mind and biological processes remain unconfirmed. However, it may be argued that it is essential to refrain from giving one form of intervention precedence over another, and to collaborate with the client to develop broad-spectrum intervention strategies that address a variety of target systems. The next section will detail how this can be carried out by targeting predispositional, biological, and interpersonal factors.

NURSING INTERVENTIONS WITH DEPRESSED WOMEN
PHENOMENA OF CONCERN TO NURSING

The following four phenomena are central in caring for the depressed woman: (1) dysregulated biological processes, (2) immobilization, (3) disrupted self-worth, and (4) social withdrawal.

Assessment of the depressed woman is a continuous process that begins with a thorough history and physical examination. A review of systems will provide baseline information and data to support biological dysregulation. Attention should be paid to reports of chronic fatigue, headaches, upper respiratory infections, and abdominal pain. Additional somatic symptoms, such as insomnia and appetite/eating changes, should also be investigated. If necessary, consultation with a primary health care provider should be sought to identify accompanying physical disorders and to secure additional diagnostic studies. In lieu of an organized nursing diagnostic framework for depression, the phenomenon of depression may be assessed by using DSM-IV criteria, or by using descriptive symptom severity measures such as the Schedule for Affective Disorders and Schizophrenia (SADS) or the Hamilton Rating Scale for Depression. Severity measures are particularly useful for the woman who does not report symptoms that meet DSM criteria (mild or early depression) or for monitoring changes in depressive symptoms over time (e.g., the SADS contains a lifetime version that organizes information about previous episodes of depression). Additional assessment should be done to determine biological and rhythm alterations, suicidal risk, self-worth and self-esteem, social support and relational adjustment, and acute and chronic stressors. Instruments that can assist in this process appear in Table 10–1. These instruments should be used in conjunction with a clinical interview and assessment process that allows the nurse to observe and interact with the client. Further information concerning each of the four key phenomena form a basic knowledge base necessary for assessment and intervention.

DYSREGULATED BIOLOGICAL PROCESSES

The hypothesis of dysregulated neurotransmitters predicts and explains the profoundly depressed mood, loss of interest and pleasure in activities, and psychomotor retardation, as well as the "vegetative symptoms" associated with depression, such as loss of energy/sense of fatigue, appetite and feeding patterns that are not in keeping with body requirements, sleep patterns that are not restorative, and constipation.

Although limited research has been done, it appears that the dysphoric mood present in depression is distinctly different from that found in sadness or grief. In one study that attempted to differentiate sadness from depression, depressed participants used terms such as "dispirited," "sluggish," "empty," and "listless." These descriptors were interpreted as not typical of sadness. Lethargy, inability to do things, and detachment from the environment also appeared to be unique to participants' depressed mood (Williams, Healy, Teasdale, White, & Paykel, 1990).

The process of grief has several observable differences from depressed mood. Grief is phasic, with periods of intense crying punctuated by other emotions. The mood of depression is monotone in nature and, except for diurnal variations, remains steady and persistent. Grief is characterized by crying and tears, whereas depression is typically empty and tearless. Grief centers on an "other" (the lost person or object), whereas the attention in depression is centered on the self. These characteristics are helpful in distinguishing depression from the process of healthy grieving.

The loss of energy associated with depression is often mystifying to the woman, who perceives herself as having many demands but lacking the energy to do them. At times, the anergy may be associated with loss of interest, and in this case the woman will express no consternation over the lost energy. However, some women may experience a sense of being very busy without accomplishing anything. Careful assessment will reveal a pattern of defocusing, where energy is not brought to bear productively. This may be related to the distractibility and difficulty in concentration associated with depression, compounded by the inability to maintain enough interest in the activities to bring them to closure.

Appetite disorders are very common in depressed women, and they may be inexorably linked to full-blown eating disorders (anorexia nervosa, bulimia, and compulsive overeating). The fusion of body appearance and self-worth in women may explain some of the intrapersonal overlay, but biological dysregulatory processes must also be considered. The central dysregulatory hypothesis would predict abnormal patterns of insulin and thyroid hormone secretion, alteration in cortical function, and dysregulation of biological rhythms, all of which affect appetite and eating behaviors (Thase et al., 1985). Loss of appetite closely parallels loss of interest and investment of energy in the pleasurable and social aspects of food. These patterns are evident and strikingly similar, but are often missed in the overeating depressed woman, who also eats without pleasure (and often has a sense of anger or self-loathing), and eats without socializing (solitary, often clandestine eating). Consistent with this, the overeating depressed woman may be able to control her eating more effectively if she eats in the company of others.

Sleep pattern disturbances in depressed persons take the form of dysregulated ultradian (e.g., rapid eye movement [REM] sleep cycles) and circadian (daily sleep-wake cycle) rhythm disruption. The central oscillator controlling sleep patterns appears to be in the suprachiasmatic nuclei (SCN) of the hypothalamus, with neural tracts linking it to the retina and the pineal gland (Wehr & Goodwin, 1981). Environmental cues such as light-dark cycles and work schedules entrain the circadian rhythm to the 24-hour clock. Artificially induced dysregulation of the sleep cycle has shown that the normal alignment of the sleep-wake cycle with temperature, cortisol secretion, and REM propensity is disrupted. Sleep becomes dissociated from the other three, which has been shown to result in poor sleep quality and short duration of sleep (Thase et al., 1985; Cartwright, 1993). Dysynchronization of the sleep-wake cycle relative to temperature, cortisol, and REM cycles and phase advancement of the latter three cycles may explain the phenomena of early morning awakening, REM abnormalities, and diurnal mood variation in depression (Wehr & Wirz-Justice, 1982). Abnormalities in REM include reduced REM latency (REM stages occur too early in the night at points when REM is normally latent), prolonged REM periods, and abnormal distribution across the entire sleep cycle (Cartwright, 1993). Because the sleep architecture is related to waking function, alterations in the rhythm of sleep cycles may result in clients reporting poor or disrupted sleep even when they have been observed to have slept a "normal" number of hours. More sophisticated technology to monitor sleep cycles is necessary to ascertain the degree to which elemental rhythms are disturbed in depression.

Constipation is the most prominent symptom associated with abnormal function of the digestive-eliminative systems in depressed persons. Not surprisingly, studies of colonic motility have demonstrated low neuromuscular tone that was associated with anergia and psychomotor retardation, again associated with neurotransmitter dysregulation (Lechin et al., 1983).

Menstrual cycle difficulties that are associated with depression include premenstrual tension, discomfort, and menstrual pain. Other forms of pain are also frequently associated with depression, such as headaches, abdominal and chest pain, and musculo-skeletal/back pain. Sometimes the literature has lumped these latter symptoms into the category of "somatization," but one should use caution in doing so because these symptoms are experienced physically by the depressed person and are never perceived as psychogenic in origin. Indeed, further research may reveal a physiological basis for the sensation. Often, the sequelae (e.g., pruritus) are as serious as the primary problem, and there is an ever-present danger of misinterpreting these manifestations as related to depression when they emanate from another disorder.

Other symptoms that have not been well-substantiated in the literature are skin disorders, including idiopathic itching, excoriation and infection related to scratching and picking at lesions, and other skin disorders related to anxiety-associated habits (e.g., nail-biting, scalp scratching, and hair pulling). Ulrich and Harms (1985) identified body touching of the face and hair as associated with depression. Bouhuys, Jansen, and van den Hoofdakker (1991) found an association of light body touching with the agitation present in depressed clients. These movements were noted to have been confounded with anxiety. Cloitre, Katz, and Van Praag (1993) noted that whereas anxiety and agitation were difficult to separate in depression, motor retardation was not associated with anxiety and hence became a better symptom to observe in depression.

IMMOBILIZATION

The phenomenon of immobilization encompasses the biological shutdown, the motor retardation, and the "mental meltdown" described by William Styron in *Darkness Visible* (1990). Studies of depressed individuals indicated that motor retardation was more indicative of depression than was agitation (Cloitre et al., 1993). Specifically, reduced looking, reduced speaking, increased pausing, and monotone voice have been associated with depression (see Cloitre et al., 1993 for discussion). Of note is a study by Katz et al. (1984) where factor analysis identified motor retardation and depressed mood as highly correlated.

In addition, the term immobilization includes the inhibition of interpersonal interactions, which takes the form of incapability to give and receive love, to act on behalf of self or other, and to express thoughts and feelings in a meaningful way (Beeber, 1989a). These aspects of immobilization are frequently the source of conflict between the depressed woman and her significant others and create the potential for an insidious decline of intimacy. This phenomenon is also the primary source of difficulty experienced by the nurse in maintaining a therapeutic relationship with the depressed woman. When the nurse experiences frustration and anger directly, or indirectly in the form of pity, oversolicitousness, and rescue fantasies, mutual withdrawal may occur, with both client and nurse engaging in an "as if" performance of a relationship. Genuine aspects of the relationship may then occur covertly, either consciously or in the form of dreams and reveries. If noted and used as information in the therapeutic process, mutual withdrawal may be therapeutic. However, unrecognized mutual withdrawal is not productive to the therapeutic process.

DISRUPTED SELF-WORTH

A profound loss of self-esteem is manifested in a continuum of behaviors ranging from minor neglectful or self-harming habits to the catastrophic act of suicide. Central to the loss of love for the self is a disturbance in self-identity, when the individual constructs the self as damaged and disadvantaged or, conversely, as idealized or perfect. Either is degrading, with idealization being the more elegant form of dehumanization. The struggle to make meaning out of profound biological alterations may create a self-constructed worldview where there is a central belief that one is powerless and incapable of change. In women, this self-construction resonates with societal messages of intrinsic devaluation and incapability to directly exert power to create desired outcomes. The woman's intimate relationships carry the potential to verify or contradict this self-view, and the health of these relationships as expressed through her roles and interactions is frequently the major measure of her worth as a person.

SOCIAL WITHDRAWAL

The combination of biological changes, immobilization, and disrupted self-worth creates a consistent pattern of social withdrawal. Social withdrawal includes isolation from the activities and day-to-day events occurring within the sustaining network of adult attachments. This may take the form of active refusal of involvement, passive neglect of connections and affiliations, and "substitutions" (Beeber, unpublished data), that is, all-encompassing involvement in an activity that is primarily nonsocial (e.g., athletic training, addictive substances or habits, solitary academic or work pursuits).

STRATEGIES IN THE THERAPEUTIC RELATIONSHIP

Addressing these four phenomena forms the structure of a comprehensive intervention initiative with the depressed woman, at the core of which is the therapeutic relationship. The goals of nursing care would be the following:

1. The restoration and protection of biological regulatory systems
2. The modulation of mood, thought, and action
3. The restoration and strengthening of self-worth
4. The restoration of social integration and enhancement of meaningful social involvement

Except for the obvious imperative of meeting basic physiologic needs and safety, no one goal is unrelated to another, nor must goals be met in any particular order. As in any holistic approach, all these goals are considered simultaneously, and interventions address several goals at once. As always, the emphasis of nursing care extends beyond mere restoration and toward the goal of a higher level of wellness and personal growth for the depressed woman.

Regardless of whether the emphasis of an intervention is biological or interpersonal, the collaboration of the client is essential to its success. Collaboration depends on the strength and viability of the therapeutic relationship. Maintaining a successful relationship with a depressed client requires vigilant attention to the interpersonal "selves" of the nurse and client because the phenomena discussed in the previous section wreak havoc on intimacy. For women, the failure of therapeutic processes to occur within the relationship not only creates a stall but also may actually create more damage to the self, which is defined in relation to significant others. That which can help can harm, and in this instance the therapeutic relationship can invalidate self, erode self-worth, and prevent the mutual growth of both client and nurse if it is not managed successfully. As already noted in this chapter's review of interpersonal processes that protect women against depression, the qualities of empathy, emotional support, feedback, advising, affection, reciprocity, physical touch, and intimacy have been demonstrated to be depression protective. Thus, while operating within a clearly defined set of limits between nurse and client, it is necessary to incorporate the qualities of affirming connections within the therapeutic relationship.

Empathy is the most central quality in the therapeutic relationship with depressed women because it provides the data for understanding, and the empathetic nurse models one of the qualities empirically supported as a stress-protective factor for women. Empathy always requires a boundary between the nurse and client, in that the client's experience is shared with the nurse but not confused with the nurse's experience. Empathy is based on an assumption that no person's experience is exactly like another's, and therefore no assumptions of understanding are ever made by the nurse. Instead, the posture of constant query as to the client's experiences, beliefs, feelings, and responses is maintained. Verification of the accurate, empathic response is made by restatement—"My understanding of your experience is . . ."—which is either validated or invalidated by the client. The reaching of consensus concretely indicates to the woman, "You are important, and you have been heard." It also allows the woman to reflect upon herself. For some women, it is their first experience hearing their own voice. This aspect is tedious and requires discipline, especially when the slowed, often disjointed thought processes of the depressed woman make interacting a predominantly nonverbal exchange. In such a moment of "verbal minimalism," it helps to attentively struggle to reflect the inner world of the woman to her. The struggle will be duly noted by the client as a measure of the nurse's interest, even if the reflection is inaccurate.

Authenticity has been described by Parse (1981) as a process in the mutual creation of meaning in a therapeutic relationship. However, creating authenticity is a tricky process in the close-in work with the depressed client because what feels to the nurse to be authentic reactions to the client may be defensive perceptions that serve to protect the nurse from discomfort. Anger, for example, is often experienced by the nurse working with the depressed client. Frequently, supervisees say, "*When is it OK to get angry at the client,*" as if anger is a given in the mutual interaction of nurse and client. Anger may, however, emanate from the complex interpersonal maneuvers of the client to withdraw from intimacy and may be the nurse's response to the frustration of being thwarted in the effort to care for the client (Beeber, 1989a). The authentic experience underlying the anger may, in fact, be the nurse's sense of powerlessness associated with the client's unclear requests for help. If so, reflection on the sense of powerlessness and clarification that this is the *client's*, not the nurse's, powerlessness are more useful to the client than the nurse's expression of anger. Supervision with a clinician who empathizes rather than directs is helpful because it allows the nurse's voice to be heard.

Interpersonal self-vigilance is required. It is critical for the nurse to take "universal emotional precautions" against depression contagion. If the nurse draws self-worth in relation to the responses and progress of the client, the blunted posture of the client may dangerously erode the nurse's efficacy and self-esteem. Recognition of the profound biological alterations associated with depression can assist in helping the nurse to maintain a living connection to the client who is interpersonally dead, or whose blunted responses are not in synch with mutuality in the relationship. To maintain attentive contact, the author imagines herself rowing across the synapse carrying vital neurotransmitters to compensate for the lost biochemicals!

Albeit silly, this type of gaming serves to neutralize the perception that the client's behavior is totally volitional and prevents the nurse from taking things personally.

Specific Strategies that Address Predispositional, Biological, and Interpersonal Factors

With a healthy therapeutic relationship established, specific strategies can be developed to (1) restore and protect biological regulatory systems; (2) modulate mood, rumination, and action; (3) restore and strengthen self-esteem; and (4) restore and enhance social integration. At the end of this section, Table 10–2 summarizes the interventions presented in the following narrative.

RESTORATION AND PROTECTION OF BIOLOGICAL REGULATORY SYSTEMS

This aspect of care centers on the biological therapies directly and requires close collaboration with other health disciplines.

Compensatory interventions to provide basic requirements for nourishment, hydration, elimination, protection from injury, and exercise must be provided. Viewing these deficits as the result of dysregulated neurotransmitters and central oscillators should remove the discomfort and worry associated with creating undue dependency by providing this care to an adult who is not physically sick. As in any basic caregiving, however, care must be taken to assure that the client is challenged to accomplish all that she can do for herself.

Psychotropic medications are potent allies in restoration of normal regulation of transmitters, and the symptomatic client must be considered a candidate for pharmacotherapy. Women are more likely than male clients to be offered, and to accept, psychotropic medication (Cooperstock, 1981). The introduction of new antidepressants has been rapid in the last decade, providing several groups that appear to exert therapeutic effects different from the original cyclic antidepressants. This advance has expanded the choices of pharmacotherapy for clients and requires ongoing updates for the psychiatric nurse, particularly in determining physiological and psychological baselines against which to detect positive and untoward responses to medication (Beeber, 1985). An excellent review of currently available antidepressants, dosages, side effects, and a discussion of clinical decision making with clients was published by the Agency for Health Care Policy and Research (AHCPR, 1993).

Further work in biological markers to identify clients who will respond to medication is necessary. In addition, promising efforts to develop MHPG, cortisol suppression, and REM sleep suppression as markers is in progress (Schildkraut, 1978, 1982; Thase et al., 1985). No matter how advanced pharmacotherapy becomes, however, the interpersonal context in which medications are given will always be a potent aspect of therapy. Weissman (Weissman, 1979; Weissman, Klerman, Prusoff, Sholomskas, & Padian, 1981) demonstrated that medications were most effective when combined with interpersonal therapy. Resistance to medication will take forms that are resonant with depression. Active (saying "no") or passive (forgetting) refusal will emanate from a sense of not being worthy of treatment or from a need to express hostility toward the caregivers. Subtle forms of hostility such as aggrandizing the effects of the medication in recovery (thereby minimizing the nurse's contribution) or emphasizing the negative effects of the medication (thereby accusing the nurse of harming) are consistent with depression and may invite nonfacilitative responses by the nurse that will undermine the therapy. Suicide must always be con-

TABLE 10–2. Nursing Intervention Strategies

STRATEGIES	RATIONALE
Biological Protection or Restoration	
Primary and Secondary Prevention	
Assist women to recognize factors in their personal histories that predispose them to dysregulatory risk; institute personal risk-reduction programs and anticipatory event interventions (e.g., securing adequate nighttime help for postpartum infant care).	Anticipatory guidance increases self-efficacy.
Develop aggregate intervention programs associated with risk factors (e.g., instituting scientifically sound shift rotation patterns in a nursing department).	The cost of such interventions is offset by their potential to prevent more severe disorders from developing.
Educate women about concomitant and prodromal disorders associated with depression (e.g., hormonal disorders); assist in developing ongoing monitoring programs in association with internists/primary care providers.	Anticipatory guidance increases self-efficacy; overall health improvement reduces vulnerability.
Prevent infradian rhythm disruption; establish history of sensitivity to seasonal light changes and depression; institute bright light therapy in early morning hours during autumn season through early spring.	Early intervention into seasonal affective disorder may prevent full development of depression.
Tertiary Prevention	
Compensate for deficits resulting from alterations in self-care/biological changes.	Compensation reduces vulnerability and may help restore neurochemical precursors.
Assess need and readiness for antidepressants; work with resistances to medication; educate and monitor response; treat side effects and intervene with adverse effects; assess readiness for cessation of pharmacotherapy; replace medications with nonmedication alterations.	Antidepressants act directly on neurochemical alterations; they are potentiated by concomitant use of nonmedication interventions.
Restore sleep pattern; assess for medications and habits that disrupt sleep or sleep cycles; readjust cycle by waking earlier or instituting sleep deprivation and reinstitution of sleep pattern; use supporting sleep-enhancing interventions (e.g., exercise program); avoid medications for sleep.	Sleep pattern restoration has a direct effect on mood and mental clarity and may assist in restoration of other neurochemical processes.
Initiate regular exercise program that is aerobic and stressful within safe limits.	Regular exercise has direct self-esteem-enhancing benefits and may assist in restoration of other neurochemical processes.
Assess nutritional patterns and institute balanced, healthy diet.	Healthy eating has direct self-esteem-enhancing benefits and may assist in restoration of neurochemical precursors.

Table continued on following page.

TABLE 10–2. Nursing Intervention Strategies *Continued*

STRATEGIES	RATIONALE
Mood-Modulating Interventions	
Primary and Secondary Prevention	
Identify factors associated with significant changes in mood; establish a personal set of baseline and altered mood patterns.	Personal pattern establishes prodromes to mood shifts and increases attention to alterations in mood that precede depressive episodes.
Tertiary Prevention	
Develop distraction through action; practice individually and with a group.	Distraction pre-empts depressive ruminative patterns that enhance negative mood.
Use progressive confrontation of stressful conditions by breaking the end goal into a series of smaller confrontations.	Progressive confrontation develops efficacy by altering the anxiety-avoiding pattern of immobility and teaching progressive skills; increased control enhances self-worth.
Self-Esteem Restoration	
Primary and Secondary Prevention	
Assist the client to build a configuration of relationships, roles, and a sense of self-efficacy supportive of self-esteem.	Relationship configuration prepares the woman for challenges to self-esteem.
Identify events that threaten these aspects; may be "positive" events (e.g., motherhood, relocation) as well as "negative" events (e.g., illness, exit of significant other).	Identification allows preparation for changes in configurations that support self-esteem.
Secondary and Tertiary Prevention	
Engage in self-reflection that does not include rumination; use journals, evocative activities (e.g., poetry, visualization, dance, play, humor).	Self-reflection places client in a position to self-know.
Focus client on delineating self-enhancing arenas from those which diminish self-esteem; configure time and energy to maximize involvement in enhancing arenas.	Self-enhancing arenas develop greater control over self-esteem.
Assist client to change interpersonal patterns to provide qualities that buffer stress (e.g., empathy, reciprocity, high-quality feedback, authenticity); use 1:1, dyad, and groups to create "laboratories" for practicing the new patterns necessary to support these qualities.	These patterns strengthen specific qualities of social support demonstrated to buffer stress.

sidered a possibility, especially in the client who is emerging from severe depression, and prodromal behaviors—such as interpersonal withdrawal and collecting medication—should be investigated.

Coining the term *ecological advocacy,* the American Nurses Association Task Force on Psychopharmacology (1994) delineated the role of nursing as engaging with the client to assure "that psychopharmacologic interventions fit with the overall style and quality of the patient's life" (p. 31). The nurse must continually collaborate with clients, significant others, and providers; educate them; and maintain rigorous legal and ethical standards. The reader is referred to the full report of the task force for additional information.

TABLE 10–2. NURSING INTERVENTION STRATEGIES *Continued*

STRATEGIES	RATIONALE
Enhancement of Social Integration *Primary and Secondary Prevention* Educate clients to consider qualities of social roles in terms of self-esteem mainte-nance; offer life-planning exercises to provide anticipatory guidance about life choices; educate clients to consider role changes as risks.	Anticipatory guidance increases sense of self-efficacy.
Tertiary Prevention Examine present roles for their contribution to self-esteem; assist client to eliminate or reduce involvement in roles that erode self-esteem; assist client to engage in long-term planning (e.g., education) to allow a shift into other roles; reduce overall number of roles if this is related to performance.	Role identification increases resources for self-esteem derivation and offers greater stress-buffering potential.

Restoration and protection of biological rhythms is a relatively new direction for nursing that is based on observations dating back to ancient times when healers were more astute about human interactions with natural changes in diurnal and sea-sonal rhythms in the environment (Wehr & Rosenthal, 1989). Two areas of rhythm restoration with preliminary evidence of effectiveness are sleep-wake interventions and phototherapy for seasonal affective disorders. In addition to overt disturbances in sleep-wake cycles (early morning awakening, hypersomnia), decreased slow-wave sleep and abnormal REM cycle distribution and onset have been documented in depressed persons (Thase et al., 1985). These disturbances have been related to central dysregulatory processes that govern serotonin and norepinephrine, as well as central oscillators that entrain sleep cycles to environmental cues and align sleep-wake with cortisol secretion and temperature cycles.

Sleep deprivation has been explored in a preliminary manner, based on the hy-pothesis that phase advancement, or misalignment of the sleep cycle, has occurred in relation to other biological rhythms. Sleep deprivation has been shown to have a tem-porary, significant mood-elevation effect in clients, and it may develop into a treat-ment that predicts response to antidepressants or potentiates antidepressants (Elsinga & Van den Hoofdakker, 1983). Experimentally, the procedure has involved either totally depriving clients of sleep one to two nights per week or awakening them early every morning to deprive them of the REM sleep that occurs more fre-quently in the morning hours (Noll et al., 1985). Research has been sparse in this area, possibly due to the technical difficulties in carrying out the protocols. However, psy-chiatric nurses who work in inpatient settings are in an ideal position to carry out in-dependent and collaborative research on the effectiveness of sleep alteration as a tech-nique to restore normal rhythmicity in depressed persons. As noted earlier, women (including nurses who rotate shifts!) encounter a variety of sleep-depriving events, which, combined with predispositional factors, may result in clinical depression.

Phototherapy has been demonstrated to be of use with persons meeting criteria for Seasonal Pattern (American Psychiatric Association, 1994). Bright light therapy (2,500 to 10,000 lux) has been demonstrated to be superior to dimmer light, with a ratio of strength to length of exposure being significant. Consequently, treatments of

10,000 lux are effective if used for only 30 minutes per day, with increasing exposure required for lower intensity lights. In addition, early morning exposure appears to have a greater effect than evening light. Exposure through the eye appears to be more effective than exposure to the skin, and it appears that although full-spectrum light is necessary, ultraviolet light (UV) does not enhance the effect. Therefore, UV light can be eliminated, which may remove the harmful effects associated with UV light (Wehr & Rosenthal, 1989). As in sleep restoration interventions, light therapy appears to offer potentiation of other treatments, or perhaps preventative possibilities. The use of light therapy is another exciting direction for developing independent and collaborative psychiatric nursing research.

Further work in psychiatric nursing research must pursue the use of aerobic conditioning exercise to restore biological dysrhythmias in depressed women. Hypothetically, there should be a relationship between physical stress, norepinephrine production, and depression. Ultimately, physical exercise combined with music and rhythmic motion may be used to restore regulation of related rhythmic processes. In addition, the more overt benefits of exercise—such as sleep pattern restoration, increased physical strength, conditioning, and weight stabilization—may be self-esteem enhancing. However, caution must be exerted not to repeat the past mistakes of confusing physical appearance with self-enhancement. The author recalls, painfully, encouraging women clients to apply makeup or to do their hair because others valued it as a measure of their recovery. Self-enhancement is a personal matter, and it is essential that the woman direct energy toward the undeveloped potentials in herself that she, not others, defines.

MODULATION OF MOOD, RUMINATION, AND ACTION

Modulation is defined as creating a proper proportion among mood, rumination, and action. A goal of intervention would be to change the disproportionate degree to which a depressed person substitutes rumination for efficacious action. Nolen-Hoeksema (1987) presented evidence that women respond to their feelings of depression by rumination, which, in turn, amplifies the depressive experience. In contrast, men use action techniques to distract themselves from the experience and, as a result, self-limit depression. Without contradicting the earlier discussion about the need to bring the woman in contact with her own internal self, this finding may be applied therapeutically through the process of preempting depressive phenomena. Preempting requires recognizing an immobilizing pattern and then inserting a cognitive or behavioral preemption. This reverses the tendency to link depressed mood and thought with inaction. Breaking this pattern often leads to new experience and insight. For example, a client who brooded about past events and ruminated about self-harm purchased razor blades and hoarded medication. The preemption consisted of going out (action) and buying a safe, symbolic object instead of the blades or pills. In one instance, these symbolic objects included a rubber rat, a package of laxatives, a belt, and a purse, each of which reminded the depressed woman of an episode where she was furious with a parent. These episodes were then processed with the nurse.

Helping the woman develop self-efficacy, or the power to influence outcomes in the direction she chooses (Beeber, 1989b), is done by progressive exposure to situations requiring action, and systematic evaluation of the actions (or lack of actions) taken. The skill of the nurse will be directed toward aborting the depressed person's capacity to avoid failure by resorting to a less meaningful level of involvement. The depressed person perceives failure as a threat to an already fragile sense of self-worth. Therefore, inactivity, including procrastination, is often a defense against imagined failure. An effective strategy is to create no-fail sequences. No-fail sequences require consensually determining a goal with the client, and then breaking the goal into a series of less energy-consuming steps until the client cannot fail to reach the first step. For example, a woman's goal of stating needs clearly and getting others to respect those needs would begin with "thinking about a need" (a small component), "practicing saying the need" (with the nurse), "trying it with a less important person," and then "trying it with the significant other." When each step is accomplished, the next agreed-upon step is tackled. These strategies may lead to new behaviors such as assertiveness or outspokenness, risk taking, or advancement into new roles. The client's actions will affect her closest relationships, and she and her significant others may require help in reconfiguring their relationship. For example, Hirsch (1980) found that families of women returning to school were not always helpful, probably due to the woman withdrawing from some of her previous functions to allow time for her own development.

Talking will not by itself change the immobility of the depressed person. Interventions to restore biological integrity also enhance the mobilization effort. These include kinesthetic therapy, massage, regular rhythmic or aerobic exercise, visualization, and other forms of doing-and-moving strategies. Physical exercise is the most useful strategy because of its self-enhancing and biological benefits. Establishing a regular aerobic outlet can become an automatic preemption that can be increased when depressed mood increases. Until recently, women were typically discouraged from developing body prowess through rough play. As a consequence, women were barred from access to the profound benefits of activities in which the total body is involved, spacial orientation is dramatically changed, and mood is modulated rapidly. This form of activity is an empowering process in itself. Catalyzed by a creative therapy aide, the author had a 4-minute, intense chase and water-balloon fight with a very depressed woman at a ward picnic. The short-term end point was much wetness and laughter, while the long-term outcome was more progress than had occurred in months.

RESTORATION AND STRENGTHENING OF SELF-WORTH

Careful assessment of the depressed woman's relationships, roles, self-efficacy, and self-image will usually reveal the portrait of her self-worth. As noted previously, the successful maintenance of relationship integrity is taken by many women as a measure of their worth and effectiveness as a person. In addition, the reflected appraisals of significant others can determine self-esteem. Roles and the sense of personal efficacy, or power to determine outcomes, are also determinants of self-worth (Beeber, 1987; 1989b), and body image is a source of reflected appraisals from significant others as well as society at large.

The preliminary step to restoration and enhancement of these elements is to place the woman in touch with herself. This requires continual reflection by the nurse to help the client enhance her inner voice. Evocative strategies that allow her access to other potentials can be used. These strategies include expressive activities and play, poetry and music, and personal journals (written and taped). The last activity is almost essential in the process of having the woman identify her own voice, but she must be ready to use it and be comfortable with writing or speaking her thoughts.

Laboratories for change in the woman's patterns of seeking and maintaining relationships include the therapeutic relationship, women's groups (Gordon & Gordon, 1987; Gordon, Matwychuk, Sachs, & Canedy, 1988), heterogeneous groups, and family strategies. Self-in-relation theory requires new scrutiny of the therapeutic relationship because of the power of this medium to convey worth or worthlessness to women and hence to shape their identity. Whereas there is a danger of being "blindsided" when the nurse and client are both women, there is also a power inherent in the recognition of the nurse-self in relation to the client-self. In addition to empathy, empirical data have identified availability, reciprocity, touch, and feedback as qualities of social support that protect women against depression. Although earlier studies indicated that these functions had to come from a male (spouse, lover), work by the author has indicated that woman-to-woman contact is efficacious as well (Beeber, 1987). The therapeutic relationship can become a learning laboratory in which the female nurse models and teaches the woman to use availability, reciprocity, touch, and feedback, and then to build them into her real-life relationships.

Incorporating these qualities into the therapeutic relationship requires aggressive examination of the nurse's conduct in the relationship. For example, the form of reciprocity most protective against depression is either equality or nurturance (taking). I have demonstrated that being a giver is correlated with depression (Beeber, unpublished results). Tilden (Tilden, 1987; Tilden & Nelson, 1988) suggested that fixed unequal relationships (such as the classical "taking" posture of the client) would diminish self-worth. The clinical problem becomes one of differentiating between authentic forms of giving by the woman-client and defensive giving that obscures her own needs. Based on this reformulation, a therapeutic relationship should promote equality and authentic nurturance by both nurse and client, and it should incorporate strategies to interrupt defensive "giving" by either the client or the nurse. This structure for the relationship models a more stress-protective form of intimacy and pushes the woman-client to acknowledge her own needs. Availability creates the material for processing day-to-day events and intricacies that are the raw material for the formation of the self in relation to others. Feedback that contains praise and useful criticism is also depression-protective in stressful conditions (Beeber, 1987; unpublished data). Criticism helps correct the course of action in the woman. However, as noted in the review of depression recidivism, criticism in some forms becomes dangerous and appears to aid chronicity. Thus, perfecting the art of delivering useful criticism that is balanced with support is a skill to develop in the therapeutic relationship. Each of these aspects represents new directions in which to develop, research, and fine-tune the technique of therapeutic use of self-in-relation as a healing-in-relation strategy in psychiatric nursing. For example, video technologies for direct feedback represent a direction for enhancing nursing strategies in the therapeutic encounter.

Groups are useful both for assessing the conduct of interpersonal relationships and for providing laboratories for the direct experience and change of interpersonal patterns. Several of the processes supported by empirical evidence—such as empathy, feedback, and equalization of reciprocity—are excellent focal points for group intervention.

Given the body of supporting evidence that marital or partner support and depression are strongly related, direct work with the marital dyad is necessary. The author has concentrated efforts on developing the qualities of empathy, availability, feedback, and physical touch with couples. Studying the woman within the context of her family is essential, as these interrelated roles and relationships form the structure of her self. An alternative view is that of the family as the unit of study, in which the roles and relationships of all members are considered simultaneously. This approach has the advantage of defocusing the "woman's depression" as the problem, as well as synergyzing the change process. Further, since heterogeneity in support structures (family and nonfamily members) has been shown to buffer the development of depression (Hirsch, 1980), developing differentiated relationships may be a helpful strategy for the woman and for others in the family.

RESTORATION AND ENHANCEMENT OF SOCIAL INTEGRATION

Relationships and roles are closely connected in women's lives. Loss or disruption of a relationship may mean the loss of multiple roles. If the woman has encountered a disruption of ties (relocation, separation from home, divorce, widowhood, transition from work to parenthood), both the lost ties and the newly developing ties should be evaluated for the relational qualities outlined previously, as well as the self-enhancing roles associated with them. Furthermore, caretaking roles—for example, *as* a parent or *of* a parent or spouse—have rhythm-disrupting elements and must be assessed for these qualities.

Lifework is a self-defined construct and is constructed from the woman's sense of identity. Indeed, defining what is meaningful work is a crucial outcome of the process of hearing her own voice. For example, nontraditional work roles may be a source of both strength and stress for women because successful functioning requires qualities that are relatively anxiety-provoking to women (e.g., separation, competition). Further, work schedules—either self-induced or institutionally induced, as noted before—can disrupt biological rhythms and relational ties. Therefore, the woman needs to achieve a balance between work and relationships. This may require validation of the need for the woman to develop an alternative work structure and expectations for achievement. Conversely, she may need support to change her own functioning within her circle of significant relationships and to ask for changes from them in return. These strategies are not exhaustive, but they should promote thoughtful synthesis by the nurse to adapt these examples to specific clients.

A great deal of intervention needs to be done so that depressive symptoms do not become severe enough to be a disorder. Nursing intervention includes identifying potential health problems and response patterns that pose health risks. Thus, it is appropriate to provide primary (removal of risks) and secondary (early intervention) prevention for clients. Table 10–2 presents examples of interventions at each of the prevention levels.

NEW DIRECTIONS FOR PRACTICE, RESEARCH, AND EDUCATION

Current restructuring of health care delivery will bring changes in the delivery of psychiatric nursing services to depressed women. Much of the emphasis in psychiatric nursing practice has been on the care of severely symptomatic clients in institutional settings. However, the material covered in this chapter indicates that there is a dynamic interaction between the environment and a woman's individual risks and predispositions for depression. Therefore, the strategy of prevention must be explored as a cost-effective alternative to tertiary or illness-related care. Because there are known predispositions for depression and known risk events that increase the likelihood of depression developing in women, individual and aggregate prevention strategies can be developed for women who are at risk. These include helping women recognize predispositional factors, both individual and social, and assisting them to engage in systematic programs to strengthen their resources and lessen their liability. The psychiatric nurse could construct continuing education offerings, collaborate with prevention programs, or offer individual initiatives as an entrepreneur. Gordon's (Gordon & Gordon, 1987) work in secondary prevention with women experiencing symptoms of depression is an excellent model of advanced practice with high-risk women.

It is this author's opinion that we have lost ground in developing the role of psychiatric nursing with severely depressed clients by failing to exploit the milieu as a theater of practice and by failing to develop models of practice that allow sustained nursing contact with clients before and after hospitalization. These limitations restrict our impact to that of episodic intervention, which does not allow enough contact to use and evaluate combined psychosocial-biological interventions. In contrast, case management models, such as those used in rehabilitation, could be applied to the care of severely depressed or moderately depressed but high-risk women.

Basic and intervention research is needed to identify high-risk events and the strategies that help women negotiate them, as well as the effect of these interventions on depression (Barnard et al., 1988). Early prodromes of depression—including the early signs of dysregulated biological processes, such as de-entrained rhythms and sluggish or inappropriate responses to environmental stimuli—must be identified to support early intervention when restorative strategies might have a greater effect. Interventions that potentiate somatic therapies and increase the client's collaboration in pharmacotherapy must be demonstrated to have clinical effectiveness. Finally, the specific impact of the relationship-as-laboratory must be studied and verified as to its effectiveness with depressed persons. These represent exciting areas for the expansion of psychiatric nursing research. Table 10–3 presents selected research questions to stimulate thinking about researchable phenomena in psychiatric nursing practice.

TABLE 10–3. RESEARCH QUESTIONS ABOUT DEPRESSION

Primary Prevention
1. What risk factors are predictors of depression in women?
2. How do identified risk factors differ over the life span of women?
3. What patterns of potentiation and interaction exist among identified risk factors?
4. What is the relationship between rhythm-disrupting factors and the development of subsequent depression?
5. What factors protect women against the effects of single and multiple risk factors?
6. What interventions are effective in reducing the impact of single and multiple risk factors?
7. What interventions restore rhythms and what is the effect of these interventions on depression?
8. How do changes along the life span of a woman affect the efficacy of interventions for depression?

Secondary Prevention
1. What prodromes and concomitant disorders are associated with depression?
2. What are the biological, behavioral, and interpersonal markers associated with the development of depressive symptoms?
3. What biological and interpersonal interventions are effective with moderate symptoms of depression?

Tertiary Prevention
1. What interventions reduce the side/adverse effects of somatic treatments for depression?
2. What interventions (biological and interpersonal) enhance somatic treatments for depression?
3. What interventions are effective with families of severely depressed women?
4. What postsuicide intervention strategies are effective in preventing subsequent suicide in survivors of suicide?
5. What biological and interpersonal interventions are effective with severely depressed women?

Data from Gross, D., Fogg, L., & Conrad, B. (1993). Designing interventions in psychosocial research. *Archives of Psychiatric Nursing, 7*(5), 259–264, and Hoffman, A. L., & Betrus, P. A. (1992). Theory and practice: Scientists' and practitioners' roles. *Archives of Psychiatric Nursing, 6*(1), 2–9.

To prepare psychiatric nurses to direct such practice, the education of psychiatric nurses must change. First, the previous emphasis on only the interpersonal has facilitated integrating away the specialty knowledge base of psychiatric nursing by creating an interpersonal curriculum thread that has been substituted for psychiatric nursing content. This has been operationalized by placing basic (and even graduate) students with moderately anxious clients to implement interpersonal interventions. Lost to the student is the experiential contact with severely symptomatic clients, as well as the exposure to somatic therapies specific to psychiatric treatment. Furthermore, the mind-body duality has been perpetuated by the association of physiologic knowledge only with the areas of medical and surgical nursing. This has virtually eliminated the study of brain biology, neurotransmission and mentation, and neurological-hormonal bases for emotion, attention, and learning. Graduate programs have emphasized models of pathology treatment and neglected mental health and prevention models. Correcting these curricular patterns is essential to changing the practice of psychiatric nursing.

In 1994, the Society for Education and Research in Psychiatric–Mental Health Nursing (SERPN) issued a position statement on the education of psychiatric nurses in which detailed knowledge and skills were delineated for undergraduate and graduate education. These included biological and psychological theories of mental health and illness, comprehensive biopsychosocial assessment, therapeutic use of self, and inclusion of families and communities in the care of populations at risk for mental illness (SERPN, 1994). Several psychiatric nursing textbooks have integrated biological and interpersonal approaches (Wilson & Kneisl, 1992; Haber, McMahon, Price-Hoskins, & Sideleau, 1992; Stuart & Sundeen, 1995; Keltner, Schwecke, & Bostrom, 1991). In addition, two conferences convened by the National Institute of Mental Health in 1989 and 1990 (Beeber, in press) produced a synthesis of biological and interpersonal knowledge that created a basic body of knowledge to incorporate into basic and advanced psychiatric nursing practice. In June 1994, the final report by the Task Force on Psychopharmacology convened by the American Nurses Association and the National Institute of Mental Health was published. This report includes guidelines for the care of clients receiving psychotropic medications and recommendations for curricular changes necessary to produce competent practitioners (American Nurses Association, 1994).

Doctoral programs must produce researchers in psychiatric nursing who have been instructed in biobehavioral methods, models of collaborative research, and clinical outcome and epidemiological methodologies that support the investigation of prevention strategies. Two notable papers have recently presented models integrating research and practice in psychiatric settings. Hoffman and Betrus (1992) presented systematic case study and representative case research methods as an alternative to large sample research, which poses a problem in psychiatric nursing practice. Gross, Fogg, and Conrad (1993) developed a model of psychiatric nursing intervention in which the linkages among theory, data, and interventions were explicit and complete. The latter model is an excellent guide for innovative programs for depressed women.

CONCLUSION

As the era of health care reform unfolds, nursing's philosophical belief in prevention, early intervention, and treatment of the human response to health problems is a cost-effective alternative to the current emphasis on tertiary treatment of advanced disease. In order to demonstrate the cost-savings and quality-of-life benefits of this approach, psychiatric–mental health nurses need to demonstrate an expanded role in provision of services to clients (Krauss, 1993). This chapter has outlined the role of advanced practice nursing with women who are at risk for or already demonstrate symptoms of depression. Psychiatric–mental health nurses must take the initiative to develop demonstration programs of care for such women. These can be done in conjunction with university schools of nursing, for example, through joint teaching, clinical care, and research programs. In addition, entrepreneurial ventures to manage the care of depressed individuals can be developed if unique services are identified and demonstrated to reduce costs—for example, home management of depressed women who are not easily mobile, for example, women with young children, elderly women, and technology-dependent women or women who are caretakers of parents or spouses.

An additional challenge of health care reform for psychiatric nurses will be to align values of client-centered caring with cost-effectiveness. Cost containment may open avenues to explore the development of quality-enhancement interventions in chronic conditions when treatment options have been exhausted. Psychiatric nurses enjoy a positive image with consumers and families and must use this alliance to advocate for mental health and illness care in a reformed health care system.

Clearly, the birthright of psychiatric–mental health nursing is in the integration of biological, developmental, psychological, social, and spiritual aspects of individuals and families who are at risk for or currently suffering depression. Innovative models of prevention and treatment of depression founded on sound science will be of great benefit to women and their significant others. Psychiatric nurses are in an excellent position to develop and implement such models.

REFERENCES

Agency for Health Care Policy and Research. (1993). *Depression in primary care: Volume 1. Detection and diagnosis* and *Volume 2. Treatment of major depression.* Rockville, MD: US Department of Health and Human Services.

American Nurses Association. (1994). *Psychiatric mental health nursing psychopharmacology project.* Washington, DC: Author.

American Psychiatric Association. (1994). *Diagnostic and statistical manual of mental disorders* (4th ed.). Washington, DC: Author.

Arieti, S., & Bemporad, J. (1978). *Severe and mild depression: The psychoanalytic approach.* New York: Basic.

Barnard, K., Magyary, D., Sumner, G., Booth, C., Mitchell, S., & Spieker, S. (1988). Prevention of parenting alterations for women with low social support. *Psychiatry, 51,* 248–253.

Barnett, P., & Gottlib, I. (1988). Psychosocial functioning and depression: Distinguishing among antecedents, concomitants and consequences. *Psychological Bulletin, 104,* 97–126.

Barrett-Lennard, G. (1962). Dimensions of therapist response as causal factors in therapeutic change. *Psychological Monographs, 76,* 1–36.

Beck, A., Rush, A., Shaw, B., & Emery, G. (1979). *Cognitive therapy of depression.* New York: Guilford.

Beck, A., Ward, C., Mendelson, M., Mock, J., & Erbaugh, J. (1961). An inventory for measuring depression. *Archives of General Psychiatry, 4,* 561–571.

Beck, A., Weissman, A., Lester, D., & Trexler, L. (1974). The measurement of pessimism: The Hopelessness Scale. *Journal of Consulting and Clinical Psychology, 42,* 861–865.

Beeber, L. S. (1980). Antidepressant medications. In S. Lego (Ed.), *The American handbook of psychiatric nursing* (pp. 568–579). Philadelphia: Lippincott.

Beeber, L. S. (1985). Psychopharmacotherapy. In D. Critchley & J. Maurin (Eds.), *The clinical nurse specialist in psychiatric–mental health nursing* (pp. 295–342). New York: Wiley.

Beeber, L. S. (1987). The relationship of self-esteem, social support and depressive symptoms in women. Unpublished dissertation, University of Rochester, Rochester, NY.

Beeber, L. S. (1989a). Enacting corrective interpersonal experiences with the depressed client: An intervention model. *Archives in Psychiatric Nursing, 3,* 211–217.

Beeber, L. S. (1989b). The role of social resources in depression: A woman's perspective. In L. Beeber (Ed.), *Depression: Old problems, new perspectives in nursing care* (pp. 1–13). Thorofare, NJ: SLACK.

Beeber, L. S. (1990). To be one of the boys: Aftershocks of the World War I nursing experience. *Advances in Nursing Science, 12,* 32–43.

Belle, D. (1982). *Lives in stress: Women and depression.* Beverly Hills, CA: Sage.

Belsher, G., & Costello, C. (1988). Relapse after recovery from unipolar depression: A contemporary review. *Psychological Bulletin, 104,* 84–96.

Bernardez, T. (1988). *Women and anger—Cultural prohibitions and the feminine ideal.* Wellesley, MA: Stone Center for Developmental Services and Studies.

Billings, A., & Moos, R. (1984). Coping, stress, and social resources among adults with unipolar depression. *Journal of Personality and Social Psychology, 46,* 877–891.

Bothwell, S., & Weissman, M. (1977). Social impairments four years after an acute depressive episode. *American Journal of Orthopsychiatry, 47,* 231–237.

Bouhuys, A., Jansen, C. J., & van den Hoofdakker, R. H. (1991). Analysis of observed behaviors displayed by depressed patients during a clinical interview: Relationships between behavioral factors and clinical concepts of activation. *Journal of Affective Disorders, 21,* 79–88.

Brown, G. (1987). Social factors and the development and course of depressive disorders in women: A review of a research programme. *British Journal of Social Work, 17,* 615–634.

Brown, G., & Harris, T. (1978). *The social origins of depression.* New York: Free Press.

Bunney, W., & Davis, J. (1965). Norepinephrine in depressive reactions: A review. *Archives of General Psychiatry, 13,* 483–494.

Carroll, B. (1982). The dexamethasone suppression test for melancholia. *British Journal of Psychiatry, 140,* 292–304.

Cartwright, R. D. (1993). Sleeping problems. In C. Costello (Ed.), *Symptoms of depression* (pp. 243–257). New York: Wiley.

Catalano, R., & Dooley, C. (1977). Economic predictors of depressed mood and stressful life events in a metropolitan community. *Journal of Health and Social Behavior, 18,* 292–301.

Chodorow, N. (1978). *The reproduction of mothering: Psychoanalysis and the sociology of gender.* Berkeley, CA: The University of California.

Chodorow, N. (1985). Gender, relation and difference in psychoanalytic perspective. In H. Eisenstein & A. Jardine (Eds.), *The future of difference* (pp. 1–19). New Brunswick, NJ: Rutgers University.

Cloitre, M., Katz, M., & van Praag, H. (1993). Psychomotor agitation and retardation. In C. Costello (Ed.), *Symptoms of depression* (pp. 207–226). New York: Wiley.

Cohen, S., & Wills, T. (1985). Stress, social support and the buffering hypothesis. *Psychological Bulletin, 98,* 310–357.

Cooperstock, R. (1981). A review of women's psychotropic drug use. In E. Howell & M. Bayes (Eds.), *Women and mental health* (pp. 131–140). New York: Basic.

Dean, A. (1985). On the epidemiology of depression. In A. Dean (Ed.), *Depression in multidisciplinary perspective* (pp. 5–31). New York: Brunner-Mazel.

Dean, A., & Ensel, W. (1982). Modeling social support, life events, competence and depression in the context of age and sex. *Journal of Community Psychology, 10,* 392–408.

Dean, A., & Ensel, W. (1983). The epidemiology of depression in young adults: The centrality of social support. *Journal of Psychiatric Treatment and Evaluation, 5,* 195–207.

Egeland, J., & Hostetter, A. (1983). Amish study: 2. Affective disorders among the Amish, 1976–83. *American Journal of Psychiatry, 140,* 56.

Elkin, I., Parloff, M., Hadley, S., & Autry, I. (1985). The NIMH treatment of depression collaborative research program. *Archives of General Psychiatry, 42,* 305–316.

Elsinga, S., & van den Hoofdakker, R. (1983). Clinical effects of sleep deprivation and clomipramine in endogenous depression. *Journal of Psychiatric Research, 17,* 361–374.

Endicott, J., & Spitzer, R. (1978). A diagnostic interview: The Schedule for Affective Disorders and Schizophrenia. *Archives of General Psychiatry, 35,* 837–844.

Ensel, W. (1985). Sex differences in the epidemiology of depression and physical illness: A sociological perspective. In A. Dean (Ed.), *Depression in multidisciplinary perspective* (pp. 83–102). New York: Brunner-Mazel.

Fagin, C. (1967; 1978). Psychotherapeutic nursing. In B. Backer, P. Dubbert, & E. Eisenman (Eds.), *Psychiatric/mental health nursing: Contemporary readings* (pp. 71–84). New York: Van Nostrand.

Field, W. (1989). Physical causes of depression. In L. Beeber (Ed.), *Depression: Old problems, new perspectives in nursing care* (pp. 47–55). Thorofare, NJ: SLACK.

Flomenbaum, N., Freedman, A., Levy, N., Simpson, G., & Talley, J. (1984). Treatment of depression in the physically ill: Multidisciplinary viewpoints in a roundtable discussion. *Emergency Medicine, 17,* 2–20.

Garcia-Sevilla, J., Guimon, J., Garcia-Vallejo, P., & Fuster, M. (1986). Biochemical and functional evidence of supersensitive platelet 2-adrenoceptors in major affective disorder. *Archives of General Psychiatry, 43,* 51–57.

Gershon, E. (1983). The genetics of affective disorders. In L. Grinspoon (Ed.), *Psychiatry update* (Vol. 2, pp. 434–456). Washington, DC: American Psychiatric Press.

Giles, D., Jarrett, R., Biggs, M., Guzick, D., & Rush, J. (1989). Clinical predictors of recurrence in depression. *American Journal of Psychiatry, 146,* 764–767.

Gilligan, C. (1982). *In a different voice.* Cambridge: Harvard University Press.

Gordon, V., & Gordon, E. (1987). Short-term treatment of depressed women: A replication study in Great Britain. *Archives of Psychiatric Nursing, 2,* 111–124.

Gordon, V., Matwychuk, A., Sachs, E., & Canedy, B. (1988). A 3-year follow-up of a cognitive-behavioral therapy intervention. *Archives of Psychiatric Nursing, 2,* 218–226.

Gortner, S. (1983). The history and philosophy of nursing science and research. *Advances in Nursing Science, 5,* 1–8.

Gotlib, H. (1986). Depression and marital interaction: A longitudinal perspective. Paper presented at the American Psychological Association, Washington, DC.

Gross, D., Fogg, L., & Conrad, B. (1993). Designing interventions in psychosocial research. *Archives of Psychiatric Nursing, 7*(5), 259–264.

Gut, E. (1989). *Productive and unproductive depression: Success or failure of a vital process.* New York: Basic.

Haber, J., McMahon, A., Price-Hoskins, P., & Sideleau, B. (1992). *Comprehensive psychiatric nursing* (4th ed.). St. Louis: Mosby Year Book.

Halbreich, U., Endicott, J., & Nee, J. (1983). Premenstrual depressive changes. *Archives of General Psychiatry, 40,* 535–542.

Hamilton, M. (1960). A rating scale for depression. *Journal of Neurology, Neurosurgery and Psychiatry, 12,* 56–62.

Hirsch, B. (1980). Natural support systems and coping with major life changes. *American Journal of Community Psychology, 8,* 159–172.

Hirschfeld, R. (1982). Epidemiology of affective disorders. *Archives of General Psychiatry, 39,* 35–46.

Hirschfeld, R., & Cross, C. (1981). Psychosocial risk factors for depression. In D. Regier & G. Allen (Eds.), *Risk factor research in the major mental disorders* (NIMH. DHHS Pub. No. [ADM] 81–1068). Washington, DC: Government Printing Office.

Hoff, L. (1989). *People in crisis: Understanding and helping* (3rd ed.). Menlo Park, CA: Addison-Wesley.

Hoffman, A. L., & Betrus, P. A. (1992). Theory and practice: Scientists' and practitioners' roles. *Archives of Psychiatric Nursing, 6*(1), 2–9.

Holsboer, F., Steiger, A., & Maier, W. (1983). Four cases of reversion to abnormal dexamethasone suppression test response as indicator of clinical relapse: A preliminary report. *Biological Psychiatry, 18,* 911–916.

Hooley, J., Orley, J., & Teasdale, J. (1986). Levels of expressed emotion and relapse in depressed patients. *British Journal of Psychiatry, 148,* 642–647.

Jack, D. (1987a). Self-in-relation theory. In R. Formanek & A. Gurian (Eds.), *Women and depression: A lifespan perspective* (pp. 41–45). New York: Springer.

Jack, D. (1987b). Silencing the self: The power of social imperatives in female depression. In R. Formanek & A. Gurian (Eds.), *Women and depression: A lifespan perspective* (pp. 161–181). New York: Springer.

Janowsky, D., Risch, S., & Gillin, J. (1983). Adrenergic-cholinergic balance and the treatment of affective disorders. *Progress in Neuro-psychopharmacology & Biological Psychiatry, 7,* 297–307.

Janowsky, D., Risch, C., Parker, D., Huey, L., & Judd, L. (1980). Increased vulnerability to cholinergic stimulation in affective disorder patients. *Psychopharmacology Bulletin, 16,* 29–31.

Kalin, N., Risch, S., & Murphy, D. (1982). Involvement of the central serotonergic system in affective illness. *Journal of Clinical Psychopharmacology, 1,* 232–237.

Kathol, R. (1985). Depression associated with physical disease. In E. Beckham & W. Leber (Eds.), *Handbook of depression: Treatment, assessment, and research* (pp. 745–762). Homewood, IL: Dorsey.

Katz, M. M., Koslow, S. H., Berman, N., Secunda, S., Mass, J. W., Casper, R., Kocsis, J., & Stokes, P. (1989). A multivantaged approach to measurement of behavioral and affect states for clinical and psychobiological research. *Psychological Reports,* Monograph Supplement 1–V55, 619–671.

Keltner, N., Schwecke, L., & Bostrom, C. (1991). *Psychiatric nursing: A psychotherapeutic management approach.* St. Louis: Mosby Year Book.

Kerr, N. (1987). Patterns of depression. In J. Haber, P. Hoskins, A. Leach, & B. Sideleau (Eds.), *Comprehensive psychiatric nursing* (3rd ed.) (pp. 647–679). New York: McGraw-Hill.

Klein, D., Taylor, E., Dickstein, S., & Harding, K. (1988). Primary early-onset dysthymia: Comparison with primary nonbipolar nonchronic major depression on demographic, clinical, familial, personality, and socioenvironmental characteristics and short-term outcome. *Journal of Abnormal Psychology, 97,* 387–398.

Kolb, B., & Whishaw, I. (1985). *Fundamentals of human neuropsychology* (2nd ed.). New York: Freeman.

Kovacs, M., Feinberg, T., Crouse-Novak, M., Paulauskas, S., & Finkelstein, R. (1984). Depressive disorders in childhood: 2. A longitudinal prospective study of characteristics and recovery. *Archives of General Psychiatry, 41,* 229–237.

Krauss, J. B. (1993). *Health care reform: Essential mental health services.* Washington, DC: American Nurses Association.

Lechin, F., van der Dijs, B., Acosta, E., Gomez, F., Lechin, E., & Arocha, L. (1983). Distal colon motility and clinical parameters in depression. *Journal of Affective Disorders, 5,* 19–26.

Lin, N., Dean, A., & Ensel, W. (1986). *Social support, life events and depression.* Orlando: Academic Press.

Lin, N., & Ensel, W. (1984). Depression mobility and its social etiology: The role of life events and social support. *Journal of Health and Social Behavior, 25,* 176–188.

Loomis, M., O'Toole, S., Brown, M., Pothier, P., West, P., & Wilson, H. (1987). Development of a classification system for psychiatric/mental health nursing: Individual response class. *Archives of Psychiatric Nursing, 1,* 16–24.

MacFarland, G., & Thomas, M. (1991). *Psychiatric mental health nursing: Application of the nursing process.* Philadelphia: Lippincott.

Mallet, J., Boni, C., Dumas, S., Faucon-Biquet, N., Grima, B., Horellou, P., & Lamouroux, A. (1987). Molecular genetics of catecholamines as an approach to the biochemistry of manic-depression. *Journal of Psychiatric Research, 21,* 559–568.

McBride, A. (1988). Mental health effects of women's multiple roles. *Image, 20,* 41–45.

McEnany, G. (1990). Psychobiological indices of bipolar mood disorder: Future trends in nursing care. *Archives of Psychiatric Nursing, 4,* 29–38.

Miller, J. (1976). *Toward a new psychology of women.* Boston: Beacon.

Miller, J. (1983). *The construction of anger in women and men.* Wellesley, MA: Stone Center for Developmental Services and Studies.

Miller, J. (1984). *The development of women's sense of self.* Wellesley, MA: Stone Center for Developmental Services and Studies.

Mitchell, R., Cronkite, R., & Moos, R. (1983). Stress, coping, and depression among married couples. *Journal of Abnormal Psychology, 92,* 433–448.

Monroe, S., Bromet, E., Connell, M., & Steiner, S. (1986). Social support, life event, depressive symptoms: A one-year prospective study. *Journal of Consulting and Clinical Psychology, 54,* 424–431.

Moos, R. (1968). The development of a menstrual distress questionnaire. *Psychosomatic Medicine, 30,* 853–867.

Moos, R., & Moos, B. (1986). *Family environment scale manual* (2nd ed.). Palo Alto, CA: Consulting Psychologists Press.

Nolen-Hoeksema, S. (1987). Sex differences in unipolar depression: Evidence and theory. *Psychological Bulletin, 101,* 259–282.

Noll, K., Davis, J., & DeLeon-Jones, F. (1985). Medication and somatic therapies in the treatment of depression. In E. Beckham & W. Leber (Eds.), *Handbook of depression* (pp. 220–315). Homewood, IL: Dorsey.

Norbeck, J., & Tilden, V. (1983). Life stress, social support, and emotional disequilibrium in complications of pregnancy: A prospective, multivariate study. *Journal of Health and Social Behavior, 24,* 30–46.

Orr, S. (1984). Maternal depression in an urban pediatric practice: Implications for health care delivery. *American Journal of Public Health, 74,* 363–365.

Parse, R. (1981). *Man-living-health: A theory of nursing.* New York: Wiley.

Paykel, E., & Weissman, M. (1973). Social adjustment and depression: A longitudinal study. *Archives of General Psychiatry, 28,* 659–663.

Pearlin, L., Menaghan, E., Lieberman, M., & Mullan, J. (1981). The stress process. *Journal of Health and Social Behavior, 22,* 337–356.

Peplau, H. (1952). *Interpersonal relations in nursing.* New York: Putnam.

Peplau, H. (1988). The art and science of nursing. *Nursing Science Quarterly, 1,* 8–15.

Perris, C., Arrindell, W., Perris, H., Eisemann, M., van Der Ende, J., & von Knorring, L. (1986). Perceived depriving parental rearing and depression. *British Journal of Psychiatry, 148,* 170–175.

Phifer, J., & Murrell, S. (1986). Etiologic factors in the onset of depressive symptoms in older adults. *Journal of Consulting and Clinical Psychology, 95,* 282–291.

Pitts, R., Schuller, B., Rich, C., & Pitts, A. (1979). Suicide among U.S. women physicians. *American Journal of Psychiatry, 136,* 694–696.

Propst, L., Pardington, A., Ostrom, R., & Watkins, P. (1986). Predictors of coping in divorced single mothers. *Journal of Divorce, 9,* 33–53.

Radloff, L. (1975). Sex differences in depression: The effects of occupation and marital status. *Sex Roles, 1,* 249–265.

Radloff, L. (1977). The CES-D scale: A self-report depression scale for research in the general population. *Applied Psychological Measurement, 1,* 385–401.

Regier, D. (1985, May). Research advances in psychiatric epidemiology—An update for the clinician. Presented at the annual meeting of the American Psychiatric Association, Dallas, TX.

Rice, J., Reich, T., Andreason, N., Lavori, P., Endicott, J., Clayton, P., Keller, M., & Hirshfield, R. (1984). Sex-related differences in depression: Familial evidence. *Journal of Affective Disorders, 7,* 199–210.

Risch, S., Cohen, R., Janowsky, D., Kalin, N., & Murphy, D. (1980). Mood and behavioral effects of physostigmine on humans are accompanied by elevations in plasma beta-endorphin and cortisol. *Science, 209,* 1545–1546.

Rosenberg, M. (1965). *Society and the adolescent self-image.* Princeton, NJ: Princeton University Press.

Rosenthal, N., Sack, D., Carpenter, C., Parry, B., Mendelson, W., & Wehr, T. (1985). Antidepressant effects of light in seasonal affective disorder. *American Journal of Psychiatry, 142,* 163–170.

Rosenthal, N., Sack, D., James, S., Parry, B., Mendelson, W., Tamarkin, L., & Wehr, T. (1985). Seasonal affective disorder and phototherapy. *Annals of the New York Academy of Sciences, 453,* 260–269.

Rosenthal, N., Sack, D., & Skwerer, R. (1988). Phototherapy for seasonal affective disorder. *Journal of Biological Rhythms, 3,* 101–120.

Schildkraut, J. (1965). The catecholamine hypothesis of affective disorder: A review of supporting evidence. *American Journal of Psychiatry, 122,* 509–522.

Schildkraut, J. (1978). Current status of the catecholamine hypothesis of affective disorders. In M. Lipton, A. DiMascio, & K. Killam (Eds.), *Psychopharmacology: A generation of progress* (pp. 1223–1234). New York: Raven.

Schildkraut, J. (1982). The biochemical discrimination of subtypes of depressive disorders: An outline of our studies on norepinephrine metabolism and psychoactive drugs in endogenous depressions since 1967. *Pharmakopsychiatria, 15,* 121–127.

Siever, L., & Davis, K. (1985). Overview: Toward a dysregulation hypothesis of depression. *American Journal of Psychiatry, 142,* 1017–1031.

Simmons-Alling, S. (1990). Genetic implications for major affective disorders. *Archives of Psychiatric Nursing, 4,* 67–71.

Society for Education and Research in Psychiatric–Mental Health Nursing (SERPN). (1994). *Position statement.* Pensacola, FL: Author.

Spanier, G. (1976). Measuring dyadic adjustment: New scales for assessing the quality of marriage and similar dyads. *Journal of Marriage and the Family, 38,* 15–28.

Stake, J., & Orlofsky, J. (1981). On the use of global and specific measures in assessing the self-esteem of males and females. *Sex Roles, 7,* 653–662.

Stephens, G. (1976). Periodicity in mood, affect, and instinctual behavior. *Nursing Clinics of North America, 11,* 595–607.

Stuart, G., Laraia, M., Ballenger, J., & Lydiard, R. (1990). Early family experiences of women with bulimia and depression. *Archives of Psychiatric Nursing, 4,* 43–52.

Stuart, G., & Sundeen, S. (1995). *Principles and practice of psychiatric nursing* (5th ed.). St. Louis: Mosby.

Styron, W. (1990). *Darkness visible.* New York: Random House.

Swanson, A. (1978). The client who generates depression. In J. Haber, A. Leach, S. Shudy, & B. Sideleau (Eds.), *Comprehensive psychiatric nursing* (pp. 306–324). New York: McGraw-Hill.

Thase, M., Frank, E., & Kupfer, D. (1985). Biological processes in major depression. In E. Beckham & W. Leber (Eds.), *Handbook of depression: Treatment, assessment and research* (pp. 816–913). Homewood, IL: Dorsey.

Thoits, P. (1985). Social support and psychological well-being: Theoretical possibilities. In I. Sarason & B. Sarason (Eds.), *Social support: Theory, research and applications* (pp. 51–72). Drodrecht: Martinus Nijhoff.

Tilden, V. (1987). Cost and conflict: The darker side of social support. *Western Journal of Nursing Research, 9,* 174–175.

Tilden V., & Nelson, C. (1988, May). Cost and reciprocity index: A measure of interpersonal exchange. Paper presented at the 21st Annual Communicating Nursing Research Conference, Western Society for Research in Nursing, Salt Lake City, Utah.

Turner, R., & Noh, S. (1988). Physical disability and depression: A longitudinal analysis. *Journal of Health and Social Behavior, 29,* 23–37.

Ulrich, G., & Harms, K. (1985). A video analysis of the nonverbal behaviour of depressed patients before and after treatment. *Journal of Affective Disorders, 9,* 63–67.

Wehr, T., & Goodwin, F. (1981). Biological rhythms and psychiatry. In S. Arieti & H. Brodie (Eds.), *American handbook of psychiatry* (pp. 46–74). New York: Basic.

Wehr, T., & Rosenthal, N. (1989). Seasonality and affective illness. *American Journal of Psychiatry, 146,* 829–839.

Wehr, T., & Wirz-Justice, A. (1982). Circadian rhythm mechanisms in affective illness and in antidepressant drug action. *Pharmacopsychiatry, 15,* 31–39.

Weissman, M. (1979). The psychological treatment of depression: Evidence for the efficacy of psychotherapy alone, in comparison with, and in combination with pharmacotherapy. *Archives of General Psychiatry, 36,* 1261–1269.

Weissman, M. (1986). Epidemiology of depression: Frequency, risk groups and risk factors. In *Perspectives on depressive disorders: A review of recent research* (pp. 1–22). Bethesda, MD: NIMH D/ART Program.

Weissman, M., Gershon, E., Kidd, K., Prusoff, B., Leckman, J., Dibble, E., Hamovit, J., Thompson, W., Pauls, D., & Guroff, J. (1984). Psychiatric disorder in relatives of probands with affective disorders: The Yale-NIMH collaborative family study. *Archives of General Psychiatry, 41,* 13–21.

Weissman, M., & Klerman, G. (1981). Sex differences and the epidemiology of depression. In E. Howell & M. Bayes (Eds.), *Women and mental health* (pp. 160–195). New York: Basic.

Weissman, M., & Klerman, G. (1985). Gender and depression. *Trends in Neurosciences, 8*(9), 416–420.

Weissman, M., Klerman, G., Prusoff, B., Sholomskas, D., & Padian, N. (1981). Depressed outpatients: Results one year after treatment with drugs and/or interpersonal therapy. *Archives of General Psychiatry, 38,* 51–55.

Weissman, M., & Paykel, E. (1974). *The depressed woman: A study of social relationships.* Chicago: The University of Chicago Press.

Williams, J. M. G., Healy, D., Teasdale, J. D., White, W., & Paykel, E. S. (1990). Dysfunctional attitudes and vulnerability to persistent depression. *Psychological Medicine, 20,* 375–381.

Wilson, H., & Kneisl, C. (1992). *Psychiatric nursing* (4th ed.). Redwood City, CA: Addison-Wesley.

Winokur, G., Tsuang, M., & Crowe, R. (1982). The Iowa 500: Affective disorders in relatives of manic-depressive patients. *American Journal of Psychiatry, 139,* 209–212.

Yesavage, J., Brink, T., Rose, T., Lum, O., Huang, V., Adey, M., & Leirer, V. (1983). Development and validation of a geriatric depression screening scale. *Journal of Psychiatric Research, 17,* 37-49.

Zimmerman, M., Coryell, W., Corenthal, C., & Wilson, S. (1986). A self-report scale to diagnose major depressive disorder. *Archives of General Psychiatry, 43,* 1076–1081.

Zis, A., & Goodwin, F. (1982). The amine hypothesis. In E. Paykel (Ed.), *Handbook of affective disorders* (pp. 175–190). New York: Guilford.

Zung, W. (1965). A self-rating depression scale. *Archives of General Psychiatry, 12,* 63–70.

BIPOLAR MOOD DISORDERS

BRAIN, BEHAVIOR, AND NURSING

Susan Simmons-Alling, MSN, RN, CS

ABSTRACT

After presenting the characteristics and epidemiology of bipolar disorder, this chapter reviews psychosocial and biological factors, asserting that they are not dualistic but should be integrated to obtain a dysfunctional gestalt of patients. Studies exploring the biological factors suggest a relationship between bipolar disorder and pathology of the limbic system, basal ganglia, and hypothalamus. The various neuronal networks connecting the limbic system and basal ganglia appear to play a major role in the production of emotions, and dysfunction of the hypothalamus—as evidenced by alterations in sleep, appetite, and libido—and biological changes in endocrine, circadian rhythms, and molecular coding systems are also prevalent in bipolar patients. Given the complex problems faced by the psychiatric nurse and client (individual and family), it is recommended that multiple assessments be used and that psychosocial and psychoeducation interventions be combined with neuropharmacology. To do so effectively, revisions in nursing curricula will need to provide a comprehensive approach to clients' needs, and nursing research must seek to further delineate the care factors with the biological data for bipolar illness so that psychiatric nurses can help reduce the dichotomy between the biomedical and care models.

Ups and downs, highs and lows—these are phenomena on a continuum ranging from normal gladness and sadness to the clinical extremes of mania and depression. Based on population prevalence, such clinical mood disruptions, known as bipolar disorders, will no doubt be encountered by psychiatric nurses at some point in their career, regardless of their setting.

Bipolar disorders are classified in the *Diagnostic and Statistical Manual of Mental Disorders* (American Psychiatric Association, 1994) under Mood Disorders, indicating the pathology of the disorder is mood. This refers to the internal emotional state of an individual, in contrast to affect, which is the external expression of emotional content (Kaplan & Sadock, 1991). This chapter will discuss bipolar (BP) mood disorders specifically and the current implications for contemporary psychiatric nursing practice. The bias that BP mood disorders are a brain disease or a neurobiological disorder as evidenced by biological variables predominating in their etiology will be emphasized; however, the psychological and social manifestations of the illness are not to be dismissed and are among the domains for nurses to manage. Etiologic factors for understanding BP illness will be identified, including psychosocial and biological factors. The chapter will also review the relationship of BP mood disorder with brain and behavior, as well as strategies to integrate biological symptoms with nursing management. The relevant behavioral theories, which are more familiar to psychiatric nurses and which have been employed in their care with clients and families, are not discussed in depth.

Psychiatric nursing has begun to mature and better differentiate its role from other health care disciplines, and now its challenge is to articulate how it can integrate into practice the biological underpinnings that influence the behaviors within nursing's domain. Nursing's clinical task is to provide outcomes that clients and their families perceive as useful and adaptive. Because stigma and lack of knowledge are lethal contributors to these disorders, it is imperative that psychiatric nurses broaden their conceptual base and critical thinking to merge the neuroanatomy and physiology of the brain with their corresponding functional behaviors to improve understanding of the pathophysiology of mental illness and treatment strategies.

CHARACTERISTICS OF BIPOLAR DISORDER
DSM-IV CATEGORIES

The diagnostic criteria for BP disorder categories are included in Table 11–1. Within each DSM-IV category of bipolar I and II disorders are course and symptom-feature modifiers. These modifiers provide for subtypes such as single, recent episode, mixed, recurrent, psychotic, seasonal pattern, rapid-cycling, and postpartum onset. The taxonomy criteria parallel the human response patterns or behaviors that are useful for focusing nursing interventions.

CLINICAL PHENOMENA

Any observable need, condition, concern, event, dilemma, difficulty, occurrence, or fact that can be described or scientifically explained and is within the target area of nursing practice is of interest to nurses (American Nurses Association, 1980). Among the clinical phenomena that nurses can assess are those shown in Table 11–2. This schema depicts the mood, cognitive and perceptual symptoms, and activity or behavior characteristics associated with BP disorders. It should be noted that the symptoms depicted vertically cross over all three phases of the illness on a continuum. These symptoms are not a complete list, but they represent the recurring presentations relevant to this population. Additionally, the DSM-IV criteria are interspersed with phenomena the psychiatric nurse can assess. The varying changes in perception, mood, attitude, cognition, and personality suggest the need for psychosocial interventions that are common in most psychiatric nurses' frameworks. Combining the psychosocial interventions with the biological variables and interventions can be of unique value to patients and families experiencing such devastating changes in the way they perceive themselves and are perceived by others. These applications will be elaborated on in the intervention section.

PATTERNS

The BP disorders are a heterogeneous group of conditions, as shown in Table 11–3, and are characterized by different symptomatology, illness course, family history, biological features, and treatment response. Most clinicians can recognize

TABLE 11-1. DSM-IV DIAGNOSTIC CRITERIA FOR BIPOLAR DISORDER CATEGORIES

Manic Episode
A. Persistent elevated, expansive, or irritable mood, lasting at least one week
B. Clusters of symptoms, including at least three of the following symptoms or four if the mood is only irritable:
   (1) Grandiosity or inflated self-esteem
   (2) Decreased need for sleep
   (3) Talkative, pressure to keep talking
   (4) Flight of ideas or subjective experience that thoughts are racing
   (5) Distractibility
   (6) Increase in goal-directed activity or psychomotor agitation
   (7) Over-involvement in pleasurable activities that have higher potential for painful consequences
C. Symptoms do not meet criteria for a mixed episode.
D. Mood disturbance causes impairment in functioning, relationship with others, or necessitates hospitalization
E. Not due to the direct effects of a substance or a general medical condition

Hypomanic Episode
A. Elevated, expansive, or irritable mood lasting at least four days
B. Same criteria of symptom clusters as manic episode
C. Episode results in change of functioning uncharacteristic of person when not symptomatic
D. Mood disturbance and change in functioning observable by others
E. Episode is not severe enough to cause impairment in social or occupational functioning, or necessitate hospitalization; there are no psychotic features
F. Mood disturbance not due to direct effect of substance or general medical condition

Cyclothymic Disorder
A. For at least 2 years, presence of periods with hypomanic symptoms and periods with depressive symptoms that do not meet criteria for manic episode or major depressive episode
B. During the above 2-year period (one-year for children and adolescents), person has not been without the symptoms in A. for more than two months at a time
C. Has never met criteria for major depression episode, manic or mixed episode
D. Symptoms in A. not accounted for by Schizoaffective Disorder and are not superimposed or Schizophrenia, Schizophreniform Disorder, Delusional Disorder, or Psychotic Disorder NOS
E. Not due to direct effects of substance or general medical disorder
F. Symptoms cause clinically significant distress or impairment in social, occupational, or other important areas of functioning

Bipolar Disorder Not Otherwise Specified (NOS)
Bipolar features that do not meet criteria for any specific bipolar disorder

Reprinted with permission from the American Psychiatric Association. (1994). *Diagnostic and Statistical Manual of Mental Disorders* (4th ed.). Washington, DC: Author.

or assess the pure or classic BP manic patient, but other atypical subtypes of BP are now being identified. Brief references to these patterns will be made to assist nurses in being more attentive in their assessments and to assist with educating patients and families to appreciate that there is no "cookie cutter" description of BP. BP I includes episodes of frank mania with psychosis or incapacitation. BP II refers to the history of major depressive disorder with a hypomanic, elevated, or irritable mood state.

TABLE 11–2. Human Responses to Bipolar Mood Disorder

MOOD			COGNITION OR PERCEPTION				ACTIVITY OR BEHAVIOR				
Depression Despair			Hopelessness Negativity Suicidal ideation Inability to problem-solve Anhedonia Decreased self-esteem Guilt Worthlessness Thought blocking Forgetful Obsessional				Decreased libido Psychomotor retardation Suicide ideation/attempts Decreased social interaction Fatigue Decreased energy Passive				
Hypomania Merriment Elation	LABILITY	IRRITABILITY	Distractibility Creativity Increased intrusiveness	PSYCHOSIS	ATTENTION DYSFUNCTION	DELUSIONS	Pressured speech Increased social interaction Increased productivity Excited Disinhibition Increased libido Expansiveness	HYPERSOMNIA OR INSOMNIA	AGITATION	APPETITE	ANXIETY
Mania Euphoria Hostility			Grandiosity Flight of ideas Hallucinations Impaired judgment No insight Confusion				Extravagance Impulsivity Hyperverbal Assertive Threatening/volatile Unreliable Excessive involvement Increased psychomotor activity				

A variety of types of BP depression have been divided by symptoms. Table 11–4 contrasts melancholic and atypical symptoms. Melancholic depressive symptoms often characterize the recurrent depressive BP phase, but atypical symptoms are also associated with anergic BP depression. Bipolar disorder most often starts with depression and then becomes a recurring illness (Wehr, Sack, Rosenthal, & Cowdry, 1988).

Hypomania refers to the beginning escalation of mania and is seen in the middle section of Table 11–2. The person experiencing the symptoms does not usually recognize the hypomanic period because subjective distress is lacking. Treatment is rarely sought, and many deny their elevated mood when directly interviewed. If left untreated, this subtype is associated with a 25% rate of suicide and often evolves into a more serious cycling pattern, suggesting the need for prophylactic treatment (Post, 1989).

Dysphoric mania is characterized by a pattern of depression switching into mania followed by an interval of wellness. This group is less likely to have a family

TABLE 11–3. BIPOLAR DISORDER PATTERNS

BP I	BP II
Single manic	Hypomanic
Mixed	Depressed
Psychotic	Chronic
Catatonic	Catatonic
Postpartum	Melancholic
Most recent episode	Atypical
Hypomanic	Postpartum
Manic	With or without interepisode recovery
Mixed	Seasonal pattern
Depressed	Rapid-cycling
Unspecified	
With or without interepisode recovery	
Seasonal pattern	
Rapid-cycling	

history of mood disorders and tends to include more females, to have fewer episodes of illness, and to present with irritability and anxious symptomatology (Post, 1989).

Secondary mania refers to those BP conditions which develop subsequent to another medical disorder or endogenous dysrhythmia. The patients present with principally manic rather than depressive behaviors and with irritability predominating over euphoria. A family history of BP illness is less often seen. An example is mania occurring in the context of substance abuse.

Rapid-cycling refers to four or more distinct episodes of mania, depression, or a mix of the two within a 12-month period. Rapid-cycling, which represents 5% to 20% of all bipolars, is more common in women, but it is not temporally related to the menstrual cycle (Potter & Bowden, 1992).

Seasonal affective disorders (SAD) are episodes of depression or mania characterized by recurring episodes of fall and winter depression that alternate with euthymia or hypomania in the spring or summer. Recently, a seasonal pattern of depression appearing in the spring and summer and resolving in the autumn or winter has been described in some patients. There is controversy among investigators whether SAD is unipolar or bipolar. Assessing if the mood changes occur at the same time each year is advantageous for treatment.

TABLE 11–4. MELANCHOLIC AND ATYPICAL DEPRESSION SYMPTOMS

MELANCHOLIC	ATYPICAL
Hyposomnia (terminal insomnia)	Hyperphagia
Anorexia	Hypersomnia
Diurnal mood	Passivity
Anxiety	Severe fatigue
Excessive guilt	Interpersonal rejection sensitivity
Obsessional preoccupation	Mood reactivity
Decreased libido	Phobic symptoms
Psychomotor agitation or retardation	

EPIDEMIOLOGY

Epidemiologic findings approximate 1 to 3 million men and women in the United States suffer from BP mood disorder. The rates of BP disorder are estimated to be about 1.2% for lifetime prevalence. Pure mania represents 5% to 9% of the BP group, while rapid-cycling persons represent 13% to 20% of the population (Goodwin & Jamison, 1990). In persons with BP disorder there are no gender differences except for dysphoric mania and rapid-cycling, which are most common in females (McElroy & Keck [1993] estimate 70% to 90%). There are no racial differences, and BP disorder is more commonly found in higher socioeconomic groups. Family history for bipolars is positively related to presenting with BP, suggesting genetic linkage.

It has been estimated that only 27% of those affected with BP illness are treated. Up to 20% of those who suffer with BP mood disorder attempt or commit suicide. An estimated 10% to 15% of untreated clients commit suicide, which is 15 to 20 times the rate of the general population (Depression Guideline Panel, 1993a).

ETIOLOGY

The critical search for the etiology of BP illness continues, and the tension between behavioral or psychosocial psychiatry and biological psychiatry misses the issue. While both factions provide tentative working hypotheses in understanding the mediating mechanisms, the psychosocial and biological factors are not dualistic. Rather, they are meant to be integrated to obtain a dysfunctional gestalt of patients. Weaving together the biopsychosocial factors and theories is necessary to provide the foundation for the holistic practice nurses strive to perform.

PSYCHOSOCIAL FACTORS

Bipolar illness is burdensome on energy and intrapsychic resources. As the state of mind becomes overwhelmed and the senses become distorted, the self-concept's value is lost. However, many of the symptoms of trying to deal with everyday life, personhood, and psychological stressors associated with the illness can be assisted by conjoint therapies, which are modeled from the following psychosocial factors.

PSYCHOANALYTIC THEORY

The psychodynamic principles primarily focus on major depressive mood defense mechanisms. Freud (1957) viewed melancholia as caused by a chronic interpersonal disappointment, or an exposure to a hypercritical or unresponsive emotional environment leading to adult love relationships marked by ambivalence. Actual or threatened interpersonal losses in adult life trigger a self-destructive struggle in the self (ego)—anger turned inward—that manifests as depression. Silber (1989) reviewed additional analytical concepts that describe depression-prone persons as needing constant reassurance, love, and maintenance of self-esteem. Frustration over their dependency needs results in low self-esteem and leads to depression. In this view, such persons generally hold contained negative feelings, which develop as a pattern throughout life. Bowlby (1960) and Spitz (1946) refer to depression as the traumatic loss or separation during childhood from significant objects of attachment and social bonding. This early separation or loss may be a predisposing factor that precipitates stress in adulthood.

Abraham (1953) characterized the manic mood as one of self-satisfaction. The ego is no longer consumed by the loved introjected object, thus having energy for eagerness in the outside world. The increasing energy leads to the euphoria of mania.

PERSONALITY FACTORS

Personality organization of mood acknowledges that a variable of self-esteem or self-concept is the underlying issue. It may be expressed as dejection or self-depreciation—as in depression—or as overcompensation with an attitude of elation or supreme confidence—as in mania (Arieti & Bemporad, 1980). Threats to self-esteem arise from perceived failure in everyday functioning, impaired or poor role performance, and absence of self-identity. The patient's interpersonal experience and attempt to adapt to environmental change and stress are factors for nursing intervention in mood disorders.

BEHAVIORAL FACTORS

Behavioral concepts emphasize the quality of rewards or reinforcements in the interactions with one's environment. A change in the rate of reinforcement is believed to be a key factor in the etiology and maintenance of depression. Ferster (1973) proposed that a social skills deficit, as evidenced in difficulty obtaining reinforcements, makes it more difficult to cope with the loss of the usual reinforcement supply. Deficits in social skills are common in mood disorder.

COGNITIVE FACTORS

The cognitive theory of depression, originated by Beck (1979), views depression as a result of the dysfunction of cognitive schemas, errors, and faulty information processing. Schemas are stable cognitive patterns through which the person interprets experience. Cognitive errors are systematic errors that lead to the persistence of negative patterns despite contradictory evidence. There is empirical evidence to support the notion that cognitive therapy assists unipolar depression, but no systematic studies have looked at its efficacy for bipolarity.

LEARNED HELPLESSNESS MODEL

Similar to Beck's cognitive model is the learned helplessness model that evolved from animal research. Seligman (1975) evolved his helplessness model of depression to propose that when individuals believe they have no control over life outcomes and their ability to reduce suffering, they do not assert for mastery in life. In other words, control and mastery of the environment are conceived to be hopeless. Because the individuals who exhibit this personality trait, this behavioral state, perceive they have lost control over important life outcomes, they refrain from adaptive responses. This tendency then leads to outcomes of hopelessness, passivity, negative cognition, attributed low self-esteem, and a depressed affect. While this model is more associated with major depression, studies are looking to support its efficacy in cognitive therapy. The theory also corresponds to some underlying neurochemical substrates that will be presented later.

Stress Factors

Stress in the form of loss and life events also provides a framework for depression. Mood disturbances may be a specific response to stress, such as the loss of physical functioning, of self-esteem, or of a significant other. In fact, the life event most associated with later development of depression is losing a parent prior to age 11 (Kaplan & Sadock, 1991). There is, however, accumulating evidence to suggest that the first episode of affective disorder, whether manic or depressive, is more associated with major psychosocial stressors than are episodes occurring later in the illness course (Post, 1992b). For example, loss of hope, which is a common stressor in suicidal persons, can take on primary importance in mood disruption. The role of stress is also correlated with neurobiological changes and will be further described with kindling and sensitization.

Bipolar illness presents via excessive behaviors. Even though each of the psychosocial factors and theories provides limited clinical explanation for the resulting behaviors summarized as BP illness, it is impossible to know whether any of them are the major etiology for the disease. Research has no definitive answer to the temperament–mood disorder origins. However, because the interrelationships with genetic alteration hold promise, biology's influence on behavior emerges as a more contemporary answer. In keeping with the premise that BP mood disorder is primarily a brain disease, basic concepts of anatomy of the brain structure and neuronal physiology are reviewed next.

Biological Factors

BRAIN STRUCTURE AND FUNCTIONING

The brain orchestrates behavior, movement, feeling, and sensing. The cerebral cortex, which contains approximately 70% of the neurons in the central nervous system, receives direct and indirect afferent input from most areas of the brain. It is divided into two hemispheres, each of which is further divided into the four main lobes—frontal, temporal, parietal, and occipital (as noted on Fig. 11–1).

The neuronal layers within the cortex are involved in the regulation of the person's internal state, including learning, memory, modulation of drives, affective coloring of experiences, hormonal regulation and autonomic functioning, and interpreting the external environment (Kaplan & Sadock, 1991).

The frontal lobe is reciprocally connected with motor, sensory, and emotional brain areas. The primary functions of the frontal lobe include attention, problem solving, memory storage, behavior regulation, learning, drive, judgment, affect, self-consciousness, planning, spontaneity, initiation, hygiene, grooming, abstract thinking, and the evaluation of sensory information.

The parietal lobe receives messages and information from the sense organs, thus analyzing gross sensory input, touch, and pressure. Orientation in space of our body parts within the environment for visual-spatial processing is also found in this lobe.

The occipital lobe is responsible for the interpretation of visual images and visual memory. Neuronal dysfunction here may give rise to visual hallucinations.

The temporal lobe's primary functions are language, memory, and emotion. Within the temporal lobe are groups of neurons known as the amygdala and hippocampus, the major components of the limbic system. The limbic system functions in primitive behavior and feeling states, mood, instincts, and self-preservation. The amygdala and hippocampus are implicated in experiencing and regulating emotions; storing, recording, and interpreting memory; and expressing

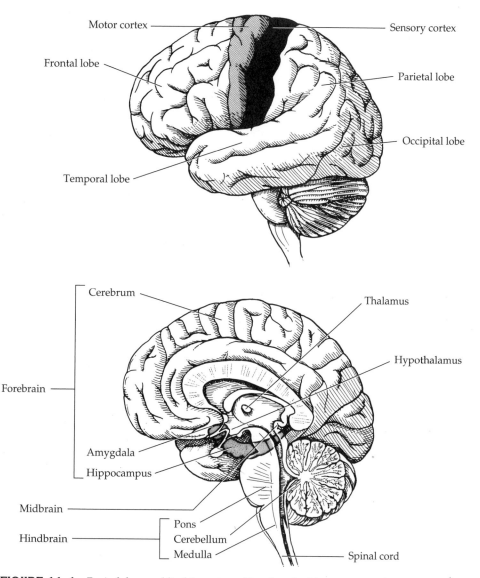

FIGURE 11–1. Brain lobes and limbic system. (Reprinted with permission from Society for Neuroscience. [1990]. *Brain facts: A primer on the brain and nervous system* [p. 3]. Washington, DC: Author.)

aggressive behavior. More specifically, connected to the thalamus, which relays information to the cortex from the senses, is the amygdala, where there are afferent nerve projections from the dopaminergic, noradrenergic, and serotonergic nuclei in the brain stem. The amygdala also gauges emotional reactions—such as anxiety, anger, elation, rage, and aggression—and modulates the starting and stopping of behaviors associated with these emotions. The hippocampus helps form new or short-term memories so they can enter permanent storage and also plays a role in learning. Much of the noradrenergic projections innervate with the hippocampus.

The limbic system also connects with the hypothalamus and the cingulate. The prefrontal cortex is the only cortical region that sends direct projections to the hypothalamus and septal regions, suggesting a major role for the prefrontal cortex in the regulation of the limbic system (Andreasen & Black, 1991). The hypothalamus regulates thirst, libido, hunger, pleasure, pain, and body temperature. Disruption in the neuronal transfer in this pathway explains the physiologic expression of vegetative symptoms of depression, so neuroendocrine dysregulation is a primary consideration in the etiology of mood disorders.

The locus coeruleus (LC), located in the pons, produces 70% of the total norepinephrine in the brain. Activation here is associated with fear, pain, and alarm. The LC also projects to the amygdala, which results in emotional and cardiovascular control.

The basal ganglia comprises the striatum (which includes the caudate nucleus), putamen and globus pallidus, the subthalamic nuclei, and the substantia nigra. Its primary functions are initiation and control of movement, but these structures also contain the neurotransmitter neurons for dopamine, acetylcholine, gamma-aminobutyric acid (GABA), and peptides, such as substance P and enkephalins. The chemical anatomy of these neurons interconnects with the limbic system and is involved in symptoms associated with depression, psychosis, and dementia. The relationship of the basal ganglia to depression is evidenced by stooped posture, motor slowness, and minor cognitive impairment.

ANATOMIC FINDINGS IN BIPOLAR DISORDER

According to Cummings (1993), five parallel segregated circuits link the frontal lobe with subcortical structures and subsume motor, oculomotor, and behavioral functions. The principal anatomic structures included in these circuits are the frontal lobe, striatum–globus pallidus or substantia nigra, and the thalamus. The three behaviorally relevant circuits originate in the dorsolateral prefrontal cortex, orbitofrontal cortex, and medial frontal or anterior cingulate cortex. The orbitofrontal cortex mediates social restraint, civil behavior, and mood stability; dysfunction results in impulsiveness, disinhibition, tactlessness, irritability, and lability—all of which may be associated with manic symptoms. The medial frontal cortex is critical to motivation and action initiation, suggesting a relationship to the behaviors of apathy, poor motivation, and disinterest in depression (p. 173).

Additionally, Aylward (1993) found male bipolar persons had significantly larger caudate volume than male controls, and Cummings (1993) saw a reduction of caudate, putamen, and temporal lobe volume on magnetic resonance imaging (MRI) in psychotically depressed patients. Those patients with hypercortisolemia evidenced enlarged ventricles, suggesting a rationale for the state-dependent cognition disturbance of decreased problem-solving ability. The frontal-subcortical circuit critical to the occurrence of depression includes reward mechanisms, set expectancy, and stress responses; their dysfunction results in anhedonia, dysphoria, and feelings of hopelessness and worthlessness.

George and his co-investigators (1993) reported blunted activation of the right cingulate and left frontal lobe using emotional recognition tasks during positron emission tomography (PET) of regional cerebral blood flow (rCBF). While this finding was on a small sample of med-free bipolars, it suggests that internal emotion recognition and possible emotion regulation in depression may be mediated in these anatomical regions. Functional imaging techniques hold promise for understanding the neurobiological changes that occur during mania and depression.

The neuroanatomy of BP disorder still lacks replicated specificity, but the limited findings to date are suggestive for depression and come from pharmacological challenges and brain imaging. The serotonergic and adrenergic neurons, which are enhanced by the antidepressant medications, project via the amygdala, hippocampus, hypothalamus, mamillary bodies, and the cerebral cortex (Kleinman & Hyde, 1993), that is, the anatomical structures associated with the affective behaviors of depressed affect, suicide, anhedonia, decreased concentration, and appetite loss.

Few postmortem studies have focused on mood disorders. However, technological advances will permit future studies to improve the understanding of the neuroanatomical mechanisms.

BRAIN NEUROTRANSMISSION

The neuron is the basic functional unit of the nervous system or the unit of transmission. The brain is known to contain 1 trillion neurons, each one interacting with the others by electrochemical means. The blood-brain barrier is a semipermeable barrier between the blood vessels and brain that shields the brain and prevents many chemical compounds from passing through the brain capillaries. The ability of a molecule to cross this blood-brain barrier is based on its molecular size, electric charge, solubility, and presence of a specific transport system for the compound.

All cells, as neurons, are encased in cell membranes, which function as complex regulatory sites. The membranes are organized by phospholipids and proteins. The proteins are enzymes and ion channels, and the synthesis of proteins is directed by genes. Hence, each neuron attains its specialized functional and structural status from genetic coding within the cell nucleus.

The neuron has four components: the cell body, or soma, containing the nucleus and cytoplasm; the axon, which conveys the electrical impulses from the cell body; the dendrite, where electrical impulses are conducted to the cell body; and the synapse. The synapse, or cleft, is the highly specialized junction between neurons where communication occurs. Reciprocal synapses—located in the dendrite, soma, axon, and between two neurons—form positive and negative feedback loops, which can be inhibitory, excitatory, or modulatory.

While neurotransmission can occur either through chemical or electrical synapses, most is known about the chemical synapses, which use a neurotransmitter as the messenger. Receptors, which are proteins located on the external surface of the neuronal membrane, detect the neurotransmitter in the vicinity of the neuron and initiate a response to it (see Fig. 11–2). Receptors on the axon are presynaptic, and receptors on the receiving dendrite are postsynaptic. Receptors are the cellular recognition sites for the specific molecular structures, and their actions select for specific chemicals. This specificity, which has been likened to a lock and key, is the basis for first messenger transmission, that is, when the neurotransmitter-receptor complex results in a rapid, direct change of the membrane potential. A first messenger transmission can, in turn, initiate a series of intracellular reactions and trigger second messenger transmissions, which cause delayed ion channel opening or closing and result in regulation of the cell.

Current research suggests a third synaptic action to explain how neurotransmitters acting through second messengers alter gene expression by protein phosphorylation (Schwartz & Kandel, 1991) and code for proteins that regulate gene expression. It is by the synthesis of proteins, composed of enzymes and ion channels, that genes produce ribonucleic acid (RNA). In this schema, changes in gene expression through the messenger ribonucleic acid (mRNA) modify the release of neurotransmitters and peptides from axons, causing inhibition or excitation of receptor synthesis. This complex cascade affects brain cells, which may, in turn, change behavior (Post, 1992b).

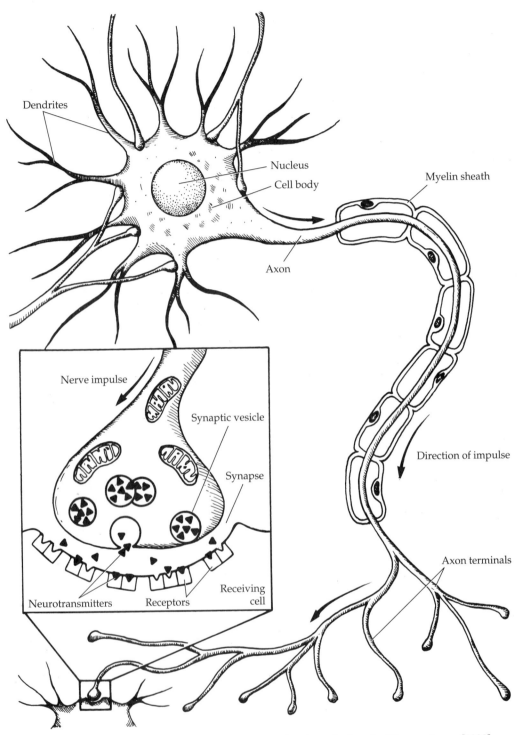

FIGURE 11–2. Neuron. (Reprinted with permission from Society for Neuroscience. [1990]. *Brain facts: A primer on the brain and nervous system* [p. 4]. Washington, DC: Author.)

Each neurotransmitter is thought to act at multiple receptor subtypes. The binding of a ligand (a drug, hormone, neurotransmitter, or any molecule that binds to a protein) does not define a receptor molecule (Dean, Kelsey, Heller, & Ciaranello, 1993); rather, compounds that bind specifically to receptors act as antagonists, agonists, or as a mixed agent. Antagonists prevent the endogenous neurotransmitter from acting at that receptor (inhibition), while agonists mimic the endogenous neurotransmitter, which is receptor activating.

Receptor activity and control are crucial in pharmacotherapy, and a better understanding of neural mechanisms underlying BP illness will provide for the synthesis of selective drug action. Therefore, psychiatric nurses in advanced practice must be familiar with the advances in molecular concepts related to medications in order to understand, and educate clients and their families regarding side effects, interactions, and behavioral response.

Neuromessengers is a generic term that includes neurotransmitters, neuromodulators, and neurohormones. Neurotransmitters are the messengers rapidly released by the presynaptic neuron upon stimulation. They have an excitatory or inhibitory effect on the postsynaptic neuron. The three classes of neurotransmitters are biogenic amines, amino acids, and peptides. The neurotransmitters most commonly associated with BP disorders are the catecholamines (dopamine and norepinephrine) and indolamine (serotonin). These neurotransmitters assist in the regulation of mood and perception, reward and pleasure, temperature and sensory regulation, sleep, and suicidal impulsivity.

Acetylcholine and histamine are additional neurotransmitters. The synthesis of these enzymes from dietary amino acids, or precursors, into metabolites is assisting researchers to refine drug therapies and understand the complex neuronal interaction in the brain. GABA and glycine are the major inhibitory amino acid neurotransmitters. GABA plays a role in decreasing neuronal excitability and restraining the firing of the LC. Electrolytes—such as sodium, calcium, potassium, and chloride—are also directly involved in neurotransmission by serving to transmit fast, discrete messages or to slow down cell excitability modulators (Kaplan & Sadock, 1991).

In the past 15 years, peptides, a whole new class of substances in nervous tissue, have been identified as having neurotransmitter or neuromodulator roles. The peptides involved in BP illness—corticotropin-releasing factor (CRF), endogenous opioids, and substance P—are cotransmitted with other neuromessengers, thus suggesting the complexity of information transmission across the synapse. However, because the brain is tremendously complex, it is not yet understood how its molecular structure results in what is normal or abnormal mental functioning.

Because the syndrome of BP illness includes physiologic changes, another area of suggested involvement is the functioning of structural areas that influence arousal, food intake, reproduction, circadian rhythms, and pituitary regulation (Gold, Goodwin, & Chrousos, 1988).

NEUROTRANSMITTER DYSFUNCTION

Early studies postulated an association between BP illness and the biogenic amine hypothesis, which suggested that too much of the neurotransmitters norepinephrine and serotonin in the synapse accounted for mania, while too little resulted in depression. These neurotransmitters remain implicated in the pathophysiology of BP illness, but new research implies the involvement of other neurotransmitters. An example is the effects of atypical antidepressants that fail to inhibit the reuptake of norepinephrine and serotonin yet produce an antidepressant effect, suggesting that receptor sensitivity is an important factor and that change is not just in the absolute number or levels of neurotransmitters, but in the capacity for them to act and be received on the postsynaptic cleft. Because BP disorders are not homogeneous but a group of disorders sharing common symptoms, each has a unique biology. Pharmacologic strategies therefore must target the bridging of chemical receptors specifically associated with behavioral correlates.

Newer studies suggest that complex interactions among neurotransmitter systems contribute to BP disorder. Studies in the second messenger functions, especially the phosphatidylinosital and calcium ion, are of particular interest in understanding the biphasic mood changes (Dubovsky, Murphy, Christian, & Lee, 1992). The changes and mixtures of affective, behavioral, and physiologic systems found in many BP states could be associated with unstable intracellular signaling related to excessive baseline calcium (Dubovsky et al., 1992). Depending upon when the cells are stimulated, a more facilitatory or inhibitory compensatory response occurs. Therefore, there is a need for thymoleptics (drugs used to treat mood disorders) that are bidirectional so they are effective for either mania or depression. As future studies clarify this hypothesis involving the second messenger system cascade response, the etiology of BP disorder and its treatment will be elucidated.

NEUROENDOCRINE DYSREGULATION

Abnormalities in the limbic-hypothalamic-pituitary axis are also reported in patients with mood disorders. These neuroendocrine regulatory mechanisms operate under the principle of closed feedback loops in which the output of the system inhibits production—a negative feedback system. Each level in the hierarchy of the endocrine system has receptors that respond to the hormones secreted by levels distal to them, and additional regulation is achieved by changes in the hormone receptor number.

Biological alterations in drug-free clients with endogenous or melancholic depression evidence the following indices during hormone challenge studies:

1. Hypothalamic-pituitary-adrenal (HPA) axis activity, which includes increased 24-hour urinary free cortisol, dexamethasone nonsuppression (seen by increased cortisol level, or hypercortisolemia), a blunted adrenocorticotropic hormone (ACTH) response to corticotropin-releasing factor (CRF), and increased cerebrospinal fluid concentrations of cortisol.
2. Hypothalamic-pituitary-thyroid (HPT) axis alterations, including exaggerated or blunted thyroid-stimulating hormone (TSH) and higher than expected rate of autoimmune thyroiditis (Altemus & Gold, 1990).

When assisting consumers to understand these test results, the psychiatric nurse must emphasize that they are state dependent, not diagnostic, and can be influenced by numerous variables, including weight change, smoking, stress, exercise, and birth control pills.

The syndrome of melancholic depression represents dysregulation of the generalized stress response. Stress or arousal in melancholic depression becomes dysphoric hyperarousal and anxiety, and vigilance is turned into hypervigilance and insomnia (Chrousos & Gold, 1992). Cognition, memory, and attention are then focused on depressive ruminations, and both the HPA axis and sympathetic nervous system are chronically activated. Because the corticotropin-releasing hormone (CRH) and LC-NE systems participate in a positive feedback loop, activation of one system tends to activate the other, and a variety of other neuropeptides also enhance central behavioral effects of CRH. This neuroendocrine stress pathophysiology is associated with the behavioral sensitization model (Post, 1992a).

KINDLING AND SENSITIZATION

The kindling-sensitization model attempts to account for the pattern of cyclicity seen in BP illness (Post, Ballenger, Uhde, Putnam, & Bunney, 1981). Kindling is the increasing behavioral and electro-physiological responsivity to repeated low level electrical stimulation to the neuron, which eventually generates an action potential. At the organ level, the repeated subthreshold stimulation, which can be the chemical cascade from stress, results in limbic seizures that are seen as affective cycling rather than convulsions. The neuron becomes sensitized, rather than tolerant of the stimuli. In this way, kindling rewires the brain, and stress can cause cell death or changes in the neural architecture.

Studies document that important psychosocial stressors and other negative life events may be related to initial manic episodes approximately 60% of the time and are less likely to be associated with later mood occurrences (Post, 1993). The sensitization model suggests that in genetically vulnerable individuals, an environmental psychosocial factor may trigger or precipitate an initial episode. In animal models, when the predisposed rat is rechallenged by a stressor, the amygdala discharges neuromessengers with increasing duration and complexity and then spreads them through the neuronal axis in synaptically related structures. Thus a process evolves in which repeated stimulations increase the brain reactivity associated with behavioral consequences and, in turn, predispose it to further episodes. According to Post (1993), this kindled seizure process is facilitated by repetition that results in a transition from requiring the triggering of key exogenous stimulation to an autonomous phase. Thus initial, regular periods of illness may trigger further mood psychopathology.

Hypothesizing a parallel process in the human neurobiology of repetitions of mood episodes, the kindling model may explain a transition to spontaneous episodes emerging in the absence of critical psychosocial triggers. A cascade of complex spatiotemporal neurobiological events in the kindling process lays down neuronal memory in the cortex-limbic-thalamic pathways that occur through altered gene transcription. Through biochemical sensitization, neurotransmitter release, and gene transcription, the individual becomes more reactive to each event. Kindling appears to be a kind of learning; it is like an emotional scar or memory of encoded emotion. Thus the pharmacology for BP illness differs with the stage or evolution of the cycle and supports the combination of drugs to stabilize the progressive course of the illness.

CHRONOBIOLOGICAL CHANGES

Seasonal mood disorders are episodes of depression or mania that recur annually at a specific season (Lewy, 1993) and appear to be related to circadian rhythmicity, which allows complex physiological systems to be internally coordinated with changes in the environment. These chronobiological changes depict the phase advance oscillator phenomenon and are seen in REM sleep, temperature, and cortisol secretion. An example is the advance timing in the initial rise in temperature (arousal) and a corresponding advance in the time of awakening; hence, early morning wakening is common in some mood disorders (Wehr & Goodwin, 1981).

Animal research suggests that many typical antidepressants are effective in changing the settings of endogenous biological clocks. For example, the hormone melatonin, which is synthesized from serotonin and secreted by the pineal gland, demonstrates a circadian rhythm with highest values at night and lowest ones during the day. Because the production of melatonin is sensitive to light, it has been suggested that light modifies the melatonin circadian pattern. Similarly, the suprachiasmic nucleus (SCN), located in the hypothalamus, is implicated in the generation and synchronization of circadian rhythms as varied by environmental light (Betrus & Elmore, 1991).

Some depressed people appear to have a desynchronization in their 24-hour internal clock rhythms. While their sleep, temperature, cortisol, and melatonin cycles may be in synchrony with each other, they may be ahead or behind the other 24-hour rhythms. They may, for example, start and stop releasing melatonin earlier—leading to early morning wakening and evening sleepiness—or start and stop releasing melatonin later than usual—resulting in difficulty awakening and initial insomnia. This is the proposed basis for persons with SAD being exposed to bright light to re-synchronize their 24-hour rhythms.

GENETIC FACTORS

For years researchers have identified an increased presence of mood disorders in the family members of patients who present with major mood disorders. Pooled data from 14 studies of BP probands show first-degree relatives have a 7.9% risk of BP disorder (Bowman & Nurnberger, 1993). In fact, the evidence for the heritability of BP disorder is stronger than that for unipolar depression. If one parent has BP disorder, there is a 27% chance that an offspring will have a mood disorder; if both parents have BP disorder, the risk goes up to 50% to 75% for the offspring. Studies of various forms of mood disorder show they appear to be related in a hierarchical manner; that is, relatives of BP probands are more likely to have BP or unipolar illness (Gershon, 1990). In a longitudinal study by Todd, Neuman, Fox, and Geller (1993) on the course of childhood onset of mood disorder, the investigators found that the probands (n = 76) originally had a diagnosis of major depression (MD). However, in follow-ups 2 to 5 years later, 22 had progressed to BP I and BP II disorder. They also found increased rates for BP and MD in the first-, second-, and third-degree relatives of childhood-onset BP and MD, as well as increased rates of suicide attempts, alcoholism, and early onset psychiatric problems in the adult relatives. Isaac (1992), in a study of 11 adolescents in a special education setting, found 9 had a first- or second-degree relative who suffered from BP disorder or an affective illness. Also noteworthy is that 7 were found to be misdiagnosed as attention deficit hyperactivity disorder.

Twin studies have shown a concordance rate of .67 for BP disorder in monozygotic twins. While the concordance for BP is higher than reported for unipolar depression, linkage studies in BP illness have not been reproducible. The Old Order Amish study that suggested chromosome 11 as the marker of the illness was not supported with the extensions of the pedigree. Recent results imply two candidate genes, a corticotropin receptor and a subunit of a G protein, on chromosome 18 increases susceptibility to BP illness (Berrettini et al., 1994). No definitive marker for heritability of BP disorder has been discovered.

In trait marker studies, however, BP individuals have been shown to be more sensitive than controls to the REM-inducing effects of arecoline, even when mèd-free and euthymic. This suggests central muscularinic cholinergic supersensitivity in the brain stem area in BP illness (Lewy et al., 1985; Nurnberger, Berrittini, Mendleson, Sack, & Gershon, 1989). As indicated earlier, BP patients are also more sensitive to the effect of light suppression of melatonin (Nurnberger et al., 1988), and these pathophysiological traits may help clinicians identify relatives at risk. In addition, even though research on the genetic contributions to response of psychotropic medications does not compare to the number of heritability studies, it may be helpful in nursing assessments to question pharmacologic efficacy of family members when choosing medicine for the proband.

SUMMARY

The biological factors combine to suggest a relationship between BP disorder and pathology of the limbic system, basal ganglia, and the hypothalamus. The limbic system and basal ganglia are connected by the various neuronal networks and provide a major role in the production of emotions. Dysfunction of the hypothalamus—as evidenced by the alterations in sleep, appetite, and libido—and the biological changes in endocrine, chronobiological rhythms, and immunological systems are all seen in the behaviors of BP patients. As yet, no one biological test will conclusively indicate a BP diagnosis; however, research is narrowing the gap for conclusive etiologies.

NURSING INTERVENTIONS FOR BP CLIENTS
ASSESSMENT

The psychiatric nurse and client (individual and family) collaborate systematically and continuously to address the client's problems. Assessments—which may employ the classical mental status framework, an institution's data base design, or the semistructured clinical interviews of the DSM-IV—are the key contribution for the expert nurse clinician. As endogenous behaviors are disrupted, a general systems review is the standard, but there is no one framework. Physical and psychosocial factors must be integrated, using such categories as respiratory, circulatory, gastrointestinal, genitourinary, endocrine, musculoskeletal, and neurologic. See Table 11–5 for examples. The examination includes assessment for predictable side effects, as well as biological disruptions resulting in physical manifestations and previous medical problems. Inclusion of the biological data would prompt the nurse to inquire about family history of medical and psychiatric disturbances. A thorough medical examination—including an electrocardiogram, computed tomography (CT) scan of the head, chemistry and hematology profiles, drug plasma levels, thyroid function tests, renal and liver function tests, electrolytes, venereal disease screen, and human immunodeficiency virus (HIV)—are the current standard parameters with which the nurse should be familiar. Observer rating scales are generally more useful

TABLE 11–5. REVIEW OF SYSTEMS

SYSTEM	EXAMINATIONS	INFLUENCING FACTORS
Respiratory	Respiration rate and pattern, dry mouth	Pharmacology, psychosis, anxiety, mood state
Circulatory	Pulse, sitting and standing blood pressure, exercise tolerance	Anxiety or panic, pharmacology, metabolic
Gastrointestinal	Appetite and nutrition patterns, weight fluctuations, nausea, pain	Pharmacology, eating disorder, mood disorder, metabolic
Genitourinary	Elimination patterns, contraception method, infectious diseases, sexual functioning	Pharmacology, mood disorder, metabolic, anxiety
Endocrine	Menses pattern, libido, sleep pattern, cold and heat tolerance, temperature patterns	Pharmacology, sleep-wake cycle, mood disorder, stress
Musculoskeletal	Tremor, gait pattern, psychomotor pattern, limb movements, muscle discomforts	Pharmacology, mood state
Neurological	Dizziness, headache pattern, mental status, blurred vision, delusions, cognitive ability, learning style	Mood state, pharmacology, metabolic, thought process disruption

TABLE 11–6. Comparison of DSM-IV Criteria and Nursing Diagnoses

DSM-IV CRITERIA	NURSING DIAGNOSIS
Human Response in Mania	
1. Increase in activity	Coping, ineffective, individual
2. Hyperverbal, pressured speech	Communication, impaired verbal
3. Racing thoughts, flight of ideas	Thought processes, alterations in
4. Grandiosity	Self-concept, disturbance in
5. Decreased need for sleep	Sleep pattern disturbance
6. Distractibility	Thought processes, alterations in
7. Poor judgment	Sensory perceptual alteration
Human Response in Depression	
1. Appetite disturbance	Nutrition, alteration in:
	Less than body requirements
	More than body requirements
2. Sleep disturbance	Sleep-pattern disturbance
3. Loss of energy	Fatigue
4. Psychomotor change	Mobility, alteration in
Retardation	
Agitation	
5. Loss of interest in usual pleasures	Coping, ineffective, individual
6. Decreased ability to concentrate	Thought processes, alteration in
7. Feelings of worthlessness, guilt	Self-concept, disturbance in
8. Recurrent thoughts of death or suicide	Potential for self-harm

in settings where the raters are skilled and experienced with the clinical phenomena of concern. Self-assessment scales are limited, as most can only be used by literate, English-reading persons. State-dependent symptoms also limit the reliability of the client to complete his or her ratings, but they can offer the clinician a current perception and the client a way of monitoring mood changes.

The phenomena of concern to psychiatric nurses working with bipolar clients could include the assessment factors cited for disrupted rhythms, disrupted moods, impaired communication, potential for self-harm, loss, powerlessness, altered coping patterns, family dysfunction, and acquisition of knowledge, to cite a few. Comparison of DSM-IV criteria and examples of nursing diagnoses for mania and depression are shown in Table 11–6.

INTERVENTIONS

PSYCHOSOCIAL MODELS

The psychodynamic, behavioral, and cognitive models all pose goals, strategies, and techniques that provide a therapeutic basis for intervention. Bipolar illnesses are most effectively treated with psychopharmacology (to stabilize the mood disruption) and adjunctive psychotherapies. Psychotherapy can help the patient and family members cope with and understand the repercussions of past and future episodes. Psychodynamic approaches may also assist with the interpersonal sequelae of BP illness, but they are insufficient as a modality as long as the patient is cycling. On the other hand, behavioral models, especially cognitive therapy, are demonstrating more efficacy when combined with thymoleptics, that is, drugs that treat mood disorders. For a comprehensive review, the reader is directed to the psychotherapy chapter in Goodwin and Jamison (1990); however, further clinical testing of psychosocial interventions in homogeneous BP populations is needed to validate their efficacy.

NEUROPHARMACOLOGY

The efficacy of various thymoleptics supports the notion that BP illness is a brain disease. Pharmacotherapy for mania includes lithium, usually efficacious for 50% of BP patients; carbamazepine, especially for rapid-cyclers; or other anticonvulsants, such as valproic acid; or neuroleptics. For depression, the class of antidepressants is specifically targeted to the patient's clinical symptom presentation, but acute depression is a treatable illness in 70% to 80% of patients. There is, however, a paucity of controlled studies in the treatment of acute BP depression. Due to the concern of inducing mania or initiating a "switch" in mood, the pharmacologic trials are targeted for unipolar persons. Individuals with a history of BP I or BP II are at risk for cycling with all antidepressants and ECT.

For those patients who are refractory to lithium, numerous combinations of drugs may be necessary to produce efficacy for the patient. Those who present with euphoric mania show a 60% to 80% response to lithium. Dysphoric mania and rapid-cycling are associated with poorer lithium responsiveness (Post, 1993). While lithium carbonate continues to be the drug of choice for acute and long-term treatment of BP illness, longitudinal studies are providing data that the efficacy changes and that alternative and/or adjunctive treatments are needed. Adolescent manics, for example, are at a high risk for relapse after lithium discontinuation and at risk for recurrent episodes during lithium maintenance (Strober, Morrell, Lampert, & Burroughs, 1990).

Carbamazepine has acute antimanic efficacy in approximately two thirds of manic individuals, and the onset and rapidity of action are equivalent with neuroleptics (Post, 1993), while valproate is effective in dysphoric mania and rapid-cycling states. Studies are under way to determine if lithium, carbamazepine, and valproate are most efficacious alone or in combination, and with which subtypes of BP conditions. The reader is referred to the Depression Guideline Panel (1993b) for a complete review of treatment guidelines for the depressive phase of the disorder.

Psychiatric nurses have an ethical responsibility to be aware of the benefits and risks of somatic and psychotherapies. Clinical management for this population requires knowledge of the illness course, realistic outcome, efficacy of medications congruent with the symptom presentations, neurobiological associations of thymoleptics, and alternatives in treatment. Until researchers understand more clearly the neuronal communication system and the pharmacokinetics of medications, somatic therapy will be based mainly on the individual and family member's response to a specific agent.

PSYCHOEDUCATION

The transition necessary for psychiatric nurses to respond to consumer demand for psychoeducation necessitates the integration of the behavioral and biological sciences with the care ethic. The framework for practice of each psychiatric nurse will determine which specific diagnostic taxonomy will initiate interventions or outcomes for the client. When care planning is beginning, the challenge is to select a label or diagnosis that has clinical utility. Because the illness is cyclic, nursing actions must be flexible, dynamic, and able to transcend the generic symptoms. Examples to demonstrate the integration of interventions utilizing the biological and psychiatric nursing concepts are shown in Table 11–7.

TABLE 11–7. NURSING INTERVENTION STRATEGIES

NURSING INTERVENTIONS	RATIONALE
Outcome: The client can expect to be taught probable biologic relationships that disrupt rhythms of the sleep-wake cycle.	
Teach client that certain dietary substances such as caffeine can alter REM sleep. Avoid heavy meals and alcohol two hours prior to bedtime. Teach client which medications can be activating and should be taken earlier in the day.	Dietary substances serve as precursors for synthesis of the neuromessengers. Food additives and chemicals in foods alter brain activity. Caffeine acts as a neuromodulator to inhibit acetylcholine release and increase NE release. This results in neuronal arousal in the limbic structure resulting in REM inhibition.
Assist the client to establish a fixed schedule for sleeping and awakening. Support the client that some persons will need long or short sleep to function adequately.	Sleep studies suggest for bipolar patients that they have shortened REM latency, decreased deep sleep, decreased total sleep. Events that disrupt sleep schedules such as staying up to study, shift work, travel, caring for a newborn infant, and social activities lead to sleep deprivation and may precipitate mania. Therefore napping should be regulated, staying up late and sudden east-west airflights avoided. Melatonin secretion from the pineal gland is inhibited by bright light, so the lowest serum melatonin concentrations occur during the day. The suprachiasmatic nucleus of the hypothalamus has been identified as the anatomical site of a circadian pacemaker that regulates melatonin secretion and the brain entrainment to a 24-hour sleep-wake cycle.
Teach the client the alternative treatments for circadian disorders. These should be done in collaboration with a psychiatric provider. Examples are manipulation of the light-dark cycle and partial sleep deprivation, especially the second half of the night. Some clients will be resistant to phase shifting as they perceive the lack of sleep is part of their problem.	Sleep and wakefulness are synchronized to the underlying phase position of the circadian clock. Shifting for shift workers is best done in a clockwise direction (day to evening to night). The natural cycle length of the circadian clock is longer than 24 hours. The use of time cues or "zeitgebers" assists in establishing the phase position of the biologic clock. The changes in timing and duration of sleep that occur during the course of bipolar illness may play a role in the pathogenesis of mania and depression (Wehr et al., 1982).

A more specific nursing intervention in working with clients is represented in Table 11–8. To plan and integrate the cycle changes, a daily structure can be formulated with the client. For example, assisting clients to have alternative goals—Plan A or Plan B—when in an altered mood allows for additional control and positive self-esteem. Thus a client who becomes depressed can schedule either a day of tasks and work—Plan A—or a day to rest and do only two tasks—Plan B. Either way, the plan is used, and the actions are not associated with failure.

The preceding examples of phenomena of concern for nursing and client outcomes are only a few of the myriad needs that can be identified with BP clients.

TABLE 11–7. NURSING INTERVENTION STRATEGIES *Continued*

NURSING INTERVENTIONS	RATIONALE

Outcome: The client will be able to identify his/her own symptoms of mood state changes.

The nurse will assist the client and family to recognize the early warning cues that signal a mood change.	Maximizing the patient's sense of control over his/her behavior diminishes the fact he/she is unable to control the illness but can control his/her behavior. The earlier symptoms are recognized, the earlier somatic therapies can be reviewed and revised to decrease the cycle severity. Sleep changes, psychomotor changes, and communication patterns are generic for most clients. Cycling can be present in a variety of ways such as irritability, hostility, dysphoria, elation, and depression—each specific for the individual. Bipolar patients often use denial to cope with the illness. In the presence of symptoms, they deny the severity, odds of recurrence, the existence of changing mood, and the fact it can recur.
Assist the client to differentiate normal, adaptive moods from prodromal symptoms.	Exploring the meaning of the illness with the client fosters collaboration and trust. The cycle symptoms are unique to each individual. Early recognition promotes mastery and decreases the learned helplessness and loss secondary to the mood state behaviors. Clients can learn to live with the failures and disappointments as well as the successes. Assisting the client to have self-recognition diminishes the preoccupation of the fear of the illness recurring. The hyperalertness and self-protection diminish as the client differentiates normal moods from abnormal changes and allows the client to incorporate the mood changes into daily living.
Assist the client and family to construct and maintain life chart of the mood episodes along with the concurrent psychopharmacological treatments, psychosocial stressors, and medical problems.	Progressive limbic kindling or sensitization, which produces a natural spontaneous cycling, has been associated with stressful life events, pharmacological, and nonpharmacological factors. Children of bipolar parents should be monitored and counseled when stressful life events occur to desensitize the possible cuing of future episodes.

Table continued on following page.

The interdependent functions were not addressed, but the obvious collaboration with psychopharmacologists is a prerequisite to successful outcomes for this cohort. Additional interventions are included in some psychiatric nursing texts, as disturbances of mood are becoming recognized as a diagnostic entity for nursing intervention (Stuart & Sundeen, 1991). The realigning of the medical and nursing model is also congruent with the consumer movement's request for information on living with the chronically and persistently mentally ill. To assist nurses currently in practice as well as future clinicians, changes in academic content must be considered.

TABLE 11–7. NURSING INTERVENTION STRATEGIES *Continued*

NURSING INTERVENTIONS	RATIONALE

Outcome: The client will be able to identify his/her own symptoms of mood state changes. *(cont.)*

The nurse teaches the suicidal client alternative strategies to use during times of suicidal ideation, recognition of psychosocial triggers, and current strengths that are effective. Assessing for suicide risk potential is done at each client contact.	Suicidal ideation is a symptom and may be a part of state-dependent cognition or a trait variable. Suicide clusters in bipolar families, suggesting a genetic factor, and can assist the client to accept its risk rather than trying to deny or avoid the feelings. Placing the ideation in a biologic context alleviates the guilt and nondisclosure many individuals present. Comorbidity of depression with anxiety is associated with higher suicide rates. Offering suicidal behaviors as illness symptoms assists the individual to plan for the symptoms, seek support, and have mastery, and provides hope.
The nurse should elicit for informed consent to use collateral informants such as family, employers, etc., to provide for feedback to the client and encourage contracting to accept and manage the mood changes. The use of Advance Directives for psychiatric episodes allows for mastery and collaboration.	Opening the communication decreases stigma, supports that the illness is not self-induced, and plans ahead for potential recurrence. The illness is cyclical, and fewer than 60% respond completely to pharmacologic management.
The nurse can reinforce that the illness is a brain disease the client is not able to control. Placing the illness in the context of a medical illness reduces the stigma, underlies the need for medication, and minimizes family and individual responsibility for the origin of the illness.	Brain imaging techniques (CT and MRI) suggest the possibility of neurobiological alterations; however, whether the changes are primary to or a result of the pathophysiology is not conclusive. A family history of mood disorder increases proband risk and is more common in first-degree relatives than the general population.

Outcome: The client will be able to independently demonstrate coping patterns to perform daily tasks.

The nurse can assist the client and family with a daily structure of achievable goals (see Table 11–8 for an example). Among the daily goals plan for activity, exercise, proper nutrition; schedule medications at times convenient with daily schedule; encourage collaboration in care with a mood diary; avoid known stressors; plan for cycle changes; review accomplishments or positive goal attainments.	These actions are supported by the behavioral approaches or self-control theory, social learning theory, and social skills training. The client can review his or her structure at the end of the day and evaluate how much was accomplished—he or she did it him/herself which leads to mastery, enhanced self-concept, and decreased negative thinking.

TABLE 11–7. NURSING INTERVENTION STRATEGIES *Continued*

NURSING INTERVENTIONS	RATIONALE

Outcome: The client will be aware of the family planning strategies and alternatives through educational counseling.

The nurse will construct a genogram to identify psychiatrically affected family members; interview first-degree relatives with patient's consent to expand data about psychiatrically ill members; ascertain client's (patient and significant other) relation to risk relative.	Biologic data to support these actions is not definitely identified, but the evidence strongly suggests genetic transmission. Relatives of people suffering from affective disorder have a higher rate of mania and depression than occurs in the general population (Simmons-Alling, 1990). Secondary prevention of an illness in a population involves reducing its morbidity by recognizing and treating cases soon after the illness develops. One fifth of diagnosed relatives have never been treated, and they constitute a high-risk population for future episodes (Gershon, 1990). Two thirds of bipolar clients have a positive family history. Taking a family history assists with an approach of pharmacologic aggressiveness if a new illness is identified. For example, if a late adolescent develops moderate depression and is the child of a parent with bipolar disorder, it is wise to begin lithium or antidepressants, or both, rather than dismiss the symptoms as a developmental crisis of late adolescence.
The nurse will assess the client's ability to assume spousal and parental role; educate female patients on the risks associated with pharmacotherapy and the need to be medication-free; provide de-escalation of anxiety and the stigma of diagnosis; and refer or provide for supportive psychotherapy for guilt and interpersonal consequences that can be secondary to the illness.	For a female bipolar client who wishes to have children, the pattern of cycling, ability to be medication free for at least the first two trimesters and precoital must be evaluated. Strategies to assist postpartum include resuming medications immediately after delivery; negating breast-feeding; providing child care workers via family, friends, and agencies to avoid sleep deprivation and exhaustion; providing interpersonal context to discuss stressors and ongoing assessment of mood with a skilled clinician. Couples seeking counseling about having children are rarely advised to refrain from having them. There is no evidence to support refraining from marriage as the bipolar client has a treatable illness. Supportive psychotherapy or family therapy in conjunction with medical management in coping with the illness and diminishing recurrences is advised.

TABLE 11–8. DAILY STRUCTURE

Depression

8:00 AM	awaken	3:00 PM	rest
8:30 AM	bathe, shave	4:00 PM	attempt to engage in hobby
9:00 AM	breakfast, take medications	5:00 PM	make schedule for next day
10:00 AM	take a walk for 15 minutes	6:00 PM	fix and eat dinner
11:00 AM	call a friend or significant other	7:00 PM	take medications
11:30 AM	sort laundry	8:00 PM	log in mood; diary
12:30 PM	do load of wash	9:00 PM	personal time—review
1:00 PM	eat lunch		accomplishments of day
1:30 PM	put laundry away	10:00 PM	take medications
2:00 PM	make bed/tidy room	10:30 PM	prepare for sleep

Mania

6:00 AM	awaken	1:00 PM	resume work
6:15 AM		2:30 PM	break
6:30 AM	jog, bike, or walk	2:45 PM	work activity
7:00 AM	shower	4:00 PM	break
7:15 AM	dress	4:15 PM	work activity
7:30 AM	breakfast	5:30 PM	depart work
7:45 AM	take medications	6:00 PM	transportation home
8:00 AM	depart for work	6:30 PM	exercise
8:30 AM	catch train or bus	7:00 PM	dinner
9:00 AM	start work or organize day	7:30 PM	schedule for next day
10:00 AM	take a break	8:00 PM	personal time—review
10:15 AM	return to work		accomplishments
10:30 AM	return calls, etc. (limit time and number)	9:00 PM	log in mood; diary
		9:30 PM	quiet down
12:00 noon	lunch	10:00 PM	medications
12:30 PM	take medications	10:30 PM	bed

FUTURE DIRECTIONS AND CURRICULUM

Academic settings must become more contemporary and congruent with consumer requests and social responsibility. Emphasis on the specialization of psychiatric–mental health nursing is essential for nursing to make a contribution toward health care. Inherent in the Joint Commission on Accreditation of Healthcare Organizations' (JCAHO) standards (1990) is the expectation of competency-based practice. For psychiatric nurses to have authority for their practice, curriculum revisions will need to provide a comprehensive approach to clients' needs.

Undergraduate programs will need to separate the psychiatric–mental health knowledge to integrate the basic and behavioral sciences with the psychiatric nursing courses. The biological basis for psychopathology integrated with pathophysiology enables the student to identify major mental disorders as physiologically based, with psychological-behavioral manifestations, just like any illness. Concurrent courses in growth and development, psychology, sociology, and communication theory provide the basis for holistic practice (Peduzzi & Simmons-Alling, 1990). Student clinical rotations in psychiatric settings would provide the student exposure to integrated biomedical and nursing models.

Graduate programs organized around the neurosciences—neuroanatomy, physiology, immunology, endocrinology, and genetics—along with advanced pharmacology will provide an improved working knowledge base for the graduate nurse to assume an accountable role in the provider marketplace. Incorporating the behavioral sciences and expanding the scope to family and group therapies would round out the expected competencies of the graduate level psychiatric nurse. The addition of basic research skills, expanding to clinically based research at the doctorate level, would result in the theory-based practice psychiatric nurses are still evolving. Sabbaticals and faculty internships in biological medical settings would assist in preparing faculty with richer learning environments.

Nursing makes a difference in the quality of life for psychiatric clients and families. The integration of knowledge from psychology, physiology, biology, neurology, and the principles of psychiatric nursing will provide interventions that are contemporary, theory based, holistic, and caring. The assimilation of the brain-body-behavior phenomena will enable psychiatric nurses a chance to educate the public and peers and to alleviate the enormous suffering and disability that result from major mental illness.

RESEARCH AGENDAS

As this is the Decade of the Brain, it is only fitting that psychiatric nurses pursue a research agenda that will further delineate the care factors with the biological data for BP illness. To date there is no biological test that can provide conclusive etiology of the illness or equate with a definitive diagnosis. Lifetime clinical symptoms with family history remain the best criteria for diagnosis, but relationships do emerge from the biological data that support contributing factors for the mood disorders.

Numerous research questions requiring additional qualitative and quantitative studies need to be addressed. Descriptive studies that attempt to identify the state phenomena of BP illness are warranted. Studies that identify factors contributing to patient noncompliance are also recommended. In addition, patterns of behavior or risk factors that lead clients to substance abuse as a form of self-medication should be explored. Phenomenological studies that explore the meaning of mood disorder to the individual might contribute to a greater understanding of the issues of stigmatization and low self-esteem that plague so many clients.

Nurse researchers have an endless opportunity to evaluate the impact of their interventions on client outcomes. The outcomes of psychoeducational, exercise, and nutritional programs on the status of these clients are among those suggested for research. The efficacy of community groups, mood charting, and daily structure programs in promoting client well-being must also be evaluated. Additionally, the benefits and empowerment of incorporating the family into the treatment program need further exploration. The role of the family in promoting adaptation through medication management, symptom monitoring, and the identification of stressors is another field of inquiry.

These generic suggestions are just a few for nurses to consider for future study. Cultural diversity, gender, and age are also variables that could contribute to the current body of knowledge regarding mood disorders. This decade will promote the opportunity for collaborative inquiry, as neuroscientists search for a more complete understanding of the neurobiological illnesses.

CONCLUSION

Psychiatric nurses are in a position to reduce the dichotomy of the biomedical and care models. If nursing's philosophy states that all persons have potential, can learn, and are open to change, then psychiatric nurses have the responsibility to teach clients as much as they can about autonomy, mastery, growth, and positive self-esteem. The collaborative model—with the nurse, patient, family, and physician—yields a contemporary, efficacious, and ethical forum for positive outcomes in the care of major mood disorders.

REFERENCES

Abraham, K. (1953). Notes on the psychoanalytical investigation and treatment of manic-depressive insanity and allied conditions. In *Selected papers on psychoanalysis* (p. 137). New York: Basic.

Altemus, M., & Gold, P. W. (1990). Neuroendocrinology and psychiatric illness. *Frontiers in Neuroendocrinology, 11*(3), 243–244.

American Nurses Association. (1980). *Nursing: A social policy statement.* Kansas City, MO: Author.

American Psychiatric Association. (1994). *Diagnostic and statistical manual of mental disorders* (4th ed.). Washington, DC: Author.

Andreasen, N. C., & Black, D. W. (1991). *Introductory textbook of psychiatry.* Washington, DC: American Psychiatric Press.

Arieti, S., & Bemporad, J. (1980). The psychological organization of depression. *American Journal of Psychiatry, 137,* 1360.

Aylward, E. H. (1993). Basal ganglia in schizophrenia and bipolar disorder [Summary]. *Proceedings of the One Hundred and Forty-sixth Annual Meeting of the American Psychiatric Association, 122.*

Beck, A. (1979). *Cognitive therapy of depression.* New York: Guilford.

Berrettini, W. H., Ferraro, T. N., Goldin, L. R., Weeks, D. E., Detera-Wadleigh, S., Nurnberger, J. I., & Gershon, E. S. (1994). Chromosome 18 DNA markers and manic-depressive illness: Evidence for a susceptibility gene. *Proceedings of the National Academy of Science, 41,* 5418–5921.

Betrus, P., & Elmore, S. K. (1991). Seasonal affective disorder: 1. A review of the neural mechanisms for psychosocial nurses. *Archives of Psychiatric Nursing, 5*(6), 357–364.

Bowlby, J. (1960). Grief and mourning in infancy and early childhood. *The Psychoanalytic Study of the Child, 15*(9), 9–52.

Bowman, E. S., & Nurnberger, J. I. (1993). Genetics of psychiatric diagnosis and treatment. In D. L. Dunner (Ed.), *Current psychiatric therapy* (p. 47). Philadelphia: Saunders.

Chrousos, G. P., & Gold, P. W. (1992). The concepts of stress and stress system disorders. *Journal of the American Medical Association, 267*(9), 1244–1252.

Cummings, J. L. (1993). Frontal-subcortical circuits and human behavior [Summary]. *Proceedings of the One Hundred and Forty-sixth Annual Meeting of the American Psychiatric Association,* 173.

Dean, R. R., Kelsey, J. E., Heller, M. R., & Ciaranello, R. D. (1993). Structural foundations of illness and treatment: Receptors. In D. L. Dunner (Ed.), *Current psychiatric therapy* (p. 7). Philadelphia: Saunders.

Depression Guideline Panel. (1993a). *Depression in primary care: Vol. 1., Detection and diagnosis* (AHCPR Publication No. 93–0550). Rockville, MD: US Department of Health and Human Services Public Health Service, Agency for Health Care Policy and Research.

Depression Guideline Panel. (1993b). *Depression in primary care: Vol. 2, Treatment of major depression* (AHCPR Publication No. 93–0551). Rockville, MD: US Department of Health and Human Services Public Health Service, Agency for Health Care Policy and Research.

Dubovsky, S. L., Murphy, J., Christian, J., & Lee, C. (1992). The calcium second messenger system in bipolar disorders: Data supporting new research directions. *Journal of Neuropsychiatry and Clinical Neurosciences, 4*(1), 3–14.

Ferster, C. B. (1973). A functional analysis of depression. *American Psychology, 10,* 857.

Freud, S. (1957). Mourning and melancholia. In *Standard edition of the complete works of Sigmund Freud* (Vol. 14, pp. 214–249). London: Hogarth.

George, M. S., Ketter, T. A., Gill, D. S., Marrengell, L. B., Pazzagglia, P. J., & Post, R. M. (1993). Blunted cerebral blood flow with emotion recognition in depression [Summary]. *Proceedings of the One Hundred and Forty-sixth Annual Meeting of the American Psychiatric Association,* 88.

Gershon, E. S. (1990). Genetics of affective illness. In F. K. Goodwin & K. R. Jamison (Eds.), *Manic-depressive illness* (pp. 369–402). New York: Oxford University Press.

Gold, P. W., Goodwin, F. K., & Chrousos, G. P. (1988). Clinical and biochemical manifestations of depression. *The New England Journal of Medicine, 319,* 413–420.

Goodwin, F. K., & Jamison, K. R. (Eds.). (1990). Psychotherapy. In *Manic-depressive illness* (pp. 725–745). New York: Oxford University Press.

Isaac, G. (1992). Misdiagnosed bipolar disorder in adolescents in a special educational school and treatment program. *Journal of Clinical Psychiatry, 53*(4), 133–136.

Joint Commission on Accreditation of Healthcare Organizations. (1990). *Accreditation manual for hospitals* (Vol. 1). Oakbrook Terrace, IL: Author.

Kaplan, H. I., & Sadock, B. J. (1991). *Synopsis of psychiatry: Behavioral sciences, clinical psychiatry* (6th ed.) (pp. 363, 366). Baltimore: Williams & Wilkins.

Kleinman, J. E., & Hyde, T. M. (1993). Structural foundations of mental illness and treatment: Neuroanatomy. In D. L. Dunner (Ed.), *Current psychiatric therapy* (pp. 5–6). Philadelphia: Saunders.

Lewy, A. J. (1993). Seasonal mood disorders. In D. L. Dunner (Ed.), *Current psychiatric therapy* (p. 220). Philadelphia: Saunders.

Lewy, A. J., Nurnberger, J. I., Wehr, T. A., Pack, D., Becker, L. E., Powell, R. L., & Newsome, D. A. (1985). Supersensitivity to light: A possible trait marker for manic-depressive illness. *American Journal of Psychiatry, 142*(4), 725–727.

McElroy, S. L., & Keck, P. E. (1993). Rapid cycling. In D. L. Dunner (Ed.), *Current psychiatric therapy* (p. 226). Philadelphia: Saunders.

Nurnberger, J. I., Berrettini, W., Mendleson, W., Sack, D., & Gershon, E. S. (1989). Measuring cholinergic sensitivity: 1. Arecoline effects in bipolar patients. *Biological Psychiatry, 25*(5), 610–617.

Nurnberger, J. I., Berrettini, W., Tamarkin, L., Hamovit, J., Norton, J., & Gershon, E. G. (1988). Supersensitivity to melatonin suppression by light in young people at high risk for affective disorder: A preliminary report. *Neuropsychopharmacology, 1,* 217–223.

Peduzzi, T., & Simmons-Alling, S. (1990, September). From education to clinical practice: Integrating biological psychiatry and psychiatric nursing. Paper presented at the meeting of the Society for Education and Research in Psychiatric Nursing, Bethesda, MD.

Post, R. M. (1989). Mood disorders: Somatic treatment. In H. I. Kaplan & S. J. Sadock (Eds.), *Comprehensive textbook of psychiatry* (5th ed.) (p. 913). Baltimore: Williams & Wilkins.

Post, R. M. (1992a, November). *Neurobiology of manic-depressive cycles.* Presented for The Foundation for Advanced Education in the Sciences, Inc., Psychopharmacology in Practice: Clinical and Research Update, Washington, DC.

Post, R. M. (1992b). Transduction of psychosocial stress into neurobiology of recurrent affective disorder. *American Journal of Psychiatry, 149*(8), 999–1010.

Post, R. M. (1993). Mood disorders: Acute mania. In D. L. Dunner (Ed.), *Current psychiatric therapy* (pp. 204–210). Philadelphia: Saunders.

Post, R. M., Ballenger, J. C., Uhde, T. W., Putnam, F. W., & Bunney, W. F. (1981). Kindling and drug sensitization: Implications for the progressive development of psychopathology and treatment with carbamazepine. In M. Sandler (Ed.), *The psychopharmacology of anticonvulsants* (pp. 27–53). Oxford: Oxford University Press.

Potter, W. Z., & Bowden, C. L. (1992, February supplement). Introduction. *Journal of Clinical Psychopharmacology, 12*(1), 25.

Schwartz, J. H., & Kandel, E. R. (1991). Synaptic transmission mediated by second messengers. In E. R. Kandel, J. H. Schwartz, & T. M. Jessell (Eds.), *Principles of neural science* (3rd ed.) (pp. 173–193). New York: Elsevier.

Seligman, M. (1975). *Helplessness: On depression, development and death.* San Francisco: Freeman.

Silber, A. (1989). Mood disorders: Psychodynamic etiology. In M. I. Kaplan & B. J. Sadock (Eds.), *Comprehensive textbook of psychiatry* (4th ed.) (Vol. 1, pp. 188–189). Baltimore: Williams & Wilkins.

Simmons-Alling, S. (1990). Genetic implications for major affective disorders. *Archives of Psychiatric Nursing, 4*(1), 67.

Spitz, R. (1946). Anaclitic depression. *Psychoanalytic Study of the Child, 2,* 313.

Strober, M. T., Morrell, W., Lampert, C., & Burroughs, J. (1990). Relapse following discontinuation of lithium maintenance therapy in adolescents with bipolar I illness: A naturalistic study. *American Journal of Psychiatry, 147,* 457–461.

Stuart, G. W., & Sundeen, S. J. (1991). Disturbance in mood. In G. W. Stuart & S. J. Sundeen (Eds.), *Principles and practice of psychiatric nursing* (4th ed.) (pp. 413–456). St. Louis: Mosby-Yearbook.

Todd, R. D., Neuman, R. J., Fox, L. W., & Geller, B. G. (1993). Transmission of childhood onset bipolar disorder [Summary]. *Proceedings of the One Hundred and Forty-sixth Annual Meeting of the American Psychiatric Association, 171.*

Wehr, T. A., & Goodwin, F. K. (1981). Biological rhythms and psychiatry. In S. L. Arieti & K. H. Brodie (Eds.), *The American handbook of psychiatry* (Vol. 2, pp. 46–74). New York: Basic.

Wehr, T. A., Goodwin, F. K., Wirz-Justice, A., Breitmaier, J., & Craig, C. (1982). 48-hour sleep-wake cycles in manic-depressive illness. *Archives of General Psychiatry, 39,* 559–565.

Wehr, T. A., Sack, D. A., Rosenthal, N. E., & Cowdry, R. W. (1988). Rapid cycling affective disorder: Contributing factors and treatment responses in 51 patients. *American Journal of Psychiatry, 145,* 179–184.

CHAPTER

12

PANIC DISORDER WITH AGORAPHOBIA

Gail W. Stuart, PhD, RN, CS, FAAN, and Michele T. Laraia, MSN, RN

ABSTRACT

Nursing has developed a holistic framework for the care of panic disorder with agoraphobia that integrates biological knowledge with behavioral and social science theory. The concept of panic disorder has undergone considerable revision, but current research most strongly supports a biopsychosocial model in which physiological, psychological, genetic, and environmental factors interact to (1) establish a vulnerability to developing panic disorder, (2) trigger the illness, (3) influence the extent of the response, and (4) guide the selection of treatment modalities. While there is a strong likelihood that patients may be misdiagnosed and have coexisting medical and psychiatric conditions, standardized instruments are now available, and psychiatric nurses can play a key role in developing and implementing a multidimensional treatment plan. The success of nurse behavior therapists in Britain is reported and recommendations made for this approach in the United States, provided appropriate preparation is incorporated into nursing curricula. More nursing research on panic disorder with agoraphobia is encouraged, particularly concerning risk factors and recognition, course of the disorder, methodological studies, and treatment strategies.

Significant advances have been made in understanding the clinical construct of anxiety over the past 40 years. During this period, it has been differentiated and defined as a personality characteristic (trait anxiety), an emotional response (state anxiety), a nursing diagnosis (anxiety), and a medical diagnosis (anxiety disorder). Early work by nurses in assessing and intervening in anxiety was articulated by Peplau (1963) and expanded by Burd (1963), who used a problem-solving and learning process approach to develop a framework for intervening with anxious patients in general health care settings. More recent nursing literature reflects an examination of the psychiatric anxiety syndromes and a holistic framework of nursing care that integrates biological knowledge with behavioral and social science theory (Boyarsky, Perone, Lee, & Goodman, 1991; Gournay, 1991b; Laraia, 1991; Laraia, Stuart, & Best, 1989; Waddell & Demi, 1993; Whitley, 1991).

In the field of psychiatry, the concept of anxiety has undergone considerable revision since the early development of the concept of the anxiety neurosis. The publication of the DSM-III (American Psychiatric Association, 1980) led to a major change in the classification of the syndrome of anxiety when two new diagnostic cat-

TABLE 12–1. History of Anxiety Syndromes

Pre-DSM-I	Anxiety neurosis
	Anxiety state
DSM-I (1952)	Anxiety reaction
DSM-II (1968)	Anxiety neurosis
DSM-III (1980)	Agoraphobia with or without panic attacks
	Panic disorder
DSM-III-R (1987)	Panic disorder with or without agoraphobia
	Agoraphobia without panic disorder
DSM-IV (1994)	Panic disorder with or without agoraphobia
	Agoraphobia without history of panic attack

egories of anxiety were identified. These were agoraphobia with or without panic attacks and panic disorder (Table 12–1). With the adoption of the DSM-III-R system (American Psychiatric Association, 1987), the anxiety categories were further refined as panic disorder with or without agoraphobia and agoraphobia without history of panic disorder. This more clearly differentiated panic disorder from generalized anxiety and from the various types of phobias. This distinction continues with the DSM-IV (American Psychiatric Association, 1994) as well.

The identification of panic, with or without agoraphobia, as a distinct disorder has sparked an exciting expansion of clinical, epidemiologic, and etiologic research in panic disorder and agoraphobia. For panic disorder in particular, pharmacologic and behavioral interventions have been introduced, thus stimulating a fertile field of research and clinical treatment opportunities. This chapter considers whether psychiatric nurses have moved forward with this evolutionary understanding of anxiety and its diagnostic categories, and what progress they have made in the integration of new knowledge about panic disorder in their practice, educational, and research settings.

DIMENSIONS OF THE PHENOMENON

A panic attack consists of an intense feeling of fear and apprehension or impending doom that is sudden in onset. It has a clear beginning and end, and it is accompanied by distressing physical sensations, such as rapid heartbeat, chest pain, choking sensation, trembling, numbness, shortness of breath, palpitations, dizziness, hot or cold flashes, sweating, and nausea or abdominal distress, as well as fears of dying, going crazy, or losing control (Table 12–2). Panic attacks can occur in feared situations (such as a crowded store), in safe situations (such as at home), or spontaneously (such as out of the blue).

Individuals with panic disorder—independent of the presence of coexisting depression, alcohol or drug abuse, or agoraphobia—have been reported to have more suicidal ideation and suicide attempts and have higher morbidity than persons with other psychiatric disorders, even the affective disorders (Weissman, Klerman, Markowitz, & Ouellette, 1989). However, not all patients who have panic attacks meet the DSM-IV criteria for panic disorder. Individuals who experience panic attacks but do not develop avoidant behaviors are considered to have panic disorder without agoraphobia.

A diagnosis of panic disorder with agoraphobia (Table 12–3) is given to those persons with panic disorder who develop significant and pervasive avoidance patterns. Approximately two thirds of individuals with panic disorder also have agora-

TABLE 12–2. DSM-IV CRITERIA FOR PANIC ATTACK

A discrete period of intense fear or discomfort, in which at least four of the following symptoms developed abruptly and reached a peak within 10 minutes:
   (1) palpitations, pounding heart, or accelerated heart rate
   (2) sweating
   (3) trembling or shaking
   (4) sensations of shortness of breath or smothering
   (5) feeling of choking
   (6) chest pain or discomfort
   (7) nausea or abdominal distress
   (8) feeling dizzy, unsteady, lightheaded, or faint
   (9) derealization (feelings of unreality) or depersonalization (being detached from oneself)
   (10) fear of losing control or going crazy
   (11) fear of dying
   (12) paresthesias (numbness or tingling sensations)
   (13) chills or hot flushes

phobia. Panic disorder with agoraphobia is a particularly disabling illness that exacts significant costs through lost workdays, increased utilization of general health care services, and considerable personal suffering. Both the severity of the illness and the avoidance behaviors may vary over time as the individual gets over a particular fear or develops new ones. These individuals avoid situations where they may have an attack and sometimes even become housebound, as their fears and avoidances begin to dominate their normal activities. Consequently, they tend to have restricted lives, deteriorated self-concepts, concurrent depression, and behavioral patterns that significantly interfere with their social functioning, career pursuits, and interpersonal relationships (Markowitz, Weissman, Ouellette, Lish, & Klerman, 1989). Thus, panic disorder with agoraphobia has a major negative impact on an individual's functional status and quality of life, making it an illness that is particularly appropriate for psychiatric nursing intervention.

   Recent community-based epidemiologic studies have reported that panic attacks are common, with a frequency ranging from recurrent in 3% of the population

TABLE 12–3. DSM-IV CRITERIA FOR PANIC DISORDER WITH AGORAPHOBIA

A. Both (1) and (2):
   (1) recurrent unexpected panic attacks
   (2) at least one of the attacks has been followed by a month (or more) of: (a) persistent concern about having additional attacks; (b) worry about the implications of the attack or its consequences (e.g., losing control, having a heart attack, "going crazy"); or (c) a significant change in behavior related to the attacks
B. The presence of agoraphobia , i.e., anxiety about being in places or situations from which escape might be difficult (or embarrassing) or in which help might not be available in the event of having an unexpected or situationally predisposed panic attack. Agoraphobic fears typically involve characteristic clusters of situations that include being outside the home alone; being in a crowd or standing in a line; being on a bridge; and traveling in a bus, train, or car.
C. The panic attacks are not due to the direct effects of a substance (e.g., drugs of abuse, medication) or a general medical condition (e.g., hyperthyroidism).
D. The anxiety or phobic avoidance is not better accounted for by another mental disorder.

to relatively isolated in 10%. Studies of college students and community residents in Canada and the United States report that 33% of respondents experienced at least one panic attack, and 11% reported three to four panic attacks in the past year (Norton, Harrison, Hauch, & Rhodes, 1985). The prevalence of panic disorder over a lifetime has been estimated to be 1.6% to 2%, and agoraphobia has been estimated to have a lifetime prevalence rate of about 5%. The most common age of onset is middle teens and early adulthood, with infrequent onset after age 40.

These illnesses are diagnosed about twice as frequently in women as in men (Weissman, 1988). Currently, there are no convincing explanations for the gender differences found in panic disorder and agoraphobia. Some have suggested that the gender difference may be partly caused by endocrine factors; the data, however, do not confirm any simple relationship between hormonal factors and the genesis and maintenance of the syndrome (Gournay, 1989).

It is obvious that these illnesses are experienced by a relatively large proportion of the population. For many sufferers, they are associated with extremely serious sequelae. Still, the magnitude of the panic attack problem in the United States is only beginning to be appreciated, and health care professionals are only starting to learn how patients with panic attacks and agoraphobia enter the health care system. Panic disorders lead the list of psychiatric conditions for which individuals seek ambulatory medical care and utilize psychotropic medications (Katon et al., 1986; Katon, Vitaliano, Anderson, Jones, & Russo, 1987), yet fewer than 25% of panic disorder patients seek psychiatric care (Weissman & Merikangas, 1986). The Epidemiological Catchment Area (ECA) Study found that subjects with panic disorder were more likely than those with major depression or other psychiatric disorders to seek health care from primary care practitioners and frequently use the services of medical emergency departments (Markowitz et al., 1989). This study also reported that in the panic disorder sample, 20% had attempted suicide at some time during their lifetime, 27% were on welfare or disability support, and 27% had misused or abused alcohol.

Finally, the panic disorders appear to be chronic disorders. Retrospective studies reveal that 50% of panic patients report impairment and 70% remain symptomatic 20 years later (NIMH, 1989). They also suffer significantly higher rates of other anxiety disorders, including generalized anxiety disorder, social phobia, simple phobia, and sexual phobias. In addition, the frequency of the comorbidity of panic disorder and agoraphobia with major depression, somatization, and substance abuse places individuals with panic disorder and agoraphobia at great risk (Michelson et al., 1990).

ETIOLOGY AND KNOWLEDGE BASES

The etiology of panic disorder is complex and controversial, with current knowledge suggesting the importance of the relationships among environment, heredity, psychology, and biology. The role of environmental and sociocultural events derives from the incidence of stressful life events reported by panic disorder patients. This hypothesis poses that in persons with an underlying predisposition, a severe environmental stressor might trigger the disease process (Reich, 1986). Studies have found a high incidence of negative life events preceding the first panic attack in people who later present with panic disorder. Life events frequently preceding the onset of the illness include marital or family conflict, birth, miscarriage, hysterectomy, and the death or illness of a significant other (Last, Barlow, & O'Brien, 1984).

Relatively little is known about familial factors, including what relationships might exist between childhood experiences of stressful events and the onset of adult anxiety disorders (Last, 1992). In a recent controlled study, Laraia, Stuart, Frye, Lydiard, and Ballenger (1994) explored the childhood environment of women with panic disorder with agoraphobia in which emphasis was placed on assessing parental rearing practices, family conflict resolution, experiences of sexual mistreatment, problematic childhood indicators, and childhood separation experiences. Study findings did not support evidence of parental overprotection, parental death, divorce, or sexual mistreatment as risk factors. Results did suggest the significance of childhood separation anxiety, a conflicted family environment, lack of parental warmth and support, and the presence of chronic physical illness and substance abuse in the childhood home of patients. In addition, patients reported more emotional, family, alcohol, and school problems as children and adolescents than normal controls.

Another psychodynamic approach has been proposed in which inborn neurophysiological irritability predisposes an individual to early fearfulness (Shear, Cooper, Klerman, Busch, & Shapiro, 1993). Exposure to parental behaviors that augment fearfulness is believed to result in disturbances in object relations and persistent conflicts between dependence and independence. This, in turn, predisposes the individual to fears of feeling trapped, suffocated, and unable to escape and/or get help. Finally, activation of a fantasy of catastrophic danger, whether conscious or unconscious, often in connection with a negative affect, is thought to trigger a panic attack.

There is also evidence that panic disorder has a high familial transmission. Torgensen (1990) found a higher concordance rate in monozygotic (MZ) than dizygotic (DZ) twins. Crowe, Noyes, Pauls, and Slymen (1982) found the rate of definite and probable panic disorder was 24.7% in panic relatives, compared with 2.2% in controls. Hopper, Judd, Derrick, and Burns (1987), who did similar studies, found that the risk of developing panic disorder increases by approximately 500% when an individual's parent or sibling is affected, and this risk is multiplied for each additional affected relative. While these findings suggest that panic disorder may be caused by dominant genetic factors, they do not diminish the importance of environmental variables (Last, 1992).

PSYCHOLOGICAL MODEL

Within the last decade, research on panic has focused on two complementary models of the disorder: the psychological, which includes cognitive and behavioral components; and the neurobiological. The primary tenet of a psychological model of panic is that people with this disorder respond to bodily sensations with an alarm reaction that has either been conditioned from prior experience or is the result of cognitive processing errors, such as extreme attention to environmental threat cues, a high tendency for catastrophic thoughts and images, or an appraisal of loss of safety (Barlow, 1988; Beck, Emery, & Greenberg, 1985; Clark, 1986). The person becomes preoccupied with stopping these physiological sensations (behavioral) or searching for their meaning (cognitive appraisal).

In this model, the search for meaning is considered a misinterpretation of the physiological symptoms, as one generates catastrophic explanations for them such as "I'm having a heart attack" or "I'm dying." Finally, a behavioral response is initiated in an attempt to relieve, flee, or avoid the anxiety experience. These three elements—physiological sensations, cognitions, and behavior—then develop into a vicious cycle (see Fig. 12–1), and the individual becomes hypervigilant for physical symptoms. Thus, panic attacks may be triggered by any one of these three factors. For example, a woman who responded to stress by blushing begins to dwell on the

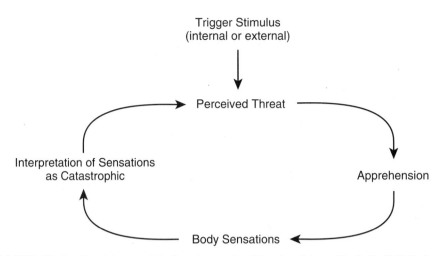

Trigger Stimulus
(internal or external)

Perceived Threat

Interpretation of Sensations
as Catastrophic

Apprehension

Body Sensations

FIGURE 12–1. Cognitive model of panic attacks. (Reprinted from Clark, D. [1986]. A cognitive approach to panic. *Behavior Research and Therapy,* 24[4], 463, with kind permission from Elsevier Science, Ltd, The Boulevard, Langford Lane, Kidlington OX5 1GB, UK.)

embarrassment this might cause her. Consequently, any sensation of warmth in her upper chest, neck, or face produces anxiety, which in turn exacerbates the blushing and further escalates her anxiety.

NEUROBIOLOGICAL MODEL

Current research has supported evidence for several neurobiological models of panic disorder. Many of these theories are based upon the actions of drugs on brain chemistry or the reactions elicited by drug administration to patients (Laraia, 1995). One model defines the pathway for panic as that of central noradrenergic stimulation, particularly the locus coeruleus, located in the pons of the brain stem, which produces 70% of the brain's norepinephrine and influences multiple autonomic systems such as the heart, lower bowel, and cerebellum (Ballenger, 1989). Neural tracks project from the locus coeruleus to other areas of the brain involved in anxiety, such as the amygdala and the hippocampus in the limbic system (the emotional brain), and the cortex. The locus coeruleus may also play a critical role in responsiveness to changes in the internal and external environment. Thus, as the neurobiological basis may explain biochemically provoked panic, the locus coeruleus might provide an explanation of the hyperactive noradrenergic system in people with panic disorder.

This theory originated in the 1960s when researchers discovered that a sodium lactate infusion increased the firing rate of the locus coeruleus and was more likely to induce panic in patients who had a history of panic attacks than in other subjects. Furthermore, certain centrally acting agents, such as imipramine, can often prevent lactate-induced panic, while peripherally acting agents do not. This difference suggests that this form of anxiety originates in the central nervous system. Attempts to document noradrenergic system hyperactivity via peripheral noradrenergic measures of plasma catecholamines remain inconclusive, and this research interest continues to be significant and controversial.

Research findings from other provoked-panic challenges have supported the hypothesis that spontaneous panic originates from biological abnormalities in serotonergic receptors and in the gamma-aminobutyric acid (GABA) system. Studies have shown that panic patients are more sensitive than controls to serotonergic stimulating agents such as fenfluramine, and that serotonin reuptake inhibitors such as fluoxetine and sertraline, which increase serotonergic tone in the central nervous system, are effective antipanic agents.

Flumazenil, a benzodiazepine receptor antagonist, also produces panic in patients with panic disorder and not in normal controls. High-potency benzodiazepines, such as alprazolam and lorazepam, enhance the effects of the inhibitory neurotransmitter, GABA, and are effective in blocking these pharmacologically induced panic attacks.

Other agents such as carbon dioxide, isoproterenol, and high-dose caffeine have also been studied for their ability to induce acute panic anxiety in patients. These agents are strong respiratory stimulants, and they provide a laboratory model for the induction of panic that may be caused by an abnormal regulation of ventilation at the brain stem level, perhaps contributing to the hyperventilation commonly experienced by panic patients.

Once it became possible to either induce or block panic and anxiety in the laboratory, imaging techniques were employed to elucidate the anatomic, neurochemical, and circulatory alterations that may serve as substrates for anxiety. For example, studies with positron emission tomography (PET) in patients who develop panic under lactate infusion sometimes show an asymmetric circulation around the hippocampus and an increased use of oxygen as compared to normal controls (Reiman et al., 1986; Reiman, 1987). These abnormalities suggest an increase in neuronal activity in the right parahippocampal area, an asymmetry in the density of cellular process innervating the hippocampal region, and an increase in the permeability of the blood-brain barrier in the right hippocampal region.

Thus, these findings suggest an abnormality in the area of the brain responsible for integrating information from all sensory modalities in order to initiate an appropriate behavioral response. Nuclear magnetic resonance imaging (MRI) studies have also shown temporal lobe abnormalities in some patients with a history of panic disorder (Fontaine, Breton, & Dery, 1990). Such studies have provided a foundation for the conceptualization of panic and anxiety as biologically based, or at least biologically mediated. This information has stimulated research directed at the discovery of pharmacologic agents that work in the central nervous system to reduce or block panic attacks in patients with panic disorder. The nurse clinician with an understanding of the differences in the action mechanisms of these agents can make informed decisions regarding selection of antipanic medication trials based on individual patient efficacy as well as side effect profiles. These decisions lead to the most efficacious utilization of psychopharmacologic agents in the treatment of panic disorder and agoraphobia (Shelton, 1993).

For example, if a patient is particularly bothered by the tachycardia associated with panic attacks, drugs such as the selective serotonin reuptake inhibitors (SSRIs) (which do not have tachycardia as a side effect), rather than the tricyclics, may be the first choice for treatment. For a patient who may not be able to take either SSRIs or tricyclics—because of cost, lack of efficacy, or side effects—it would make sense to change to an antipanic drug of a different class. A benzodiazepine, such as alprazolam, or a monoamine oxidase inhibitor, such as phenelzine, would provide different mechanisms of action, thereby increasing the chance of finding a drug suitable for the patient. Yet again, if a patient has been self-medicating with alcohol for anxiety symptoms or has a severe secondary depression, use of a benzodiazepine may be contraindicated. Thus the type of drug, dosing schedule, and rate of dose titration are examples of drug differences that can be used to minimize side effects and maximize efficacy for individual patients with panic disorder.

TABLE 12–4. Variables of Importance in a Biopsychosocial Model

---

Biological Factors
Central and autonomic functions
Internal biological conditioning
Biological abnormalities
Effects of medication and other biological treatments
Comorbid medical illness

Psychological Factors
Life-style issues
Cognitive processing skills
Conditioned responses
Self-appraisal
Goals and values
Emotional arousal and stability
Previous experiences with illness
Coping mechanisms
Attitudes toward psychiatric illness
Help-seeking behavior

Sociocultural Factors
Living conditions
Coping resources
Cultural norms and values
Social supports
Environmental and developmental stressors
Structure of the health care system

BIOPSYCHOSOCIAL MODEL

Taken together, current research most strongly supports a holistic biopsychoso-cial model in which physiological, psychological, genetic, and environmental factors interact in (1) establishing a vulnerability to developing panic disorder; (2) triggering the illness; (3) influencing the extent of one's response; and (4) determining one's prognosis for recovery. Such a model would take into consideration the multidimensional and individualized relationships among social, cultural, environmental, psychological, and biological factors that may affect the development, course, and outcome of panic disorder and agoraphobia (Table 12–4). Such an integrated approach also suggests the necessity for psychiatric nurses working with these patients to have a firm knowledge base in neurobiological, behavioral, cognitive, and social theories.

TREATMENT CONSIDERATIONS

Accurate assessment and diagnosis is a critical issue in working with patients with panic disorder. Because panic symptoms are similar to those of medical illness, patients most often present numerous times to primary care practitioners and emergency rooms prior to receiving a diagnosis of panic disorder. There they undergo repeated physical examinations and laboratory tests that reflect normal findings, but they do not feel reassured that theirs is not a serious, life-threatening illness.

Much is known about the presenting complaints of these patients, as well as where they seek care. Pain complaints, notably chest pain, epigastric distress, and headaches were found to be the presenting symptoms of 80% of primary care patients who met DSM-III criteria for panic disorder (Katon, 1984). Sheehan (1982) re-

TABLE 12–5. INSTRUMENTS FOR THE ASSESSMENT OF PANIC DISORDER

Diagnostic Assessments

Structured Clinical Interview for the DSM-III-R (SCID)
Comprehensive semistructured interview guide that definitively yields the major Axis I diagnoses for all the DSM categories when utilized by trained clinicians (Spitzer, Williams, & Gibbon, 1988)

Anxiety Disorders Interview Schedule (ADIS)
Structured interview that includes specific questions concerning the presence or absence of DSM-III criteria for each of the anxiety disorders and affective disorders, as well as anxiety cues, avoidance, precipitants, and history (DiNardo & Barlow, 1988)

Treatment Assessments

Panic Attack Questionnaire
23-item clinician-rated inventory that provides a retrospective description of the characteristics of attacks and cognitions typically experienced during a panic attack, as well as lifestyle change or avoidance, and family history (Norton, Dorward, & Cox, 1986)

Mobility Inventory for Agoraphobia (MIA)
30-item self-report measure that indicates the degree to which patients avoid a number of potentially phobic situations or places due to anxiety, both when alone and when accompanied by others (Chambless, Caputo, Jasin, Gracely, & Williams, 1985)

Fear Questionnaire
17-item self-report inventory that provides a total phobia score; subscale scores for agoraphobia, social phobia, and blood-injury phobia; ratings of the main phobia and global phobic symptoms; and a composite anxiety-depression score (Marks & Matthews, 1979)

Hamilton Anxiety Scale (HAM-A)
14-item clinician scale that factors into somatic anxiety (muscular, sensory, cardiovascular, respiratory, GI, GU, and autonomic) and psychic anxiety (mood, tension, fears, sleep, cognition, and behavior at interview); it places great emphasis on the patient's subjective state (Hamilton, 1956)

Symptom Checklist (SCL-90)
90-item multidimensional self-report inventory that factors into nine subscales (somatization, obsessive-compulsive, interpersonal sensitivity, depression, anxiety, anger-hostility, phobic anxiety, paranoid ideation, psychoticism) as well as providing an overall general index of symptomatology (Derogatis, 1983)

Phobia Scale
20-item self-report inventory that identifies and measures specific phobias targeted for treatment. A spectrum of phobias associated with anxiety disorders is presented, as well as assessment of the four main phobias experienced by patients. Phobias are measured separately on two dimensions: fear of the identified situation and avoidance of that situation.

Agoraphobic Cognitions and Body Sensations Questionnaire
32-item self-report inventory that assists in the assessment of cognitions and bodily sensations when agoraphobics are nervous or frightened (Chambless, Caputo, Bright, & Gallagher, 1984)

Panic Attack and Homework Diary
Patient's ongoing record of panic parameters and real-life exposure activities, which tracks the frequency of attacks as well as the following: type (spontaneous vs. situational), duration (in minutes), intensity (scale of 1-10), symptoms (listed from the DSM-III-R), time of day, and circumstances of practice homework (Thyer, 1987)

Fear and Avoidance Hierarchy
Detailed list of at least 10 feared situations or events that are specific to an individual patient (Walker, Norton, & Ross, 1991). Activities could be performed relatively easily in these situations or events if it were not for fear and avoidance, and these items become the focus for behavioral desensitization treatment.

ported that 70% of panic disorder patients had consulted at least 10 physicians, and 95% had seen a psychiatrist without the correct diagnosis being made. Overall, 44% of them go to neurologists, 39% to cardiologists, and 33% to gastroenterologists (Katon, 1984).

Research also suggests certain factors that predict the patient's decision to seek care. These variables that affect entry into the health care system, for whatever reason, include being white, having panic-related symptoms, having a higher level of education, and, most important, feeling free to discuss panic. Gender, marital status, age, phobic avoidance, limited symptom attacks, and fear during panic were not found to be significant factors in the decision to seek care (Katerndahl, 1990).

Psychiatric nurses should consider the strong likelihood that these patients may be misdiagnosed and that they might have coexisting medical conditions. Medical disorders that occur more commonly in patients with panic disorder include atypical chest pain, irritable bowel syndrome, asthma, and migraine. For this patient population, appropriate case finding is an important function of the psychiatric nurse. Another critical responsibility is the education of primary care practitioners and emergency room staffs about their need to be aware of panic attacks and actively look for them in patients with chest pain, shortness of breath, nervousness, and dizziness, particularly if medical workups are negative and recidivism is high.

Standardized instruments have been developed both to diagnose panic disorder and to assess treatment of the panic patient over time. A listing of some of these tools is presented in Table 12–5. Space considerations do not allow for discussion of the strengths and limitations of each of these various assessment tools, but the source document for each scale can be reviewed for more detailed information. In addition, a nursing assessment of the patient should include attention to the time, cost, and distress that the disorder has exacted. Specific questions should be asked about the symptoms of first-degree relatives, as well as the patient's undiagnosed but classic avoidant behaviors. Psychiatric comorbidity should be explored in detail, particularly substance abuse and depression (Maser & Cloniger, 1990). Finally, life-style changes that reflect creative but dysfunctional coping mechanisms of the panic patient need to be assessed to exchange them for more functional methods of handling panic anxiety during the course of treatment.

Upon completion of a thorough assessment, the nurse will be able to identify the range of possible maladaptive responses evidenced by the individual with panic disorder. Because of the somatic nature of the illness, as well as its considerable concomitant psychosocial impairment, many nursing diagnoses may be appropriate. Table 12–6 lists some of the North American Nursing Diagnostic Association

TABLE 12–6. NANDA Nursing Diagnoses Related to Panic Disorder

Anxiety	Powerlessness
Breathing patterns, ineffective	Role performance, altered
Coping, ineffective individual	Self-esteem disturbance
Diarrhea	Sensory/perceptual alterations (specify)
Family processes, altered	Sleep pattern disturbance
Fatigue	Social isolation
Fear	Spiritual distress
Home maintenance management, impaired	Swallowing, impaired
Hopelessness	Thought processes, altered
Knowledge deficit (specify)	Urinary elimination, altered
Pain	Violence, potential for self-directed

(NANDA) nursing diagnoses that may be used by the psychiatric nurse in working with a patient with panic disorder. As is evident from this list, the panic patient presents a treatment challenge for the caregiver.

NURSING CARE INTERVENTIONS

Psychiatric nurses may function as primary clinicians in working with patients with panic disorder, or they may be in collaborative practice arrangements with other mental health care professionals. Regardless of the organizational structure, panic disorder patients need an individualized treatment plan that addresses primary and secondary psychiatric symptomatology, as well as any comorbid physical conditions. In addition to symptom reduction, goals of treatment should include enhancing the individual's quality of life and overall psychosocial functioning. As with many other medical illnesses, treatment of panic disorder precedes a full understanding of etiology and pathophysiology, but effective treatment strategies are well known for this disorder (Klerman et al., 1993). Specific caregiving principles for nurses working with patients with panic disorders should take into consideration the interaction of biopsychosocial factors and include the following: (1) education about the illness, remission, and relapse; (2) pharmacologic blockade of the panic attacks; (3) cognitive-behavioral treatment directed toward sensations, cognitions, and behaviors; (4) psychotherapy focused on residual psychosocial problems or psychologic vulnerabilities; and (5) support of sociocultural coping resources. Which treatment or combination of treatments are selected and in what order it is introduced depends on the patient's presenting symptoms, goals for treatment, treatment preference, and tolerance of specific interventions.

The nurse's approach to diagnosis and choice of treatments begins with a thorough assessment of the patient, including history (medical, psychiatric, and family); past treatment-seeking efforts; efficacy of prior treatments; specific characteristics of panic attacks and avoidances; cognitions; comorbidities; current coping strategies and level of functioning; support systems; knowledge base; degree of treatment urgency; and treatment goals, expectations, and preferences. Specific interventions are then selected that are directed at defined target symptoms and also are sensitive to the patient's circumstances as an active architect and participant in the treatment program. Well-designed measurement tools at baseline and throughout the course of treatment are an invaluable component of the treatment approach. These measures will document success, support the decision to alter a treatment strategy that seems ineffective, and provide the patient with a quantifiable approach to an illness that has seemed hopelessly perplexing and out of control.

EDUCATIONAL STRATEGIES

The somatic symptoms of panic disorder are extremely frightening to the patient, and the cultural stigma associated with mental illness prevents many people from considering seeking psychiatric care. In addition, many patients believe they have a severe physical illness that is causing their symptoms of panic. They also often feel, however, that their illness eludes diagnosis; they begin to wonder what exactly is wrong with them; and they may fear that they are truly "crazy." Thus, the first level of intervention involves eliciting patients' beliefs about their illness. Specifically, this involves asking them what they believe is wrong; what treatment they expect to receive; and what they would like to gain or what outcomes they expect to see from appropriate care. This exchange forms the basis of a beginning partnership between the patient and the clinician and engages the patient's active participation in the treatment process.

The next intervention involves educating the patient about the illness itself, emphasizing two basic but very important points. First, the individual has an illness that can be diagnosed and is experienced by many people throughout the world. Second, this illness, panic disorder with or without agoraphobia, is a treatable condition. Because many patients are quite demoralized about their symptoms, it is important to convey confidence and hope in the treatment process. The discussion can then be focused more specifically on the following:

- known and hypothesized causes of the illness
- nature and extent of panic disorder with an emphasis on its prevalence and ability to be correctly diagnosed
- familial and environmental vulnerability
- reasons for the onset of symptoms at a particular time
- biological knowledge, including current understanding of brain changes and hypersensitivity to stimuli
- severity and course of the illness
- treatments that are safe and effective and appear to calm a hypersensitive brain alarm system.

Underlying these interventions is the assumption that the nurse demonstrates the responsive and active dimensions of a therapeutic relationship, including respect, empathic understanding, concreteness, and emotional catharsis (Stuart & Sundeen, 1995). All of these clinician qualities are essential for the establishment of a therapeutic alliance with the panic disorder patient.

The educational component of the treatment plan for panic disorder has been identified by patients as one of the most important (Gitlin et al., 1985). These strategies can be further enhanced by providing or suggesting reading materials on panic disorder for individuals who would like to learn more about this disorder (Gold, 1989; Sheehan, 1986). Patient education materials are also available through NIMH, The Phobia Society of America, The Anxiety Disorders Association of America, and the National Panic/Anxiety Disorders Newsletter. In addition, self-help groups are available throughout the country and provide an important source of support and information on panic disorder.

Psychopharmacologic Strategies

The goal of psychopharmacologic treatment is to block spontaneous and situational panic attacks. Recent double-blind, placebo-controlled studies have shown that three classes of medication are equally effective for the treatment of panic disorder: (1) tricyclic antidepressants (TCAs), (2) monoamine oxidase inhibitors (MAOIs), and (3) high-potency benzodiazepines (BZs). In addition, there is emerging evidence of the efficacy of SSRIs.

Tricyclic Antidepressants

TCAs are quite safe when taken as prescribed. They are also the most extensively studied medications in the treatment of panic disorder. Perhaps the most rigorously studied of the TCAs is imipramine, which has been proven to be superior to placebo in over a dozen controlled studies and in a number of open trials. With this medication, improvement usually requires at least 4 to 6 weeks of treatment, although 12 to 24 weeks may be necessary for significant symptomatic improvement. Dosing should be very slow (some patients require a starting dose as low as 20 mg per day) during the first 3 weeks to minimize side effects that may seem like panic symptoms to the patient. Generally, 70% to 90% of patients who stay on the medicine experience moderate or marked improvement (Ballenger, 1986). Other studies have shown a comparable efficacy in the treatment of panic disorder for clomipramine, nortriptyline, amitriptyline, and doxepin (Lydiard & Ballenger, 1988).

Advantages of the TCAs are that they only require once daily dosing after steady state is reached, and, unlike the MAOIs, they have no dietary restrictions. In addition, they may provide increased protection against depression and do not pose a dependency risk for the patient. The major disadvantages are their delayed onset of action and their hyperstimulatory and anticholinergic side-effect profile. They are also dangerous in overdose. Other less common adverse effects include weight gain, orthostatic hypotension, and sexual dysfunction.

MONOAMINE OXIDASE INHIBITORS

MAOIs have been extensively studied, particularly phenelzine, and there is compelling evidence of their usefulness in the treatment of panic disorder (Buiges & Vallejo, 1987). Dosing for panic is the same as the regimen used for depression. Like the TCAs, the MAOIs appear to help the patient with depression and pose no risk for medication dependency, but most require dietary restrictions. In fact, the major disadvantage of the currently available MAOIs is the dietary restrictions that are necessary to minimize the chance of a tyramine-induced hypertensive episode. Foods that must be avoided while taking MAOIs include some cheeses, aged meats, red wine, and caffeine products. These restrictions are problematic for some patients and have limited the usefulness of the MAOIs. However, there are at least two reversible MAOIs currently being studied in the United States for the treatment of panic disorder, and these MAOIs will not require the usual dietary restrictions. Another disadvantage of MAOIs, as with TCAs, is the delayed onset of action. They are also associated with the side effects of insomnia, weight gain, postural hypotension, and sexual difficulties.

BENZODIAZEPINES

Recent studies have been done on the high-potency benzodiazepines, particularly alprazolam, which has been found to be as effective as imipramine and phenelzine in the treatment of panic disorder (Ballenger et al., 1988). For the treatment of panic disorder, it is not unusual to require 2 to 8 mg of alprazolam per day, in divided doses, for 6 months or longer, to obtain antipanic effects. Two other high-potency benzodiazepines, clonazepam and lorazepam, also appear to be comparably effective antianxiety drugs.

The advantages of these medications include a rapid onset of action and the tendency to be well tolerated with few side effects. The main side effects include sedation, psychomotor impairment, fatigue, ataxia, slurred speech, and amnesia. Another disadvantage is the fact that they can cause physiological dependence—seizures can result with abrupt discontinuation. Thus, patients should be slowly tapered off these medications. An additional reason for slowly tapering patients is to minimize rebound anxiety, a phenomenon characterized by a rapid return of anxiety that is initially worse than the level of anxiety experienced pretreatment. Finally, several types of patients should not be treated with benzodiazepines because of their likelihood to abuse them. These include patients with a history of polydrug or alcohol abuse, personality disorders, and chronic benign pain conditions (Marks, 1983).

SELECTIVE SEROTONIN REUPTAKE INHIBITORS

The newest antidepressant class of drugs to come on the market, the SSRIs, is attracting much attention for the treatment of panic disorder and agoraphobia. These drugs, such as fluoxetine and sertraline, are now widely accepted for their low side-effect profile, safety profile, and efficacy in the psychopharmacologic treatment of depression. Like the tricyclics and the MAOIs, they are also reported to be effective antipanic agents, while retaining their advantages over other antidepressants.

Their mechanism of action takes place at the presynaptic membrane in the serotonin tracts of the central nervous system, where they prevent an efficient re-absorption of serotonin back into the axon, thus making more serotonin available in the synapse and toning the efficiency of the serotonin system. While the majority of the clinical research studies documenting the efficacy of the SSRIs in panic are taking place at this time, there are numerous anecdotal reports verifying the use of these drugs in the treatment of panic disorder, with the same dosing regimens as in depression. Unfortunately, as with many newly marketed medications, they tend to be more expensive than the older tricyclics. But if cost is not an issue, or if the patient is unable to take the other antipanic drugs because of either side effects or lack of efficacy, the SSRIs provide a good treatment option for the panic patient.

NURSING IMPLICATIONS

Patients with panic disorder are often difficult to treat with medications for a variety of reasons. Some patients have self-esteem problems associated with the perceived need for medication and their feeling out of control with regard to the symptomatology of their illness. They may be reluctant to begin or continue medication and express concern over becoming addicted to it. They may also initially feel worse because all these medicines have side effects and these patients are already hypervigilant about bodily symptoms (Stuart & Sundeen, 1995). Thus education, reassurance, and support are critical nursing interventions for enhancing patient compliance with pharmacological treatment.

In addition, several useful treatment approaches to increase compliance have been suggested (NIMH, 1989). These include the following:

1. Inform all patients that they might have side effects from the medication, but if they can endure the first few weeks of side effects, the panic attacks can be blocked. In this way, the temporary discomfort of the side effects can be re-framed as evidence that the medication is working.
2. Meet with these patients at least once a week initially and be available by telephone to answer questions that arise. Emphasize that they should not stop the medicine without first calling.
3. Continue increasing the dose of the medication until the patient is entirely free of panic attacks or until recommended upper limits are reached, or the patient experiences dose limiting effects. The effective therapeutic dose is usually several times the starting dose. The most common mistake is medicating to partially relieve symptoms, rather than titrating to full dosage and the amelioration of anxiety attacks.

4. Describe the approximate dosage of medication that the patient will need to obtain relief, but allow the patient as much control as possible over how fast the dosage is increased in order to minimize side effects.

COGNITIVE BEHAVIORAL STRATEGIES

Although there continues to be debate over the theoretical underpinnings that would explain the use of cognitive behavioral strategies in the treatment of panic and phobias, the obvious success of these approaches over many years, whether utilized singly or more often in treatment combinations, is well documented. There is a growing body of empirical evidence indicating that cognitive behavioral strategies are very effective for the treatment of panic as well as agoraphobic avoidance (Craske & Barlow, 1987). These strategies appear to be as effective as pharmacological treatments in the short term and superior to them in the long term (Klosko, Barlow, Tassinari, & Cerny, 1987). Thus, the nonpharmacological treatments of panic with or without agoraphobia are regarded as crucial ingredients when determining the individualized multifaceted treatment plan required for this complex and diverse illness. While most of the well-tested pharmacological approaches are considered to effect a direct chemical intervention at the location of the synapse that blocks the panic response, the cognitive behavioral approach includes interventions directed at diminishing physiological sensations, restructuring cognitions, and changing avoidance behaviors.

The process of selecting a cognitive behavioral component to the treatment plan begins after the diagnosis and assessment have provided clearly defined target symptoms and the clinician and the patient have established realistic treatment goals. Additionally, the patient should be as engaged as possible to maximize the potential for success. The cognitive behavioral approach requires considerable effort, commitment, and motivation on the part of the patient, as well as a trusting, therapeutic alliance with the clinician. In addition, because any comorbid problems (such as marked depression or substance abuse) or intervening issues (such as the dynamic of secondary gain) may inhibit motivation and compromise success, these may need to be the initial focus of treatment. The most effective cognitive behavioral techniques include exposure therapy, cognitive restructuring, breathing control, and relaxation.

EXPOSURE TECHNIQUES

Behavioral approaches to reduce fear and agoraphobic avoidances have traditionally used exposure techniques—systematic confrontation by the patient, in imagination or in reality, accompanied or alone, of the feared objects or events. Exposure-based techniques are well studied and widely accepted in their application to agoraphobic avoidance (Bandura, 1977; Marks, 1981) and have been shown in some studies to be a necessary component of behavioral treatment approaches to this disorder (Emmelkamp, Kuipers, & Eggeraat, 1978; Michelson, Mavissakalian, Marchione, Dancu, & Greenwald, 1986).

It is hypothesized that exposure effectively halts the expectation of panic, reduces the avoidance behavior by dissociating the panic from the situations and somatic cues, produces habituation to or extinction of the conditioned fear responses, and enhances the development of self-efficacy or confidence (Craske, Street, & Barlow, 1989). Although the rates of exposure can vary, the predominant approach at this time holds that what is necessary for exposure is simply to ensure that individuals stay long enough in the feared situation to disconfirm their earlier expectations of harm (Walker, Norton, & Ross, 1991).

Systematic desensitization is an extensively utilized exposure strategy. It employs a hierarchy of fears specific to a patient who is then exposed to them in a gradual, minimally threatening, repetitive fashion, at a rate that avoids extreme levels of anxiety. The patient keeps a diary of daily activities to document progress. The level of involvement of the clinician can range from full participation to simply handing out directions. This choice depends upon the clinician's preference and the patient's ability to be self-motivated and to attend or pay for regular sessions with a therapist. Research supports both approaches (Walker et al., 1991). The hierarchy and the diary become invaluable tools that the patient can call upon long after the acute treatment phase is completed.

Recently, these techniques have been extended to include reduction of panic attacks through exposure to internal cues. Thus, interoceptive exposure is aimed at teaching the individual that somatic sensations are not harmful and can be experienced without fear. This technique is effective even if there are no phobic avoidances. Techniques such as voluntary hyperventilation, running up a flight of stairs, or spinning in a chair provide the stimuli needed to reduce the fear they provoke through exposure.

Cognitive Restructuring

Panic disorder is characterized by dramatically negative interpretations and predictive consequences of bodily stimuli that usually are normal responses to anxiety. For example, the patient will think: "I am going to have a heart attack" when experiencing palpitations; "I am going crazy" when experiencing confusion; or "I am going to lose control of myself" when experiencing depersonalization. Descriptive studies have found that panic patients report more catastrophic cognitions than patients with other anxiety disorders (Sanderson, Rapee, & Barlow, 1987). The hypothesis that these irrational modes of thinking result in or exacerbate panic attacks and thus support avoidance behaviors is the basis for the use of cognitive restructuring in this patient population. Several studies have demonstrated the efficacy of this technique in panic patients and in normal controls under controlled laboratory conditions (Rapee, Mattick, & Murrell, 1986; Sanderson et al., 1987) and in controlled and uncontrolled clinical trials (Michelson & Marchione, 1991; Sokal, Beck, Greenberg, Wright, & Berchick, 1989).

Cognitive restructuring emphasizes the discrepancy between the patient's catastrophic predictions and the reality of events, experiences, and outcomes. Patients are helped to monitor their thoughts by assessing the evidence of their consistently erroneous predictions, placing doubts on these predictions, determining alternative explanations for the symptoms, and desensitizing themselves to their worst fears. Thus the patient tests specific distortions of reality and recognizes the connection between cognition, affect, and behavior. Additionally, the patient is assisted in constructing cue cards, usually 3 × 5 file cards, each with a positive, potent, reality-based statement countering common negative thoughts. Patients then keep these cards with them and read them when negative thoughts begin. Although cards are individualized based on patient assessment, Beck et al. (1985) note some common examples of card statements:

> "This is a panic attack, not a heart attack."
> "My worst fear has never really happened."
> "Relax, I can do it." (Stand in line at the store, etc.)
> "Remember, this attack will go away in just a few minutes."

Cue cards are tangible tools for the patient to gain better control of the panic disorder.

BREATHING CONTROL

Symptoms of respiratory alkalosis (dizziness, breathlessness, faintness, choking, and paresthesia) caused by hyperventilation, whether occurring as a prelude to or consequence of stress, are reported more by patients with panic than by those with other anxiety disorders (Rapee, 1985; Sanderson et al., 1987). Panic patients may have a hypersensitive CO_2 chemoreceptor system (Papp, Klein, & Gorman, 1993). Research has shown that challenge studies using CO_2 inhalation cause panic attacks in panic-prone individuals (Gorman & Papp, 1990). Whether panic patients are more inclined to overbreathe or more internally cued to their normal bodily sensations, evidence suggests that breathing control is useful in decreasing the frequency of panic attacks and resetting the pCO_2 levels to normal for panic patients (Bonn, Readhead, & Timmons, 1984; Salkovskis, Jones, & Clark, 1986). When combined with cognitive techniques, breathing control can assist the patient in the accurate identification and reattribution of sensations that are due to hyperventilation as part of normal physiology and therefore not dangerous (Sholomskas & Woods, 1992). This technique gives the patient a tool with which to gain some measure of control over the condition.

Breathing control is accomplished by teaching the patient to recognize overbreathing and to utilize methods of diaphragmatic breathing to control hyperventilation. The patient should be taught to practice conscious control of slow, deep, even abdominal breaths, rather than shallow, rapid, thoracic ones. Breathing into a paper bag, the "cure" for most cases of hyperventilation, is contraindicated for the panic patient because rebreathing exhaled CO_2 may make the panic attack worse.

RELAXATION TRAINING

Relaxation training for the panic patient is assumed to be useful because of its effectiveness in reducing muscle tension, the body's response to anxiety-producing thoughts and events. Muscle tension, in turn, intensifies the subjective experience of anxiety, and a feedback cycle develops, potentially precipitating or exacerbating a panic attack. Deep muscle relaxation counters this effect and provides a tool for some panic patients to gain control over their bodily sensations.

Only a few studies have provided preliminary evidence that applied deep muscle relaxation is beneficial in the reduction of panic attacks (Ost, 1988; Walker et al., 1991) or in generalized anxiety disorder (Michelson & Marchione, 1991). Still, the technique remains in common use. The individual is instructed to sit comfortably with eyes closed, focus attention on one muscle group at a time, and systematically tense and release one of seven body muscle groups (Davis, Eshelman, & McKay, 1988; Wolpe & Lazarus, 1966). Although there are various anecdotal reports that guided imagery and biofeedback are also useful techniques for panic patients, controlled clinical trials are needed to support these observations.

In summary, there are a variety of cognitive behavioral strategies directed at specific target symptoms to treat panic disorder with or without agoraphobia. When these are combined, as needed, with each other, as well as with education, pharmacotherapy, and psychotherapy, the patient is afforded an appropriate, holistic, and comprehensive treatment approach with a very high rate of success.

PSYCHOTHERAPEUTIC STRATEGIES

Patients with panic disorder vary widely in their use of adaptive coping mechanisms, the strength of their social support systems, and their baseline self-esteem and ego competencies. Once the panic symptoms and avoidance behaviors are

TABLE 12–7. Presenting Problems and Treatment Approaches

PRESENTING PROBLEMS	TREATMENT STRATEGIES
Knowledge deficit	Patient education
	Reading materials
	Self-help support groups
Panic attacks	Breathing control
	Cognitive restructuring
	Interoceptive exposure
	Psychopharmacology
Agoraphobic avoidance	Exposure
	Cognitive restructuring
	Breathing control
	Relaxation training
Negative cognitions	Cognitive restructuring
Anticipatory anxiety	Relaxation training
	Cognitive restructuring
	Exposure techniques
Sensitivity to body sensations	Interoceptive exposure
	Cognitive restructuring
Numbness and tingling	Breathing control
Shortness of breath	Breathing control
Psychosocial problems	Psychotherapy
Marital discord	Marital therapy
Skills deficit	Skills training
Lack of treatment efficacy	Re-evaluation of treatment plan
	Compliance counseling

under control, any remaining problems may be appropriate targets for additional intervention. Life stressors or chronic daily hassles may place the individual at increased risk of developing symptoms of panic disorder. Thus it is useful to determine the vulnerability to stressful life events by exploring experiences in the patient's family of origin, such as early loss of parents, lack of parental warmth and support, childhood physical or sexual abuse, parental chronic illness or substance abuse, and personal and family history of anxiety or depressive disorders. Current adult intimate relationships may also be reviewed to assess the presence of marital or family problems. Chronic problems with low self-esteem, difficulty expressing anger, lack of assertiveness, or prolonged feelings of rejection and unhappiness would be appropriate for psychotherapeutic intervention. Marital therapy might also be indicated for patients experiencing marital conflict or discord.

These psychodynamic interventions, however, attempt to treat the residual symptoms of the illness and chronic problem areas of the patient, rather than the primary somatic and behavioral manifestations of panic disorder. There are no studies that examine the efficacy of psychodynamic, family, or marital therapy as primary treatments in patients with panic disorder, either alone or in combination with psychopharmacology (Roy-Byrne & Katon, 1987). However, such interventions may serve to decrease social and psychological distress and enhance self-esteem. They can also provide the patient with more adaptive problem-solving coping mechanisms and thus may decrease both the tendency to relapse and the morbidity should the panic attacks recur. A combination of treatment strategies is the most effective way to treat both primary and secondary symptoms of the panic disorder patient (Table 12–7).

RECOMMENDATIONS FOR NURSING EDUCATION

Anxiety disorders are the number one mental health problem among women and are second only to drug and alcohol abuse among men. Panic symptoms are extremely common, affecting 10% of adults at some point during their lives. Thus, they represent a significant health care problem in this country that is accompanied by great social and economic disability. Furthermore, patients with panic disorder with agoraphobia present unique treatment challenges that require a sophisticated understanding of complex interactions among somatizations, cognitions, and behaviors.

Interestingly, there are few reports in the literature of nurses in this country giving clinical care to patients with diagnosed anxiety disorders. One 5-week partial hospitalization program for the treatment of anxiety disorders is described by Waddell and Demi (1993). It was based on an integration of biological, cognitive, and behavioral theories, including behavioral therapy, pharmacotherapy, anxiety management skills, psychoeducation, cognitive therapy, group therapy, social skills, family therapy, and discharge planning.

Yet the concept of nurse behavior therapists is a common phenomenon in Britain (Gournay, 1991b; Hume, 1990; Marks, Hallam, Connelly, & Philpott, 1977). Hume (1990) believes this may be because Britain has been pragmatic in its approach to nursing care and somewhat skeptical of the therapeutic rationale of such "fuzzy concepts" in America as caring for and looking after the patient—concepts that are commonly taught but poorly defined in many nursing programs in this country. The British also more quickly acted upon the research data that demonstrated the clinical effectiveness of behavior therapy.

In recognition that nurses were eminently positioned to contribute to the increased demand for behavioral services, training programs were established in Britain for nurses to become competent as behavior therapists. The first training program for nurses to function as independent practitioners of care was established by Isaac Marks at the Maudsley Hospital in London in 1975, and his subsequent work clearly demonstrates the clinical effectiveness of nurses practicing in this advanced clinical role in Britain (Marks et al., 1977; Marks, 1985). A similar training course for nurses was also developed in Scotland. For more information on this topic, Deakin (1989) outlines the development, curricula, and implementation of nurse behavior training in Britain. When one examines the educational programs available to psychiatric nurses in England and Scotland, the large deficits in the current educational curricula of nursing programs in this country with regard to behavioral training become obvious.

In this country, most nursing students at the undergraduate level are exposed to general theories of anxiety (many of which were developed over 30 years ago) and presented basic knowledge of pathophysiology. These conceptualizations are important because they are foundational, but they are insufficient for addressing current treatment strategies appropriate for individuals diagnosed with anxiety disorders. Given the prevalence and disability associated with psychiatric illnesses such as anxiety disorders and their significant interaction with physical illnesses, it is clear that additional content needs to be presented in undergraduate nursing programs related to contemporary treatments of psychiatric illness. Recent years have seen these programs focusing almost exclusively on psychosocial phenomena rather than psychiatric disorders, suggesting that these are comparable areas of study when they clearly are not (Pothier, Stuart, Puskar, & Babich, 1990). In reality, undergraduate nursing programs often fail to provide nursing students with the information and skills they need to intervene with patients who present with psychiatric health care problems. Additionally, greater emphasis needs to be placed on case finding in general health care settings and appropriately referring patients with psychiatric disorders.

Graduate psychiatric nursing education provides more depth in assessing, diagnosing, and intervening in psychiatric illness, and faculty should be updating this content continuously to ensure that it is current with clinical and research developments in the field of psychiatry. Programs that restrict content to state or trait anxiety, psychosocial manifestations of anxiety, or anxiety in relation to stress-adaptation models are not preparing their graduates for clinical care of the most prevalent of psychiatric illnesses, anxiety disorders. Specifically, graduate students in psychiatric nursing need substantive course content addressing neurobiology, psychopharmacology, cognitive and behavioral therapies, supportive psychotherapy, patient education, and treatment compliance. Most important, increased emphasis must be placed on current treatment strategies with documented efficacy in treating psychiatric illness, rather than on global therapeutic approaches that are either too vague or general to be useful, have primarily historical significance, or are not supported by current research.

AN AGENDA FOR FUTURE NURSING RESEARCH

A review of the literature on panic disorder with agoraphobia reveals very few nursing studies related to this clinical condition. The studies that have been done examine the childhood environment of women with panic disorder (Laraia et al., 1994); the effects of a nurse therapist behavioral treatment program on medical utilization (Bowen, D'Arcy, South, & Hawkes, 1990); and whether patients seen in the home or in outpatient clinics by nurse behavior therapists experience better treatment outcomes (Gournay, 1991a). This last study is the only controlled study of treatment by nurses of patients with agoraphobia and it was done in Great Britain. One may assume that nurses contribute to research endeavors with other professionals and share authorship on related publications, but it is difficult to determine the nature or extent of their interdisciplinary participation. Nonetheless, in this relatively new field many research questions remain unanswered, and each new finding is likely to stimulate additional questions. The following are areas amenable to an agenda for nursing research.

RISK FACTORS AND RECOGNITION. Little is known about risk factors associated with the development of panic disorder. Inquiry is needed into family and genetic patterns, developmental indicators, and personality characteristics. Then the study of children of high-risk families and prospective population studies are needed to answer these questions. The rate of primary care recognition of panic disorder and the consequences of nonrecognition need to be investigated, as well as the cultural and gender factors and social stigmatization that impact on the incidence, prevalence, and help-seeking behavior of individuals with panic disorder symptoms. Finally, additional research is needed in genetic transmission, as well as the biological, psychological, and environmental etiology of the disorder.

COURSE OF THE DISORDER. Most current research is cross-sectional in study design or provides primarily short-term follow-up. More information is needed on the occurrence of the illness over time, the development of comorbid conditions, treatment-seeking behavior, medical care utilization costs associated with the illness and its effective treatment, and the impact of treatment on psychosocial functioning and quality of life. Quantitative and qualitative methods need to be applied to better understand the panic patient's experience.

METHODOLOGICAL STUDIES. More valid and reliable tools are needed for diagnosis, description of clinical features, and outcome measurements. Sensitive screening instruments need to be developed that can be utilized in primary care settings by a variety of health care professionals.

TREATMENT RESEARCH. Present studies do not allow for satisfactory comparison across treatment strategies. More controlled clinical studies are needed on combination therapies, the placebo response, the optimal length of treatment, and indications for maintenance therapy. Analyzing patient beliefs and preferences with treatment strategy, the importance of the clinician-patient therapeutic alliance, and the efficacy of educational strategies are important research questions, as is following up on those individuals who drop out of treatment initiatives or show lack of treatment efficacy. Finally, increased emphasis should be placed on prevention strategies for those at risk for the disorder and on the effectiveness of nurse therapists.

Thus, many areas of inquiry are open for psychiatric nursing research in panic disorder. Additionally, the prospects for identifying funding sources are good. Both the National Institute of Mental Health and the Agency for Health Care Policy and Research have identified strong interest in this area and can provide psychiatric nurses with valuable resources for carving out their contribution to this expanding area of psychiatric research.

REFERENCES

American Psychiatric Association. (1980). *Diagnostic and statistical manual of mental disorders* (3rd ed.). Washington, DC: Author.

American Psychiatric Association. (1987). *Diagnostic and statistical manual of mental disorders* (3rd ed. rev.). Washington, DC: Author.

American Psychiatric Association. (1994). *Diagnostic and statistical manual of mental disorders* (4th ed.). Washington, DC: Author.

Ballenger, J. C. (1986). Pharmacotherapy of the panic disorders. *Journal of Clinical Psychiatry, 47*(6), 27–32.

Ballenger, J. C. (1989). Toward an integrated model of panic disorder. *American Journal of Orthopsychiatry, 59*(2), 284–293.

Ballenger, J. C., Burrows, R. L., Dupont, R. L., Jr., Lesser, I. M., Noyes, R., Pecknold, J. C., Rifkin, A., & Swinson, R. P. (1988). Alprazolam in panic disorder and agoraphobia: Results from a multicenter trial. 1. Efficacy in short-term treatment. *Archives of General Psychiatry, 45,* 413–422.

Bandura, A. (1977). *Social learning theory.* Englewood Cliffs, NJ: Prentice-Hall.

Barlow, D. H. (1988). Current models of panic disorder and a view from emotion theory. In A. J. Frances & R. E. Hales (Eds.), *Review of psychiatry* (Vol. 7, pp. 342–420). Washington, DC: American Psychiatric Press.

Beck, A. T., Emery, G., & Greenberg, R. L. (1985). *Anxiety disorders and phobias: A cognitive perspective.* New York: Basic.

Bonn, J. A., Readhead, C. P. A., & Timmons, B. H. (1984). Enhanced adaptive behavioral response in agoraphobic patients pretreated with breathing retraining. *Lancet, 2,* 665–669.

Bowen, R. C., D'Arcy, C., South, M., & Hawkes, J. E. (1990). The effects of a nurse therapist conducted behavioral agoraphobia treatment program on medical utilization. *Journal of Anxiety Disorders, 4,* 341–349.

Boyarsky, B. K., Perone, L. A., Lee, N. C., & Goodman, W. K. (1991). Current treatment approaches to obsessive compulsive disorder. *Archives of Psychiatric Nursing, 5*(5), 299–306.

Buiges, J., & Vallejo, J. (1987). Therapeutic response to phenelzine in patients with panic disorder and agoraphobia with panic attacks. *Journal of Clinical Psychiatry, 48,* 55–59.

Burd, S. F. (1963). Effects of nursing intervention in anxiety of patients. In S. F. Burd & M. A. Marshall (Eds.), *Some clinical approaches to psychiatric nursing* (pp. 307–320). New York: Macmillan.

Chambless, D. L., Caputo, G. C., Bright, P., & Gallagher, R. (1984). Assessment of fear in agoraphobics: The Body Sensations Questionnaire and the Agoraphobic Cognitions Questionnaire. *Journal of Consulting and Clinical Psychology, 52,* 1090–1097.

Chambless, D. L., Caputo, G. C., Jasin, S. E., Gracely, E. J., & Williams, C. (1985). The Mobility Inventory for Agoraphobia. *Behavior Research and Therapy, 23,* 35–44.

Clark, D. (1986). A cognitive approach to panic. *Behavior Research and Therapy, 24*(4), 461–470.

Craske, M. G., & Barlow, D. H. (1987). *Behavioral treatment of panic: A controlled study.* Paper presented at the annual meeting of the Association for the Advancement of Behavior Therapy, Boston, MA.

Craske, M. G., Street, L., & Barlow, D. H. (1989). Instructions to focus upon or distract from internal cues during exposure treatment of agoraphobic avoidance. *Behavior Research and Therapy, 27*(6), 663–672.

Crowe, R. R., Noyes, R., Pauls, D. L., & Slymen, D. (1982). A family study of panic disorders. *Archives of General Psychiatry, 40,* 1065–1069.

Davis, M., Eshelman, E. R., & McKay, M. (Eds.). (1988). *Relaxation and stress reduction handbook.* Oakland, CA: New Harbinger.

Deakin, H. (1989). The treatment of agoraphobia by nurse therapists: Practice and training. In K. Gournay (Ed.), *Agoraphobia: Current perspectives on theory and treatment.* London: Routledge.

Derogatis, L. R. (1983). *SCL-90 administration, scoring and procedures manual.* Towson, MD: Clinical Psychometric Research.

DiNardo, P. A., & Barlow, D. H. (1988). *Anxiety Disorders Interview Schedule, Revised.* Phobia and Anxiety Disorders Clinic, 1535 Western Avenue, Albany, NY 12203.

Emmelkamp, P. M. G., Kuipers, A. C. M., & Eggeraat, J. G. (1978). Cognitive modification versus prolonged exposure in vivo: A comparison with agoraphobics as subjects. *Behavior Research and Therapy, 16,* 33–41.

Fontaine, R., Breton, G., & Dery, R. (1990). Temporal lobe abnormalities in panic disorder: An MRI study. *Biological Psychiatry, 27,* 304–310.

Gitlin, B., Martin, J., Shear, M. K., Frances, A., Ball, G., & Josephson, S. (1985). Behavior therapy for panic disorder. *The Journal of Nervous and Mental Disease, 173,* 742–743.

Gold, M. (1989). *The good news about panic, anxiety and phobias.* New York: Villard.

Gorman, J. M., & Papp, L. A. (1990). Respiratory physiology of panic. In J. Ballenger (Ed.), *Neurobiology of panic disorder* (pp. 187–203). New York: Alan R. Liss.

Gournay, K. J. M. (1991a). The base for exposure treatment in agoraphobia: Some indicators for nurse therapists and community psychiatric nurses. *Journal of Advanced Nursing, 16,* 82–91.

Gournay, K. J. M. (1991b). The failure of exposure treatment in agoraphobia: Implications for the practice of nurse therapists and community psychiatric nurses. *Journal of Advanced Nursing, 16,* 1099–1109.

Gournay, K. (1989). *Agoraphobia: Current perspectives on theory and treatment.* London: Routledge.

Hamilton, M. (1956). The assessment of anxiety states by rating. *British Journal of Medical Psychology, 32,* 50–55.

Hopper, J. L., Judd, F. K., Derrick, P. L., & Burns, G. O. (1987). A family study of panic disorder. *Genetic Epidemiology, 4*(1), 33–41.

Hume, A. (1990). Behavior therapy model: Principles and general application. In W. Reynolds & D. Cormack (Eds.), *Psychiatric and mental health nursing.* London: Chapman and Hall.

Katerndahl, A. A. (1990). Factors associated with persons with panic attacks seeking medical care. *Family Medicine, 22,* 462–466.

Katon, W. (1984). Panic disorder and somatizations: Review of 55 cases. *American Journal of Medicine, 77,* 101–106.

Katon, W., Vitaliano, P. P., Russo, J., Cormier, L., Anderson, K., & Jones, M. (1986). Panic disorder: Epidemiology in primary care. *The Journal of Family Practice, 23*(3), 233–239.

Katon, W., Vitaliano, P. P., Anderson, K., Jones, M., & Russo, J. (1987). Panic disorder: Residual symptoms after the acute attacks abate. *Comprehensive Psychiatry, 28*(2), 151–158.

Klerman, G., Hirschfeld, R., Weissman, M., Pelicier, Y., Ballenger, J., Silva, J., Judd, L., & Keller, M. (1993). *Panic anxiety and its treatment.* Washington, DC: American Psychiatric Press.

Klosko, J. S., Barlow, D. H., Tassinari, R. B., & Cerny, J. A. (1987). *Comparison of alprazolam and cognitive behavior therapy in the treatment of panic disorder: A preliminary report.* Paper presented at the annual convention of the Association for the Advancement of Behavior Therapy, Boston, MA.

Laraia, M. T. (1991). Biological correlates of panic disorder with agoraphobia: Practice perspectives for nurses. *Archives of Psychiatric Nursing, 5*(6), 373–381.

Laraia, M. T. (1995). Biological context of psychiatric nursing care. In G. Stuart & S. Sundeen (Eds.), *Principles and practice of psychiatric nursing* (5th ed.). St. Louis: Mosby–Year Book.

Laraia, M. T., Stuart, G. W., & Best, C. L. (1989). Behavioral treatment of panic-related disorders: A review. *Archives of Psychiatric Nursing, 3*(3), 125–133.

Laraia, M. T., Stuart, G. W., Frye, L., Lydiard, R. B., & Ballenger, J. C. (1994). Childhood environment of women having panic disorder with agoraphobia. *Journal of Anxiety Disorders, 8*, 1–17.

Last, C. G. (1992). *Anxiety across the lifespan.* New York: Springer.

Last, C. G., Barlow, D .H., & O'Brien, D. (1984). Precipitants of agoraphobia: Role of stressful life events. *Psychological Reports, 54*, 567–570.

Lydiard, R. B., & Ballenger, J. C. (1988). Panic-related disorders: Evidence for efficacy of the antidepressants. *Journal of Anxiety Disorders, 2*, 77–94.

Markowitz, J. S., Weissman, M. M., Ouellette, R., Lish, J. D., & Klerman, G. L. (1989). Quality of life in panic disorder. *Archives of General Psychiatry, 46*, 984–992.

Marks, I. M. (1981). New developments in psychological treatments of phobias. In M. Mavissakalian & D. H. Barlow (Eds.), *Phobia: Psychological and pharmacological treatment.* New York: Guilford.

Marks, I. (1983). The benzodiazepines—for good or evil. *Neuropsychobiology, 10*, 115–126.

Marks, I. (1985). *Psychiatric nurse therapists in primary care: The expansion of advanced clinical roles in nursing.* London: Royal College of Nursing.

Marks, I., Hallam, R. S., Connelly, J., & Philpott, R. (1977). *Nursing in behavioral psychotherapy.* London: Royal College of Nursing.

Marks, I. M., & Mathews, A. M. (1979). Brief standard rating scale for phobic patients. *Behavior Research and Therapy, 17*, 263–267.

Maser, J. D., & Cloniger, C. R. (Eds). (1990). *Comorbidity of mood and anxiety disorders.* Washington, DC: American Psychiatric Press.

Michelson, L., & Marchione, K. (1991). Behavioral, cognitive and pharmacological treatments of panic disorder with agoraphobia: Critique and synthesis. *Journal of Consulting and Clinical Psychology, 59*(1), 100–114.

Michelson, L., Marchione, K., Greenwald, M., Glanz, L., Testa, S., & Marchione, N. (1990). Panic disorder: Cognitive-behavioral treatment. *Behavior Research and Therapy, 28*(2), 141–151.

Michelson, L., Mavissakalian, M., Marchione, K., Dancu, C., & Greenwald, M. (1986). The role of self-directed *in vivo* exposure practice in cognitive, behavioral, and psychophysiological treatments of agoraphobia. *Behavior Therapy, 17*, 91–108.

National Institute of Mental Health (NIMH). (1989). *Panic disorder in the medical setting.* DHHS Pub. No. (ADM) 89-1629. Washington, DC: Superintendent of Documents, U.S. Government Printing Office.

Norton, G. R., Dorward, J., & Cox, B. J. (1986). Factors associated with panic attacks in nonclinical subjects. *Behavior Therapy, 17*, 239–252.

Norton, G. R., Harrison, B., Hauch, J., & Rhodes, L. (1985). Characteristics of people with infrequent panic attacks. *Journal of Abnormal Psychology, 94*(2), 216–221.

Ost, G. L. (1988). Applied relaxation versus progressive relaxation in the treatment of panic disorders. *Behavior Therapy and Research, 26*(1), 13–22.

Papp, L. A., Klein, D. F., & Gorman, J. M. (1993). Carbon dioxide hypersensitivity, hyperventilation, and panic disorder. *American Journal of Psychiatry, 150*(8), 1149–1157.

Peplau, H. (1963). A working definition of anxiety. In S. F. Burd & M. A. Marshall (Eds.), *Some clinical approaches to psychiatric nursing* (pp. 323–327). New York: Macmillan.

Pothier, P., Stuart, G., Puskar, K., & Babich, K. (1990). Dilemmas and directions for psychiatric nursing in the 1990s. *Archives of Psychiatric Nursing, 4*(5), 284.

Rapee, R. (1985). Distinctions between panic disorder and generalized anxiety disorder: Clinical presentation. *Australian and New Zealand Journal of Psychiatry, 19*, 227–232.

Rapee, R., Mattick, R., & Murrell, E. (1986). Cognitive mediation in the affective component of spontaneous panic attacks. *Journal of Behavior Therapy and Experimental Psychiatry, 17,* 245–253.

Reich, J. (1986). The epidemiology of anxiety. *Journal of Nervous and Mental Disorders, 174*(3), 129–136.

Reiman, E. M. (1987). The study of panic disorder using positron emission tomography. *Psychiatric Developments, 1,* 63–78.

Reiman, E., Raichle, M., Robins, E., Butler, F., Herscovitch, P., Fox, P., & Perlmutter, J. (1986). The application of positron emission tomography to the study of panic disorder. *American Journal of Psychiatry, 143*(4), 469–477.

Roy-Byrne, P. P., & Katon, W. (1987). An update on treatment of the anxiety disorders. *Hospital and Community Psychiatry, 38,* 835–843.

Salkovskis, P. M., Jones, D. R. O., & Clark, D. M. (1986). Respiratory control in the treatment of panic attacks: Replication and extension with concurrent measurement of behavior and pCO_2. *British Journal of Psychiatry, 148,* 526–532.

Sanderson, W. C., Rapee, R. M., & Barlow, D. H. (1987). *The phenomenon of panic across the DSM-III-R anxiety disorder categories.* Paper presented at the 21st Annual Meeting of the Association for the Advancement of Behavior Therapy, Boston, MA.

Shear, M., Cooper, A., Klerman, G., Busch, F., & Shapiro, T. (1993). A psychodynamic model of panic disorder. *American Journal of Psychiatry, 150*(6), 859–866.

Sheehan, D. V. (1982). Panic attacks and phobias. *New England Journal of Medicine, 307,* 156–158.

Sheehan, D. V. (1986). *The anxiety disease.* New York: Bantam.

Shelton, R. C. (1993) Pharmacotherapy of panic disorder. *Hospital and Community Psychiatry, 44*(8), 725–726.

Sholomskas, D. E., & Woods, S. (1992). Anxiety disorders: Structured psychotherapy. *New Directions for Mental Services, 55* (p. 85). San Francisco: Jossey-Bass.

Sokal, L., Beck, A. T., Greenberg, R. L., Wright, F. D., & Berchick, R. J. (1989). Cognitive therapy of panic disorder: A non-pharmacological alternative. *Journal of Nervous and Mental Disease, 177*(12), 711–716.

Spitzer, R. L., Williams, J. B. W., & Gibbon, M. (1988). *Structured Clinical Interview for DSM-III-R.* Biometrics Research Department, New York State Psychiatric Institute, 722 West 168th Street, New York, NY 10032.

Stuart, G. W., & Sundeen, S. J. (1995). *Principles and practice of psychiatric nursing* (5th ed.). St. Louis: Mosby–Year Book.

Thyer, B. A. (1987). *Treating anxiety disorders: A guide for human services.* Sage Human Services Guides, Vol. 45. Newbury Park, CA: Sage.

Torgersen, S. (1990). Twin studies in panic disorder. In J. Ballenger (Ed.), *Neurobiology of panic disorder* (pp. 51–58). New York: Wiley Liss.

Treatment of Panic Disorder. (1991, September). *Consensus statement.* Presented at NIH Consensus Development Conference, Washington, DC.

Waddell, K., & Demi, A. (1993). Effectiveness of an intensive partial hospitalization program for treatment of anxiety disorders. *Archives of Psychiatric Nursing, 7*(1), 2–10.

Walker, J. R., Norton, G. R., & Ross, C. A. (1991). *Panic disorder and agoraphobia: A comprehensive guide for the practitioner.* Pacific Grove, CA: Brooks/Cole.

Weissman, M., & Merikangas, K. R. (1986). The epidemiology of anxiety and panic disorders: An update. *Journal of Clinical Psychiatry, 47,* 11–17.

Weissman, M. M. (1988). The epidemiology of panic disorder and agoraphobia. In R. E. Hales & A. J. Frances (Eds.), *Review of psychiatry* (Vol. 7, pp. 54–66). Washington, DC: American Psychiatric Press.

Weissman, M. M., Klerman, G. L., Markowitz, J. S., & Ouellette, R. (1989). Suicidal ideation and suicide attempts in panic disorder and attacks. *The New England Journal of Medicine, 321*(18), 1209–1214.

Whitley, G. G. (1991). Ritualistic behavior: Breaking the cycle. *Journal of Psychosocial Nursing, 29*(10), 31–35.

Wolpe, J., & Lazarus, A. A. (1966). *Behavior therapy techniques.* Elmsford, NY: Pergamon.

CHAPTER

13

Information Processing Deficits in Schizophrenia

Jeanne C. Fox, PhD, RN, FAAN, and Catherine F. Kane, PhD, RN

ABSTRACT

   This chapter describes recent research findings that are important for psychiatric nurses to know in diagnosing and treating clients with schizophrenia. It outlines the complexity of processes—genetic, neurostructural, neurochemical, cognitive, and behavioral—that have been implicated in brain dysfunctions characteristic of schizophrenics, focusing especially on Patterson's information processing model. Topics include the processing of experience, failures in automaticity, and attentional-perceptual deficits. Based on this biopsychosocial information, the chapter describes the treatment implications of the model—for example, cognitive training, links between dysfunction and everyday coping, skills training, self-monitoring of prodromal symptoms, and the role of families, including the construct of expressed emotion. It also raises questions for further nursing research and reviews implications for psychiatric nursing practice.

   Schizophrenia, undeniably the most disabling of all mental illnesses, has been diagnosed in over 2 million Americans and approximately 1% of the total world population. It is five times more common than multiple sclerosis and six times more common than insulin-dependent diabetes. Onset most commonly occurs in late adolescence or early adulthood, and the disorder is found approximately equally in men and women. The very poor are at greatest risk for being diagnosed with this disorder (eight times higher than the highest socioeconomic group). More than 40% of the nation's mental hospital beds are occupied by patients diagnosed with schizophrenia.

   The illness associated with schizophrenia has been described as an assault on everything distinctly human. All mental processes—sensation, perception, cognition, language, emotion, and interpersonal relationships—are seriously disrupted. Further, patients describe the disorder as devastatingly terrorizing, inescapably lonely, and so distressing that as many as 10% commit suicide within 10 years of the onset of symptoms (Keith, Regier, & Lewis, 1988).

   While brain pathophysiology, genetic vulnerability, and socioenvironmental stressors are all implicated in both the interpersonal and mental process disruption characteristic of schizophrenia, information processing deficits provide an avenue both for understanding these disruptions and for modifying treatment/nursing interventions to accommodate the everyday disabilities and dysfunction experienced by persons with this devastating disease. To provide high-quality psychiatric nursing interventions, sensitivity and the art of human relatedness must be grounded in scientific understanding of the genetic and physiologic vulnerabilities associated with schizophrenia. The humane and compassionate care characteristic of psychiatric nursing develops from professionals' capacity to access and apply the most accurate knowledge of schizophrenia to individual and family responses to the disorder.

REVIEW OF SCHIZOPHRENIA RESEARCH

The search for causes of schizophrenia has been stimulated significantly by efforts of the National Institute of Mental Health (NIMH) and the National Alliance for the Mentally Ill (NAMI), a national advocacy group made up of family members, persons with schizophrenia, and other concerned individuals. Research on schizophrenia has been a priority for NIMH since its establishment in 1948, and much of the seminal work on brain pathology and genetics of schizophrenia conducted betweeb 1950 and 1985 was directly supported by NIMH. In 1985, a renewed emphasis on schizophrenia research was highlighted by NAMI and the National Advisory Mental Health Council, the primary advisory board to NIMH. Since that time, many contributions of the United States to the science of schizophrenia are the result of the NIMH's efforts, financial support, and commitment. Additionally, the World Health Organization (WHO) has supported worldwide epidemiologic studies that have contributed to an understanding of the incidence and prevalence of this disorder, and numerous international investigators have contributed to current scientific knowledge about causation and neuropathological deficits of the disorder.

It is not possible within the scope of this chapter to provide a comprehensive review of the current status of research on the genetics, brain structure, and neurochemical hypotheses relevant to the etiology of schizophrenia. Furthermore, current published reports of research are more appropriate, timely, and accurate sources than textbooks. Therefore, the reader is referred to major journals—such as *Schizophrenia Bulletin, The American Journal of Psychiatry, British Journal of Psychiatry, Journal of Abnormal Psychology, Biological Psychiatry, Archives of General Psychiatry, Schizophrenia Research*, and *The Journal of Nervous and Mental Disorders*—for a thorough and critical exposure to this information. For this chapter, however, a limited number of genetic, neurostructural, and neurochemical findings will be reported to introduce the reader to the specific phenomenon of information processing deficits accompanying schizophrenia. Because psychiatric nursing interventions are directly related to information processing of persons with psychiatric disorders and their families, an understanding of information processing deficits is essential for psychiatric nursing practice.

GENETIC FACTORS

The definitive study documenting the exact location of the genetic defect is yet to be conducted, but general evidence for substantiated genetic involvement in schizophrenia has been widely reported. Crow (1990) suggested there is strong evidence that schizophrenia is the result of a rapid increase in brain weight related to evolution and that this rapid increase in brain weight is associated with specific genetic aberrations. Reporting molecular evidence of a linkage to a pseudoautosomal probe in a 1989 sibling pair study, Crow (1990) proposed that schizophrenia and manic depressive psychoses are reflections of a continuum of brain dysfunction that originates in the pseudoautosomal region of sex chromosomes, and this is clearly related to the cerebral dominance gene. Curtis and Gurling (1990), however, suggested that chromosome 5 is the more likely site of the genetic aberration associated with schizophrenia.

Gottesman and Bertelsen (1989) reported that 20 family studies of schizophrenia over the past 62 years have demonstrated lifetime morbid risks (age corrected) of about 13% in children of schizophrenics, 9% in siblings, and 6% in parents, in comparison with a general population risk of 1%. Further, the risk for schizophrenia and related disorders in the offspring of schizophrenic identical twins is 16.8%, while the risk in normal co-twin offspring is 17.4%. Risk for fraternal schizophrenic offspring is 17.4%, while in normal co-twin offspring the risk is 2.1%. These investigators proposed that discordance in identical twins may be explained primarily by the capacity of a schizophrenic genotype or diathesis to remain unexpressed unless it is released by some kind of environmental stressor, including a nonfamilial one. Gottesman and Bertelsen (1989) also suggested that cerebral abnormalities, diseases, and viruses may not serve as necessary or sufficient causes of schizophrenia, but may account for remaining discordance. This position is not incongruent with Jablensky's (Jablensky et al., 1992) suggestion that schizophrenia is not a single disease but a common final pathway for a number of cerebral disorders and neurodevelopmental lesions.

Delisi (1992) proposed that the interaction of genes and other factors controlling brain development and differentiation lead to poor premorbid language and cognitive development. This interaction contributes to one component of the illness process for adult schizophrenia, a disturbance in the development of specific brain pathways leading to subtle language processing deficits from early childhood onward. Timing of the activity of these genes and their interaction, coupled with neuronal toxicity, results in a second and more toxic process that occurs in early adulthood. This progressive process may lead to chronic illness and subsequently prevent some individuals from ever regaining premorbid levels of functioning (Delisi, 1992).

NEUROFETAL DEVELOPMENT

It has been hypothesized that some structural and functional deviations in the brains of schizophrenics result from disrupted neurofetal development, probably during the second trimester. Neurostructural and neurochemical factors believed to contribute to schizophrenia include dysfunction in the frontal, parieto-occipital, neocortex, basal ganglia, hippocampus, and amygdala regions of the brain. Basal ganglia defects and neocortical disturbances have been related to aberrations in normal dopamine transmission (Lyon, Barr, Cannon, Mednick, & Shore, 1989).

McNeil (1987) reported a greater frequency of pre- and perinatal complications among schizophrenics than among normal controls; similarly, Green, Satz, Garer, Ganzell, and Kharabi (1989) suggested that an increased incidence of minor physical congenital anomalies—commonly associated with disrupted fetal neural development of schizophrenic patients—lends evidence to the hypothesis that some disruption in fetal neural development may be responsible for brain abnormalities common among schizophrenics. Studies related to enlarged lateral and third ventricles among these individuals also tend to implicate disrupted fetal neural development or delivery complications as contributors to ventricular disorders. In addition, decreased cranial, cerebral, and frontal brain areas in schizophrenics (as measured by MRI scans) have suggested fetal or perinatal disruption (Andreasen et al., 1986; Nasrallah, Schwarzkopf, Olson, & Coffman, 1990; Katz, 1989).

Gender differences in schizophrenia may be related to genetic influences that differentially affect normal sexual dimorphism of the brain resulting in deviations (Goldstein & Tsuang, 1990). Nasrallah et al. (1990) reported that smaller total cranial, cerebral, and frontal areas occurred primarily in males with a family history of schizophrenia. Katz (1989) has proposed that male brains are more susceptible to developmental complications than are female brains. Flor-Henry (1983) and Kopala and Campbell (1990) also proposed that males may be more susceptible than females to brain abnormalities in certain regions. Seeman and Lang (1990) discussed hormonal influences on earlier neural ionization in women and brain lateralization differences in men.

Nowakowski, in a workshop on fetal neural development and schizophrenia, presented evidence of how genetically controlled cell migration in the hippocampus and hippocampal gyrus in mice resulted in specifically located, partially migrated cells and in divergent growth of cell processes and immunocompetence (Lyon, Barr, Cannon, Mednick, & Shore, 1989). This investigator proposed the "two hit hypothesis," that is, interaction between genetic and environmental factors affecting the inheritance of susceptibility to an adult-onset neurological disease (see Fig. 13–1).

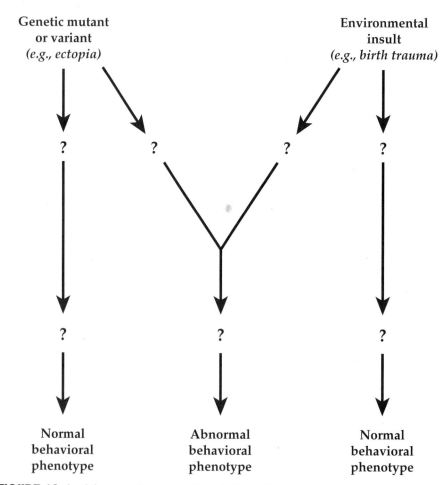

FIGURE 13–1. Schematic diagram of "two-hit hypothesis" suggesting a possible biological basis for the inheritance of susceptibility to an adult-onset neurological disease. (From Lyon, M., Barr, C., Cannon, T., Mednick, S., & Shore, D. [1989]. Fetal neural development and schizophrenia. *Schizophrenia Bulletin, 15,* 155.)

There is a strong possibility that an important component of the phenotypic expression of genetic disorder in schizophrenia consists of a specific gene defect controlling the migration and interconnection of young neurons (Lyon et al., 1989). Cortical malformations induced by these developmental disorders may be partially responsible for certain cognitive defects observed in schizophrenic patients. Genetic liability appears to provide a predisposition for elevated levels of periventricular damage associated with delivery complications in those at high genetic risk for schizophrenia (Lyon et al., 1989).

To summarize, abnormalities in neurofetal development are well documented and appear to precede onset of the disorder. Certain structural aberrations observed in the brains of schizophrenic individuals (e.g., in hippocampus and parahippocampal areas, dorsolateral and frontal cortex, globus pallidus, and amygdala) are most likely due to disorders occurring during fetal neural development (Lyon et al., 1989), but Nasrallah et al. (1990) highlighted gaps in knowledge about the significance of disruption of different neurodevelopmental processes. According to Nasrallah et al. (1990), genetic and perinatal factors produce different cortical and subcortical changes in schizophrenia. He suggested that controlled animal studies to determine "the neuropathological cascade resulting from adverse prenatal and perinatal factors (such as hypoxia) at a series of different developmental stages are necessary. Also, combined neurochemical/neuropathologic correlations in the same sample could provide information on the effect of neurodevelopmental lesions on neurotransmitter function" (Lyon et al., 1989, p.152).

Neurochemical Disturbances

The original dopamine hypothesis related to schizophrenia suggested that schizophrenia was caused by a primary disruption in dopamine metabolism or transmission resulting in an increase in dopaminergic function (Meltzer & Stahl, 1976; Snyder, 1976). While the dopamine hypothesis is widely published (Lee, 1988; Carlsson, 1988), numerous investigations have also focused on disturbances of the norepinephrine system (Stein & Wise, 1971; Mason, 1981; Van Kammen & Antelman, 1984) or dysregulation of the dopamine system. It has also been hypothesized that dysfunctions in both of these systems may interact to cause defects in memory, attention, information processing, and affect, which in turn lead to negative symptoms, increased disturbances in the autonomic nervous system, increased neuroleptic side effects, cortical metabolic activity, and change in brain blood flow (Van Kammen & Slawsky, 1988). As these authors maintain, multiple disturbances in both dopamine and norepinephrine activity observed in schizophrenics probably result from different factors, such as genetic vulnerability (Zubin, Steinhauer, Kay, & Van Kammen, 1985), a membrane disorder (Stevens, 1972; Rotrosen, Miller, Mandio, Traficante, & Gershon, 1980; Henn & Henn, 1982; Tolbert et al., 1983), or pre- or perinatal disruption (Rieder, Rosenthal, Wender, & Blumenthal, 1975; Schulsinger et al., 1984; Van Kammen & Slawsky, 1988).

Results of serotonin studies in schizophrenics were reviewed by Stahl et al. (1988). These authors concluded that whole blood serotonin (5HT) levels are elevated in chronic schizophrenics as a group, and that these elevated levels are not an artifact of age, sex, or medication. Rather, the elevated 5HT is associated with decreased monoamine oxidase (MAO) activity and with the storage and release of normal platelet 5HT uptake. However, the clinical significance of these findings is not yet understood. Bleich, Brown, and van Praag (1991) proposed that dopamine pathophysiology may be related more to Crow's (1980, 1981) type I schizophrenia (increased dopaminergic function, primarily positive symptoms, and good response to neuroleptics), while 5HT dysfunction and postsynaptic receptor hypersensitivity may be more directly associated with type II schizophrenia (cortical atrophy or ventricular enlargement, accompanied by negative symptoms and limited response to antipsychotics).

There is also considerable evidence of neurochemical abnormality in the temporal lobes of schizophrenics (Kerwin & Murray, 1992). Glutamate, cholecystokinin (CCK), and interaction with sigma/phencyclidine and GABA systems may result in the dopaminergic hyperactivity characteristic of schizophrenia. Kerwin and Murray (1992) concluded that the abnormalities of neurotransmitters commonly found in the temporal lobe (excitatory amino acids and CCK) may be the residue of abnormalities and play a role in control of hippocampal development. While the mechanism for this linkage is not yet clear, this hypothesis holds considerable promise for future important findings.

In summary, research on neurostructural and neurochemical defects in schizophrenia has progressed rapidly in the past quarter-century, as brain imaging technologies (MRI, PET, SPECT) have greatly enhanced our capacity to accurately describe brain structure and function. The combination of these methodologies with neuropsychological testing and behavioral mapping studies should result in major scientific advances related to schizophrenia in the near future.

PATTERSON'S INFORMATION PROCESSING MODEL

Because of the complexity of the processes (genetic, neurostructural, neurochemical, cognitive, and behavioral) characteristic of schizophrenia, Patterson's information processing model will be discussed in an effort to provide a framework for considering the effects of neurostructural and neurochemical deficits on cognition and information processing occurring with this disorder.* Patterson (1987) explained that information used in cognitive processes is actually created and assembled by brain structures. Lower order bits of information from the retina and other sensory organs ascend through the brain stem and through progressively higher order structures until the highest order bits are contributed by the neurointegrating structures (such as the hippocampus, amygdala, and thalamic nuclei) in complex interaction with the cortex, frontal lobes, and cerebellum. Flaws or defects in any part of the hardware or the functioning of the system may contribute to cognitive and information processing deficits.

The barrage of upward information from the external world to the cerebral cortex contains codes of information generated by brain nuclei at many different levels. Significance codes are generated by the neurointegrating structures of the limbic, thalamic, and striatal nuclei in conjunction with the cortex. Neurointegration results in content that contains codes about where the information will be directed in the cortex and the affective or emotional significance of the information (Patterson, 1987).

PROCESSING OF EXPERIENCE

Throughout childhood, experiences are integrated through the process of neurointegration, which promotes simultaneous recreation and parallel processing of

---

*In this section we directly use Patterson's ideas and his discussions of these. Any possible incorrect interpretations of these are our responsibility.

stimuli. Limbic, thalamic, striatal, cingulate, and cerebellar structures form a complicated set of systems that control much of the subcortical interaction with the cortex, and specific developmental aspects of cortical column differentiation may depend on the nature of subcortical relay. It is probable that defects in this cortical relay system may be responsible for some abnormal behaviors of schizophrenia. For example, automaticity (the ability to rapidly compare incoming stimuli with previously experienced stimuli) is frequently defective and results in slowness, inconsistency, and inaccuracy in rapidly understanding a current behavioral context. Further, if expectancies based on current contextual understanding cannot be generated, this deficit has even more damaging behavioral consequences.

PET scanning studies of Gur and associates (1987a, 1987b) suggest that subcortical to cortical relay may, in fact, be defective in schizophrenics and that defective structure and function in the lower brain may result in some of the information processing deficits accompanying schizophrenia. In mechanistic terms, the neurointegrating structures of the hippocampus and thalamus fail to provide high-order assembly of ongoing information processing; this failure leads to inappropriate affective and significance assessments of ongoing stimulation; thalamic and limbic dysfunction may also participate directly, for example, in failures of timing in relation to speech processes, in failures in temporal mapping of pictorial information generation, and in motor and linguistic and speech mechanisms (Patterson, 1987).

Patterson further hypothesized that onset of schizophrenia and course of the illness are related to ontogenetic or developmental genetic failures in cell migration, when the hippocampus itself is being formed. This hypothesis is supported by the work of Conrad and Scheibel (1987) and Jakob and Beckmann (1986), who suggested a similar mechanism in the limbic cortex. Information processing is continual from birth to death. Therefore, learning interacts with neural development to form many aspects of the functioning brain. Memory is integrally involved with brain function and structure (Patterson, 1987).

Thus, a maldeveloped limbic brain gives rise to an information assembly that is subtly defective (because high-order bits derived from the functioning of these neurointegrative structures are not correctly assembled). With continuing experience throughout childhood, lower order bits of information do not seem to be disturbed, but higher order neurointegration is variably defective (as dictated by the degree of developmental deficit) (Patterson, 1987). The psychological significance of this defective neurointegration is that the affective or significance tagging of each experience is continually abnormal relative to the normally developing brain. Neurologically, there are inconsistencies in the mapping that directs a given and repeated information assembly to cortical columns. Alterations in limbic and thalamic nuclei determine this mapping of upward stimuli. Even more important, differentiation within the cortical columns, and therefore communication between them, may be affected. These deficits may produce very subtle effects that are not obvious during childhood but are critical as adolescence begins (Patterson, 1987).

A defective assembly of the neurointegrative processing of instantaneous experience is expressed when the preschizophrenic adolescent has difficulty identifying appropriate affective interpretations. Perception may be largely learned, as aspects of a previous experience must be recreated in parallel with current stimulus input, and neurointegrative structures probably play an important part in this recreation or automatic categorization (as described by Schneider & Schiffrin, 1977). Any failures in this automaticity will lead to instabilities in perception within a temporal context; that is, deficits in experience from the earliest years accumulate and produce a defective internalized conceptualization or inadequate model of the world.

A young adult achieves independence from parents presumably when the individual has developed an internalized world consistent with reality and the individual's frontal cortex has developed enough to interact with the vertical world, thereby directing intraspecies behavior and communication. The capacity for executing future planning, based on re-creation of vectors through experience, depends on frontal cortices as well as the limbic-thalamic systems. The limbic system and thalamus, as well as the frontal cortices interacting with the limbic and thalamic nuclei, actually influence the frontal growth and development through consistent patterns of neurointegration, thereby producing the mapping of experience to cortical columns. Indeed, the structural interconnectivity and development of later columns is probably strongly dependent on the consistency with which they receive relevant and similar input.

Adolescence brings on the demand for planning for future behavioral ramifications. This planning is set in motion by the mature frontal lobes' ablility to stimulate a firing pattern in the limbic and thalamic nuclei, which activates specific cortical columns and re-creates aspects of previous experience. Any experience that generates a particular neurointegration from the limbic and thalamic nuclei will also automatically activate cortical columns, which have been activated by similar neurointegration in the past. This activation provides the neurological base for the capacity of any given stimulus input to be able to generate rapid contextual understanding and expectations.

So, in schizophrenia, there may be what Patterson describes as a double-sided malaise: first, ontogenetic defects in the limbic and thalamic nuclei may lead directly to defects in frontal lobe development and to the limbic and thalamic nuclei providing abnormal neurointegration of experience; second, abnormally developed frontal lobes may not be able to successfully access the neurointegrating limbic and thalamic nuclei to effectively re-create previous experience. This dysfunction produces a fundamental incapacity to plan for the ramifications of behavior (Patterson, 1987).

FAILURES IN AUTOMATICITY

The most disturbed aspects of schizophrenia may occur when prior experience must be re-created in parallel with current stimulus input to achieve an accurate understanding of the current behavioral context. The experience may be neurologically subtly flawed, so the capacity to re-create becomes inconsistent and inaccurate; therefore, future orientation becomes seriously distorted. All this becomes obvious when the young adult reaches a stage of expected behavioral independence but cannot meet expectations because abnormalities of affective tagging stimulation over a long period lead to failures in automaticity among schizophrenics. These failures in automaticity do not allow the subject's past experience to be rapidly and appropriately brought to bear upon present stimulation. Thus, there is no base in experientially rooted understanding for the present context.

This failure in automaticity is most apparent behaviorally when contextually generated expectation is distorted, inaccurate, or absent, and where comparative capacity is critical—such as in speech, behavior, and other communication. Patterson (1987) described the schizophrenic as stimulus-bound with no past or future to provide guidance within short, temporal duration. This limitation occurs because of neurostructural and neurochemical abnormalities developing from early stages of fetal neurogenesis—abnormalities that contribute to a disrupted hardware for processing stimuli and forming cognitions. Histologic studies and MRI, CT, and PET scanning are beginning to corroborate some of these propositions.

Attentional-Perceptual Deficits

Patterson's model also refers to attentional-perceptual deficits in cognition, including the following: (1) deficits of selective and sustained attention; (2) nonresponding to innocuous stimuli; (3) difficulty overcoming distractive or interruptive efforts that occur at the same time stimuli are presented in rapid succession (sensorimotor gating); (4) inability to filter out extraneous noise from meaningful stimuli; (5) deficits in tasks that require active, effortful, attentional manipulation of materials, such as maintaining a set (continuous task performance), scanning memory (forced choice span of apprehension), and active recall (serial recall); (6) high vulnerability to interference and memory recall in consciously controlled cognitive processes; and (7) deficits in assimilating new information with background knowledge.*

Some of these deficits can be demonstrated with neurobehavioral, neuropsychological studies. In general, individuals diagnosed with schizophrenia perform poorly on complex cognitive and perceptual tests, especially those which pose high demands on information processing systems involved in maintenance of attention and rapid psychomotor speed. The Wisconsin Card Sort (Grant & Berg, 1980) and the Halstead Category Test (Golden, 1977) have been used to document involvement of anterior brain systems (especially frontal lobe) and therefore possible deficits in higher level abstraction and mental flexibility. Further, low verbal IQ (relative to performance IQ) and impairment on language tests suggest the involvement of the left hemisphere, which is implicated by deficits in verbal cognitive functions. Subcortical and cortical dysfunction are implicated by studies of attention and information processing.

The disruption of attentional processes because of impaired selective gating of information may occur at the level of interconnectivity between frontal lobes and diencephalic limbic and reticular structures. A neural network for attention, which involves the temporal and frontal cortex as well as the cingulate gyros and subcortical limbic regions, has been proposed, but no single neurobehavioral measure has yet been developed to assess this deficit.

Batteries of tests are, however, available to measure a range of behavioral dysfunctions and implicated brain regions. Therefore, it is possible to test a hypothesis of impairment in the frontal lobe relative to the temporal lobe by contrasting performance of some patients on functions associated with these brain regions, that is, the frontal lobe hypothesis would predict that patients are more impaired on the Wisconsin Card Sort Test (WCST) than on the memory and learning tests, whereas the temporal lobe hypothesis would predict the reverse. Weinberger (1992) reported a comparative study of memory and abstraction (as assessed by WCST) for 36 normal and 36 schizophrenic patients. Schizophrenic subjects demonstrated significantly greater impairment on memory and learning than on abstraction, thus supporting a selective temporal lobe deficit hypothesis. This effect occurred across sexes and ages.

Using a profile analysis to compare abstraction and memory with other functions, researchers found that abstraction was significantly better in patients relative to their neuropsychological performance, while memory and learning were significantly worse. However, given the available data supporting the temporal lobe hypothesis, it can only be concluded that schizophrenia is a complex illness involving neurotransmitter systems, with distributed psychological effects not limited to one

---

*A review of research about the neurostructural and neurochemical bases for these deficits is in the Second Annual State of the Art and Science of Psychiatric Nursing Conference report (Fox, 1990).

brain region. Therefore, it is necessary to combine neuropsychological testing with hypothesis testing to sort out areas of cortical dysfunction.

Gur et al. (1987a, 1987b) described this analysis as neurobehavioral imagery. They emphasized that neuropsychological testing of mental disorders is aimed at assessing and characterizing the pattern of behavioral impairment and preserved abilities. It quantifies the pervasiveness of impairment and can help determine the degree of brain dysfunction, which is important in assessing progression, effect of medication, and rehabilitation status. Additionally, exploration of the relationship between cognition, brain regional activity, brain structure, and schizophrenia is greatly facilitated by collecting physiological data while individual subjects are involved in neurobehavioral tasks known to activate certain brain regions, simultaneously with data gathered through the use of brain imaging, thereby permitting visualization of this process. If Mason (1981) is correct in suggesting that lesions in the norepinephrine system are responsible for schizophrenic attentional deficits, inability to adjust to novel stimuli, and limited capacity to ignore irrelevant stimuli (Van Kammen & Slawsky, 1988), these advancing methods of examining brain activity and cognition should encourage more specific rather than generalized hypotheses. However, our current incapacity to monitor intrabrain dopamine systems still presents a significant barrier to accessing the norepinephrine system.

While there is no definitive understanding of biological dysfunctions associated with schizophrenia and their linkages to attentional, cognitive, information processing, behavioral, and social disabilities, there is still a need to use what *is* known to explore applications of this knowledge in psychiatric care. Levin, Yurgelun-Todd, and Craft (1989) provide a comprehensive discussion of neuropsychological test findings relevant to schizophrenia, and many of these assessments could be modified for use by psychiatric nurses.

Investigators have proposed that differential deficits in attention appear to be a marker of schizophrenia (Spring, Lemon, Weinstein, & Haskell, 1989). Furthermore, Andres and Brenner (1989) reported that schizophrenic responders to innocuous stimuli tended to be hyperaroused relative to controls, while nonresponders exhibited disassociation of the autonomic subsystem. Electrodermally, these nonresponders were hypoaroused with accompanying cardiac hyperarousal. This disassociation of the autonomic system highlights the complexity of schizophrenia and further emphasizes the need to develop intervention strategies that address more than one aspect of attentional, cognitive, behavioral, or interactional functioning.

Andres and Brenner (1989) also argued for the development of cognitive measures that can differentiate between vulnerabilities and impairments in the premorbid, prodromal, acute, and residual phases of schizophrenia. They suggest that for information about perception, cognition, and information processing to be used appropriately in psychiatric care, we must be able to identify and quantify deficits that are amenable to treatment (care) and monitor them as treatment proceeds. These investigators proposed that to achieve therapeutic relevance, a systematic approach to improving attentional performance in schizophrenics must involve integrative training of cognitive, communicative, and social skills.

INFORMATION PROCESSING DEFICITS: TREATMENT IMPLICATIONS

Brenner (1989) reviewed treatment of the basic psychological dysfunctions associated with schizophrenia. He suggested that from a systems point of view, specific informational processing dysfunctions should not be defined as structural characteristics of vulnerability leading to increased susceptibility, but instead as moderating factors in the positive feedback processes that exist between the biological dysfunctions and psychosocial stressors. Information processing deficits therefore may lead through vicious circles that exacerbate one another, so that deficits continually worsen, eventually going out of control to produce psychotic behavior. Brenner (1989) emphasized that impairments of processes (such as attention) that operate at the interface of biological abnormalities and external stressors pervasively affect macrosocial and microsocial functioning.

Brenner proposed that it is necessary to examine interactions of neural systems (dopaminergic activity) with cognitive and emotional processes of behavioral control. The pathway from biological abnormalities, through perceptual, conceptual, and behavioral processes related to information processing in schizophrenia, to symptom expression is represented schematically by Brenner in Figure 13–2. According to Brenner, schizophrenia produces dysfunction, or deficits, at all stages of information processing (attention, perception, conceptualization, memory, and recall). For individuals with schizophrenia, the characteristic difficulties of selecting relevant stimuli and rejecting irrelevant stimuli, maintaining focused attention, and relating current stimuli to previous experience occur within the various stages of this schematic representation of information processing.

COGNITIVE TRAINING

To intervene in the complex informational processing deficits of schizophrenia, Brenner developed integrated psychological therapy (IPT) (Brenner, Roder, Kienzel, & Hodel, 1991). IPT comprises five subprograms (cognitive differentiation, social perception, verbal communication, social skills, and interpersonal problem solving) designed to progressively ameliorate the cognitive dysfunctions and social-behavioral deficits of schizophrenia. The subprograms are arranged hierarchically; early interventions target basic cognitive skills, middle interventions shape cognitive skills into verbal and social responses, and later interventions prepare patients to solve more complex and arousing interpersonal problems. Each subprogram contains discrete steps that prescribe therapeutic tasks for improving social and cognitive skills. IPT is presented to groups of five to seven patients for 30- to 60-minute sessions three times a week for approximately 3 months. Evaluations of the program suggest that IPT has favorable outcomes in affecting elementary cognitive processes that can be detected within the first few weeks of treatment; however, evidence has been mixed regarding IPT's effect on more complex cognitive skills that coordinate and integrate information (Brenner, Hodel, Roder, & Corrigan, 1992).

LINKS BETWEEN DYSFUNCTION AND EVERYDAY COPING

According to Brenner (1989), two vicious cycles must be interrupted in the treatment of information processing dysfunction in schizophrenia. The first is the linkage between perceptual and conceptual processes and their integration, and the second consists of positive feedback loops between cognitive dysfunctions and psychosocial stressors. Brenner concluded that the treatment and rehabilitation of attentional-perceptual and cognitive dysfunctions must be connected with simultaneous, direct intervention with the corresponding emotional and activation processes, and the treatment must be carried out in situations relevant to everyday life. Further, these situations must be much more specific than our common sense approaches of the past. It is necessary to link information about identification of discrete emotions and percep-

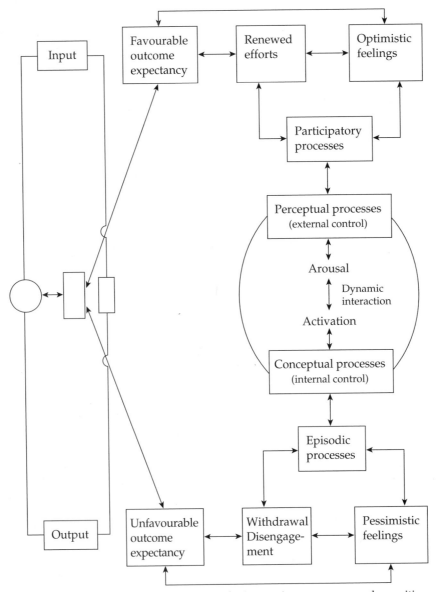

FIGURE 13–2. Heuristic model representing the interactions among neural, cognitive, and emotional processes of behavior control. (From Brenner, H. D. [1989]. The treatment of basic psychological dysfunctions from a systematic point of view. *British Journal of Psychiatry, 155*[Suppl. 5], 79.)

tual information to the discrete emotions and inherent adaptive functions of individuals' experience of sensory and motor characteristics. Treatment and rehabilitation for basic cognitive dysfunction must be tied to the activation processes associated with coping in natural life situations. For instance, teaching an individual to recognize a smiling face in a photograph must be tied to the individual's experience of smiling and to identifying situations and feelings that evoke smiling. Then the smile recognition task must be practiced in actual social situations, with opportunities for the client to verify an identification of smiling behavior with the person smiling.

Understanding patients' patterns of coping with attentional disorder through adaptive regulation or self-regulation of psychophysiologic responsiveness is another essential component and is absolutely necessary for successful treatment. For instance, patients frequently have difficulty focusing on a single topic in a conversation. Therefore, to enable development of appropriate interventions, the therapist must assess what occurs when the patient switches to another topic, thereby determining what effective and ineffective strategies a patient uses to deal with challenging situations. This assessment can then give the therapist options for helping the individual learn new coping behaviors. For example, in conversation, if environmental noise is distracting, the patient can learn ways to decrease the noise. If other activity in the room is distracting, the patient can be helped to engage in strategies to ignore or avoid the distractions. If lack of conversational skill is the problem, the patient can be given simple phrases and questions to use in conversations. Then, as the individual gains expertise in attending to topics, the more complex aspects of conversation can be addressed. The hierarchical and integrated organization of elementary cognitive levels of functioning in the direction of complex levels of behavior can be seen as a balancing act in which efforts are made to cope with the accumulating and circularly linked internal and external stressors.

The IPT model, based as it is on increasing task complexity, can be seen as providing repetitive practice through exercises that make challenging tasks—such as social perception, problem solving, and verbal communication—more automatic. When tasks become automatic, coping with them takes less effort and subsequently reduces stress.

Cost-effectiveness of intensive cognitive rehabilitation therapies will eventually determine their utility. Presently these strategies are labor-intensive and lengthy (Liberman & Green, 1992). Further, research in cognitive rehabilitation for brain injuries indicates that training individuals in self-care skills and instrumental role activities is substantially more effective in promoting clinical gains than focal cognitive rehabilitation strategies. For instance, if an individual must learn to navigate a wheelchair through crowded areas, it is more efficient to teach the individual in actual crowded settings than to use computer simulations. If future research does not demonstrate clinical generalizability of focal cognitive training, then more experiential and practical forms of training may prove effective (Liberman & Green, 1992).

SKILLS TRAINING

A skills training methodology has also been developed. It uses modules that focus on practical skills building to improve individual functioning in social learning situations. This approach—aimed at fostering sustained attention, problem solving, and goal setting—is demonstrated in the Social and Independent Living Skills Series developed by the UCLA Clinical Research Center for Schizophrenia and Psychiatric Rehabilitation. Modules on medication management, symptom management, leisure activity, and basic conversation skills incorporate learning activities that enhance cognitive and behavioral performance. The curriculum involves goal setting, video demonstrations, role playing, problem-solving exercises, and in vivo and homework exercises. The involvement of the trainer in exercises is gradually reduced over time to encourage independence and self-confidence in engaging in newly acquired skills.

Research has documented the efficacy of these methods for individuals with schizophrenia (Eckman, Liberman, Phipps, & Blair, 1990; Wallace, Liberman, MacKain, Blackwell, & Eckman, 1992). The theoretical and curricular framework for the social skills model has been well documented, and the techniques have been applied in a variety of settings (Liberman, DeRisi, & Mueser, 1989; Liberman, 1988). In addition, promising modifications of this model have been developed for nursing application during acute hospitalization (Mann et al., 1993).

Clearly, applying cognitive rehabilitation strategies in the psychosocial treatment of schizophrenia has produced promising outcomes, and the variety of new techniques and procedures being developed bodes well for continuing achievements in the field. Application and testing of cognitive rehabilitation techniques not only demonstrate clinical treatment effects but also contribute to understanding the nature of cognitive and information processing dysfunctions in schizophrenia.

PRODROMAL SYMPTOMS

One dimension of coping with the deficits and disabilities of schizophrenia is the recognition of prodromal symptoms. Marder et al. (1984), Herz and Melville (1980), Herz, Glazer, Mirza, Mostert, and Hafez (1989), and McCandless-Glimcher et al. (1986) reported that prodromal nonpsychotic signs of insomnia, tension, anxiety, social withdrawal, and inability to concentrate occur over days or weeks before a full-blown psychotic episode. The Early Signs Questionnaire, Problem Appraisal Scale, and Global Assessment Scale (Endicott, Spitzer, Fleiss, & Cohen, 1976), as well as the Social Stress and Functioning Inventory for Psychotic Disorder (SSFIPD) (Serban, 1978) and Expanded Brief Psychiatric Rating Scale (Lukoff, Nuechterlein, & Ventura, 1986), are examples of assessment scales that can be used to monitor impaired role function or an increase of nonpsychotic symptoms prior to acute episodes of schizophrenia.

Most investigators reported that prodromal symptoms are generally intraindividually specific and stable across time. Mendel (1976) developed a program where patients carried a list of specific warning signs and were taught to telephone for help if they experienced these symptoms. Herz and Melville (1980) reported that while there is considerable variation in the length of time prodromal symptoms are experienced before an acute exacerbation, over 50% of clients reported noticing symptoms for less than 1 week before acute psychotic episodes (Lukoff, Liberman, & Nuechterlein, 1986). All these studies document the importance of monitoring client-specific prodromal symptoms as a method for early identification of increasing vulnerability to psychotic episodes and potential avoidance of unnecessary decompensation and hospitalization.

Nursing studies in this area have validated and expanded upon the findings regarding symptom self-monitoring by schizophrenics (McCandless-Glimcher et al., 1986; Hamera, Peterson, Handley, Plumlee, & Frank-Ragan, 1991). Based on a symptom self-regulation model adapted from illness representation (Leventhal, Norenz, & Strauss, 1982) and control theory (Carver & Scheier, 1981), the model in these studies proposes that individuals are continually comparing their current experience to their standard of reference, that is, the way they usually feel. When discrepancies occur, some individuals interpret these discrepancies as symptoms, associate them with schizophrenia, and take actions to alter the symptoms. In studying these phenomena, clients were found to identify readily nonpsychotic signs and symptoms of illness exacerbation (McCandless-Glimcher et al., 1986), including indicators such as nervousness, difficulty in sleeping, increased fatigue, and depression. Two thirds of the sample took action to prevent relapse by resuming or increasing medications and seeking psychiatric treatment. Further, Hamera et al. (1991) determined that client functional level was indicative of prodromal symptoms: lower functioning clients identified psychotic symptoms, whereas higher functioning clients identified depression and anxiety as indicators of impending relapse, and follow-up of these clients demonstrated the relative stability of relapse indicators. Because such findings suggest that individuals with schizophrenia can identify symptom indicators of relapse, so that interventions can be instituted to prevent a full-blown episode, facilitating symptom identification and regulation is a primary nursing intervention; it should be a standard modality incorporated into psychiatric nursing practice.

Cognitive processing is involved in symptom monitoring in two ways. First, cognition enables awareness of bodily sensation and ability to identify the sensation as different from familiar experience. Second, cognition is involved in interpreting the sensation as a symptom indicative of relapse. Therefore, deficits in cognition can interfere with symptom monitoring. Hamera, Peterson, Young, and Schaumloffel (1992) found that some individuals with schizophrenia identified experiences that were quite idiosyncratic; they did not fall neatly into generally accepted symptom categories.

Since these idiosyncracies may be related to cognitive deficits and distortions, nurses need to assess and understand the internal states of individuals with schizophrenia and the unique ways they process information. Response to symptoms can be evaluated in conjunction with the meanings of the symptoms. For individuals to share these symptom beliefs, nurses need to develop ongoing supportive relationships that enable their clients to describe how they attempt to cope with their illness indicators. Nurses can then help them use problem solving to identify the most effective actions to take when illness indicators are present (Hamera et al., 1992). As this client-nurse collaboration continues, individual symptom monitoring will become more accurate and more easily practiced (O'Connor, 1991).

THE ROLE OF FAMILIES

Schizophrenia has been described as a diathesis-type disorder in which a constitutional predisposition or tendency makes one vulnerable to the disease, but environmental factors (such as psychosocial or physical stress) may influence the course or episodes of illness. Within this framework, family interaction has been conceptualized as one environmental factor that can influence the course of illness. Unfortunately, for many families with schizophrenic members, this conceptualization appears similar to the family genesis models of schizophrenia predominant in the 1960s. In fact, Hatfield, Spaniol, and Zipple (1987) suggested that this family environment focus simply reflects a resurgence of such family-blaming.

Brown, Birley, and Wing (1972), Vaughn and Leff (1976), and Hogarty et al. (1979) defended their research on family environment by arguing that their concern was identification of stressors and changes that predict relapse or onset of symptoms. From this work, the construct of expressed emotion (EE) was developed. High EE families are defined as those with marked emotional overinvolvement, hostility, or criticism (defined as six or more critical comments about the schizophrenic family member during a structured interview). In contrast, low EE families show minimal or no overinvolvement, no hostility, and make fewer than six critical comments. Mintz, Liberman, Miklowitz, and Mintz (1987) reported higher rates of relapse among schizophrenics residing with high EE families in the 9 months following discharge; in addition, investigators have reported that decreasing the contact of high EE family members with schizophrenic patients, coupled with regular medication use, was associated with lower relapse rates (Vaughn & Leff, 1981; Vaughn, Sorensen-Snyder, Jones, Freeman, & Falloon, 1984). However, other investigators (Kottgen, Sonnichsen, & Mollenhauer, 1984; MacMillan, Gold, Crow, Johnson, & Johnstone, 1986; McReadie & Phillips, 1988; Parker, Johnston, & Hayward, 1988) have not found support for the relationship between high EE family environments and relapse. Still, Hogarty et al. (1986) reported that whatever the cause, when high EE families adopted characteristics consistent with low EE families, relapse rates decreased significantly.

As with many other derived psychosocial constructs, expressed emotion is neither specific nor exclusive, so the construct may lead to misinterpretations regarding causality and correlation. Furthermore, Hatfield and other authors (Hatfield et al., 1987; Kanter, Lamb, & Loeper, 1987; Koenigsberg & Handley, 1986) suggested that hostility, criticism, and overinvolvement do not consistently appear together, and the construct therefore does not validly represent emotional tone in the families under study. Other investigators (Hooley, 1985; Miklowitz, Goldstein, & Falloon, 1983) suggested that a stressful family environment may reflect family members' attempts to cope with the experience of schizophrenia. Support for this model has been reported by Cole, Kane, Zastowny, Grolnick, and Lehman (1993), who concluded that families are attempting to cope with patient behaviors and ambitions, which the family has learned from experience to be dysfunctional. They proposed that the family's simultaneous efforts to establish limits and be supportive interfere with the family's communication and problem solving, leading to escalating conflict and criticism. This pattern appears to be stronger with patients who remain symptomatic but relatively high functioning.

Findings about attentional and information processing deficits accompanying schizophrenia would suggest that individuals with schizophrenia experience distortions of attention and information processing that are likely to disrupt normal social interactions within families. Consonant with Cole et al. (1993), it could be assumed that some family members may react with anxiety, anger, or other emotions in their attempts to control distorted family interactions. Hahlweg, Feinstein, Muller, and Dose (1989) propose that high EE seems to be related to hyperarousal of patients. Thus, decreasing involvement and criticism may act to decrease the information-overload status that hyperaroused schizophrenic patients are believed to experience.

Hahlweg et al. (1989) reported that 25% of families that rated high in EE over time became low in EE without any intervention. Clearly, families learn from experience what to expect from their relative with schizophrenia (Cole et al., 1993), and many learn from trial and error what strategies are effective in managing the situation (Kane, DiMartino, & Jimenez, 1990). Family understanding of this interactive effect and subsequent modification of family intensity and involvement may act to interrupt the runaway cycle of disturbed information processing that individuals with schizophrenia experience.

While some families learn effectively through a specific intervention, others may benefit from psychoeducational programs and psychosocial interventions developed to inform families about schizophrenia. The latter approach of providing strategies to enable families to cope has been quite successful in reducing family upset and patient relapse (see Kane [1994] and Strachan [1992] for reviews). These programs indicate that increasing the problem-solving and communication skills in families coping with schizophrenia reduces the sick relative's stress from external life stressors and family conflict. Programs that address the social skills of the patient as well as the family may have positive additive effects for long-term patient outcome.

A major concern of family members is the attitude of professional care providers about collaboration with them. Frequent reports in the literature highlight family members' negative experiences with professional providers. Katschnig and Konieczna (1989) emphasized that successful work with families involves professionals' partial giving up of the expert role and a willingness to work with families in educational groups. Group education for families is aimed at increasing competence, autonomy, information, and self-confidence, not at interpersonal or intrapsychic change. Kane (1994) emphasized that high-quality treatment programs for schizophrenia should include educational programs for families, and applications of psychoeducational programming for both patients and families are uniquely appropriate for psychiatric nursing. In fact, there is a growing literature addressing the implementation of such strategies by psychiatric nurses (Kane et al., 1990; Malone, 1992).

PSYCHIATRIC NURSING RESEARCH

Increasing knowledge about the information processing deficits experienced by schizophrenics, as well as the development of psychoeducational and environmental strategies and interventions that promote specific compensation for specific deficits, is a promising field for psychiatric nursing research. The effectiveness and evolution of psychiatric nursing practice is clearly dependent on linking new knowledge with psychiatric nursing's rich practice experience in caring for mentally ill individuals and their families.

Ciompi (1989) discussed the linkage of biological and psychosocial systems, arguing that between these two systems we must build conceptually valid bridges that will allow us to test hypotheses; otherwise, a disastrous splitting of our understanding and treatment of schizophrenia into biological or psychosocial reductionism will result. Ciompi's proposed model of the long-term evolution of schizophrenia stresses the interaction of vulnerability, stressors, biological reactivity, social responsiveness, and the nature of complex systems (see Fig. 13–3).

Ciompi related these ideas to the long-term course of schizophrenia and presented the following data on the course of illness for 228 and 289 schizophrenics. The beginning phase, considered the premorbid phase, is from conception until the outbreak of psychosis. This phase is the period when combinations of unfavorable biological and psychosocial conditions combine to increase susceptibility. The second phase, often occurring in adolescence, produces a progressive overtaxation and final psychotic decompensation of the vulnerable information processing system, where

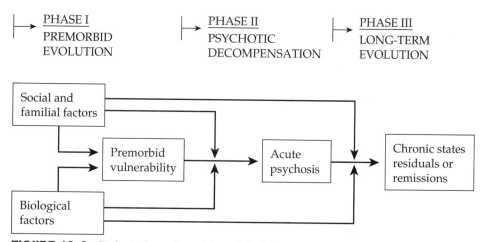

FIGURE 13–3. Biological-psychosocial model of the long-term evolution of schizophrenia in three phases. (From Ciompi, L. [1989]. The dynamics of complex biological-psychosocial systems: Four fundamental psycho-biological mediators in the long-term evolution of schizophrenia. *British Journal of Psychiatry, 155*[Suppl. 5], 15.)

escalating interactions between vulnerability, inadequate environmental conditions, and other unfavorable situational influences contribute to switching from a functional system to a psychotic regime. The third phase, long-term evolution, is open and variable.

Nursing research questions arising from such a model include, but are not limited to, determining (1) what factors protect vulnerable individuals from the deterioration in cognitive functioning associated with onset of psychotic processes; (2) what interventions are most suitable to different phases of the illness; and (3) what interventions are additive to psychopharmacological treatment. Empirical research into these questions requires an ongoing familiarity with current neuropsychiatric findings, further development of relevant research methods, application and evaluation of existing interventions in various phases of the illness progression, and subsequent improvement of selected interventions based on empirical outcomes.

Ciompi's model presents a schematic for understanding the variety of illness presentations observed in schizophrenia, but research is needed to explicate the antecedents of the various types of schizophrenic illness and to determine what strategies most effectively treat each type. For instance, when paranoid ideation is part of the presentation, are cognitive interventions most effective? When negative symptoms predominate, do behavioral programs have more successful outcomes? Future research must be directed toward discriminating symptom clusters and refining interventions that will effect the most successful outcomes.

The application of valid and reliable measurement instruments for assessing symptom patterns in schizophrenia is another crucial area for further investigation. Instruments that can be useful in nursing studies (e.g., those presented in Table 13–1) indicate symptom and diagnostic measures that enable discrete characterizations of illness presentations, as well as measures of functioning, thereby allowing the researcher to quantify social, role, self-care, and work abilities. Such measures can be used to guide selection of appropriate interventions and to determine resulting changes, both improvements and deterioration.

Psychosocial factors such as family environment and individual attitudes also significantly affect the course of the illness. Psychiatric nursing research can address questions related to the burden of care on families—specifically, what types of cognitive dysfunction are most burdensome to families and what programs are most appropriate to help families learn effective strategies to deal with cognitive deficits. Programs that focus on families' coping with cognitive dysfunction can also be examined for subsequent reduction in EE. For example, the Camberwell Family Interview (CFI) (Rutter & Brown, 1966) is a semistructured interview that takes a few hours to complete; it measures EE, and that construct has been found to be associated with relapse. Alternatively, Kreisman, Blumenthal, Johnson, Dushay, and Haas (1990) have developed measures of criticism and emotional overinvolvement that are Likert-type questionnaires that seem to approximate the CFI.

Knowing that family caregiving in serious mental illness can present a serious burden to family members, nurses can use interventions that address cognitive dysfunction for clients and families and then evaluate them for a consequent reduction in family burden. The Social Behavior Assessment Scale (Platt, Weyman, Hirsch, & Hewett, 1980), for example, has a section that evaluates the objective and subjective burden experienced by family members in caring for their mentally ill relative. Understanding the impact of cognitive interventions for the natural family environment can then lead to further development of programs that foster the maintenance of individuals with schizophrenia in the community and promote the continuing support of their natural social networks.

TABLE 13–1. RESOURCES/INSTRUMENTS FOR ASSESSMENT IN SCHIZOPHRENIA

FACTORS	RESOURCES/INSTRUMENTS
Prodromal symptoms	Self-Regulation Interview for Schizophrenia (Hamera et al., 1992)
	Early Signs Questionnaire (Herz & Melville, 1980)
Symptoms	NOSIE—Nurses Observational Scale for Inpatient Environments (Honigfeld, Gillis, & Klett, 1966)
	BPRS—Expanded Brief Psychiatric Rating Scale (Lukoff, Nuechterlein, & Ventura, 1986)
	PANSS—Positive and Negative Symptom Scale (Kay, Fiszbein, & Opler, 1987).
	SAPS—Scale for Assessment of Positive Symptoms (Andreasen, 1984)
	SANS—Scale for Assessment of Negative Symptoms (Andreasen, 1982)
Diagnoses	DSM-IV—Diagnostic and statistical manual of mental disorders (American Psychiatric Association, 1994)
	SCID—Structured Clinical Interview for DSM-III-R (Spitzer, Williams, Gibbon, & First, 1992)
	SADS—Schedule for Affective Disorders and Schizophrenia (Endicott & Spitzer, 1978)
	DIS—Diagnostic Interview Schedule (Robins, Helzer, Croughan, & Ratcliff, 1981)
Functioning	GAS—Global Assessment Scale (Endicott, Spitzer, Fleiss, & Cohen, 1976)
	SAS—Social Adjustment Scale (Paykel, Weissman, Prusoff, & Tonks, 1971)
	SBAS—Social Behavior Assessment Scale (Platt, Weyman, Hirsch, & Hewett, 1980)
	SSFIPD—Social Stress and Functioning Inventory for Psychotic Disorder (Serban, 1978).
	Problem Appraisal Scale (Spitzer & Endicott, 1971)
	Disability Assessment Rating Scale (Hoyle, Nietzel, Guthrie, Baker-Prewitt, & Heine, 1992)
	Independent Living Skills Survey (Wallace, 1986)
Family environment	CFI—Camberwell Family Interview (Rutter & Brown, 1966)
	Patient Rejection Scale (Kreisman, Simmens, & Joy, 1979)
	POPS—Patient Overprotection Scale (Kreisman, Blumenthal, Johnson, Dushay, & Haas, 1990)
	SBAS—Social Behavior Assessment Scale (Platt, Weyman, Hirsch, & Hewett, 1980)

The knowledge base and tools exist to determine the antecedents and consequences of neuropsychiatric dysfunction, to develop innovative nursing interventions, and to evaluate outcomes. It is incumbent on psychiatric nursing to contribute to the research base necessary for developing effective, phase-specific interventions that demonstrate improved outcomes both in inpatient and outpatient settings.

IMPLICATIONS FOR PSYCHIATRIC NURSING PRACTICE

What is the role of therapy in psychiatric nursing as we begin to change our concepts, our focus of intervention, and our practice? Zubin (1989) described the complexity of linking therapeutic intervention and scientific models of etiology. He highlighted the continuing tension between a focus on natural healing of the patient and the more aggressive trend for treatment of the disease, as well as the clash of qualitative versus quantitative approaches to describing the phenomena or measuring affects.

Zubin's discussion is highly recommended for psychiatric nurses. It raises issues that many psychiatric care providers educated as psychotherapists are now struggling with, as we attempt to assimilate new biological knowledge and responsibly participate in the evolution of professional psychiatric nursing practice. Zubin—relating the theory of vulnerability models, ecological models, developmental models, learning theory models, genetic models, neurophysiologic-neuroanatomy models, and internal environment models—argued that a good therapist is really a teacher who opens new options for individuals, who helps people find their own coping strategies.

Scientific advances related to genetic, neurobiological, cognitive, and behavioral factors associated with psychiatric disorders are important for professional psychiatric nursing practice. While Liaschenko (1989) and other nursing authors express skepticism about expanding the focus of psychiatric nursing interventions to include constructs implicated by neurobiological dysfunction, Lowery (1992), McBride (1990), Fox (1989, 1990, 1991), Abraham, Fox, and Cohen (1992) and others proposed that this information, appropriately integrated with nursing principles, greatly enhances the potential benefit of psychiatric nursing interventions.

As Coursey (1989) and Katz (1989) proposed, the personal loss, tragedy, and grief accompanying a chronic debilitated condition—as schizophrenia often is—demand sensitive, skillful caring. Certainly the distortions of perception described by many schizophrenics require attention to the person experiencing such altered realities. Indeed, there is no doubt that individuals diagnosed with schizophrenia need support with the experiences and pain associated with their illness, with their distorted perceptions and altered cognitions; what *is* in question, however, is how, given what we have learned about the neuropathology of schizophrenia, this support can be soundly, scientifically, cost-effectively, and humanely delivered. To determine the how's, it is important that psychiatric nurses aggressively pursue new biological knowledge and work with other care providers who understand the effects of the neuropathology of schizophrenia on perceptions, cognitions, behaviors, and emotions. This knowledge must then be applied in practice as we support individuals coping with this complex illness.

Neurochemical-neuroanatomic disabilities underlying the information processing deficits of schizophrenic patients affect stress vulnerability, perception, cognition, language, emotion, and social relationships. New rehabilitation and care models that link this information with treatment and environmental strategies, as well as the daily life of psychiatric clients, are critically needed (see Table 13–2 for examples of some suggested nursing interventions). Increased knowledge about information processing deficits will need to be applied to home and daily life patterns to decrease vulnerability to relapse. Psychiatric nursing investigators must explore when and how specific environmental conditions and interventions decrease the negative effects of these disabilities. The effects of neurostructural, neurochemical disabilities resulting in disturbed perception and cognition greatly influence daily adaptation and coping. Further, these disabilities interact with physical health strengths, predisposing weaknesses, and compromises experienced by individuals. Therefore, psychiatric nursing researchers and clinicians must work together to integrate this information in assessing, monitoring, intervening with, and caring for schizophrenic patients.

TABLE 13–2. NURSING INTERVENTION STRATEGIES

NURSING INTERVENTION	RATIONALE
Communication Problems	
Teach the client to clarify communications from others by repeating statements, paraphrasing, and questioning. Emphasize that the client should slow down and take the time to get the correct information and meaning from communications.	Information processing deficits may cause the client to misinterpret communications from others and to misread their facial expressions and body language.
Teach the client to recognize facial expressions and to check with the person to make sure the interpretations are correct.	
Stress Management	
Teach the client problem-solving strategies so that stressful situations can be anticipated and contingency plans developed.	Failures in automaticity make it difficult for the client to respond to stressful circumstances appropriately and to learn from them. Clients tend to get overstimulated in certain environments. Using problem-solving approaches and relaxation techniques enables clients to exert some control over stressful circumstances.
Teach families to problem-solve with their relative and to avoid "surprises."	
Teach the client relaxation techniques and strategies to avoid overstimulation.	
Teach the client and family to break down complicated tasks into smaller tasks.	Impaired selective gating and associated attention deficits prevent clients from organizing and focusing their thought processes and actions. Clients can get "lost" performing complex tasks.
Teach clients to give themselves verbal prompts during tasks to remind themselves what they are doing and enable them to keep to the task.	
Symptom Monitoring	
Teach clients and families the definitions of symptoms of schizophrenia and their biological basis. Work with the client and family to identify and monitor specific symptoms and behaviors that precede relapse.	When clients and families understand the symptoms of schizophrenia and their causes, misinterpretations can be prevented and treatment compliance enhanced. Recognition of prodromal symptoms can enable early intervention to prevent relapse.

The knowledge explosion about schizophrenia, particularly in the biological and psychosocial sciences, requires that psychiatric nurses invest in knowledge acquisition and clinical research related to care applications of this knowledge. High-quality psychiatric nursing care represents successful adaptation of biological knowledge to social intervention and caring. The specialty must update psychiatric nursing knowledge and engage in clinical research to assure appropriate, efficacious, ethical, and humane transfer of knowledge in the care of schizophrenic individuals.

Changes in psychiatric nursing educational content, research, and practice must reflect the increasing scientific knowledge base contributing to our understanding of the disorder, disabilities, and life experiences associated with schizophrenia. The capacity to compassionately provide nursing care depends not only on the art of sensitive human relatedness but also on a comprehensive understanding of the causes and disabilities that disrupt the schizophrenic individual's information processing.

REFERENCES

Abraham, I. L., Fox, J. C., & Cohen, B. T. (1992). Integrating the bio into the bio-psychosocial: Understanding and treating biological phenomena in psychiatric–mental health nursing. *Archives of Psychiatric Nursing, 6,* 296–305.

American Psychiatric Association. (1994). *Diagnostic and statistical manual of mental disorders* (4th ed.). Washington, DC: Author.

Andreasen, N. C. (1982). Negative symptoms in schizophrenia: Definition and reliability. *Archives of General Psychiatry, 39,* 784–788.

Andreasen, N. C. (1984). *Scale for assessment of positive symptoms of schizophrenia.* Manuscript. University of Iowa.

Andreasen, N. C., Nasrallah, H. A., Dunn, V., Olson, S. C., Grove, W. M., Ehrhardt, J. C., Coffman, J. A., & Crossett, J. H. W. (1986). Structural abnormalities at the frontal system in schizophrenia: A magnetic resonance imaging study. *Archives of General Psychiatry, 43,* 136–144.

Andres, K., & Brenner, H. (1989). Coping with attentional disorders as a systematic process in schizophrenic patients. *British Journal of Psychiatry, 155*(Suppl. 5), 57–62.

Bleich, A., Brown, S., & van Praag, H. (1991). A serotonergic theory of schizophrenia. In S. Brown & H. van Praag (Eds.), *The role of serotonin in psychiatric disorders* (pp. 183–214). New York: Brunner/Mazel.

Brenner, H. D. (1989). The treatment of basic psychological dysfunctions from a systematic point of view. *British Journal of Psychiatry, 155*(Suppl. 5), 79.

Brenner, H. D., Hodel, B., Roder, V., & Corrigan, P. (1992). Treatment of cognitive dysfunctions and behavioral deficits in schizophrenia. *Schizophrenia Bulletin, 18,* 21–26.

Brenner, H. D., Roder, V., Kienzel, N., & Hodel, B. (1991). *Treatment and rehabilitation of schizophrenic patients: An integrated psychological therapy program.* Toronto: Hans Huber.

Brown, G. W., Birley, J. L. T., & Wing, J. K. (1972). Influence of family life on the course of schizophrenic disorders: A replication. *British Journal of Psychiatry, 121,* 241–258.

Carlsson, A. (1988). Dopamine autoreceptors and schizophrenia. In A. Sen & T. Lee (Eds.), *Receptors and ligands in psychiatry* (pp. 1–10). Cambridge: Cambridge University Press.

Carver, C. S., & Scheier, M. F. (1981). *Attention and self-regulation: A control-theory approach to human behavior.* New York: Springer.

Ciompi, L. (1989). The dynamics of complex biological-psychosocial systems: Four fundamental psycho-biological mediators in the long-term evolution of schizophrenia. *British Journal of Psychiatry, 155*(Suppl. 5), 15–21.

Cole, R., Kane, C. F., Zastowny, T., Grolnick, W., & Lehman, A. (1993). Expressed emotion, communication and problem solving in the families of chronic schizophrenic young adults. In R. E. Cole & D. Reiss (Eds.), *How do families cope with chronic illness?* (pp. 141–172). Hillsdale, NJ: Lawrence Erlbaum.

Conrad, A., & Scheibel, A. (1987). Schizophrenia and the hippocampus: The embryological hypothesis extended. *Schizophrenia Bulletin, 13*(4), 577–587.

Coursey, R. (1989). Psychotherapy with persons suffering from schizophrenia: The need for a new agenda. *Schizophrenia Bulletin, 15,* 349–354.

Crow, T. J. (1980). Positive and negative schizophrenia and the role of dopamine: 2. *British Journal of Psychiatry, 137,* 383–385.

Crow, T. J. (1981). Positive and negative schizophrenia symptoms and the role of dopamine. *British Journal of Psychiatry, 139,* 251–254.

Crow, T. J. (1990). The continuum of psychoses and its genetic origins: The sixty-fifth Maudsley Lecture. *British Journal of Psychiatry, 156,* 788–797.

Curtis, D., & Gurling, H. (1990). Unsound methodology in investigating a pseudoautosomal locus in schizophrenia. *British Journal of Psychiatry, 155,* 415–416.

Delisi, L. (1992). The significance of age of onset for schizophrenia. *Schizophrenia Bulletin, 18,* 209–215.

Eckman, T. A., Liberman, R. P., Phipps, C. C., & Blair, K. E. (1990). Teaching medication management skills to schizophrenic patients. *Journal of Clinical Psychopharmacology, 10,* 33–38.

Endicott, J., & Spitzer, R. (1978). A diagnostic interview: The schedule for affective disorders and schizophrenia. *Archives of General Psychiatry, 35,* 837–844.

Endicott, J., Spitzer, R., Fleiss, J., & Cohen, J. (1976). The global assessment scale—A procedure for measuring overall severity of psychiatric disturbance. *Archives of General Psychiatry, 33,* 766–771.

Flor-Henry, P. (1983). Determinants of psychosis in epilepsy: Laterality and forced normalization. *Biological Psychiatry, 18,* 1045–1057.

Fox, J. (1989). *The Galt visiting scholar chair in public mental health final report.* Richmond, VA: Virginia DMHMRSAS.

Fox, J. (1990, November). *Etiologic factors and information processing deficits associated with schizophrenia: A review of findings.* Paper presented at NIMH, Washington, DC.

Fox, J. (1991). Psychiatric nursing, directions for the future. In L. Aiken & C. Fagin (Eds.), *Charting nursing's future: Agenda for the 1990s* (pp. 216–234). Philadelphia, Lippincott.

Golden, C. J. (1977). Validity of the Halstead-Reitan neuropsychological battery in a mixed psychiatric and brain-injured population. *Journal of Consulting and Clinical Psychology, 45,* 1043–1051.

Goldstein, J., & Tsuang, M. T. (1990). Gender and schizophrenia: An introduction and synthesis of findings. *Schizophrenia Bulletin, 16*(2), 179–183.

Gottesman, I., & Bertelsen, A. (1989). Confirming unexpressed genotypes for schizophrenia. *Archives of General Psychiatry, 46,* 867–872.

Grant, D. A., & Berg, E. A. (1980). *The Wisconsin Card Sort Test random layout: Directions for administration and scoring.* Madison, WI: Wells Printing.

Green, M. F., Satz, P., Garer, D. J., Ganzell, S., & Kharabi, F. (1989). Minor physical anomalies in schizophrenia. *Schizophrenia Bulletin, 15,* 91–99.

Gur, R. E., Resnick, S. M., Alavi, A., Gur, R. C., Caroff, S., Donn, R., Silver, F. L., Saykin, A. J., Chawluk, J. B., Kushner, M., & Reivich, M. (1987a). Regional brain function in schizophrenia: 2. A positron emission tomography study. *Archives of General Psychiatry, 44,* 119–125.

Gur, R. E., Resnick, S. M., Gur, R. C., Alavi, A., Caroff, S., Kushner, M., & Reivich, M. (1987b). Regional brain function in schizophrenia: 2. Repeated evaluation with positron emission tomography. *Archives of General Psychiatry, 44,* 126–129.

Hahlweg, K., Feinstein, E., Muller, U., & Dose, M. (1989). Family management programmes for schizophrenic patients. *British Journal of Psychiatry, 155*(Suppl. 5), 112–116.

Hamera, E., Peterson, K., Handley, S., Plumlee, A., & Frank-Ragan, E. (1991). Patient self-regulation and functioning in schizophrenia. *Hospital and Community Psychiatry, 42*(6), 630–631.

Hamera, E. K., Peterson, K. A., Young, L. M., & Schaumloffel, M. M. (1992). Symptom monitoring in schizophrenia: Potential for enhancing self-care. *Archives of Psychiatric Nursing, 6,* 324–330.

Hatfield, A. B., Spaniol, L., & Zipple, A. M. (1987). Expressed emotion: A family perspective. *Schizophrenia Bulletin, 13*(2), 221–226.

Henn, F., & Henn. S. (1982). Phospholipids as markers for schizophrenia. In E. Usdin & T. Hanin (Eds.), *Biological markers in psychiatry and neurology* (pp. 183–185). New York: Pergammon.

Herz, M., Glazer, W., Mirza, M., Mostert, H., & Hafez, H. (1989). Treating prodromal episodes to prevent relapse in schizophrenia. *British Journal of Psychiatry, 155*(Suppl. 5), 123–127.

Herz, M., & Melville, C. (1980). Relapse in schizophrenia. *American Journal of Psychiatry, 137,* 801–805.

Hogarty, G., Schooler, N., Ulrich, R., Mussare, F., Ferro, P., & Herron, E. (1979). Fluphenazine and social therapy in the aftercare of schizophrenic patients. *Archives of General Psychiatry, 36,* 1283–1294.

Hogarty, G. E., Anderson, C. M., Reiss, D. J., Kornblatt, S., Greenwald, D., Javna, C., & Madonia, M. (1986). Family psychoeducation, social skills training and maintenance chemotherapy in the aftercare treatment of schizophrenia. *Archives of General Psychiatry, 43,* 633–642.

Honigfeld, G., Gillis, R. D., & Klett, C. J. (1966). NOSIE-30: A treatment-sensitive ward behavior scale. *Psychological Reports, 19,* 180.

Hooley, J. M. (1985). Expressed emotion: A review of the critical literature. *Clinical Psychology Review, 5,* 119–139.

Hoyle, R. H., Nietzel, M. T., Guthrie, P. R., Baker-Prewitt, J. L., & Heine, R. (1992). The Disability Rating Form: A brief schedule for rating disability associated with severe mental illness. *Psychosocial Rehabilitation Journal, 16*(1), 77–94.

Jablensky, A., Sartorius, N., Ernberg, G., Anker, M., Korten A., Cooper, J. E., Day, R., & Bertelsen, A. (1992). Schizophrenia: Manifestations, incidence and course in different cultures. A WHO ten-country study. *Psychological Medicine,* Monograph Supplement 20, 1–97.

Jakob, H., & Beckmann, H. (1986). Prenatal developmental disturbances in the limbic allocortex in schizophrenics. *Journal of Neural Transmission, 65,* 303–326.

Kane, C. F. (1994). Psychoeducational programs for families of the mentally ill: From blaming to caring. In E. Kahana, D. E. Biegel, & M. Wykle (Eds.), *Family caregiving across the lifespan* (pp. 219–239). Beverly Hills: Sage.

Kane, C. F., DiMartino, E., & Jimenez, M. (1990). Short-term multifamily groups for relatives coping with chronic schizophrenia. *Archives of Psychiatric Nursing, 6*(6), 343–353.

Kanter, J., Lamb, R., & Loeper, R. (1987). Expressed emotion in families: A critical review. *Hospital and Community Psychiatry, 38,* 374–380.

Katschnig, H., & Konieczna, T. (1989). What works with relatives—A hypothesis. *British Journal of Psychiatry, 155*(Suppl. 5), 144–150.

Katz, H. (1989). A new agenda for psychotherapy of schizophrenia. *Schizophrenia Bulletin, 15,* 355–357.

Kay, S. R., Fiszbein, A., & Opler, L. A. (1987). The Positive and Negative Syndrome Scale (PANSS) for schizophrenia. *Schizophrenia Bulletin, 13,* 261–276.

Keith, S., Regier, D., & Lewis, J. (Eds.). (1988). *A national plan for schizophrenia research.* Report of the National Advisory Mental Health Council, NIMH U.S. Dept. of Health and Human Services, Public Health Services, ADAMHA DHHS Publication No. (ADM) 88-1571.

Kerwin, R., & Murray, R. (1992). A developmental perspective in the pathology and neurochemistry of the temporal lobe in schizophrenia. *Schizophrenia Research, 7,* 1–12.

Koenigsberg, H. W., & Handley, R. (1986). Expressed emotion: From predictive index to clinical construct. *American Journal of Psychiatry, 143,* 1363–1373.

Kopala, L., & Campbell, C. (1990). Implications of olfactory agnosia for understanding sex differences in schizophrenia. *Schizophrenia Bulletin, 25,* 5–260.

Kottgen, C., Sonnichsen, I., & Mollenhauer, K. (1984). Families' high expressed emotion and relapses in young schizophrenic patients. *International Journal of Family Psychiatry, 5,* 71–82.

Kreisman, D. E., Blumenthal, R. L., Johnson, J., Dushay, R., & Haas, G. (1990). Measuring emotional overinvolvement: A multi-factorial construct [manuscript]. New York: New York State Psychiatric Institute.

Kreisman, D. E., Simmens, S. J., & Joy, V. D. (1979). Rejecting the patient: Preliminary validation of a self-report scale. *Schizophrenia Bulletin, 5,* 220–222.

Lee, T. (1988). Postmortem studies of dopamine receptors in schizophrenia. In A. Sen & T. Lee (Eds.), *Receptors and ligands in psychiatry* (pp. 11–28). Cambridge: Cambridge University Press.

Levanthal, H., Norenz, D., & Strauss, A. (1982). Self-regulation and the mechanism for symptoms appraisal. In D. Mechanic (Ed.), *Psychological epidemiology* (pp. 55–86). New York: Neale Watson Academic Press.

Levin, S., Yurgelun-Todd, D., & Craft, S. (1989). Contributions of clinical neuropsychology to the study of schizophrenia. *Journal of Abnormal Psychology, 98,* 341–356.

Liaschenko, J. (1989). Changing paradigms within psychiatry: Implications for nursing research. *Archives of Psychiatric Nursing, 3,* 153–158.

Liberman, R. P. (Ed.). (1988). *Psychiatric rehabilitation of chronic mental patients.* Washington, DC: American Psychiatric Press.

Liberman, R. P., DeRisi, W. J., & Mueser, K. T. (1989). *Social skills training for psychiatric patients.* New York: Pergamon.

Liberman, R. P., & Green, M. F. (1992). Whither cognitive-behavioral therapy for schizophrenia. *Schizophrenia Bulletin, 18*(1), 27–35.

Lowery, B. (1992). Psychiatric nursing in the 1990s and beyond. *Journal of Psychosocial Nursing, 30,* 7–13.

Lukoff, D., Liberman, P., & Nuechterlein, K. (1986). Symptom monitoring in the rehabilitation of schizophrenic patients. *Schizophrenia Bulletin, 12,* 578–593.

Lukoff, D., Nuechterlein, K., & Ventura, J. (1986). Appendix A manual for expanded BPRS. *Schizophrenia Bulletin, 12,* 594–602.

Lyon, M., Barr, C., Cannon, T., Mednick, S., & Shore, D. (1989). Fetal neural development and schizophrenia. *Schizophrenia Bulletin, 15,* 149–160.

MacMillan, J., Gold, A., Crow, T., Johnson, A., & Johnstone, E. (1986). Expressed emotion and relapse. *British Journal of Psychiatry, 148,* 133–143.

Malone, J. (1992). *Schizophrenia: Handbook for clinical care.* Thorofare, NJ: SLACK.

Mann, N. A., Tandon, R. J., Butler, J., Boyd, M., Eisner, W. H., & Lewis, M. (1993). Psychosocial rehabilitation in schizophrenia: Beginnings in acute hospitalization. *Archives of Psychiatric Nursing, 7,* 154–162.

Marder, S., Van Putten, T., Mintz, J., Labell, M., McKenzie, J., & May, P. R. A. (1984). Low and conventional dose therapy with fluphenazine decanoate: Two-year outcome. *Archives of General Psychiatry, 44,* 518–521.

Mason, S. (1981). Noradrenaline in the brain: Progress in theories of behavioral function. *Progress in Neurobiology, 17,* 263–303.

McBride, A. B. (1990). Psychiatric nursing in the 1990s. *Archives of Psychiatric Nursing, 4,* 21–28.

McCandless-Glimcher, L., McKnight, S., Hamera, E., Smith, B. I., Peterson, K. A., & Plumlee, A. A. (1986). Use of symptoms by schizophrenics to monitor and regulate their illness. *Hospital and Community Psychiatry, 37,* 929–933.

McNeil, T. F. (1987). Perinatal influences in the development of schizophrenia. In H. Helmchen and F. A. Henn (Eds.), *Biological perspectives in schizophrenia* (pp. 125–138). London: Wiley.

McReadie, R. G., & Phillips, K. (1988). The Nithsdale schizophrenia survey: 7. Does relatives' high EE predict relapse? *British Journal of Psychiatry, 152,* 477–481.

Meltzer, H. Y., & Stahl, S. M. (1976). The dopamine hypothesis of schizophrenia: A review. *Schizophrenia Bulletin, 2*(1), 19–76.

Mendel, W. (1976). *Schizophrenia: The experience and the treatment.* San Francisco: Jossey Bass.

Miklowitz, E., Goldstein, J., & Falloon, I. (1983). Premorbid and symptomatic characteristics of schizophrenics from families with high and low levels of expressed emotion. *Journal of Abnormal Psychology, 92,* 359–367.

Mintz, L. I., Liberman, R. P., Miklowitz, D. J., & Mintz, J. (1987). Expressed emotion: A call for partnership among relatives, patients and professionals. *Schizophrenia Bulletin, 13*(2), 227–236.

Nasrallah, H. A., Schwarzkopf, S. B., Olson, S. C., Coffman, J. A.. (1990). Gender differences in schizophrenia on MRI brain scans. *Schizophrenia Bulletin, 16,* 205–210.

O'Connor, F. W. (1991). Symptom monitoring for relapse prevention in schizophrenia. *Archives of Psychiatric Nursing, 5,* 193–201.

Parker, G., Johnston, P., & Hayward, L. (1988). Parental "expressed emotion" as a predictor of schizophrenic relapse. *Archives of General Psychiatry, 45,* 806–813.

Patterson, T. (1987). Studies toward the subcortical pathogenesis of schizophrenia. *Schizophrenia Bulletin, 13*(4), 559–576.

Paykel, E. S., Weissman, M., Prusoff, B. A., & Tonks, C. M. (1971). Dimensions of social adjustment in depressed women. *Journal of Nervous and Mental Disease, 152*(3), 158–172.

Platt, S., Weyman, A., Hirsch, S., & Hewett, S. (1980). The social behavior assessment schedule (SBAS): Rationale, contents, scoring, and reliability of a new interview schedule. *Social Psychiatry, 15,* 43–55.

Rieder, R., Rosenthal, D., Wender, P., & Blumenthal, H. (1975). The offspring of schizophrenic fetal and neonatal death. *Archives in General Psychiatry, 32,* 200–204.

Robins, L. N., Helzer, J. E., Croughan, J., & Ratcliff, K. (1981). NIMH diagnostic interview schedule: Its history, characteristics and validity. *Archives of General Psychiatry, 38,* 381–389.

Rotrosen, J., Miller, A., Mandio, D., Traficante, L., & Gershon, S. (1980). Prostaglandins, platelets and schizophrenia. *Archives in General Psychiatry, 37,* 1047–1054.

Rutter, M., & Brown, G. W. (1966). The reliability and validity of measures of family life and relationships in families containing a psychiatric patient. *Social Psychiatry, 1,* 38–53.

Schneider, W., & Schiffrin, R. M. (1977). Controlled and automatic human information processing: 1. Detection, search and attention. *Psychological Review, 84,* 1–66.

Schulsinger, F., Parnas, J., Petersen, E., Schulsinger, H., Teasdale, T., Mednick, S., Moller, L., & Silverton, L. (1984). Cerebral ventricular size in offspring of schizophrenic mothers. *Archives of General Psychiatry, 41,* 602–606.

Seeman, M. V., & Lang, M. (1990). The role of estrogens in schizophrenia gender differences. *Schizophrenia Bulletin, 16,* 185–194.

Serban, G. (1978). Social stress and functioning inventory for psychotic disorders (SSFID): Measurement and prediction of schizophrenics' community adjustment. *Comprehensive Psychiatry, 19,* 337–347.

Snyder, S. H. (1976). The dopamine hypothesis of schizophrenia: Focus on the dopamine receptor. *American Journal of Psychiatry, 133,* 197–202.

Spitzer, R. L., & Endicott, J. (1971). An integrated group of forms for automated psychiatric case records: A progress report. *Archives of General Psychiatry, 24,* 448–453.

Spitzer, R. L., Williams, J. B., Gibbon, M., & First, M. B. (1992). The Structured Clinical Interview for DSM-III-R (SCID): 1. History, rationale, and description. *Archives of General Psychiatry, 49,* 624–629.

Spring, B., Lemon, M., Weinstein, L., & Haskell, A. (1989). Distractibility in schizophrenia: State and trait aspects. *British Journal of Psychiatry, 155*(Suppl. 5), 63–68.

Stahl, S., Berger, P., Benson, K., Zarcone, V., Barchas, J., King, R., Faull, I. K., Uhr, S., & Thiemann, S. (1988). Serotonin studies in schizophrenia. In A. Sen & T. Lee (Eds.), *Receptors and ligands in psychiatry* (pp. 64–92). Cambridge: Cambridge University Press.

Stein, L., & Wise, C. (1971). Possible etiology of schizophrenia: Progressive damage to the noradrenergic reward system by G-hydroxydopamine. *Science, 171,* 1032–1036.

Stevens, J. D. (1972). Membrane abnormalities in schizophrenia. *Schizophrenia Bulletin, 6,* 60–61.

Strachan, A. S. (1992). Family management. In R. P. Liberman (Ed.), *Handbook of psychiatric rehabilitation* (pp. 183–212). New York: Macmillan.

Tolbert, L., Monti, J., O'Shields, H., Walter-Ryan, W., Medows, D., & Smythies, J. (1983). Deficits in transmethylation and membrane lipids in schizophrenia. *Psychopharmacology Bulletin, 19,* 594–599.

Van Kammen, D., & Antelman, S. (1984). Impaired noradrenergic transmission in schizophrenia. *Life Sciences, 34,* 1403–1413.

Van Kammen, D., & Slawsky, R. (1988). State dependence and dysregulation of norepinephrine activity in schizophrenia. In A. Sen & T. Lee (Eds.), *Receptors and ligands in psychiatry* (pp. 93–126). Cambridge: Cambridge University Press.

Vaughn, C. E., & Leff, J. P. (1976). The influence of family and social factors in the course of psychiatric illness. *British Journal of Psychiatry, 129,* 125–137.

Vaughn, C. E., Sorensen-Snyder, K. S., Jones, S., Freeman, W. B., & Falloon, I. R. H. (1984). Family factors in schizophrenic relapses: Replication in California of British research on expressed emotions. *Archives of General Psychiatry, 41,* 1169–1177.

Wallace, C. J. (1986). Functional assessment in rehabilitation. *Schizophrenia Bulletin, 12,* 604–630.

Wallace, C. J., Liberman, R. P., MacKain, S. J., Blackwell, G., & Eckman, T. A. (1992). Effectiveness and replicability of modules for teaching social and instrumental skills to the severely mentally ill. *American Journal of Psychiatry, 149,* 654–658.

Weinberger, D. R. (1992). Presentation to National Advisory Mental Health Council, National Institute of Mental Health, Bethesda, MD.

Zubin, J. (1989). Suiting therapeutic intervention to the scientific models of aetiology. *British Journal of Psychiatry, 155*(Suppl. 5), 9–14.

Zubin, J., Steinhauer, S., Kay, R., & Van Kammen, D. (1985). Schizophrenia of the cross roads: A blueprint for the '80s. *Comprehensive Psychiatry, 26,* 217–240.

CHAPTER

14

ALZHEIMER'S DISEASE

Kathleen Coen Buckwalter, PhD, RN, FAAN, and Geri Richards Hall, PhD(c), ARNP, CS

ABSTRACT

This chapter first reviews the rapid advances that have been made in solving the mystery of Alzheimer's disease (AD) and future needs in the area of biomedical and epidemiological research. Biological, and especially genetic and pharmacological, research on AD has been progressing at an astounding pace since the mid-1980s, in part because of emerging technologies and methods of study. In the next section, the chapter examines the etiologies and neuropathologies of AD as they relate to impairments of memory and intellectual abilities, personality changes, and behavioral symptoms (such as wandering and catastrophic reactions) that are so consuming of nursing time and resources. Next, specific assessment parameters and nursing interventions for persons with AD are set forth, based upon Hall and Buckwalter's (1987, 1991) progressively lowered stress threshold and whole disease care planning models. Caregivers of persons with AD are also discussed, including issues related to burden and stress, the physical and psychosocial morbidity associated with caregiving, and social and financial responses. Cultural and ethnic issues, the continuum of care, and nursing intervention studies related to caregivers are then briefly highlighted. This chapter concludes with a discussion of implications for nursing education and research.

The dementing disorders, of which Alzheimer's disease (AD) is the most prevalent, are brain diseases that lead to the eventual loss of mental functions and self-care abilities. Onset of AD reduces an individual's remaining life expectancy by at least one half. However, death usually results not from the brain pathology itself, but rather from physical deterioration and the secondary effects of immobility that accompany the profound cognitive changes (Burns & Buckwalter, 1988). As noted by the Advisory Panel on Alzheimer's Disease in their 1989 report:

> The peculiar tragedy of Alzheimer's disease and other related dementias (ADRD) is that they dissolve the mind and steal the humanity of the victim, leaving a body from which the person has largely been removed. Simultaneously, these disorders devastate the lives of spouses and other family members, who must endure this deterioration of their loved ones and the loss of the person and relationship that is implied. (Executive Summary, p. x)

The number of persons with AD is increasing because of demographic shifts to an ever older population. Recent epidemiological data from Evans and colleagues

(1989) suggest that approximately 10% of persons between the ages of 65 and 75 suffer from some form of dementia. Among persons over age 85, the fastest growing cohort in the United States, the prevalence rate reaches 50% (Evans et al., 1989). Projections suggest that by the year 2040 there will be more than 6 million cases of AD. These statistics, while impressive, in no way reflect the human costs of this devastating illness. Further, the projections have enormous implications for scientists, health care professionals, and policymakers, who must respond to "an epidemic of long-term, currently incurable illness" (Report of the Advisory Panel on Alzheimer's Disease, 1989, p. i).

Care of persons with Alzheimer's disease and their family members offers an ideal opportunity to integrate the biological and behavioral sciences in the practice of psychiatric nursing (McBride, 1990). Nurses are assuming increasing responsibilities in the assessment, diagnosis, and management of nursing problems associated with AD along the care continuum from medical diagnosis to death, although at present prescriptions for care are not always theoretically or empirically based (Maas & Buckwalter, 1991).

CURRENT BIOMEDICAL-EPIDEMIOLOGICAL KNOWLEDGE OF ALZHEIMER'S DISEASE

The development of effective treatments and preventive strategies is dependent upon our understanding of the etiology and biological processes of AD (Office of Technology Assessment, 1987). It is known that a number of pathological changes occur in the brains of persons with AD, including damage to neurons that integrate complex information from a variety of sensory systems and damage to cells in the hippocampus that moderate memory functions. The degree of cognitive impairment, which varies considerably among affected individuals, has been found to be a function of the loss of critical neurons, their processes, and intercell connections (neocortical synapses) (Advisory Panel on Alzheimer's Disease, 1990), but there are still many unanswered questions. For example, it is quite possible that AD is really a group of related disorders, each of which may have a different etiology. Scientists are beginning to identify subtypes of patients with AD, characterized by age of onset, familial incidence, development of psychiatric disorders, abnormal movement, and disturbances in communication (Mayeux, Stern, & Spanton, 1985).

Biomedical research (basic, clinical, and epidemiological) offers promise for discovering the cause(s) and cure(s) of AD, which at present cannot be prevented (see Fig. 14–1 for an overview of possible leads). Although there is much exciting research activity in this area, at present the progressive, devastating, and chronic course (average length of disease is 8 to 10 years) cannot be reversed or retarded. For purposes of this chapter, advances in three major areas of basic research are examined: (1) investigations of the sequence of pathophysiological changes that take place in the brain; (2) research on the etiology of AD; and (3) development of diagnostic screens for early detection. The reader interested in a more detailed description of the morphologic, neurochemical, neuroendocrine, and physiologic alterations in aging and in AD is referred to Burns and Buckwalter (1988).

BASIC RESEARCH IN ALZHEIMER'S DISEASE

Molecular genetics and biochemistry are among the most exciting and promising areas in the biomedical research effort. Aided by technological advances in techniques such as brain imaging and cell staining, understanding of diseased sites

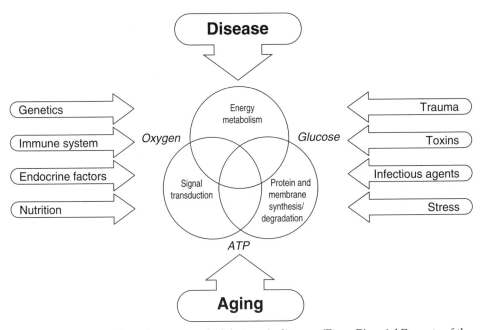

FIGURE 14–1. Leads to the causes of Alzheimer's disease. (From Biennial Reports of the NIH Institutes, Centers and Division, 1991, p. 37.)

within the brain and the process of cellular degeneration is progressing rapidly. The technique of positron emission tomography (PET), for example, has made it possible for researchers to map metabolic functions in the brain during cognitive processes and to discover metabolic changes in the parietal lobes in the early stages of Alzheimer's disease. Importantly, nurses (Algase, 1991) have used this information on parietal lobe pathology (DeLeon, Potegal, & Gurland, 1984) in their investigation of the problem of wandering. Other sensitive instrumentation, such as magnetic resonance spectroscopy and single positron emission computerized tomography (SPECT) should soon be generally available to enhance diagnostic precision, increase our understanding of related behavioral phenomena, and guide interventions.

Alzheimer's disease involves several chemically specific neural systems, or networks of nerve cells in the brain, that produce neurotransmitters. Research has shown that nerve cells in selected parts of the brain are particularly vulnerable to AD. The greatest neurotransmitter losses occur in the cholinergic system, which produces acetylcholine (ACh) and affects learning and memory functions. In fact, a 75% reduction in ACh cells in the nucleus basalis of Meynert and a 50% reduction of norepinephrine cells in the locus coeruleus have been reported in persons with AD (Coyle, Price, & DeLong, 1983). The degree of deficit in choline acetyltransferase (CHAT) correlates with the degree of impairment and the extent of cortical neuritic plaque formation (Davies, 1983). Research also suggests that excitotoxins, such as the amino acids glutamate and aspartate, may be related to Alzheimer's disease, in that they can damage or even destroy brain cells. Nerve growth factors may thus be significant in the treatment of AD in that they preserve or restore the integrity of neurons. Although other neurotransmitters and neurohormones are altered in AD, at this time the cholinergic system deficiency in the brain of persons with AD is the most significant and consistent neurotransmitter abnormality.

Other investigators have focused their studies on an abnormal fibrous protein called amyloid that accumulates in the neuritic plaques that are characteristic of

Alzheimer's disease. There are several known steps in the process by which a normal brain cell protein degenerates into beta amyloid fragments, which form the core of the neuritic plaques. Investigation is now under way to determine how other brain proteins undergo phosphorylation, producing the molecular changes that form neurofibrillary tangles (Advisory Panel on Alzheimer's Disease, 1991).

Neuritic plaques are an important target of research because they cluster near the brain's communication points, and the number of plaques has been shown to be positively correlated with disturbances in memory and intellectual functioning. Scientists are looking at both the function of amyloid and the mechanism(s) causing its breakdown in AD (Advisory Panel on Alzheimer's Disease, 1991). This area of research has potentially important clinical applications in that the abnormal metabolism and breakdown of amyloid might be amenable to medical intervention with pharmacological agents that block abnormal protein degradation (Advisory Panel on Alzheimer's Disease, 1990). Of note is the recent finding that the gene that codes for the amyloid precursor protein is located on chromosome 21, near the region of trisomy 21 (see Fig. 14–2). Interestingly, in Down's syndrome, AD-like pathological changes occur in the brain by middle age, and this pathology is attributed to triplication of chromosome 21. Diffuse amyloid plaques have also been noted in adolescents with Down's syndrome.

Researchers have reported that genes on chromosomes 19 (Roses et al., 1990) and 21 may be associated with a familial (hereditary) type of AD that affects 5% to 10% of persons with AD and is characterized by early onset (St. George-Hyslop et al., 1987). While the exact mechanism of gene action in familial-type AD is as yet unknown, population genetic studies have offered strong evidence of a familial factor in some cases of AD (Huff, Auerback, Chakravarti, & Boller, 1988). However, studies of AD in identical twins indicate that environmental as well as genetic factors contribute to the onset of the disorder.

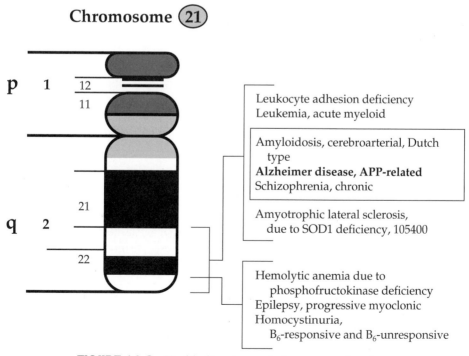

FIGURE 14–2. Health disorders and chromosome location.

Recent discoveries related to the gene that codes for the amyloid precursor protein (APP) and genetic mutations on chromosomes 14, 19, and 21 have attracted widespread scientific and public interest. Stirring even more excitement are findings that were first reported in April 1993 related to apolipoprotein E (APOE), which has three forms: APOE2, APOE3, and APOE4 (Advisory Panel on Alzheimer's Disease, 1993). APOE, a normal cholesterol-carrying protein produced by a gene on chromosome 19, has been linked to late-onset AD and appears to play a significant role in susceptibility to the development of AD (Morrison-Bogorad, 1993). For example, persons with the E2/E3 genotype have as little as one fourth the risk of developing the disease as those who have E3/E3. High-risk individuals include those with the E4/E4 combination, who are about 15 times more likely to develop AD than those with E3/E3 and 60 times more likely to develop the disease compared to those with E2/E3. Interestingly, researchers have found that persons with the E2/E4 genotype have "neutral" risk similar to those with E2/E3, as the effects of E2 and E4 appear to cancel each other out (Twombly, 1994). Researchers claim to have found a possible mechanism by which APOE2 protects against abnormal changes in proteins that lead to tangles associated with dementia, whereas APOE4 appears to leave these proteins unprotected. Genetic research in this area may lead to development of a protective anti-Alzheimer's drug that mimics the action of APOE2.

PHARMACOLOGICAL DEVELOPMENTS

Causing an even greater public furor and promoting inquiries from desperate family members was the recent Food and Drug Administration approval of the first specific medication for the treatment of Alzheimer's disease: tacrine hydrochloride (now commercially available as Cognex). This medication increases the amount of acetylcholine (a neurotransmitter affected in AD) in the brain. Tacrine also has been found to reduce some of the cognitive problems associated with AD in some (25% to 30%) patients. Other promising drugs that target cognitive deficits in AD are expected on the market in the near future.

TACRINE

Tacrine hydrochloride was approved by the Food and Drug Administration in September 1992 as the first drug for use in the treatment of mild-to-moderate Alzheimer's disease. Tacrine (Cognex) elevates acetycholine concentrations in the cerebral cortex by slowing the degradation of acetylcholine released by still-intact cholinergic neurons. Based on this mode of action, the effects of tacrine are expected to diminish as the number of intact cholinergic neurons decreases. Another caution is that elevations of liver enzymes (ALT/SGPT) occur in approximately 50% of patients taking Cognex. Nursing considerations include the following (Miller, 1994):

- Liver function (specifically ALT/SGPT) should be assessed prior to initiating treatment and then weekly for the first 18 weeks of treatment. Assessment should continue every 3 months thereafter. Weekly monitoring should be resumed for 6 weeks following an increase in dosage. If the treatment has been suspended for more than 4 weeks and then reinstated, monitoring should occur on a weekly basis for 18 weeks.
- Nicotine can reduce plasma concentrations of tacrine to one third the concentrations of nonsmokers. Tacrine can double the elimination half-life and average plasma concentrations of theophylline.
- To obtain maximum benefit, tacrine should be taken between meals on an empty stomach.

EXPERIMENTAL DRUGS

Other drugs are currently being studied with the hope that they may increase existing cognitive abilities in persons with AD. The Alzheimer's Association reports that the following drugs are being tested in multicenter clinical trials throughout the United States:

- Physostigmine (Synapton) inhibits an enzyme that breaks down acetylcholine. Research has shown a deficit of acetylcholine in the brains of individuals with AD. The action of physostigmine results in an increase in acetylcholine, which may serve to alleviate cognitive impairment associated with AD.
- Nimodipine (a calcium channel blocker) is another drug that is currently being researched. Calcium is essential for the proper function of all cells, and its role in the nerve cell degeneration that occurs in AD is being studied. It is predicted that nimodipines will reduce the amount of calcium entering nerve cells, thus preventing calcium overload, which in turn may prolong nerve cell survival.
- Research has shown that acetylcholine, norepinephrine, and other neurotransmitters are deficient in the brains of persons with AD. Besipirdine hydrochloride (HP749) mimics the action of acetylcholine and enhances the release of norepinephrine. Testing is currently being conducted to determine if this action will improve nerve cell communication in the brains of persons with AD.
- E2020 is a specific inhibitor of acetylcholinesterase, which limits the amount of acetylcholine. It is hoped that by inhibiting the enzyme that limits acetylcholine, higher concentrations will be available in the brain, alleviating many of the symptoms associated with AD. Studies in animals have shown that E2020 improves performance in tests of learning and memory. A small preliminary study in patients with AD suggests that E2020 is worthy of further evaluation.

OTHER EXPERIMENTAL TREATMENTS

Restorative therapy is used to enhance the survival and function of neurons that are prone to degeneration. One of the most direct ways to restore neuronal function is the administration of neurotrophins. Nerve growth factor is the best-characterized neurotrophin and, because of its action on cholinergic cells, the one most relevant to AD. Most of the acetylcholine in the cerebral cortex and hippocampus comes from cholinergic cells located in the ventral forebrain, but these cholinergic forebrain neurons, which degenerate early in the course of the disease, are also highly responsive to nerve growth factor. Another possible way to stimulate nerve cell growth in persons with AD is tissue transplantation, and this treatment is currently being studied in animals. However, both these approaches require careful study before they can be tested in humans.

CLINICAL RESEARCH IN ALZHEIMER'S DISEASE

In the area of clinical research, development of specific diagnostic criteria (McKhann et al., 1984) has brought accuracy rates close to 90%. Researchers continue to look for a specific biological marker or diagnostic test, however, to aid identification before the onset of clinical symptoms. Recent efforts to identify a diagnostic blood or skin test for AD have suggested that metabolic changes may occur in other body tissues in AD (Blass & Zemcov, 1984). Further research in this area should provide greater understanding of the pathophysiology of AD and may lead to the development of strategies to correct metabolic abnormalities early in the course of the disease. Gross structural changes also occur in the brains of persons with AD, including a decrease in brain weight and thickness of the cortical ribbon (Terry, Peck, DeTeresa, Schechter, & Houroupian, 1981). Increasing ventricular dilation has been correlated with increasing intellectual impairment, and physical measurement of the third ventricle is the single most powerful linear correlate of cognitive impairment (DeLeon, Ferris, & George, 1980).

Epidemiological and cross-cultural research efforts are also important to our understanding of the etiology of AD and have potentially significant societal implications, particularly with regard to risk factors. In addition to hereditary factors discussed earlier, environmental factors have been implicated in the onset of AD. In particular, brain trauma has been postulated as a major risk factor for AD (Graves et al., 1990). It is thought that head trauma, anoxia, or other insults to the brain, such as alcohol, may lead to the production of excess amounts of the amyloid precursor protein discussed above and to the development of neuritic plaques. For example, the brains of prize fighters who suffer from dementia pugilistica contain diffuse plaques and neurofibrillary tangles, although the latter are distributed differently than in AD.

Cross-cultural research conducted by five groups of researchers (Alzheimer's Association, 1994; Yu et al., 1989) has found that people with dementia are more likely to have lower levels of education than those without dementia. Some scientists have hypothesized that increased educational level leads to increased brain reserve that may delay onset of symptoms by up to 5 years in persons with AD. This theory is based on the notion that there is a threshold of brain activity below which a person must fall before symptoms appear. Others have speculated that "exercising the brain," through maintaining additional outside interests, such as using puzzles and games, may be a factor. Much more research is clearly needed to understand the role that level of education plays in AD. From a diagnostic and clinical perspective, it is essential to consider educational level in the interpretation of mental status exams. However, level of education may be confounded by other factors, such as access to medical care, occupational and recreational activities, income, chronic illnesses, nutrition, and life-style factors (such as alcohol intake and smoking), making the precise contribution of this variable to the risk of developing AD unclear (Alzheimer's Association, 1994).

Another study has linked myocardial infarctions to AD in the very old (Aronson et al., 1990), but this finding requires further investigation. Also, because several dementing disorders (e.g., Kuru, Creutzfeldt-Jacob disease) are caused by viral or infectious agents, it has been suggested that AD may also be caused by a virus or infection (Prusiner, 1984). At present no specific virus has been consistently associated with AD, although scientists are searching for viral DNA in the brains of persons with AD. Finally, theories related to exogenous toxins, especially through environmental exposure to aluminum and silicon, are plausible in that the neurofibrillary tangles and neuritic plaques found in the brains of persons with AD have been associated with high levels of aluminum (Perl & Brody, 1980). However, research in this area is quite inconsistent, and it may be that aluminum and silicon deposits are the result of cell degradation and death, rather than the cause. Clearly, more research is needed to determine which is the antecedent condition and to investigate the role of dietary metals such as calcium and magnesium (Burns & Buckwalter, 1988).

In summary, biomedical research in Alzheimer's disease is progressing at a rapid pace, and these basic and clinical research advances will have numerous direct applications to the care of persons with AD (Advisory Panel on Alzheimer's Disease, 1989). During the past decade important new discoveries have been reported almost monthly; therefore, the reader is urged to continue the pursuit of new information, as much of what is reported below will be "old" by the time this chapter is in print. We can expect that scientists will soon understand the etiology and pathophysiology of AD, that early and precise diagnosis will be widespread, and that clinicians will be able to identify individuals with precursors of AD and intervene to arrest or retard progress of the disease from the earliest stages. It is anticipated that within the next decade, the preventive and restorative effects of pharmacologic agents, environmental factors, and treatments such as infusion of nerve growth factor and cholinergic nerve cell implantation (Shapira, 1994; Fishman, 1986) will revolutionize care of the person with AD. Genetic engineering may also play a vital role in future treatment strategies. But until such time as a breakthrough in the cause and cure of Alzheimer's disease occurs, nurses continue to play an essential role in the education, support, and management of patients with AD and their families. It is also important for nurses to be able to advise families of the validity of proposed treatments, as desperate loved ones are often quick to latch on to the false hope of a miracle drug to cure the inexorably progressive course of AD (Burns & Buckwalter, 1988).

THE RELATIONSHIP BETWEEN BRAIN PATHOLOGY AND BEHAVIOR IN ALZHEIMER'S DISEASE

The very fabric of which the human brain is built is the substrate of cognition, emotion, and all of our faculties and, therefore, is also the substrate of the cognitive changes that occur in aging and in AD. (Burns & Buckwalter, 1988, p. 23)

COGNITIVE CHANGES

The brain is an organ, and like other organs of the body, it sometimes fails because of the influence of genetic and/or environmental factors. Brain aging involves a loss over time of the biophysiologic substrate of homeostatic and integrative neurologic mechanisms. The effects of this loss are then reflected at the behavioral level (Burns & Buckwalter, 1988). The work of DeLeon and colleagues (1980) cited earlier demonstrates this brain-behavior relationship in vivo in AD. Regression analyses conducted by these investigators indicated that global cognitive assessments (such as the Global Deterioration Scale and a mental status questionnaire) are the best predictors of both ventricular and cortical pathology (Burns & Buckwalter, 1988).

In Alzheimer's disease, memory impairment eventually becomes so marked that the affected individual is unable to follow a line of thought; converse; or recognize familiar objects, places, and persons. The inability to remember, calculate, concentrate, discriminate, and make decisions leads, in many cases, to a number of altered emotional states and behaviors, including anxiety and depression, irritability, agitation, and withdrawal. These behavioral aberrations, together with loss of ability to control motor functions (e.g., apraxia, incontinence) and deteriorating physical condition, often result in institutional placement (Burns & Buckwalter, 1988).

While most nurses are aware of these cognitive and behavioral changes, few appreciate the underlying pathophysiology. For example, memory dysfunction and emotional and personality changes in AD correlate with lesions in the limbic system. Agnosia, aphasia, and apraxia appear to be related to lesions of the temporoparietooccipital association cortex. Interestingly, the sparing of frontal lobes and the anterior cingulate gyrus may be related to the preservation of habitual personality traits, even late into the course of the disease (Burns & Buckwalter, 1988). This may lead to better relationships with caregivers as social skills are preserved for participation in social activities, such as dining; it also allows patients to maintain self-control at ap-

TABLE 14–1. RELATIONSHIP OF AREAS OF THE BRAIN TO BEHAVIOR CHANGE

Limbic system	Memory dysfunction, personality and emotional changes
Temporo-parietal lobes and neocortex	Agnosia, aphasia, apraxia, visual-spatial and perceptual alterations, loss of executive functions, hallucinations, delusions
Hippocampus	Memory loss
Temporal lobe	Alterations in speech
Frontal lobe	Personality traits, behavior, judgment
Cholinergic basal forebrain	Some relationship with severity of AD
Noradrenergic locus coeruleus and serotonic raphe nuclei	May relate to depressed affect
Amygdala and entorhinal cortex	Relationship to behavior unclear; possible decreases in learning and memory

From Whitehouse, P., Tabaton, M., & Lanska, D. (1991). Pathological and chemical correlates of dementia. In F. Corkin (Ed.), *Handbook of neuropsychology of aging* (Vol. 5, pp. 29–37). Amsterdam: Elsevier Science Publisher B.V.

propriate stimulus levels. It has even been hypothesized that an altered microenvironment and/or damaged neuronal membranes, secondary to a compromised blood-brain barrier, may be causally related to the manifestation of behavioral abnormalities in AD (Burns & Buckwalter, 1988). Table 14–1 demonstrates the relationship of brain pathology to behavioral alterations.

Sleep changes have been observed during all stages of AD and represent one of the most clear-cut relationships between biological and behavioral phenomena. There is a positive correlation between neuronal degeneration and sleep-wake disturbances; that is, more sleep-wake changes are noted in patients with more advanced disease (Poceta, 1991). This is not surprising, in that AD affects the brain stem region and neural pathways that regulate sleep-wake patterns in the cortical tissues. Research has shown that more severely impaired patients spend more time awake, awaken more often, and spend less time in short-wave and REM sleep than less severely impaired individuals, supporting the hypothesis that changes in sleep-wake variables parallel neuronal degeneration in AD. In an effort to compensate for lack of nighttime sleep, many patients with advanced AD take daytime naps, indicating a generalized disturbance in their circadian sleep-wake rhythm. At present, sleep-wake changes are not a discriminating biomarker for AD, but EEG variables obtained during sleep may be useful diagnostically (Poceta, 1991).

A compelling argument for psychiatric nurses to become more knowledgeable of brain pathophysiology in AD was set forth by Butcher and Woolf (1986), who noted that only when we fully understand how the brain is wired neurochemically will we be able to make meaningful correlations between structure and function. And only then will we be able to appreciate the behavioral consequences of the structural and functional alterations that result from the process of normal aging and from diseases such as AD (Burns & Buckwalter, 1988).

BEHAVIORAL CHANGES ASSOCIATED WITH ALZHEIMER'S DISEASE

Persons with Alzheimer's disease present with a variety of symptoms, although memory impairment, especially for recent events, is considered the hallmark. These symptoms may be conceptualized as clustering into four groups. The first three reflect losses in the intellectual, affective, and conative (planning) domains, as shown in Table 14–2, and represent the major nursing care problems associated with AD. The fourth symptom cluster, progressively lowered stress threshold (Hall & Buckwalter, 1987), refers to the fact that persons with dementia experience mounting frustration because of deficits in planning ability, intolerance to multiple and competing stimuli, and increased fatigue from the need to constantly process new information from the environment (Dawson, Kline, Wiancko, & Wells, 1986; Mace & Rabins, 1981). Not surprisingly, their tolerance for stress diminishes over the course of the disease, compounded by negative and restrictive feedback from caregivers and the environment. When the stress threshold is exceeded, behaviors such as purposeful wandering, agitated night awakening, and repetitive behaviors are manifested (Hall, 1988).

TABLE 14–2. CLUSTERS OF BEHAVIORAL SYMPTOMS AND ALTERATIONS IN THOUGHT PROCESSES DUE TO PROGRESSIVE DEGENERATION OF THE CEREBRAL CORTEX

1. Cognitive or intellectual losses
   A. Loss of memory, initially for recent events
   B. Loss of time sense
   C. Inability to abstract, such as understanding safety needs
   D. Inability to make choices and decisions
   E. Inability to reason and problem solve
   F. Poor judgment
   G. Altered perceptions
   H. Loss of language abilities
2. Affective or personality losses
   A. Loss of affect
   B. Diminished inhibitions, characterized by emotional lability, spontaneous conversation and loss of tact, loss of control of temper, and inability to delay gratifications
   C. Decreased attention span
   D. Social withdrawal
   E. Loss of recognition of others, environment, and, eventually, self (agnosia)
   F. Increasing self-preoccupation
   G. Antisocial behavior
   H. Confabulation, perseveration
   I. Psychotic features, such as paranoid ideation, delusions, and pseudohallucinations
   J. Increased fatigue with exertion or cognition, loss of energy reserve
3. Conative or planning losses
   A. Loss of general ability to plan activities
   B. Inability to carry out voluntary activities or those activities requiring thought to set goal, organize, and carry out
   C. Functional loss starting with high-level maintenance activities, such as money and legal management, shopping, and transportation; as the condition progresses, losses in activities of daily living, generally in the following order: bathing, grooming, choosing clothing, dressing, mobility, toileting, communicating, and eating
   D. Motor apraxia (the inability to plan and coordinate voluntary motor activity)
4. Progressively lowered stress threshold
   A. Catastrophic behaviors (sudden changes in behavior characterized by cognitive and social inaccessibility)
   B. Purposeful wandering
   C. Violent, agitated, or anxious behavior
   D. Purposeless behavior
   E. Withdrawal or avoidance behavior
   F. Compulsive repetitive behavior
   G. Other cognitively and socially inaccessible behaviors

Hall (1988) explicated three levels of patient behavior (baseline, anxious, and dysfunctional) that are important to understanding the concept of lowered stress threshold in AD. This concept is critical to management of the symptoms that result in this disorder.

- Baseline or normative behavior is a calm state incorporating the intellectual, affective, and planning losses noted in Table 14–2. Persons are cognitively and socially accessible (Wolanin & Phillips, 1981) and are able to function within the limits of neurologic capacity.
- Anxious behavior occurs when patients with AD experience internal or external stress. They attempt to avoid the offending stimuli but still react appropriately within the environment and remain open to communication. However, if the stress level continues or increases, the next level of behavior ensues.
- Dysfunctional or catastrophic behaviors (abrupt changes from normative behavior that are both cognitively and socially inaccessible) occur when the patient's stress threshold is crossed. This level of behavior is characterized by the patient's inability to communicate effectively and to respond appropriately to the environment. Dysfunctional behaviors are usually sudden in onset and of short duration, and episodes tend to increase as fatigue and stress increase throughout the day.

Both the symptoms listed in Table 14–2 and the levels of behavior described above are related to the progression or stage of the disease (Hall & Buckwalter, 1987). That is, baseline behaviors tend to diminish as the disease progresses, whereas anxious and dysfunctional behaviors increase in frequency, at least until the terminal stage. Concurrently, the stress threshold of the person with AD continues to decrease over the course of the illness.

MANAGEMENT OF BEHAVIORAL PROBLEMS ASSOCIATED WITH AD: UNDERSTANDING THE MANAGEABLE CAUSES

ASSESSMENT

Initial assessment of the person with AD should be a diagnostic evaluation. At this time, definitive diagnosis of AD is accomplished only by autopsy or biopsy, and the latter is not generally done. Diagnostic evaluations are therefore a process of excluding reversible causes of dementia by posing three primary questions (Hall, 1991b):

1. Is memory/cognitive loss present?
2. What could be causing the cognitive changes?
3. Are the findings consistent with what is known about AD?

The presence of memory loss is established by taking a thorough history of both cognitive and functional decline from patient and caregiver, often separately. The nurse should ask about changes in higher level functions, such as managing money and driving. Care must be taken to establish whether the person has a history of depression or other mental health problems. Historical findings should then be confirmed using a standardized mental status assessment, such as one listed in Table 14–3. The remainder of the diagnostic assessment consists of comprehensive physical, serologic, and imaging examinations to rule out treatable causes of dementia.

TABLE 14–3. SELECTED ASSESSMENT INSTRUMENTS FOR USE IN PERSONS WITH DEMENTIA

FACTORS	SELECTED INSTRUMENTS
Level of cognitive functioning (Includes factors such as orientation, recent and remote memory, perceptual ability, attention span/concentration, learning ability, problem solving, and judgment)	Short Portable Mental Status Questionnaire (Pfeiffer, 1975) Set Test (Isaacs & Kennie, 1973) Face-Hand Test (Kahn, Goldfarb, Pollack, & Peck, 1960). Alzheimer's Disease Assessment Scale (ADAS) Rosen, Mohs, & Davis, 1984) Blessed Dementia Rating Scale (Blessed, Tomlinson, & Roth, 1968) Cognitive Capacity Screening Examination (Jacobs, Bernard, Delgado, & Strain, 1977) Consortium to Establish a Registry in Alzheimer's Disease (CERAD) Neuropsychological Battery, including Mini Mental State Exam (Folstein, Folstein, & McHugh, 1975), Modified Boston Naming Test, Verbal Fluency Test, word list memory, word list recall, word list recognition, and testing of constructional praxis (McKhann et al., 1984) Clock Drawing Test (visual-spatial ability in AD) (Sunderland et al., 1989)
Stage of dementia	Global Deterioration Scale (Reisberg, Ferris, DeLeon, & Crook, 1982)
Multi-infarct dementia (differentiating vascular dementias from Alzheimer's disease)	Ischemic Score (Hachinski, Iliff, Zilhka, et al., 1975)
Functional abilities (Note: Some of these tools are for geriatric patients in general, not specific to AD.)	Geriatric Rating Scale (Plutchik et al., 1970) Multidimensional Functional Assessment: The OARS Methodology (Duke University, 1978) Direct Assessment of Functional Status (DAFS) Scale for Older Adults (Loewenstein et al., 1989)
Agitation/disruptive-aggressive behaviors (including measures of aggressive, physically nonaggressive, and verbally agitated behaviors)	Cohen-Mansfield Agitation Inventory (Cohen-Mansfield, 1986). Aggressive Behavior Scale (Ryden, 1988) Assessment of Behavioral Problems in Dementia: The Revised Memory and Behavior Problems Checklist (Teri et al., 1991)
Institutional behaviors (useful for evaluating residents with AD, but not necessarily specific to this population)	Nursing Home Behavior Problem Scale (NHBPS) (Ray, Taylor, Lichtenstein, & Meador, 1992) Multidimensional Observation Scale for Elderly Subjects (MOSES) (Helmes, 1988)
Activities of daily living for AD patients	Bathing Behaviors Observation Scale (Sloane, 1992) Beck Dressing Performance Scale (Beck, Heacock, Mercer, Walton, & Shook, 1991)
Caregiver burden and appraisal	Philadelphia Geriatric Center Caregiving Appraisal Scales (Lawton, Kleban, Moss, Rovine, & Glickman, 1989) Memory and Behavior Problems Checklist—Revised (Zarit, Todd, & Zarit, 1986)
Suitability for low-stimulus environment	Behavioral Assessment for Low Stimulus Care Plan (Hall, 1986)
Depression (not specific to AD)	Geriatric Depression Rating Scale (Yesavage et al., 1983) The Center for Epidemiological Studies Depression (CES-D) Scale (Radloff, 1977)
Social support (not specific to AD)	Social Provisions Scale (Cutrona & Russell, 1987)
Elder abuse and neglect (not specific to AD)	Elder Assessment Instrument (EAI) (Fulmer & Ashley, 1989) H.A.L.F. (Ferguson & Beck, 1983)

In planning care, the health care team should consider additional assessment criteria, such as patterns of behavior. How does the patient spend the day? How does that behavior change over the course of the day? What happens when the patient becomes fatigued or stressed? How does the family manage behavioral complications? It is also important to look for behaviors that suggest impulsivity, poor judgment, or lack of insight and to observe the patient navigating the environment. Does the patient overreach or underreach for items? Clues to visual-spatial perception will help to determine whether the patient is at risk for falls (Hall, 1991b).

Another area to evaluate is the patient's language abilities, for example, by having the patient write a sentence. Can the patient think of a phrase and write it down? Another approach is to find a humorous anecdote in large print and watch for a response when the patient reads it to you. Does the patient understand the humor? Can the patient explain the story to you? A patient who is unable to comprehend simple written materials will probably not respond to written signs, reminders, clocks, and calendars. Can the patient find words, or does the patient talk in generalities or describe objects? If this is occurring, it is usually safe to assume some receptive impairments also exist (Hall, 1991b).

It is often difficult to determine which interventions will work for which clients. Care of persons with AD should begin with longitudinal assessment covering a variety of factors, such as predisease personality, interests, activities, cultural identity, and level of social participation. This knowledge enables the nurse to better understand the client's spiritual and personal care needs, as well as the client's coping mechanisms and preferences for food, activities, and so on (Hall & Buckwalter, 1991). Functional assessment is also essential to the development of a sound plan of care. As the abilities of the client with AD change, progressing from a state of forgetfulness to impairment in activities of daily living (ADLs) and then on to immobility, the focus of care also changes. Thus, social and activity interventions common in the early states of the disease are eventually replaced by more skilled nursing care needs (Hall & Buckwalter, 1991). Throughout the illness, nurses must assess the environment for subtle cues (e.g., an open door that signals the client to leave) and then modify the environment to provide the message intended (e.g., strategic placement of a comfortable chair that invites the client to sit and rest), since clients may continue to respond to logical stimuli even after they are incapable of explaining what motivates them.

Many valid assessment instruments assist nurses with identifying clients suffering from chronic dementia, and each has a specific purpose. Table 14–3 identifies some of the more common assessment tools and the purpose of each.

Nurses must also continually assess for and deal with five basic categories of stressors that potentiate the likelihood of behavioral problems in clients with Alzheimer's disease: change of routine, physical stressors, fatigue, inappropriate stimuli, and excessive demands. Because of the complexity of symptom presentation and care, a conceptual model can prove useful in helping nurses and other caretakers to understand behavioral alterations (Hall, 1988). According to Hall and Buckwalter's (1987) Progressively Lowered Stress Threshold (PLST) Model, the above five factors temporarily heighten stress and thus may cause impaired individuals to exceed their stress threshold, thereby producing dysfunctional and catastrophic behaviors and leading to excess disability (Brody, Kleban, Lawton, & Moss, 1974; Dawson et al., 1986). The concept of excess disability refers to a situation in which functional limitations are greater than those directly attributable to the disease process itself. Fortunately, when the precipitating stressors are removed, the dysfunctional behaviors also tend to disappear. Monitoring, preventing, and managing these five factors, as discussed below, is critically important to care of the client with AD (Hall, 1988).

Change of Routine, Caregiver, or Environment

A consistent, highly structured routine (e.g., activities performed in the same way at about the same time of day) is preferable for care of the individual with AD, as this approach makes functioning more automatic and requires less thought. Any change in the environment or care routine, be it a new roommate, reconfiguration of furniture, or moving art therapy from mornings to midafternoon, can be problematic, in that the cognitively impaired individual must now rethink every new situation, which may lead to stress, frustration, and occasionally incapacity.

Physical Stressors

Because individuals with dementia are cognitively impaired, it is sometimes easy to forget that they are also vulnerable to acute and chronic illnesses or other factors such as adverse reactions to medications, pain, and/or discomfort. Thus, it is important for nurses to continually evaluate the presence of a variety of physical stressors that the client may not be able to articulate but that may cause dysfunctional behavior. Common examples include constipation, infections (especially of the upper respiratory and urinary tracts), ingrown toenails, full bladder, or arthritic joints.

Fatigue

Just as the ability to tolerate stress diminishes over the course of the illness, so, too, does the ability to tolerate activities. Persons with Alzheimer's disease tend to fatigue rapidly, and their program of care and the planning of special events should compensate for increased fatigability. For example, it is recommended that important activities (e.g., visiting the doctor) be scheduled in the morning hours, as the ability to tolerate activities tends to decrease over the course of the day; further, activities can be shortened (e.g., 45 minutes of music therapy versus 2 hours) to reflect principles of energy conservation. In particular, frequent breaks or rest periods are advised, especially in the midmorning and midafternoon and between potentially stressful activities.

Excess Demands

One of the most tragic features of Alzheimer's disease is that many affected individuals still appreciate that they were once able to undertake various tasks and functions, and they may continue to push themselves to perform despite current limitations. When confronted with their lack of ability and loss of function, or challenged to perform by well-meaning but misinformed caretakers, they often become anxious and stressed (Hall, 1988). Thus any internal or external demands to function that exceed the limits posed by cortical deterioration, such as caretaker demands to "just try harder to remember the names of your grandchildren," should be eliminated and replaced by the caregiver acting in a supportive role and serving as a memory prosthesis. In order to relieve stress and prevent the onset of dysfunctional behavior, caretakers must help rather than challenge the client who is unable to function; compensate for the client's losses, rather than test them; and distract clients when they are trying too hard.

Inappropriate Stimuli

Over the course of Alzheimer's disease, affected individuals lose the ability to process stimuli and to tolerate too much sensory input. Thus, in later stages, visual stimuli are commonly misinterpreted. Common examples include thinking people on television are in the room or avoiding use of the bathroom because the mirror represents a stranger in the room. Perceptual alterations of visual and auditory stimuli, together with normal age-related changes that make the older adult less able to manage distractions and background noise, become overwhelming. Therefore, nurses must continuously evaluate, and simplify as necessary, levels of sensory input. Particular attention should be paid to noise levels and sizes of groups. For example, is the crowded congregate dining hall, with its flurry of mealtime activities and noises from the kitchen, loud speakers, and so on, too much for the demented client to tolerate, so that the client attempts to avoid the situation and flee back to the room? Nurses can observe and record comfort or discomfort with a particular group size for future activity planning. The verbal and nonverbal behavior of the client serves as a barometer of tolerable levels of stimuli, and the wise caregiver heeds these cues. If these cues are ignored—so that intolerable levels of overwhelming, misleading, and competing stimuli are allowed to continue—hours of dysfunctional behavior may ensue, or the staff may find themselves dealing with a client who is awake, agitated, and pacing all night long.

Nurses should strive to control the factors of change of routine, physical stressors, fatigue, demands to exceed function, and overwhelming stimuli, for by so doing they can maximize the client's level of function. But the care approach does vary according to stage of the disease. Early on, most clients with AD can be taught to structure their own schedule and environment, for example, by using memory aids. Later, as they become increasingly susceptible to stressors, either family or staff caregivers must assume a more active role in monitoring and structuring the client's environment, using the client's response to evaluate the need for adjustment of the environment or simplification of routine (Hall, 1988). At all times, safety precautions must also be reinforced, and cognitively impaired clients must be protected from such hazards as wandering, getting burned by a stove, being scalded in a too-hot bath, or cutting themselves with sharp utensils.

CARE INTERVENTIONS IN ALZHEIMER'S DISEASE: WHOLE DISEASE CARE PLANNING

Hall and Buckwalter (1991) have set forth a model of care, whole disease care planning, based on nursing management of the client with AD according to stage of the disease. In the earliest, or forgetful, stage, the client loses things but compensates for the losses, attributing them to a variety of factors such as fatigue, stress, or illness. Depression is common in this stage. Few clients are identified at this stage, and most are living relatively normal lifestyles. Therefore, no care plan is identified at this point in the disease, although nurses should conduct careful assessment for common signs of depression, for example, alterations in sleep, appetite, and expressions of guilt or sadness. Once assessed, troubled individuals or family members should be encouraged to seek medical and/or psychological evaluation and treatment.

In the second stage, the confused stage, difficulties with instrumental activities of daily living—such as money management, transportation, home maintenance, shopping, and cooking—become obvious. Although overlearned skills are usually retained, individuals with AD gradually begin to withdraw from large social groups, as it becomes more difficult for them to manage outside the home environment. Clients may acknowledge that something untoward is happening to them and may complain of increasing anxiety and fatigue. Depressive feelings often persist into this stage, accompanied by disturbances in eating and sleep patterns.

During this stage, the client may lose perceptions of risk to safety or potential harm. It is not uncommon for second-stage clients to suffer from closed cranial trauma, burns, traumatic amputations, fractures, and cuts from accidents resulting from poor judgment. Automobile accidents, problems with lawnmowers or snow-blowers, smoking while using flammable substances, improper use of power tools, and accidents with kitchen equipment are common, as both client and family fail to recognize the danger and attempt to maintain function as long as possible.

At this point in the disease trajectory, family members begin to recognize that they are dealing with a problem beyond simple forgetfulness, and they initiate the diagnostic process. After diagnosis, nurses must begin a long-term counseling effort to assist clients and their families to cope with their grief and with the realities of this devastating, inexorably progressive illness. Support groups for families and victims of Alzheimer's disease may prove helpful.

The next stage, ambulatory dementia, is characterized by functional losses in basic ADLs progressing from problems with bathing, grooming, choosing attire, dressing, toileting, and ambulating to pushing a wheelchair. As ADLs become impaired, caretakers are advised to simplify the routine by breaking activities into basic components. For example, clients who are unable to completely bathe themselves may still be able to wash their hands and face and should be allowed and encouraged to do so.

Communication is an area that dramatically illustrates the integration of biological and behavioral changes in AD. Over the course of the disease, communication becomes increasingly problematic, and the affected individual experiences more difficulty understanding both written cues and spoken language. As higher order cortical processes degenerate, linguistic cues appear to be among the first affected; the pattern of deterioration apparently follows, in reverse order, that of language development (Emery, 1986). Table 14–4 demonstrates the approximate order of language loss.

A growing body of knowledge suggests that clinicians will be able to use specific alterations in verbal output to differentiate diagnostically between Alzheimer's-type dementia and other disorders with cognitive impairment (Murdoch, Chenery, Wilks, & Boyle, 1987). An excellent review of language changes in AD by Lee (1991) notes that there is variation in the effects of Alzheimer's disease on specific subsystems of language at different stages of the disease. Moreover, bicultural clients may return to their primary language before becoming aphasic. As basic communication skills diminish, nurses must pay particular attention to nonverbal communication, striving to interpret the client's body language and to send appropriate signals themselves, reinforcing verbal messages with gestures, illustrations, and other physical cues. Good eye contact is essential, and environmental distractors should be minimized. Ques-

TABLE 14–4. PROGRESSION OF LANGUAGE LOSS

Complex
    Loss of writing skills
    Loss of reading comprehension
    Inability to read
    Word-finding problems as demonstrated by circumlocution, loss of ability to name
        people and objects, poverty of thought
    Return to primary language
    Receptive and expressive aphasia
    Nonverbal communication
Simple

tions should be short and simple. The use of pronouns should be minimized because clients may not be able to grasp the reference. Similarly, requests or statements should be short, simple, and direct, avoiding, whenever possible, abstractions, analogies, or long-winded logical explanations. Further, because it takes persons with AD longer to process information, the nurse should allow adequate time for a response and be prepared to repeat the question or statement in exactly the same manner (Lee, 1991).

Behavioral and personality changes also become apparent in this stage, as the client becomes increasingly withdrawn and self-absorbed, with a flattened affect. Many of the behaviors noted earlier in Table 14–1 now emerge and tend to become worse later in the day. Perceptual difficulties compromise the ability to accurately interpret visual, auditory, and tactile stimuli. The ability to reason, recognize others, and use sound judgment with respect to safety is also impaired. Pseudohallucinations, in which the client mistakes common visual stimuli for something else, often develop in this stage. Some clients also begin to interpret the environment through past experiences—for example, thinking that the nursing home dining room is a truck stop—and behave accordingly. Reminiscence and validation approaches can assist persons with AD to better communicate their needs and feelings and to interpret the perceived environment. These therapeutic activities may also boost self-esteem.

In the ambulatory dementia stage the client becomes increasingly fearful of seeing anyone but the primary caretaker (usually still a family member early in this stage of the disease) and may become totally dependent on that individual for cueing and other forms of assistance. Despite this dependence, the client with AD may express feelings of anger, frustration, and ambivalence toward the caretaker, leading to feelings of helplessness and burnout on the part of the family care provider and precipitating institutionalization. Therefore, the family, and not just the identified client, should be considered in the nurse's plan of care. Family members should be listened to empathetically, referred for supportive community services such as respite care or ADRDA support groups, and encouraged to obtain legal and financial counseling (Weiler & Buckwalter, 1988). When the person with AD is institutionalized, the family should be viewed as a resource and ally and actively involved in programming, care conferences, and so on (Buckwalter & Hall, 1987).

In the end stage, or terminal stage, of the disease little purposeful activity or recognition of others is apparent. Once the client is immobile, physical nursing care intensifies. During this final stage, persons with AD are incapable of self-care activities and often forget how to eat, chew, and swallow. They lose weight and become vulnerable to infections and skin breakdown. Primitive reflexes that disappeared during infancy—for example, sucking and rooting reflexes and primitive grasp—return. These reflexes may enhance feeding function as the nurse may try squeeze bottles with straws or bottle feedings with enlarged nipples. Some clients are mute at this point in the disease, whereas others scream spontaneously. Clients who scream or call out spontaneously should be evaluated carefully for the presence of pain, discomfort, depressive symptoms, and seizure activity.

Although the care plan at this stage is primarily focused on hygienic measures and physiologic requirements (e.g., adequate hydration and nutrition, repositioning, bowel and bladder regimens), clients should be closely monitored for signs of discomfort, fear, and isolation. There are few well-developed and rigorously tested care interventions for the terminal stage, and more research is clearly needed in this area. Selected activities, such as music, massage, and video or audio tapes of family members, are often soothing and communicate caring.

There is a growing body of research and clinical literature on nutritional needs during the end stage. However, it is critical that the nurse understand the family's wishes and state laws regarding parenteral feeding, life support measures, and so on and be knowledgeable of legal issues such as living wills and other forms of advance directives that may influence practice at this stage of the disease (Hall, 1991a).

Care Interventions in Alzheimer's Disease: The Progressively Lowered Stress Threshold (PLST) Model

The PLST model (Hall & Buckwalter, 1987) offers assistance to nurses in managing care of demented clients in the confused and ambulatory dementia stages of the disease. The model emphasizes the need for individualized interventions, based on the unique needs and abilities of the client with Alzheimer's disease and family member(s), although some basic principles are applicable to various clients and care settings. The following interventions flow logically from the PLST model and form the basis of the nursing plan of care (Buckwalter & Smith, 1991).

REDUCE ENVIRONMENTAL STRESS

As noted earlier, stress in the environment often contributes to dysfunctional behavior in persons with AD. Relatively easy and yet important interventions that contribute to managing environmental stress include the elimination of caffeine, of potentially frightening and misleading stimuli (such as television, artwork with large eyes or animal figures, mirrors), of unending spaces, of unnecessary noise (such as public address systems, radios), of extra people, and of large groups. Other successful environmental modifications include eating in small groups rather than large congregate settings and serving only one food at a time.

Pleasant decor and personal items enhance the client's sense of well-being and provide links to the past to cue desired socially appropriate behavior. Care should be taken to personalize the environment with objects such as a favorite chair, letters from home, video visits from absent family members, pillows, pictures, afghans, and albums of family photographs that have been reproduced to prevent loss.

COMPENSATE FOR CLIENT'S PLANNING DEFICITS

Excess disability may be minimized by compensating for the client's lost abilities. Interventions to promote optimal functioning include providing a calm, consistent routine; eliminating changes of pace and environment; and keeping choices only to those the client can handle. It is best not to ask the client to "try harder," attempt to teach new routines, or encourage trying to recover lost skills. Occupational therapists can assist with task analysis to simplify new activities and preserve remaining skills.

PROVIDE UNCONDITIONAL POSITIVE REGARD

Although clients with AD have difficulty communicating their needs and desires (Lee, 1991), nurses and other caretakers must resist the temptation to treat them as objects or children rather than as the adult persons they are. Interpersonal respect is communicated in a variety of ways, including using touch to reassure, allowing the client to use remaining social skills, using reminiscence and validation rather than forcing "reality orientation," eliminating the negative (e.g., "you're wrong!") messages from the environment, promoting one-to-one communication, and distracting, rather than confronting, the client. Reassuring therapies such as music, validation, reminiscence groups, and therapeutic recreation have also been used successfully with this population.

ALLOW FOR LOWERED STRESS THRESHOLD AND DIMINISHED ENERGY RESERVE

A number of nursing interventions can help the client with AD to better manage fatigue and other anxiety-provoking stimuli. Examples of such interventions are providing rest periods midmorning and midafternoon and alternating high stimulus activities with quiet ones or rest periods. If catastrophic reactions occur, the nurse should immediately decrease the amount of environmental stimuli and reevaluate stressors, including conducting a physical assessment. If future episodes are to be prevented, it is essential to keep detailed records that suggest possible cause-and-effect relationships between environmental stressors and dysfunctional behavior.

Whether the client remains in the home or is institutionalized, record keeping of catastrophic events will help caregivers develop a sense of mastery in managing care. When a catastrophic event occurs, the caregiver should record the time of day, antecedent or precipitating events, a description of observed behavior, the length of the event, and management techniques. Antecedent events may occur up to 24 hours prior to a catastrophic episode and may include a large group activity, a children's birthday party, a trip, remodeling or redecorating the client's environment, holiday decorations and activities, a visit to a shopping mall, a tiring day, or lunch at a buffet restaurant. Appendix 14-1 demonstrates a log for in-home caregivers to record catastrophic events.

Education on catastrophic events is especially important for in-home caregivers, as these episodes are often frightening and may involve physical aggression. Caregivers need to understand the antecedent-behavior link, realize that episodes are time-limited but may recur, be familiar with management strategies, and know that clients are most vulnerable to injury during a catastrophic event. Nurses may serve as an ongoing resource in helping in-home caregivers identify antecedents and prevent catastrophic events, thereby limiting the caregivers' feelings of isolation and frustration.

In addition to limiting stressors, the nurse should assist caregivers to develop care strategies that use the customs, life-style preferences, and activities developed over a lifetime. Emphasis should be placed on preserved abilities. Occupational therapists are very helpful in identifying these skills. Care planning should be highly individualized and flow logically throughout the disease process. For example, clients in the confused stage often enjoy highly stimulating activities they have always found meaningful. They can often rely on written cues, clocks, and calendars. In the third stage, the previous activities are simplified, noise and group size are decreased, and the client must rely on people for cueing.

Table 14–5 sets forth a care plan for clients with chronic dementia of the Alzheimer's type.

In summary, care of persons with Alzheimer's disease is complex and changes over the course of the illness. Therefore, nursing strategies are best developed from a conceptual perspective, such as the whole disease care planning and PLST models presented. Using these models, new interventions can easily be evaluated in terms of behavioral outcomes, and the care individualized. Care is also logically derived from the nurse's understanding of the client's premorbid characteristics, sociocultural background, and level of functional loss(es). Intervention strategies arise from the client's daily routine, which is modified as the disease progresses. As noted by Hall and Buckwalter (1991):

> The desired outcomes at all levels of care are to maximize the potential for safe function by controlling for excess disability and providing appropriate levels of assis-

TABLE 14–5. NURSING INTERVENTION STRATEGIES

NURSING INTERVENTION	RATIONALE
Loss of Cognition Collect baseline data on client behavior. Train staff and family caregivers to prevent fearfulness. Individualize care plans. If admitted to a facility, match stimulus level to that of home.	Persons with dementia lose cognitive abilities and can become easily overstimulated, withdrawn, or anxious.
Loss of Planning Develop a schedule client can follow daily. Post schedule where it can be easily seen (e.g., Kardex, room), so other caregivers will not vary from it.	Persons with dementia lose conative abilities and function better with a routine (i.e., with a routine, they don't have to plan activities).
Loss of Stress Tolerance Have client rest in recliner or spend quiet time in room for about 40 minutes midmorning and midafternoon. Use afghans and other environmental cues to define rest periods. Avoid caffeine, activities, and visitors during the rest periods. Train staff and family caregivers to recognize mounting tension and anxiety. When anxiety is noted, remove client to quiet area. Do not restrain unless injury to client will result. In nursing homes, avoid communal dining in favor of two or three residents at a table in a quiet area.	As dementia progresses, the client's stress threshold becomes progressively lower; clients become increasingly unable to tolerate stress.
Loss of Recent Memory Avoid reality testing and reality orientation, unless client requests it or safety is threatened. Use reminiscence and validation approaches instead. Recognize that behavior may be rooted in past perceptions.	Clients with dementia experience memory loss with destruction of brain cells in the hippocampal region. Challenging them to recall forgotten data and remember current events only leads to frustration for both the client and the caregiver.
Decreased Ability to Perceive Multiple Stimuli Avoid misleading and frightening stimuli, such as TVs, mirror images, art work representing animals or humans, and some geometric images. Use easy listening music, music from the person's era, or favorite music prior to the onset of dementia. Avoid large group activities in favor of one-to-one or small group activities. Simplify activities (e.g., sorting, stacking, gross motor activities). Encourage activities that appeal to basic senses of touch, taste, and smell. Remove glare and shine from highly waxed floors and, if possible, avoid use of public address systems.	As dementia progresses, the client's ability to accurately perceive environmental stimuli decreases. Sounds and images that are misperceived can be extremely frightening and often lead to wandering and other agitated/aggressive behaviors.

Table continued on following page.

TABLE 14–5. Nursing Intervention Strategies *Continued*

NURSING INTERVENTION	RATIONALE
Loss of Ability to Choose and Decide Lay out clothing for client and promote similarity in attire. Keep choices and decisions simple and at a level client can handle. Do not force client to make choices. Minimize options and need to choose if client becomes frustrated or is unable to respond. Also simplify mealtime with fewer utensils and food choices.	Loss of ability to make choices and decisions is characteristic of Alzheimer's disease. Forcing clients to make choices, or providing them with too many options only frustrates them and prevents them from participating at an optimal level in activities of daily living such as eating and dressing.
Loss of Sense of Time If client awakens at night, increase the number or duration of daytime rest periods. Provide a bedtime snack. When client awakens, take him/her to the toilet and then allow the client to remain in a safe, common area. Engage in quiet activity and provide snack. Do not restrain in bed. Use photosensitive night lights rather than turning on lights, as normal lighting cues the client that it is morning.	In Alzheimer's disease, day-night disorientation is a common phenomenon and troubling to caregivers and other residents whom the demented client may disturb. Increasing rest periods during the day helps to diminish the cumulative effects of stress and promotes better nighttime sleep. Feeding and toileting the client with dementia may alleviate the drive that awoke him/her in the first place, so that the client can return to sleep. Restraining or forcing the demented client back to bed will only increase agitation and level of disruption.
Weight Loss Avoid group dining areas. Provide extra time and quiet with one or two other clients when eating. Have family provide favorite foods, snacks, especially foods from the client's culture. Use punch bowl in activity areas to encourage consumption of fluids, and provide high caloric "finger food" snacks that may be carried around in paper bag by clients who wander.	As dementia progresses, clients may become more anorexic and suffer from dysphagia, while still remaining physically active. Also, communal dining experiences often prove too stressful for the client with dementia, who, in the process of trying to avoid the stimuli, does not consume adequate amounts of food and fluids. Eating in small groups preserves the normative social experience of dining without the chaos of a congregate dining hall. All these factors can lead to compromised nutritional status and weight loss in persons with dementia.

tance; encourage participation in activities as desired by the client; minimize discomfort caused from physical and emotional stressors; and maximize expressions of comfort. (p. 41)

CAREGIVERS

The family is the primary health care provider for persons with AD and related disorders (ADRD) (Daniels & Irwin, 1989; Miller, McFall, & Montgomery, 1991). Approximately 70% of all dementia patients are cared for at home by family members,

TABLE 14–5. NURSING INTERVENTION STRATEGIES *Continued*

NURSING INTERVENTION	RATIONALE
Communication Loss Assess client's ability to read, write, comprehend, and express self. Use touch to reassure when communicating and voice inflection, facial expression, and gentle gestures to add meaning. If message is not understood, repeat it exactly. Stand directly in front of client, your face at eye level or below. Use one-to-one communication, and provide plenty of time for a response. Allow client the comfort of using any preserved social graces. Use title and last name when addressing the client, unless he/she invites you to do otherwise.	In Alzheimer's disease, clients lose the ability to communicate verbally and to understand the communication of others in a meaningful manner. Therefore, nonverbal communication, especially gestures and touch, assume a major role in efforts to communicate with demented clients, along with other principles of good communication. Even if the clients are unable to communicate meaningfully, they should be talked to with respect and dignity.
Fearfulness Allow increased time for all activities. Use reminiscence and validation approaches and remaining social skills to give client a sense of control in fearful situations. If client is confused or agitated, decrease environmental stimuli and simplify routine. Provide soft, reassuring objects and colors. Verbally reassure clients that they are safe and that you will help them.	With progressive memory loss as the hallmark of Alzheimer's disease, every activity is potentially new and frightening and every person encountered may be regarded as a "stranger." Caregivers must therefore assist the demented client to feel as safe and in control of situations as possible, through environmental management and verbal reassurance. Validation and reminiscence techniques serve to increase the clients' self-esteem, rather than to challenge their abilities and highlight their losses.
Incontinence Provide a regular schedule of bathroom visits. Avoid use of oral laxatives and enemas— use high-fiber diet, fluids, and exercise instead. If client is chronically constipated, use a stimulant suppository (such as Dulcolax) immediately prior to the first meal every day or every other day. Limit fluids after 6 p.m.	Loss of control of bowel and bladder occurs commonly in Alzheimer's disease and is a major precipitant of institutionalization. Oral laxatives and enemas decrease the client's control and are therefore to be avoided. Judicious use of stimulant suppositories, on the other hand, incorporates the gastro-colic reflex, insuring complete evacuation.

Table continued on following page.

and spouses typically are the primary caregivers. This trend is expected to continue with projected cutbacks in services, such as respite for this population (Grant, Patterson, Hauger, & Irwin, 1992; Neundorfer, 1991), so the associated burdens of care placed on families and society at large have emerged as one of the most serious issues facing our society today (Buckwalter, 1989).

The costs associated with ADRD are staggering, and with anticipated increases in the age of our population, the cost of care is expected to rise dramatically. Ernst and Hays (1994) estimated the costs of caring for 1.6 million victims at $82.7 billion this

TABLE 14–5. Nursing Intervention Strategies *Continued*

NURSING INTERVENTION	RATIONALE
Safety Concerns	
Supervise client when bathing, while eating, and during activities. Stairways and doors should always be monitored, including the use of some type of door-alarming device whenever possible. Clients should not be allowed access to hot objects, such as coffee pots, radiators, or hot water taps, without supervision. Medications and potentially hazardous substances, such as shaving lotion, should be carefully administered. All sharp or potentially dangerous materials should be kept out of the patient's reach. Spills must be wiped up when discovered. Clients who use adaptive devices, such as canes, for weapons should be supervised in their use. Other residents, staff, and visitors should be reminded not to confront confused residents who are in the wrong area. Take agitated residents to a quiet area. Residents who can no longer walk, but continue to try and are in danger of injuring themselves, should be restrained in the least restrictive manner possible, and only after other alternatives have been tried and failed.	Persons with dementia lose "semantic memory" for such things as rules that govern behavior and activities. Thus, concepts such as "no right turn on red" or "caution—do not enter" become meaningless. This is compounded by the fact that as the disease progresses, persons with dementia experience increasing difficulty interpreting the written word (signs), and their judgment and ability to anticipate danger become markedly impaired. Moreover, residents whose reality is altered and who may believe, for example, that they are "going to work " or "home to take care of their children" are at great risk for elopement and must be monitored carefully and continuously. Confronting them with reality (e.g., "stay right here, your children are dead") may lead to physical and verbal aggression. Thus clients with dementia are at great risk for injuring themselves or others in their immediate environment. With the passage of OBRA '87, there has been diminished use of physical and chemical restraints with this population and more emphasis on alternative management approaches.
With institutionalization, families should be oriented to the safety policies and procedures of the facility in order to understand that the client will not be unduly restrained and that the staff will not be able to prevent all episodes of wandering. Families must understand that clients with dementia may have injuries which are not preventable without severely restricting the resident's movement and mobility.	Families may feel that freedom to wander represents a lack of concern or insufficient staff attention. They should be informed of the reasons behind less restrictive environmental controls, as well as conditions under which restraint may be necessary to prevent injury and harm.

year. Using the same formula, the Alzheimer's Association (1994) projects future costs of caring for an estmated 4 to 5 million victims of dementing illness will be $1.75 trillion. Direct medical costs are a nominal expense (approximately $14,140 over a 4-year period) (Ernst & Hays, 1994). In 1994, the total cost to care for a loved one over a 4-year period—from diagnosis to death—was estimated at $213,700, which represents a $39,800 increase since 1991 (Ernst & Hays, 1994), and only about 10% of these expenses are covered by third-party payers, or federal and state governments. Federal agencies pay for less than 4% of care provided (Doty, Liu, & Wiener, 1985). Therefore, containment of long-term care costs will depend on American families.

TABLE 14–5. NURSING INTERVENTION STRATEGIES *Continued*

NURSING INTERVENTION	RATIONALE
Family Concerns	
The nurse and social worker should, whenever possible, conduct a preadmission assessment to meet the resident and family, assess needs, and explain programs of care. If the resident has been transferred from another facility, the assessors should gain permission to visit the potential client and family in that facility.	Alzheimer's disease affects more than the victim—the entire family constellation is affected. In many cases families approach a placement decision with despair, feeling as though they have somehow failed in their ability to provide care, or have abandoned their loved one. Family members need an opportunity to discuss these concerns and fears with staff and other family members in a supportive environment. Often the family has been caring for the person with dementia for many years and has become the "expert." Staff should encourage and value this input and should help recreate, whenever possible, the routines and behavioral approaches the family used before placement.
Family members should be encouraged to choose a time for visiting, to be included in the resident's consistent schedule. Visitors should be encouraged to visit in small groups and recognize resident fatigue, limiting their visit when fatigue occurs. Family should anticipate the first visits to be emotional or difficult, understanding that they can discuss this with the nurse, social worker, or peer counselor. Visitors should be discouraged from visiting during rest hours.	If families are not adequately prepared to visit their loved one, it can be a time of high stress for both the resident and family member—resulting in agitation and disruptive behaviors for the staff to contend with following the visit. This unfortunate event can foster an adversarial rather than complementary relationship between families and staff.
Visitors should be encouraged to bring a small indication of celebration when they visit, such as flowers, food, pictures, or an object from the past to talk about. Families can make anecdotal booklets of reminiscences to help them visit. Teach the family to participate in simple activities or administer simple adult games. Minimize visits outside the facility if the resident becomes agitated, wanders, or is up at night following an outside visit.	It is important for staff to work in partnership with family members, to teach them about the disease, the care plan, factors that can precipitate stress, and how they can best be involved in the care of their loved one. Families can very effectively continue in a modified caregiving role after institutionalization; they should feel satisfied with the care their family member receives and feel that they are an important part of the care delivery team. Too often, however, families are a "neglected resource" in long-term care facilities.

Table continued on following page.

The average American family spends about $20,900 per year on in-home care services or about $40,000 per year for a loved one in a nursing home (Ernst & Hays, 1994). Two thirds of the expenses are out-of-pocket (Ernst & Hays, 1994). The length of the illness, behavioral symptoms, and often overwhelming expense have resulted in family crises. Families are often ill-equipped to understand

TABLE 14–5. NURSING INTERVENTION STRATEGIES *Continued*

NURSING INTERVENTION	RATIONALE

Family Concerns (cont.)

Have family members attend a monthly support group where they can voice their concerns about care and receive feedback from other families. This also provides opportunities for continuing education. Have family members who express social isolation or the need for more contact perform volunteer activities in the facility (e.g., assist with meals, bathing, co-lead reminiscence or music/movement groups). Encourage families to attend care planning sessions, communicating that they are an important part of the care process and can come to staff with any concerns they may have. Provide ongoing feedback until all concerns are resolved.

Wandering

Tactile Wanderers

The nurse should redirect the client away from hallways and doors. For chronic elopement, door knobs may be modified and alarm systems used. Clients can often be redirected to other tactile objects. The staff can also supervise client walking.

There are several different types of "wanderers" for whom different nursing interventions may be appropriate. Some persons with dementia who are nearing the end of the ambulatory dementia phase may spend time using their hands to explore the environment. Some may appear to be blind and unable to interpret visual cues consistently. They remain calm and appear to elope by accident as they continue to feel their way through doorways and down halls. These tactile wanderers have often lost the ability to communicate verbally as well.

Environmentally Cued Wanderers

Some facilities build tracks or identify wandering pathways in halls for these clients. Other facilities provide cues to stop (e.g., shortening hallways, providing chairs, locating stop signs at doors, disguising doors with pictures and mirrors to provide a new set of environmental cues).

Environmentally cued wanderers appear calm and tend to follow cues within the environment. If they see a window, they look out it; a chair may cue them to sit; or a door may indicate an exit. Hallways provide cues to keep pacing. These clients elope on a regular basis and may appear to be searching. They respond well to nonrestrictive environmental barriers and concrete indicators of territory. They are usually in the mid- to late-ambulatory dementia phase, requiring assistance for at least bathing and dressing.

TABLE 14–5. NURSING INTERVENTION STRATEGIES *Continued*

NURSING INTERVENTION	RATIONALE
Environmentally Cued Wanderers (cont.) The nurse should assess the environment for cues to wander. Doors may be disguised with wall coverings that either conceal or divert clients. Door windows can be curtained or covered with "mirror plastic" so the client will try to avoid contact. Special closures can be fitted to the door so that the demented client is unable to open it. Chairs and other cues to stop and rest should be provided. When no barrier is present, one may be created by adhering a double line of brightly colored tape (red or yellow) to the floor. Diversionary activities, such as music therapy, are useful in keeping the client's attention.	
Reminiscent/Fantasy Wanderers The nurse should gently remind the client that he/she does not have to go to work, do chores, or see parents at this time. A fantasy area might be created, such as a desk with papers on it, an area for the housewife to clean up, or stacks of foam for the person to restack.	These residents are calm and in the ambulatory dementia phase of the illness. The desire to elope stems from a delusion or fantasy, usually based in the person's past (e.g., a person going to work, seeing parents, or doing chores). Frequently, the client announces that he/she is leaving and is reassured that there is a specific place to go.
The nurse may also find that validation of the meaning of the delusion, for example, the feelings of worth associated with work, will distract the client. Use of the term "later" and diversional activities also help.	
Recreational Wanderers The nurse should plan for a staff member to take the client for a walk each day at the same time. Walks should follow exactly the same route each day, beginning and ending at the same place. This will help staff to locate clients should they elope. Walking the clients is an excellent way for staff to interact on a one-to-one basis and reminisce with clients.	Recreational wanderers may be in the confused or ambulatory dementia phases of the illness. They may have a history of an active life-style prior to becoming ill or may have been taken for walks regularly by a caregiver. The wandering is purposeful, recurs regularly, usually at the same time, and appears to serve a need for exercise. The client is calm, unless stopped.

Table continued on following page.

symptoms and progression of the disease, basic care and behavioral management techniques, crisis intervention strategies, long-term care planning, and strategies for self-preservation. As discussed in this section, overburdened, ill-prepared families suffer consequences such as social isolation, stress-related illness, adult abuse, financial ruin, mental health problems, and even suicide. Support of caregiving families through education, research, and provision of innovative AD-ca-

TABLE 14–5. Nursing Intervention Strategies *Continued*

NURSING INTERVENTION	RATIONALE
Agitated Purposeful Wanderers IMMEDIATE INTERVENTIONS The staff should not confront the resident but try to diffuse the situation. Tell the client about staff fear and concerns. Offer suggestions, such as waiting for a glass of juice, that will buy time to allow the client to regain composure. Use preserved social skills to allow client maximum control of the situation. Remove offending stressors.	These clients are upset, fearful, agitated, and/or exhibiting stress-related dysfunctional behavior. They are cognitively and socially inaccessible. Preoccupied with leaving, the client may pack suitcases to take home. Staff will be generally unable to reason with the client and may recognize the client's fear of them. Staff who attempt to remove control from the resident may be assaulted as the resident attempts to maintain control by fleeing and panics. Once recognized, agitated purposeful wandering can be prevented.
If the client leaves, accompany or follow, with a coat when appropriate. Bring back as quickly as possible, providing measures to decrease stress. This may include tranquilizing medications. Assure safety and security. PREVENTION OF FURTHER EPISODES Evaluate the cause of the incident. Reduce the amount of stimulus client is exposed to; increase rest periods or attempt to decrease stressors from others, such as negative feedback from visitors. These clients may benefit from a protected environment where unconditional positive regard is provided and environmental stimuli reduced.	

pable and friendly services becomes a primary mission in the care of persons with dementia and their families.

Although, as noted above, the financial costs of caring for a person with dementia are staggering, the human costs of this devastating illness may be even more overwhelming and cannot be overestimated. The effects on caretakers are both financially and personally devastating, as they watch their loved ones become increasingly confused, incapable of communicating or carrying out everyday activities, undergoing personality and emotional changes, and losing control of elementary physical functions over an unpredictable clinical course that often lasts 8 to 10 years.

A number of converging trends suggest that demands on family caregivers will only continue. These include increased longevity, geographic dispersion of the family, the need for many caregivers (especially women) to enter the work force, and changing patterns of marriage and child care (Advisory Panel on Alzheimer's Disease, 1989). There is an ever increasing number of "old-old," who require care from adult children and spouses who themselves may be elderly and infirm. The increasing mobility of our society also diminishes access to family care, and increases in maternal age at the birth of the first child mean that more and more caregivers are experiencing "double dependency," that is, caring for both a parent and child simultaneously, a situation Brody (1985) has labeled "the Sandwich Generation."

The growing volume of caregiver literature has identified a number of factors that affect the functioning of the caretaker. Among the most prominent are coping styles of the caretaker, past relationship with the patient, gender, socioeconomic status, and the accessibility of support networks, both formal and informal (Brody, 1985; Cantor, 1983; George & Gwyther, 1986; Zarit & Zarit, 1982). Caretakers report they need assistance obtaining information regarding community resources and dealing with their feelings of grief, depression, and anger (Grunow, 1988).

Geographic location also appears to have an impact on the caregiving process in terms of different patterns of health service utilization and use of informal versus formal support systems (Blieszner, McAuley, Newhouse, & Mancim, 1987; Scott & Roberto, 1985). In general, caretakers in rural environments tend to rely more on informal support networks, whereas their urban counterparts utilize formal organizations more frequently for tasks such as homemaking, personal care, and meal preparation.

Although caring for a relative with AD is among the most difficult forms of family responsibility, caretakers often receive inadequate support and training for the task. Thus, they may become physically and emotionally exhausted and face social deprivation and financial ruin. Dementia is unquestionably a family affair, as families today provide more care to a greater number of older people than at any other time in our history (Advisory Panel on Alzheimer's Disease, 1989).

A vast amount of research and literature, including entire books, has been written on the caregiving experience (see, for example, a comprehensive evaluation of the literature by Kuhlman, Wilson, Hutchinson, and Wallhagen [1991]; Light and Lebowitz's 1989 book *Alzheimer's Disease Treatment and Family Stress: Directions for Research;* and a review of the psychiatric and physical morbidity effects of caregiving by Schultz, Visintainer, and Williamson, [1990]). However, few studies, with the notable exception of the work of Vitaliano, Maiuro, Ochs, and Russo (1989), have examined caregiver burden using theoretical models of distress to guide the research effort. Fewer still have examined in detail the cultural and ethnic issues related to Alzheimer's disease (Valle, 1989). Despite these gaps in the literature and inconsistencies in the research methods used, studies overwhelmingly point to the adverse effects of caregiving for a person with dementia. Of particular note are the large number of methodologically rigorous studies citing caregiver depression as a major outcome. Other replicated findings include high levels of caregiver hostility; caregiver ill health and physical and emotional strain; increased psychotropic drug use and stress-related symptoms among caregivers; higher rates of health care utilization, including more physician visits and prescription medications; and development of asocial behaviors (Rabins, Mace, & Lucas, 1982; Schultz et al., 1990). Space limitations of this chapter preclude a thorough review of the literature in this domain. Therefore, the following sections will provide an abbreviated overview of caregiver burden and stress, the physical and psychosocial morbidity associated with caregiving, social and financial responses, cultural and ethnic issues, the continuum of care, and nursing intervention studies related to caregiving.

CAREGIVER BURDEN AND STRESS: OVERVIEW

The notion of burden or stress has emerged as an important concept in caregiver research and has been defined as "the physical, psychological or emotional, social and financial problems that can be experienced by family members caring for impaired older adults" (George & Gwyther, 1986, p. 243). Spouses of AD patients may be at greatest risk for caregiver stress as they are often themselves elderly and may have physical problems that limit their ability to respond to caregiving demands (Pruchno & Resch, 1989; Kuhlman et al., 1991). Major findings from the current literature on caregiver stress suggest that psychological morbidity (especially depression) is a frequent negative outcome associated with the caregiving experience. Decline in health status as a result of caregiving is also frequently reported by caregivers, but data on the physical health consequences of caregiving are inconclusive (Schultz et al., 1990).

CARE-RECIPIENT BEHAVIORS THAT PROMOTE STRESS

A number of investigators have concluded that catastrophic reactions, waking at night, incontinence, suspiciousness, and poor communication are most problematic for caregivers of persons with AD (Chenoweth & Spencer, 1986; Gmeiner, 1987; Rabins et al., 1982). Other reported troublesome behaviors include repetitive questions; wandering; embarrassing, dangerous, and hostile behaviors; and difficulty in bathing, cooking, and managing money (Grunow, 1988; Quayhagen & Quayhagen, 1988). A number of variables—for example, the more rapid the perceived rate of the AD patient's decline, the older the spouse caregiver, the greater the reported level of fatigue, and the more restless and less verbal the patient—are related to whether the caretaker is more likely to institutionalize. In fact, those variables, along with ease of food preparation, were predictive of institutional versus home-based care in the vast majority of AD patients and their families studied (Maas & Buckwalter, 1991).

FACTORS THAT PROMOTE ASSISTANCE-SEEKING AND INSTITUTIONALIZATION

The level of cognitive dysfunction in the patient with AD is not the only factor in the family's decision to institutionalize. Importantly, many researchers have cited the demands associated with the constant care of a person with dementia as a precipitating factor in the decision to place someone in an institution (Stevens, Walsh, & Baldwin, 1993), although the role of patient disability or severity of patient problems has only been weakly correlated with burden among dementia caregivers (George & Gwyther, 1986; Zarit, Todd, & Zarit, 1986). Chenoweth and Spencer (1986) found that the most common symptoms that prompted over half of the family members surveyed to seek assistance included memory loss and problems related to personality changes; physical functional losses; and problems with work, driving, money management, and drinking. The inadequate response of the health care professions to families at the time of diagnosis is reflected in the fact that 54% of family members were told that the situation is hopeless and that nothing could be done for them, while another 20% received no explanation or information. Only 28% of those surveyed reported they received a factual, adequate explanation of the disease, and a mere 16% received any advice on caregiving needs or how to cope with the stressful behavioral problems associated with AD. Family members also noted that they sought and found most helpful a physician's advice regarding institutional placement of their loved one. Wilson (1989) identified the primary social-psychological problem experienced by family caretakers as confronting negative choices, which she defined as "different degrees of impossibility" and "undesirable alternatives" (p. 95).

RELATIONSHIP BETWEEN PSYCHOLOGICAL STRESS AND PHYSICAL MORBIDITY

Alterations in physiological functioning as a result of exposure to stress have been found to increase the probability of disease or illness (Brantley & Garrett, 1993).

Similarly, psychological stress and major life events can increase vulnerability to illness by compromising the integrity of the immune system (Kiecolt-Glaser & Glaser, 1987). The exact mechanism by which immunologic function moderates the effects of stress on health is not known. Most of the caregiving literature that examines the physical effects of caregiving has used one or more of the following indicators of caregiver health: (1) self-reported health status, (2) self-reported incidence of illness-related symptoms; (3) self-reported utilization of health care services, (4) self-reported medication use, and (5) biological indicators as a measure of susceptibility to disease (Garand, 1993). Findings from these studies are summarized briefly below.

Numerous studies (Haley, Levine, Brown, Berry, & Hughes, 1987; Stone, Cafferata, & Sangl, 1987) have found that both male and female caregivers perceive themselves in poorer health and report more chronic illness than age-matched peers. Interestingly, these same caregivers also reported lower family incomes than controls, which may explain, in part, the lower reported health level. Similarly, Baumgarten and associates (1992) found that caregivers in their study reported lower levels of well-being on all measures of health status and higher levels of depression than matched controls, suggesting that the consequences of caring for a person with dementia are expressed in a number of somatic symptoms frequently associated with stress (e.g., chronic fatigue, headache, etc.).

MENTAL HEALTH RESPONSES

The chronic stresses associated with taking care of persons with AD have significant consequences for the caretakers' mental health. As noted earlier, caretakers are particularly at risk for developing depression (Crook & Miller, 1985; Eisdorfer & Cohen, 1983). Several studies (Cohen & Eisdorfer, 1988; Coppel, Burton, Becker, & Fiore, 1985; Fiore, Becker, & Coppel, 1983) have established high rates of depression among caregivers using stringent diagnostic criteria. In addition, Goldman and Luchins (1984) documented three cases of severe clinical depression requiring hospitalization, which they attributed directly to the caregiving relationship. Barusch (1988) reported that 67% of the caregivers surveyed responded that they had been depressed during their caregiving careers and that of these, most had coped fairly well with the depression. However, 16% of those questioned were unable to cope with their depressive feelings.

Gallagher and colleagues (1989) at the Palo Alto Veterans Administration Medical Center have extensively studied depression and other negative emotions such as anxiety, anger, and hostility in family caregivers. Their research supports previous work that has identified depressive disorders as common among caregivers but differs in that they identified anger as the most common negative affect among AD caregivers, with 67% of their sample expressing frequent feelings of anger.

A growing number of studies (Anthony-Bergstone, Zarit, & Gatz, 1988; Fitting, Rabins, Lucas, & Eastham, 1986) found that wives were significantly more likely to report symptoms of depression than husbands. The wives attributed the symptoms to demoralization and a sense of powerlessness over the disease rather than to true depression.

As noted earlier, some of the most complex and interesting research in this area has been conducted by Kiecolt-Glaser and associates at Ohio State, who have examined depression and distress as immunological modifiers. These researchers have documented poorer immune response, in particular changes in the percentages of helper T-lymphocytes and natural killer (NK) cells, in caregivers of persons with dementia, while controlling for nutritional intake and illness-related variables (Kiecolt-Glaser et al., 1987). Caretakers in their study reported about three times as many stress symptoms and higher rates of psychotropic drug use than controls, especially those caretakers living with the patient.

In summary, although depression is consistently reported as a consequence of caregiving, it is often difficult to ascertain if many of the symptoms associated with depression are, in fact, a response to physical illness, a direct manifestation of an illness, or represent a co-existing psychological illness. Research by Pruchno, Kleban, Michaels, and Dempsey (1990) supported a model that suggests a "wearing out" of caregivers, such that high levels of depression left them vulnerable to decline in physical health over time. This finding makes intuitive sense, as many persons who are depressed fail to eat and sleep well; they ignore their health status in general, thus increasing their vulnerability to illness. Interestingly, studies comparing caregivers of persons with dementia and caregivers of persons with other diagnoses continue to support a pattern of poorer perceived health among the dementia caregivers and more use of psychotropic medications (Grafstom, Fratiglioni, Sandman, & Winbald, 1992).

Not all family outcomes are negative or burdensome. A few studies have identified variables related to positive well-being rather than strain among caretakers. For example, Gilhooly (1984) found that none of the caregivers in her study exhibited psychiatric impairments and that perceived satisfaction with social support, which was associated with good mental health and high morale, was common in her sample of caregivers. The nature of the relationship between the AD patient and the caretaker may be a critical factor, in that those relationships defined as very close seemed to have more negative impact on the caretaker's mental health and overall well-being. Many caregivers feel useful, competent, and proud as a result of their caretaking role; for some, caregiving improved their sense of self-worth and sense of meaning and provided an important source of companionship (Gwyther, 1990). At this time, however, not enough is known about the positive consequences of caregiving and the relationship between a positive experience and caretaker health outcomes.

Thus, characteristics of the caretaker—such as age, gender, and the nature of the relationship with the care recipient—may be more important in our understanding of caregiver burden and well-being than symptoms manifested by the patient with Alzheimer's disease. The relationship between caregiver coping and health outcomes clearly deserves more investigation focusing on differences in physical, psychological, and physiologic (immune and neuroendocrine) differences. Comparisons of AD caretakers and caregivers of persons with other chronic conditions are also warranted (Daniels & Irwin, 1989).

SOCIAL AND FINANCIAL RESPONSES

A chronic illness like Alzheimer's disease taxes the family's emotional and financial resources. Caregivers consistently report less time for their own activities and interests as care demands increase over time with progression of the disease. George and Gwyther (1986) also reported that caregivers who provided continuous at-home care over a 1-year period experienced decreased satisfaction with the amount of time available for social participation. Further, although caretakers need supportive relationships to ease their burden, the time available for such relationships often diminishes in relation to the increasing time devoted to care management. Friends and family may stop visiting because the AD patient insults them or engages in bizarre behaviors. For similar reasons, as well as for considerations of safety, caretakers may stop taking their loved one outside the home for programs, activities, and social events (Barnes, Raskind, Scott, & Murphy, 1981).

In addition, the financial resources of the caretaker frequently become seriously strained by the caregiving experience. Older caretakers are often particularly reluctant to spend their limited reserves on home-care services or respite care, preferring instead to save what little they have to be eligible for "a good nursing home" and to support institutionalization, which lasts on average 3 years.

There is a great need for multidisciplinary longitudinal studies if we are to better understand caregiver burden and strain. These studies must be broad-based and take into account a variety of immunological, social, and psychological variables.

CULTURAL AND ETHNIC ISSUES

The culturally diverse ethnic minority elderly population is estimated to be growing at least twice as rapidly as the general elderly population (Manuel, 1982), and many of these culturally diverse elderly are presenting with dementia. The NIMH Epidemiological Catchment Area Studies reported relatively high levels of cognitive impairment among African-American and Hispanic populations, almost double the level found among the general Anglo population. However, insufficient attention has been paid to the role of culture in the area of family care and related research in Alzheimer's disease, especially in light of the fact that help-seeking and help-accepting behaviors, caretaking practices, and responses to the disease itself vary based on culturally normative outlooks (Valle, 1989). For example, African-American caregivers emphasize religiosity as a coping mechanism and report higher use of internal cognitive coping strategies, whereas Anglos are more likely to attend support groups and take action-oriented problem-solving approaches (Wykle & Segal, 1991). African-Americans also tend to maintain larger caregiver households and to use a broader range of informal social supports than their Anglo counterparts (Wood & Parham, 1990).

THE CONTINUUM OF CARE

Patients with Alzheimer's disease and their caretakers require assistance at several levels, including the opportunity to receive a clear diagnosis and explanation of the problem, help in assessing changing care needs throughout an unpredictable and changing clinical course, and assistance in sorting through various care options, including when home care is no longer appropriate (Advisory Panel on Alzheimer's Disease, 1989). The long-term care system must reflect a multiplicity of entry points for care along the continuum from diagnosis to death. Most studies indicate that families prefer in-home care (OTA, 1987), yet current federal policies and financing mechanisms clearly favor institutional care.

NURSING INTERVENTION STUDIES ON CAREGIVING

Nurses are making substantial contributions to caregiving research in general as well as in the area of caregiving and Alzheimer's disease (Archbold, 1983; Bowers, 1987; Phillips & Rempusheski, 1986; Stommel, Given, & Given, 1990). Because the space limitations of this chapter prohibit a comprehensive analysis of the extensive caregiver intervention literature, this review will be limited to selected caregiver intervention research conducted by nurses. One example is the promising program of research on caregiving in AD conducted by Farran and Keane-Hagerty and colleagues at Rush Medical Center in Chicago (Buckwalter, 1988). The caregiver model they postulate is comprehensive and takes into consideration caregiver characteristics and resources; stages of the disease; care-receiver functional levels; and impact on the caregiver in terms of functioning, health, psychological reactions, stress, and help-seeking behaviors. The model makes several assumptions: (1) changes in patient functional levels have a direct impact on the caregiver; (2) caregiver characteristics and resources are interactive and act as mediating variables in their influence upon caregiver functioning; (3) caregiving, whether it is a positive or negative experience, is stressful and impacts on the caregiver's lifestyle; and (4) the amount, type, and timing of assistance or support determine whether the caregiver is able to manage the stress of caregiving at a tolerable level.

SUPPORT GROUPS

During the first 3 years of their research, with funding from NIMH and the Alzheimer's Association, the Farran research team developed and refined an educational support group program to be tested in both urban and rural settings. The educational support group was limited to 10 caregivers, lasted for 2 hours over an 8-week period, and was led by professionals. The weekly topics were predetermined by the group leaders. Each session included both didactic content and written handouts, which were compiled into a caregiver manual at the end of the group. Group members could also receive observational and problem-solving assignments. Data suggest that there may be a natural sequence of service use for caregivers, dictated by stage of the disease. For example, in the earlier stages, caretakers may need educational interventions to develop the skills necessary to provide adequate care. Later on, as the AD patient begins to withdraw and become less disruptive, ongoing support may be a more critical factor in reducing caregiver burden.

Other professionally led support groups have been reported in the literature. They vary in format—for example, structured versus unstructured, time-limited versus ongoing—and differ in the amount of education and support provided. For example, using controlled clinical trials, Chiverton and Caine (1989) examined the effects of a time-limited educational support group on the coping skills of spouses of persons with AD. Although some spouses were noted to become distressed or overwhelmed by the information presented in the groups, most spouses who received the educational intervention increased in their feelings of competency and functioned more independently. The investigators also found no relationship between gender of the spouse and coping ability.

Another study by Baldwin, Kleeman, Stevens, and Rasin (1989) examined caregivers of persons with AD who were randomly assigned to either a didactic/educative group or a support/psychotherapeutic program. The former intervention featured a defined curriculum in a classroom format that focused on family systems and dynamics, stress and stress management, and differentiating normal from pathological aging. The latter intervention resembled a psychotherapy group in that the topics for discussion were introduced by the family members. Group leaders provided clarification, guidance, and direction. Although both interventions proved effective in reducing caregiver strain, the support/psychotherapeutic intervention had the greatest and most lasting impact on participants.

Studies of support groups for husbands of victims of AD describe bonding among the participants to enhance self-help and deal with the caregiver issues (Moseley, Davies, & Priddy, 1988). Themes of pride, role changes, grieving, and frustration were identified by the all-male group, which tended to avoid overt expression.

In sum, educational support groups appear to be an effective mechanism for reducing caretaker stress. Those components most often associated with reduced stress include information regarding management of behavioral problems; types of assistance available; discussion of the disease process; discussion of caregiver responses, such as anger, fear, depression, and social isolation; provision of legal and financial information; advice on taking care of the caregiver; and guilt related to in-stitutional placement decisions (Fruehwirth, 1989; Glosser & Wexler, 1985; Niederhe & Fruge, 1984; Schmidt & Keyes, 1985; Zarit & Zarit, 1982). There is some evidence to suggest that family members benefit most from work on their coping skills earlier in the course of the caregiving trajectory and require more emotional support later on in the process (Gallagher, 1985). The work of Archbold, Stewart, Greenlick, and Harvarth (1990) indicates that the more skilled the caregiver, the less traumatic the caregiving process for both care recipients and care providers.

Self-help-styled support groups, such as those run by the Alzheimer's Associa-tion, have also helped caregivers by providing support and sharing practical tips on caregiving and behavioral management. Participants in self-help groups use both in-formal and formal resources more widely than caregivers who do not participate in these groups.

A successful variation of the support group intervention was reported by Ebbitt, Burns, and Christensen (1989). It consisted of work therapy for community-based AD patients and their spouses. The sheltered work program was available for 2 days per week over a 6-month period, during which all work was supervised and the assigned tasks specially adapted to the patients' abilities. Although some anxi-ety was noted for both patients and family members at the beginning of the pro-gram, caregiver burden scores decreased by the end of the program, as did patient depression scores.

IN-HOME INTERVENTIONS

Quayhagen and Quayhagen (1989) evaluated a home-based program of cogni-tive stimulation for both AD patients and their caregivers. In addition to patients in the early stages of the disease maintaining their levels of cognitive and behavioral functioning and improving emotionally, the investigators found that the stimulation program positively affected the well-being of family members and enhanced their coping resources.

Often caregivers are unable to attend support groups because of geographic in-accessibility, their loved one's limitations, or their own impaired health. The Farran research team has also developed and is testing an in-home intervention consisting of evaluation of caregiver needs, information sharing, provision of support, prob-lem-solving exercises, and referrals for needed services (Buckwalter, 1988).

RESPITE

Nurses have also investigated the effects of respite programs on family care-givers. Miller, Gulle, and McCue (1986) examined a program for AD patients re-quiring constant attention as well as a residential program for those who only required companion and housekeeping services in a nursing home setting. Results indicated that seven of the family caregivers were enthusiastic about the respite in-tervention, and another seven were satisfied and more open to long-term placement, but four family members expressed dissatisfaction with the respite program. The in-vestigators suggested that the latter group was unable to relinquish caregiving con-trol. Moreover, family members also cited problems associated with excessive costs and processing in relation to the relatively short patient stays.

In Australia, Johnson and Maguire (1989) evaluated the effects of a day away center on a variety of patient variables and caregiver stress. Although caregivers were positive in their evaluation of the center, no significant decrease in stress scores was noted.

FAMILY MEMBERS IN THE INSTITUTIONAL SETTING

The vast majority of research on family caregivers focuses on family members providing care in the home. Relatively little is known about what happens to family members vis-à-vis their caretaking role when institutionalization takes place. One longitudinal descriptive study by Maas, Buckwalter, and Kelley (1991) found that most family members continued to visit on a regular basis and were overall quite satisfied with the care their AD relative received in a long-term care facility over time. Interestingly, the study revealed that family members were less satisfied with nursing care than with the care provided by other members of the health care team. Family members also had the most contact with nurses, which the investigators interpreted as providing more opportunity for role conflict and ambiguity. They reasoned that diminished satisfaction with care by nurses might reflect family members' discomfort in the transition from their role as primary caretaker to visitors with relatively little control. In addition, family members reported low satisfaction with resources available for the care of their loved one, which may reflect the low levels of funding and the high proportion of nonprofessional caregiver staff found in most nursing homes.

Nursing research in this area has emphasized the caretaker-patient relationship and caretaker feelings of stress and burden. Although a number of studies have evaluated support groups, more research is needed to determine effective leadership styles, group composition, and ways to facilitate access of family members to different types of available support, such as in the home and maximizing use of natural support systems in the community. More controlled intervention studies are called for. Despite anecdotal evidence of the merits of respite and day care programs for this population, little empirical evidence exists to suggest that these interventions actually reduce caregiver stress or delay institutionalization. Finally, more research should be directed to the special needs of caregivers in rural environments, ethnic minorities, and those with intact family units as well as without family.

IMPLICATIONS FOR NURSING RESEARCH

In the past decade, nursing has made excellent progress in describing and examining the needs of patients with AD and their families. The focus of this research effort has thus far been primarily on patient characteristics and problem behaviors and on the experiences and needs of family caregivers. Certainly, work in these important areas must continue, but it is time that nurses expanded their theoretical and research efforts in this domain. For example, explanatory theories and interventions designed to maintain optimal function of patients with AD should be devised and tested. More evaluation research is also needed to examine the cost effectiveness of various care programs (e.g., home-based, institutional) and to determine the impact of care strategies such as special care units on staff, patients, and their family members.

At present, culturally and geographically diverse subjects are notably underrepresented in research on AD, and this situation must be rectified. Nurses are called upon to develop and refine assessment tools that are culturally sensitive and effective for use with minority populations and those residing outside urban areas.

Maas and Buckwalter (1991) have set forth several areas of promising research related to Alzheimer's disease. These include the identification of functional strengths of persons with AD over the course of the illness, which will serve as the basis for nursing management of specific behavioral problems, such as wandering and agitation. More studies addressing disordered person-environment interaction are also needed, such as those which investigate the value of physical or social environmental cues. In addition, more research on treatment modalities relevant to the wide variety of problems noted in Table 14–2 is called for, particularly studies that identify and test approaches designed to alleviate excess or reversible disabilities. Assessment and remediation of cognitive skills also warrant further investigation to determine if certain subgroups of clients with AD may benefit more from particular interventions.

Clearly, much more needs to be known about the relationship of client behaviors to types and levels of caregiver, both formal (e.g., nursing home staff) and informal (e.g., family and friends). Factors that promote positive caregiving experiences and types of assistance required by family caregivers must be examined in more detail. Finally, there is a need for more research in institutional settings, including the development and testing of effective roles for family members following institutionalization. More research is also needed that targets administrative, educational, and ethical issues, such as optimum levels of staffing, staff preparation and training needs, and sources of both satisfaction and conflict in the caregiver role.

In summary, the potential for nursing research is almost limitless throughout the entire continuum of care. Examples of research might include studies of family help-seeking behavior, behavioral descriptions, testing specific nursing interventions, and service utilization patterns of minority clients. The following are examples of potential research questions:

1. What events prompt families to seek diagnostic evaluations and alternative treatments?
2. How are functional strengths identified and maintained in clients with AD?
3. What are the characteristics of clients with terminal AD?
4. What are the effects of therapeutic touch, massage, relaxation, and other stress-reduction techniques on persons at various stages of dementing illness?
5. What are the characteristics of clients with specific behavioral problems, for example, those who yell or scream spontaneously or those who pace continuously?
6. What is the relationship between specific behaviors and the presence of pain in clients with limited communication skills?
7. What is the relationship between specific nursing techniques and resident participation in daily activities (e.g., bathing)?
8. What are the best methods for teaching families to care for loved ones with AD?
9. What is the relationship between different methods for selecting and training nursing assistants to care for residents with AD and dysfunctional resident behavior?
10. What is the influence of environmental factors on resident behavior (e.g., do characteristics of bathroom decor affect willingness to bathe)?

IMPLICATIONS FOR NURSING EDUCATION

Most educational programs for health care professionals, including nurses, stress acute rather than chronic care (Institute of Medicine, 1986) and provide little education or training related to the care of persons with Alzheimer's disease, the chronically mentally ill, or the elderly in general. Student nurses may be exposed to some of the behaviors and care problems of clients with AD through practicum experiences in long-term care facilities (LTCFs) or hospitals but are provided with little theoretical background regarding effective nursing care. Because so few nursing programs offer specific coursework regarding care of the cognitively impaired individual, interested students must often pursue knowledge through elective or continuing education courses, as they are available. Thus many nurses are often not equipped with the knowledge and skills required to care for clients with AD (Stolley, Buckwalter, & Shannon, 1991). This, in turn, promotes work dissatisfaction, resulting in high turnover rates (Chambers, 1990; Sbordone & Sterman, 1983).

This problem has not, however, gone unrecognized. Organizations such as the National League for Nursing are examining the specific educational content and competencies of many specialty areas in gerontological nursing. And the Division of Nursing supports programs for developing nurse practitioners and clinical nurse specialists in gerontology. Other sources of federal support include the National Institute on Aging, which supports Alzheimer's research centers that also develop curricula for training nursing staff in the care of persons with AD. Despite these efforts, there is an ongoing need for even more support for curriculum development and educational opportunities for nurses who work with demented clients (Stolley et al., 1991).

The Office of Technological Assessment's important volume *Losing a Million Minds* (1987) suggested modifications in basic nursing curriculum to improve preparation of nurses to care for the elderly in general and for clients with AD in particular. The curricular revisions include the following:

- Differentiation of acute and chronic illness, including management of the chronically ill and rehabilitation potential
- Assessment skills, including assessment of self-care abilities, cognitive skills, living environment, and social interactions, in addition to physical assessment
- Case management
- Patient and family education
- Training and supervising paraprofessionals
- Working within a multidisciplinary team
- Administrative and supervisory skills

Nurses who work with persons with Alzheimer's disease and related disorders must receive specific training related to their care. Stolley and colleagues (1991) have proposed a curriculum for nurses in this regard, as set forth in Table 14–6.

In summary, there are too few nurses caring for persons with AD, and many of those providing care are inadequately trained. Nurses need specific preparation to care for clients with Alzheimer's disease. Regrettably, at present few incentives exist for nurses to become expert in the care of this complex population, and too few funding opportunities are available to finance educational preparation in this area. To correct the current situation generic curricula must be altered to include more specific content on AD. Additional funding is also needed for advanced education, for the preparation of clinical specialists and geriatric nurse practitioners who will serve as role models in the care of the cognitively impaired. However, this is not a problem of nursing education alone. On a broader scale, the poor image of nursing homes and the low wages and benefits received by nurses who work in them also contribute to the instability and short supply of nurses willing to work with demented clients. Thus, sweeping efforts are needed to enhance the image and prestige of long-term care in particular. Promoting educational preparation should help increase motivation and interest both in gerontological nursing and care of clients with AD (Stolley et al., 1991).

TABLE 14–6. CURRICULUM FOR NURSES

Introduction to Aging, with Foci on the Biological and Psychological Aspects of Aging
Included would be content on normal aging, theories of aging, psychosocial aspects of aging, age-associated losses, reactions to loss, and ethnic or cultural issues.

Cognitive Functioning in the Aged
Normal cognitive functioning versus abnormal functioning and progression of the disease process should be outlined. Included would be physiological changes associated with Alzheimer's disease (AD), with accompanying reasons for corresponding cognitive deficits. Changes associated with reversible and irreversible dementias should be examined. Nurses should also be trained in the use, scoring, and interpretation of various assessment tools to measure cognitive function.

Behavior and Nursing Care Problems, including Dressing, Bathing, and Grooming, Problems with Incontinence, Immobility, and Eating
Assessment and identification of concomitant diseases and disorders should be stressed. Techniques and interventions regarding behavior problems—such as catastrophic behaviors, wandering, withdrawal, depression, sundowning, agitation, and combativeness—must be described.

Use of Psychotropic Drugs
Included should be an in-depth view of types of medications, their appropriate use and side effects, and the implications of polypharmacy. Nurses should be trained to identify both the need for a particular drug as well as inappropriate prescribing. Attention should be paid to changes associated with dementing illness that may change the intended drug actions (e.g., diminished circulation and weight loss). Side effects (especially of neuroleptics) must be outlined, and alternative therapies discussed.

Restructuring the Environment
The need for structure, consistency, and modified stimuli must be reviewed, and methods for providing a safe and secure environment set forth.

Social and Emotional Aspects of AD
Providing support for the family and the AD patient should be highlighted. Interventions, community resources, and institutionalization can be discussed, along with possible reactions of the patient and family members to various care options. The importance of obtaining information about the social support network and social history of the patient must be emphasized, and ways to facilitate continuity of care between various levels of care (home to the hospital or long-term care facility) presented.

Methods for Recognizing and Preventing Excess Disability
The causes of excess—e.g., disability, fatigue, physical causes (pain, infection), medications, change in environment or caregiver, stressors, sensory impairment, and psychological causes (such as depression)—should be considered. Alternatives to using physical and chemical restraints must be included.

Methods for Training, Supervising, and Evaluating Nursing Assistants Caring for Patients with AD

From Stolley, J. M., Buckwalter, K. C., & Shannon, M. D. (1991). Caring for patients with Alzheimer's disease: Recommendations for nursing education. *Journal of Gerontological Nursing, 17*(6), 37.

CONCLUSION

The development, implementation, and testing of appropriate, safe, and effective services for the care and support of person with AD and their caregivers in both community-based and institutional settings is a particular challenge because of the complexity of the disease process (Buckwalter, Abraham, & Neundorfer, 1988). Nurses who care for this population must therefore be able to integrate knowledge from both the biomedical and behavioral sciences if they are to deal effectively with the many care problems that arise over the long, unpredictable, and changing clinical course of this devastating brain disease.

REFERENCES

Advisory Panel on Alzheimer's Disease. (1989). *First Report of the Advisory Panel on Alzheimer's Disease.* DHHS Pub. No. (ADM) 89-1644. Washington, DC: Superintendent of Documents, US Government Printing Office.

Advisory Panel on Alzheimer's Disease. (1990). *Second Report of the Advisory Panel on Alzheimer's Disease.* DHHS Pub. No. (ADM) 91-1791. Washington, DC: Superintendent of Documents, US Government Printing Office.

Advisory Panel on Alzheimer's Disease. (1991). *Third Report of the Advisory Panel on Alzheimer's Disease.* DHHS Pub. No. (ADM) 92-1917. Washington, DC: Superintendent of Documents, US Government Printing Office.

Advisory Panel on Alzheimer's Disease. (1993). *Biomedical Update to Congress: Special Report.* Washington, DC: National Institute on Aging.

Algase, D. L. (1991). *Cognitive discriminants of wandering.* Unpublished paper, University of Michigan.

Alzheimer's Association. (1994). Newsletter. *Advances in Alzheimer's Research, 4*(1), 4.

Anthony-Bergstone, C. R., Zarit, S. H., & Gatz, M. (1988). Symptoms of psychological distress among caregivers of dementia patients. *Psychology and Aging, 3,* 245–248.

Archbold, P. G. (1983). Impact of patient-caring on women. *Family Relations, 32,* 39–45.

Archbold, P., Stewart, B., Greenlick, M., & Harvarth, T. (1990). Mutuality and preparedness as predictors of caregiver role strain. *Research in Nursing and Health, 37,* 217–222.

Aronson, M., Ooi, W. L., Morgenstern, H., Hafner, A., Masur, D., Crystal, H., Frishman, W. H., Fisher, D., & Katzman, R. (1990). Women, myocardial infarction, and dementia in the very old. *Neurology, 40,* 1102–1106.

Baldwin, B., Kleeman, K., Stevens, G., & Rasin, J. (1989). Family caregiver stress: Clinical assessment and management. *International Psychogeriatrics, 1,* 185–194.

Barnes, R. F., Raskind, M. A., Scott, M. A., & Murphy, C. (1981). Problems of families caring for Alzheimer's patients: Use of a support group. *Journal of the American Geriatrics Society, 29*(2), 80–85.

Barusch, A. S. (1988). Problems and coping strategies of elderly spouse caregivers. *Gerontologist, 28,* 677–685.

Baumgarten, M., Battista, R. N., Infante-Rivard, C., Hanley, J. A., Becker, R., & Gauther, S. (1992). The psychological and physical health of family members caring for an elderly person with dementia. *Journal of Clinical Epidemiology, 45*(1), 61–70.

Beck, C., Heacock, P., Mercer, S., Walton, C. G., & Shook, J. (1991). Dressing for success: Promoting independence among cognitively impaired elderly. *Journal of Psychosocial Nursing and Mental Health Services, 29*(7), 39–40.

Blass, J. P., & Zemcov, A. (1984). Alzheimer's disease: A metabolic systems degeneration? *Neurochemistry and Pathology, 2,* 103–114.

Blessed, G., Tomlinson, B. E., & Roth, M. (1968). Association between quantitative measures of dementia and senile changes in the cerebral grey matter of elderly subjects. *British Journal of Psychiatry, 114,* 797–811.

Blieszner, F., McAuley, W., Newhouse, J., & Mancim, J. (1987). Rural-urban differences in service use by older adults. In T. H. Brubaker (Ed.), *Aging, health and the family: Long-term care* (pp. 162–176). Newbury Park, CA: Sage.

Bowers, B. J. (1987). Intergenerational caregiving: Adult caregivers and their aging parents. *Advances in Nursing Science, 9*(2), 20–31.

Brantley, P. J., & Garrett, V. D. (1993). Psychobiological approaches to health and disease. In P. B. Sutker & H. E. Adams (Eds.), *Comprehensive handbook of psychopathology* (2nd ed.) (pp. 647–670). New York: Plenum.

Brody, E. M. (1985). Parent care as a normative family stress. *The Gerontologist, 25,* 19–29.

Brody, E. M., Kleban, M., Lawton, M. P., & Moss, M. (1974). A longitudinal look at excess disabilities in the mentally impaired aged. *Journal of Gerontology, 29*(1), 79–84.

Buckwalter, K. C. (Ed.). (1988). *Intervention strategies for maintaining control thoughout the caregiving trajectory.* Iowa City, IA: Iowa Geriatric Education Center Monograph Series.

Buckwalter, K. C. (1989). Report of the advisory panel on Alzheimer's disease. *Archives of Psychiatric Nursing, 3*(6), 358–362.

Buckwalter, K. C., Abraham, I. L., & Neundorfer, M. M. (1988). Alzheimer's disease: Involving nursing in the development and implementation of health care for patients and families. *Nursing Clinics of North America, 23*(1), 1–11.

Buckwalter, K. C., & Hall, G. R. (1987). Families of the institutionalized older adult: A neglected resource. In T. Brubaker (Ed.), *Aging, health and the family: Long-term care* (pp. 176–196). Newbury Park, CA: Sage.

Buckwalter, K. C., & Smith, M. (1991). Special needs of the elderly. In K. S. Babich (Ed.), *Discharge planning: A manual for psychiatric nurses* (pp. 146–158). Thorofare, NJ: Slack.

Burns, E. M., & Buckwalter, K. C. (1988). Pathophysiology and etiology of Alzheimer's disease. *Nursing Clinics of North America, 23*(1), 11–29.

Butcher, L. L., & Woolf, N. J. (1986). Central cholinergic systems: Synopsis of anatomy and overview of physiology and pathology. In A. B. Scheibel, A. F. Wechsler, & M. A. B. Brazier (Eds.), *The biological substrates of Alzheimer's disease* (p. 73). Orlando, FL: Academic.

Cantor, M. H. (1983). Strain among caregivers: A study of experience in the U.S. *The Gerontologist, 23,* 597–604.

Chambers, J. D. (1990). Predicting licensed nurse turnover in skilled long-term care. *Nursing and Health Care, 11,* 474–477.

Chenoweth, B., & Spencer, B. (1986). Dementia: The experience of family caregivers. *The Gerontologist, 26,* 267–272.

Chiverton, P., & Caine, E. D. (1989). Education to assist spouses coping with Alzheimer's disease: A controlled trial. *Journal of the American Geriatric Society, 37,* 593–598.

Cohen, D., & Eisdorfer, C. (1988). Depression in family members caring for a relative with Alzheimer's disease. *Journal of the American Geriatric Society, 36,* 885–889.

Cohen-Mansfield, J. (1986). Agitated behaviors in the elderly. II. Preliminary results in the cognitively deteriorated. *Journal of American Geriatrics Society, 34*(10), 722–727.

Coppel, D. B., Burton, C., Becker, J., & Fiore, J. (1985). Relationships of cognitions associated with coping reactions to depression in spousal caregivers of Alzheimer's disease patients. *Cognitive Therapy and Research, 9,* 253–266.

Coyle, J. T., Price, D. L., & DeLong, M. R. (1983). Alzheimer's disease: A disorder of cortical cholinergic innervation. *Science, 219,* 1184.

Crook, T. H., & Miller, N. E. (1985). The challenge of Alzheimer's disease. *American Psychologist, 40,* 1245–1250.

Cutrona, C. E., & Russell, D. (1987). The provisions of social relationships and adaptation to stress. In W. H. Jones & D. Perlman (Eds.), *Advances in personal relationships* (Vol. 1, pp. 37–67). Greenwich, CT: JAI Press.

Daniels, M., & Irwin, M. (1989). Caregiver stress and well-being. In E. Light & B. D. Lebowitz (Eds.), *Alzheimer's disease treatment and family stress: Directions for research* (pp. 292–309). Rockville, MD: National Institute of Mental Health.

Davies, P. (1983). The neurochemistry of Alzheimer's disease and senile dementia. *Medical Research Review, 3*(3), 221–226.

Dawson, P., Kline, K., Wiancko, D., & Wells, D. (1986). Preventing excess disability in patients with Alzheimer's disease. *Geriatric Nursing, 7*(6), 298–330.

DeLeon, M. J., Ferris, S. H., & George, A. E. (1980). Computed tomography evaluations of brain-behavior relationships in senile dementia of the Alzheimer type. *Neurobiology of Aging, 1,* 69–79.

DeLeon, M. J., Potegal, M., & Gurland, B. (1984). Wandering and parietal lobe signs in senile dementia of the Alzheimer's type. *Neuropsychobiology, 11,* 155–157.

Doty, P., Liu, K., & Wiener, J. (1985). An overview of long-term care. *Health Care Financing Review, 6,* 69–78.

Duke University. (1978). *Multidimensional functional assessment: The OARS methodology.* Durham, NC: Duke University Press.

Ebbitt, B., Burns, T., & Christensen, R. (1989). Work therapy: Intervention for community-based Alzheimer's patients. *American Journal of Alzheimer's Care and Related Disorders, 4*(5), 7–15.

Eisdorfer, C., & Cohen, D. (1983). Management of the patient and family coping with dementing illness. In H. Cox (Ed.), *Aging* (3rd ed.). Guilford, CT: Bushkin.

Emery, O. (1986). Linguistic cues in the differential diagnosis of Alzheimer's disease. *Clinical Gerontologist, 6*(1), 59–61.

Ernst, R. L., & Hays, J. W. (1994). The U.S. economic and social costs of Alzheimer's disease revisited. *American Journal of Public Health, 84*(8), 1261–1264.

Evans, D. A., Funckenstein, H. H., Albert, M. S., Scherr, P. A., Cook, N. R., & Chown, M. J. (1989). Prevalence of Alzheimer's disease in a community population of older persons. *Journal of the American Medical Association, 262,* 2551–2556.

Ferguson, D., & Beck, C. (1983). H.A.L.F.—A Tool to assess elder abuse within the family. *Journal of Gerontological Nursing, 4*(5), 301–304.

Fiore, J., Becker, J., & Coppel, D. B. (1983). Social network interactions: A buffer to stress. *American Journal of Community Psychology, 11,* 423–439.

Fishman, P. S. (1986). Neural transplantation: Scientific gains and clinical perspectives. *Neurology* (NY), *36,* 389–392.

Fitting, M., Rabins, P., Lucas, M. J., & Eastham, J. (1986). Caregivers for dementia patients: A comparison of husbands and wives. *The Gerontologist, 26,* 248–252.

Folstein, M. F., Folstein, S. E., & McHugh, P. R. (1975). Mini mental state: A practical method for grading the cognitive state of patients for the clinician. *Journal of Psychiatry Research, 12,* 189–198.

Fruehwirth, S. S. (1989). An application of Johnson's behavioral model: A case study. *Journal of Community Health Nursing, 6,* 61–71.

Fulmer, T. T., & Ashley, J. (1989). Clinical indicators of elder neglect. *Applied Nursing Research, 2*(4), 161–167.

Gallagher, D. E. (1985). Intervention strategies to assist caregivers of frail elders: Current research status and future research directions. In M. P. Lawton & G. Maddox (Eds.), *Annual Review of Gerontology and Geriatrics* (Vol. 5, pp. 249–283). New York: Springer.

Gallagher, D., Wrabetz, A., Lovett, S., DelMaestro, S., & Rose, J. (1989). Depression and other negative affects in family caregivers. In E. Light & B. Lebowitz (Eds.), *Alzheimer's disease treatment and family stress: Directions for research* (pp. 218–245). Rockville, MD: National Institute of Mental Health.

Garand, L. (1993). *Physical morbidity associated with giving care to a person with dementia.* Unpublished paper, University of Iowa College of Nursing, Iowa City, Iowa.

George, L. K., & Gwyther, L. P. (1986). Caregiver well-being: A multidimensional examination of family caregivers of demented adults. *The Gerontologist, 26*(3), 253–259.

Gilhooly, M. (1984). The impact of caregiving on care-givers: Factors associated with the psychological well-being of people supporting a dementing relative in the community. *British Journal of Medical Psychology, 57,* 35–44.

Glosser, G., & Wexler, D. (1985). Participants' evaluation of educational/support groups for families of patients with Alzheimer's disease and other dementia. *Gerontologist, 25,* 232–236.

Gmeiner, C. (1987). Patient behavior, care needs, personalized community resources of both institutionalized and non-institutionalized Alzheimer's patients. In H. J. Altman (Ed.), *Alzheimer's disease: Problems, prospects, and perspectives. Proceedings of a National Conference on AD and Dementia* (April, 1986) (pp. 271–278). New York: Plenum.

Goldman, L. S., & Luchins, D. (1984). Depression in spouses of demented patients. *American Journal of Psychiatry, 141*(11), 1467–1468.

Grafstom, M., Fratiglioni, L., Sandman, P. O., & Winbald, B. (1992). Health and social consequences for relatives of demented and non-demented elderly. A population-based study. *Journal of Clinical Epidemiology, 45*(8), 861–870.

Grant, I., Patterson, T., Hauger, R., & Irwin, M. (1992). Current research on dementia and Alzheimer's disease [Special issue]. *Archives of Psychiatry, 4*(Suppl.), 77–80.

Graves, A. B., White, E., Koepsell, T. D., Reifler, B. V., Belle, G. V., Larson, E. B., & Raskind, M. (1990). The association between head trauma and Alzheimer's disease. *American Journal of Epidemiology, 131,* 491.

Grunow, J. L. (1988). *An in-home intervention program for caregivers of persons with dementia.* Iowa City, IA: Iowa Geriatric Education Center Interdisciplinary Monograph Series.

Gwyther, L. P. (1990). Clinician and family: A partnership for support. In N. L. Mace (Ed.), *Dementia care: Patient, family, and community.* Baltimore, MD: The Johns Hopkins University Press.

Hachinski, V. C., Iliff, L. E., Zilhka, E., et al. (1975). Cerebral blood flow in dementia. *Archives of Neurology, 32,* 632–637.

Haley, W. E., Levine, E. G., Brown, S. L., Berry, J. W., & Hughes, G. H. (1987). Psychological, social, and health consequences of caring for a relative with senile dementia. *Journal of the American Geriatrics Society, 35,* 405–411.

Hall, G. R. (1986). *Development of an assessment instrument: Behavioral assessment for alterations in thought process due to cognitive loss.* Unpublished manuscript, University of Iowa Hospitals and Clinics, Department of Neurology.

Hall, G. R. (1988). Care of the patient with Alzheimer's disease living at home. *Nursing Clinics of North America, 23*(1), 31–46.

Hall, G. R. (1991a). Challenges in feeding a patient with chronic dementia. *Clinics in Applied Nutrition, 1*(2), 81–89.

Hall, G. R. (1991b). This hospital patient has Alzheimer's. *American Journal of Nursing, 91*(10), 44–53.

Hall, G. R., & Buckwalter, K. C. (1987). Progressively lowered stress threshold: A conceptual model for care of adults with Alzheimer's disease. *Archives of Psychiatric Nursing, 1*(6), 399–406.

Hall, G. R., & Buckwalter, K. C. (1991). Whole disease care planning: Fitting the program to the client with Alzheimer's disease. *Journal of Gerontological Nursing, 17*(3), 38–41.

Helmes, E. (1988). Multidimensional Observation Scale for Elderly Subjects (MOSES). *Psychopharmacology Bulletin, 24*(2), 733–745.

Huff, F. J., Auerback, J., Chakravarti, A., & Boller, F. (1988). Risk of dementia in relatives of patients with Alzheimer's disease. *Neurology, 38,* 786–790.

Institute of Medicine. (1986). *Improving the quality of care in nursing homes.* Washington, DC: National Academy Press.

Isaacs, B., & Kennie, A. T. (1973). The set test as an aid to the detection of dementia in old people. *British Journal of Psychiatry, 132,* 467–470.

Jacobs, J. W., Bernard, M. R., Delgado, A, & Strain, J. J. (1977). Screening for organic mental syndromes in the medically ill. *Annals of Internal Medicine, 86,* 40–46.

Johnson, M., & Maguire, M. (1989). Give me a break: Benefits of a caregiver support service. *Journal of Gerontological Nursing, 15*(11), 22–26.

Kahn, R. L., Goldfarb, A. I., Pollock, M., & Peck, A. (1960). Brief objective measure for the determination of mental status in the aged. *American Journal of Psychiatry, 117,* 326–328.

Kiecolt-Glaser, J. K., & Glaser, R. (1987). Psychosocial moderators of immune function. *Annals of Behavioral Medicine, 9,* 16–20.

Kiecolt-Glaser, J. K., Glaser, R., Shuttleworth, E. C., Dyer, C. S., Orocki, P., & Speicher, C. E. (1987). Chronic stress and immunity in family caregivers of Alzheimer's disease victims. *Psychosomatic Medicine, 49,* 523–535.

Kuhlman, G. J., Wilson, H. S., Hutchinson, S. A., & Wallhagen, M. (1991). Alzheimer's disease and family caregiving: Critical synthesis of the literature and research agenda. *Nursing Research, 40*(6), 331–337.

Lawton, M. P., Kleban, M. H., Moss, M., Rovine, M., & Glickman, A. (1989). Measuring caregiving appraisal. *Journal of Gerontology, 44*(3), 61–71.

Lee, V. K. (1991). Language changes and Alzheimer's disease: A literature review. *Journal of Gerontological Nursing, 17*(1), 16–20.

Light, E., & Lebowitz, B. D. (Eds.). (1989). *Alzheimer's disease treatment and family stress: Directions for research.* Rockville, MD: National Institute of Mental Health.

Loewenstein, D. A., Amigo, E., Duara, R., Guterman, A., Hurwitz, D., Berkowitz, N., Wilkie, F., Weinberg, G., Black, B., Gittelman, B., & Eisdorfer, C. (1989). A new scale for the assessment of functional status in Alzheimer's disease and related disorders. *Journal of Gerontology, 44*(4), P114–121.

Maas, M., & Buckwalter, K. C. (1991). Nursing research in Alzheimer's disease. *Annual Review of Nursing Research.* New York: Springer.

Maas, M., Buckwalter, K., & Kelley, L. (1991). Characteristics and perceptions of family members of institutionalized Alzheimer's patients. *Applied Nursing Research, 4*(3), 135–140.

Mace, N., & Rabins, P. V. (1981). *The 36-hour day.* Baltimore: Johns Hopkins University Press.

Manuel, R. C. (Ed.). (1982). *Minority aging: Sociological and social psychological perspectives.* Westport, CT: Greenwood.

Mayeux, R., Stern, Y., & Spanton, S. (1985). Heterogeneity in dementia of the Alzheimer's type: Evidence of subgroups. *Neurology, 35,* 435–461.

McBride, A. B. (1990). Psychiatric nursing in the 1990s. *Archives of Psychiatric Nursing, 4*(1), 21–28.

McKhann, G., Drachman, D., Folstein, M., Katzman, R., Price, D., & Stadlan, E. (1984). Clinical diagnosis of Alzheimer's disease: Report of the NINCDS-ADRDA work group under the auspices of Department of Health and Human Services Task Force on Alzheimer's Disease. *Neurology, 34,* 939–944.

Miller, B., McFall, S., & Montgomery, A. (1991). The impact of elder health, caregiver involvement, and global stress on two dimensions of caregiver burden. *Journal of Gerontology, 46*(1), 59–69.

Miller, C. A. (1994). Drugs in development for Alzheimer's disease. *Geriatric Nursing, 15*(1), 53–54.

Miller, D. B., Gulle, N., & McCue, F. (1986). The realities of respite for families, clients, and sponsors. *The Gerontologist, 26,* 467–470.

Morrison-Bogorad, M. (1993). Scientists discover possible risk factor for Alzheimer's disease [press release]. Seattle, WA: Alzeimer's Disease Research Center, University of Washington.

Moseley, P. W., Davies, H. D., & Priddy, J. M. (1988). Support groups for male caregivers of Alzheimer's patients: A follow-up. *Clinical Gerontologist, 7,* 127–136.

Murdoch, B., Chenery, H., Wilks, V., & Boyle, R. S. (1987). Language disorders in dementia of the Alzheimer's type. *Brain Language, 31,* 122–137.

Neundorfer, M. (1991). Coping and health outcomes in spouse caregivers of persons with dementia. *Nursing Research, 40*(5), 260–265.

Niederhe, G., & Fruge, E. (1984). Dementia and family dynamics: Clinical research issues. *Journal of Geriatric Psychiatry, 17*(1), 21–60.

Office of Technology Assessment (OTA). (1987). *Losing a million minds: Confronting the tragedy of Alzheimer's disease and other dementias.* Washington, DC: US Congress.

Perl, D. P., & Brody, A. R. (1980). Alzheimer's disease: X-ray spectrometric evidence of aluminum accumulation in neurofibrillary tangle-bearing neurons. *Science, 208,* 297–299.

Pfeiffer, E. (1975). A short portable mental status questionnaire for the assessment of organic brain deficit in elderly patients. *Journal of the American Geriatrics Society, 23,* 433–441.

Phillips, L. R., & Rempusheski, V. F. (1986). Caring for the frail elderly at home: Toward a theoretical explanation of the dynamics of poor quality family caregiving. *Advances in Nursing Science, 8*(4), 62–84.

Plutchik, R., Conte, H., Lieberman, M., Bakur, M., Grossman, J., & Lehman, N. (1970). Reliability and validity of a scale for assessing the functioning of geriatric patients. *Journal of the American Geriatrics Society, 18*(6), 491–500.

Poceta, S. (1991). Sleep changes in Alzheimer's: Parallel neuronal degeneration. *Aging Research and Training News, 4*(3), 24.

Pruchno, R. A., Kleban, M. H., Michaels, J. E., & Dempsey, N. P. (1990). Mental and physical health of caregiving spouses: Development of a causal model. *Journal of Gerontology, 45*(5), 192–199.

Pruchno, R. A., & Resch, N. L. (1989). Aberrant behaviors and Alzheimer's disease: Mental health effects on spouse caregivers. *Journal of Gerontology, 44,* S177–S182.

Prusiner, S. B. (1984). Prions. *Scientific American, 251,* 50–59.

Quayhagen, M. P., & Quayhagen, M. (1988). Alzheimer's stress: Coping with the caregiving role. *The Gerontologist, 28,* 391–396.

Quayhagen, M. P., & Quayhagen, M. (1989). Differential effects of family-based strategies on Alzheimer's disease. *The Gerontologist, 29,* 150–155.

Rabins, P. V., Mace, H. L., & Lucas, M. S. (1982). The impact of dementia on the family. *Journal of the American Medical Association, 248,* 333–335.

Radloff, L. S. (1977). A self-report depression scale for research in the general population. *Applied Psychological Measurement, 3,* 85–40.

Ray, W. A., Taylor, J. A., Lichtenstein, M. J., & Meador, K. G. (1992). The nursing home behavior problem scale. *Journal of Gerontology, 47*(1), M9–16.

Reisberg, B., Ferris, S. H., DeLeon, M. J., & Crook, T. (1982). The global deterioration scale for assessment of primary degenerative dementia. *American Journal of Psychiatry, 139*(9), 1136–1139.

Rosen, W. G., Mohs, R. C., & Davis, K. L. (1984). A new rating scale for Alzheimer's disease. *American Journal of Psychiatry, 41*(11), 1356–1364.

Roses, A. D., Bebout, J., Yamaoka, L. H., Gaskell, P. C., Hung, W-Y., Walker, A. P., Alberts, M. J., Clark, C., Welch, K., Earl, N. L., Heyman, A. L., & Pericak-Vance, M. A. (1990). Linkage of late-onset familial Alzheimer's disease on chromosome 19. *Society of Neuroscience Abstracts, 16,* 149.

Ryden, M. B. (1988). Aggressive behavior in persons with dementia who live in the community. *Alzheimer's Disease and Associated Disorders: An International Journal, 2,* 342–355.

Sbordone, R. J., & Sterman, L. T. (1983). The psychologist as a consult in a nursing home: Effect on staff morale and turnover. *Professional Psychology: Research and Practice, 14,* 240–250.

Schmidt, G. L., & Keyes, B. (1985). Group psychotherapy with family caregivers of demented patients. *The Gerontologist, 25,* 347–349.

Schultz, R., Visintainer, P., & Williamson, G. M. (1990). Psychiatric and physical morbidity effects of caregiving. *Journal of Gerontology, 45,* 181–191.

Scott, J. P., & Roberto, K. A. (1985). Use of informal and formal support networks by rural elderly poor. *The Gerontologist, 25*(6), 624–630.

Shapira, J. (1994). Research trends in Alzheimer's disease. *Journal of Gerontological Nursing, 20*(4), 4–10.

Sloane, P. D. (1992). Bathing behaviors observational scale. Instrument developed to measure disruptive behaviors during bathing through direct observation. Reducing Disruptive Behavior During Bathing in Dementia grant application to the National Institute on Aging.

Stevens, G. L., Walsh, R. A., & Baldwin, B. A. (1993). Family caregivers of institutionalized and noninstitutionalized elderly individuals. *Advances in Clinical Nursing Research, 28*(2), 349–362.

St. George-Hyslop, P. H., Tanzi, R. E., Polinsky, R. J., Haines, J. L., Nee, L., Watkins, P. C., Myers, R. H., Feldman, R. G., Pollen, D., Drachman, D., Growdon, J., Bruni, A., Foncin, J-F., Salmon, D., Frommelt, P., Amaducci, L., Sorbi, S., Piacentini, S., Stewart, G. D., Hobbs, W. J., Conneally, P. M., & Gusella, J. F. (1987). The genetic defect causing familial Alzheimer's disease maps on chromosome 21. *Science, 235,* 885–890.

Stolley, J. M., Buckwalter, K. C., & Shannon, M. D. (1991). Caring for patients with Alzheimer's disease: Recommendations for nursing education. *Journal of Gerontological Nursing, 17*(6), 34–38.

Stommel, M., Given, C. W., & Given, B. (1990). Depression as an overriding variable explaining caregiver burdens. *Journal of Aging and Health, 2,* 81–102.

Stone, R., Cafferata, G. L., & Sangl, J. (1987). Caregivers of the frail elderly: A national profile. *The Gerontologist, 27*(5), 616–626.

Sunderland, T., Hill, J. L., Mellow, A. M., Lawlor, B. A., Gundersheimer, J., Newhouse, P. A., & Grafman, J. H. (1989). Clock drawing in Alzheimer's disease: A novel measure of dementia severity. *Journal of American Geriatric Society, 37*(8), 765–729.

Teri, L., Truax, P., Logsdon, R., Uomoto, J., Zarit, S., & Vitaliano, P. P. (1991). *Assessment of behavioral problems in dementia: The revised memory and behavior problems checklist.* Unpublished manuscript, the University of Washington, Seattle.

Terry, R. D., Peck, A., DeTeresa, R., Schechter, R., & Houroupian, D. (1981). Some morphometric aspects of the brain in senile dementia of the Alzheimer's type. *Annals of Neurology, 10,* 184.

Twombly, R. (1994) Gene found to reduce risk of Alzheimer's disease. *The Caregiver* (Duke University Medical Center Release), 5–6.

Valle, R. (1989). Cultural and ethnic issues in Alzheimer's disease family research. In E. Light & B. D. Lebowitz (Eds.), *Alzheimer's disease treatment and family stress: Directions for research* (pp. 122–154). Rockville, MD: National Institute of Mental Health.

Vitaliano, P., Maiuro, R. D., Ochs, H., & Russo, J. (1989). A model of burden in caregivers of DAT patients. In E. Light & B. D. Lebowitz (Eds.), *Alzheimer's disease treatment and family stress: Directions for research* (pp. 267–292). Rockville, MD: National Institute of Mental Health.

Weiler, K., & Buckwalter, K. C. (1988). Care of the demented client. *Journal of Gerontological Nursing, 14*(7), 26–31.

Whitehouse, P., Tabaton, M., & Lanska, D. (1991). Pathological and chemical correlates of dementia. In F. Corkin (Ed.), *Handbook of neuropsychology of aging* (Vol. 5, pp. 29–37). New York: Elsevier.

Wilson, H. S. (1989). Family caregivers: The experience of Alzheimer's disease. *Applied Nursing Research, 2,* 40–45.

Wolanin, M., & Phillips, L. (1981). *Confusion: Prevention and care.* St. Louis: Mosby.

Wood, J. B., & Parham, I. A. (1990). Coping with perceived burden: Ethnic and cultural issues in Alzheimer's family caregiving. *The Journal of Applied Gerontology, 9*(3), 325–339.

Wykle, M., & Segal, M. (1991). A comparison of black and white family caregivers' experience with dementia. *Journal of the Black Nurses Association, 5*(1), 29–41.

Yesavage, J., Brink, T., Rose, T., Lum, O., Huang, O., Adey, V., & Leier, V. (1983). Development and validation of a geriatric depression screening scale: A preliminary report. *Journal of Psychiatric Research, 17,* 37–49.

Yu, E. S. H., Liu, W. T., Levy, P., Shang, M. Y., Katzman, R., Lung, C. T., Wong, S. C., Wang, Z. Y., & Qu, G. Y. (1989). Cognitive impairment among elderly adults in Shanghai, China. *Journal of Gerontology, 44,* 97–106.

Zarit, S. H., Todd, P. A., & Zarit, J. M. (1986). Subjective burden of husbands and wives as caregivers; A longitudinal study. *The Gerontologist, 29,* 260–266.

Zarit, S. H., & Zarit, J. M. (1982). Familes under stress: Interventions for caregivers of senile dementia patients. *Psychotherapy, Theory, Research and Practice, 19,* 461–471.

APPENDIX 14-1

BEHAVIOR LOG

Instructions: The Behavior Log on the following pages provides information on what behaviors your Alzheimer's patient experiences and how frequently and how much these behaviors bother or trouble you. Please fill in the number of times each behavior occurs *each* day for the next two weeks, starting at Day 1 and going through Day 14 on the form. Then check the answer that tells how much that behavior bothers you and describe how you managed the problem and how well it worked. Please include any other details below under care notes.

CARE NOTES

Date & Time:

Description of behavior:

Strategy used by caregiver:

Response by the care recipient:

Date & Time:

Description of behavior:

Strategy used by caregiver:

Response by the care recipient:

DEFINITIONS

Falls: Any incident where the patient loses balance and/or trips and falls to the floor or on some other object (even if a person partially breaks their fall) or if a patient is found lying on the floor.

Physical restraints: Any physical mechanism that is used to curtail freedom of a patient's movement (e.g., locking doors, tying in bed or chair, tying patient to self, siderails on bed).

Participation in activities: Engaging in spontaneous or planned activities at home or away from home with one or more persons.

Other incidents: Incidents other than falls that result in injury or potential injury (e.g., choking, skin tears, abrasions, hitting another person, wandering away from house, getting lost).

Mail back every two weeks.

DAILY TOTALS

BEHAVIOR	1	2	3	4	5	6	7	8	9	10	11	12	13	14
Wakes up confused at night														
Becomes agitated, irritable late in the day (sundowning)														
Refuses to help or participate in care. Is belligerent, yells, curses														
Wets or soils clothing														
Has purposeful wandering, tries to leave home														
Violent, hits, or strikes out														
Repeats a word or behavior over and over														
Withdraws, unsociable, refuses to participate in activities														
Paces, fidgets														
Increased social interaction or participation in activities														
Falls														
Restraints														
Other incidents (please describe)														

HOW MUCH DOES THIS BOTHER
OR UPSET YOU?   HOW WELL DOES IT WORK?

NONE 0	NOT MUCH 1	SOME 2	VERY MUCH 3	WHAT DO YOU DO TO COPE WITH OR HANDLE THIS? (DESCRIBE)	NONE 0	NOT MUCH 1	SOME 2	VERY MUCH 3

CHAPTER

15

Fluid Imbalance and Water Intoxication
The Elusive Syndrome

Mary Ann Boyd, PhD, DSN, RN, CS, and Ernest D. Lapierre, DSN, RN, CS, CNAA

ABSTRACT

The chapter focuses primarily on disordered water balance in persons with long-term mental illness, primarily schizophrenia, although water intoxication has also been identified as a complication of urine drug testing, in individuals with mental retardation, and among the homeless and bottle-fed infants of poor families. After reviewing the difficulties of determining the prevalence of the disorder, the chapter provides a brief history of views about water intoxication and the varying terminology used to describe this condition. The etiology in persons with mental illness, which is likely to be multidimensional, is currently unknown, but there is some initial support for an underlying neurobiological dysfunction that affects the ADH-thirst and the salt appetite mechanisms. The chapter then suggests a three-stage process as a way to categorize the progression of clinical manifestations of the disorder—simple polydipsia, water intoxication, and physical complications secondary to long-term hyponatremia—and describes the changes that may occur in individuals' cognitive functioning, behavioral features, and emotional characteristics, as well as the physiological manifestations of disordered water balance (e.g., lowered serum sodium levels and urinary dilution). Nursing management of the condition generally aims to prevent water intoxication, for example, by using a target weight procedure, and to help polydipsic individuals develop self-monitoring skills and intervention strategies to control fluid balance. Finally, the chapter considers curriculum implications for nursing education and a research agenda.

Chronic fluid imbalance often occurs in individuals with mental retardation and persons with severe and persistent mental disorders, primarily schizophrenia, who are chronically psychotic. This form of water dysregulation is described in the medical, psychiatric, and nursing literature by numerous and often confusing names and has as yet an unexplained etiology. Chronic fluid imbalance has a wide range of reported prevalence, continues to baffle and create nonconcurrence among clinicians regarding treatment practices, and if undetected and untreated can quickly lead to water intoxication and death.

The typical symptom pattern of this syndrome consists of polydipsia, intermittent afternoon hyponatremia, and nocturnal diuresis. It is a daily pattern beginning with compulsive polydipsia during the day, with the client reaching a state of hyponatremia by late afternoon and then polyuria during the night. Accompanying the physical alterations are cognitive, emotional, and behavioral changes. The person becomes irritable, hostile, and psychotic along with being restless, unable to relax, and agitated. When hyponatremia becomes severe, seizures, coma, and death can follow. Besides the physical dangers related to the intoxication, the short-term problems for the individual are a compulsion to drink fluids, a decrease in cognitive functioning, and emotional lability. Rehabilitation efforts are usually stymied because of the individual's inability to concentrate on intervention strategies. The long-term effects of the chronic hyponatremia and excessive fluid ingestion are just beginning to be understood.

Nursing care of the patient with a chronic psychotic disorder who is experiencing fluid imbalance leading to water intoxication is challenging and complex. The physiological status of the individual must be constantly monitored in an attempt to prevent water intoxication. The monitoring tools are inexact, and the nurse is required to rely upon interpretation of subtle physical changes that accompany the emotional and behavioral symptoms and are often difficult to differentiate from the psychiatric disorder itself. However, the real challenge of the nursing care is to help the individual who is impaired with a severe and persistent mental illness to develop the self-monitoring skills and intervention strategies that control fluid balance.

OVERVIEW OF WATER INTOXICATION
WATER INTOXICATION: A MEDICAL EMERGENCY

Water intoxication is the sudden and/or severe hyponatremia that leads to brain edema causing neurological and psychiatric symptoms (deLeon, Verghese, Tracy, Josiassen, & Simpson, 1994). The development of severe hypotonicity leads to the rapid expansion of the brain and increased intracranial pressure. In some instances the brain can herniate into the foramen magnum.

Water intoxication is now known to be a complication of several illness states, but it was not until 1923 that Rowntree identified it and introduced the term in the medical literature. He identified the symptoms of water intoxication, recognized that it could lead to death if not treated, and suggested that it was caused, in part, by increased intracerebral pressure due to disturbance of the salt/water equilibrium. From animal experiments, Rowntree (1923) also concluded that water intoxication occurred when water was ingested in excess of the ability of the organism to excrete it and recommended intravenous hypertonic sodium chloride solution for treatment.

One disorder that can lead to water intoxication is the syndrome of inappropriate secretion of the antidiuretic hormone (SIADH). This syndrome is caused by a failure to repress the antidiuretic hormone (ADH), vasopressin. The increase in ADH causes a decrease in the sodium concentration (and the osmolality) of the extracellular fluid and only a slight increase in extracellular fluid volume. The mechanism begins with ADH causing a decrease in urine output and a simultaneous slight increase in blood volume that causes a slight rise in arterial pressure. This in turn causes a secondary increase in urinary output that is very concentrated because ADH is still causing the excessive reabsorption of water by the kidney tubules. Consequently, the kidney excretes extreme amounts of sodium and other ions into the urine but keeps the water in the extracellular fluid. The sodium concentration becomes seriously reduced, sometimes falling as low as 110 to 120 mEq/L.

Water intoxication has also been reported as a complication of urine drug testing in the workplace (Klonoff & Jurow, 1991). In one report a 40-year-old flight attendant was admitted to an emergency room in a state of water intoxication after being randomly selected for a urine drug test 8 hours earlier. She forced fluids upon instruction and consumed 3 L (thirty 100 ml cups) of tap water over 3 hours in an attempt to void, but she could not and was sent home. She was unable to void freely until after she arrived at the emergency room that evening. She had no other medical history, and her inability to void was attributed to paruresis or hesitancy (inability to initiate micturition because of lack of privacy encountered in public restroom); this condition occurs occasionally in 25% of women and 30% of men and results in delay in the initiation of urination or complete inhibition of voiding (Rees & Leach, 1975). This case was one of eight instances reported where there was acute voluntary water intoxication in the absence of psychiatric or neurologic disorders. It was concluded that water intoxication in these persons was caused by excessive water intake and impaired renal water excretion (Klonoff & Jurow, 1991).

Recently, Keating, Schears, and Dodge (1991) published an alarming report that water intoxication is an American epidemic among bottle-fed infants of poor families. Their study indicated that in this population of poor American families, water becomes the staple when formula is not readily available due to financial restraints. Unfortunately, brain damage or death of these bottle-fed infants may result. Education about the dangers of supplementing formula with water and revamping the federal Women, Infants, and Children (WIC) food program to make formula available at no charge to these parents are important options for preventing or reducing the possible incidences of brain damage or death for these infants. Water intoxication has also been reported in infants when beta-adrenergics are used in combination with steroids as a treatment of premature labor (Reimann & Frolich, 1981) and in hypernatremic mothers who had been given intravenous fluids during labor (Tarnow-Mordi, Shaw, Liu, Gardner, & Flynn, 1981).

Another population recently identified as at risk for water intoxication is the homeless. As with infants, the most probable cause of water intoxication for the homeless is poor nutrition. Again, fluids, such as water from public fountains, are often less costly and more readily available than solid forms of food.

WATER INTOXICATION IN INDIVIDUALS WITH PSYCHIATRIC AND DEVELOPMENTAL DISORDERS

A fascination with water has long been noted in persons with psychiatric disorders. In Shakespeare's *King Lear*, Act III, scene 4, Tom O'Bedlam, an inmate of the Bethlehem Asylum, was described drinking "the green mantle of the standing pool." It was not reported in the scientific literature until 1938, when Barahal described water intoxication in a female diagnosed with dementia praecox, paranoid type; her acute state included seizures and coma. Throughout the years, there have been many other case reports of individuals with mental disorders being admitted to emergency rooms for treatment of water intoxication (Bewley, 1964; Chinn, 1974; Emsley & Taljaard, 1987; Jos, 1984; Jose & Evenson, 1980; Khamnei, 1983; Rae, 1976; Roberge et al., 1984). The symptoms have been similar in that most of the persons were admitted in a state of intoxication following ingestion of large amounts of water (see Case Study 1). In some instances, deaths were reported (Blotcky, Grossman, & Looney, 1980; Rendell, McGrane, & Cuesta, 1978; Raskind, 1974; Vieweg et al., 1985b; Peh, Devan, & Low, 1990).

CASE STUDY 1

Tom T. was diagnosed in 1956 with schizophrenia. He was 17 years old and was hospitalized for hallucinations and paranoid thinking. He was rehospitalized during his freshman year at college for similar symptoms and never returned to school. For the next 40 years, Tom was hospitalized in a long-term care institution with occasional periods of community living. He received all the usual treatments for schizophrenia, including psychotropic medications, electroconvulsive therapy, psychotherapy, and psychoeducation.

His first recognized episode of water intoxication occurred at age 26 when he was admitted to a general hospital following seizures. However, he had been having seizures for 2 to 3 years prior to the first acknowledged episode of water intoxication. When admitted to the emergency room, his serum sodium level was 120 mEq/L. Within the next 12 hours, Tom excreted 4 L of urine with a urine specific gravity of 1.000.

This was one of many episodes of water intoxication for Tom. He believed that water was good for him and that he should be able to drink as much as possible.

Water intoxication is reported less often in persons with mental retardation, but it is relevant because of its severe complications, which include hyponatremia, hypo-osmolality, hypocalcemia, cerebral edema, delirium, psychosis, generalized seizures, coma, polyuria, bowel and bladder dilation, hypotonicity, hydronephrosis, urinary incontinence, renal failure, congestive heart failure, and death (Vieweg et al., 1989). There have been no studies determining the prevalence of water intoxication in this population.

PREVALENCE OF WATER INTOXICATION IN PERSONS WITH MENTAL DISORDERS

The prevalence of water intoxication in patients in psychiatric hospitals remains unclear. In 1979 Jose and Perez-Cruet's survey of 239 patients found that 16 (6.6%) had a consistent history of compulsive water drinking and, of these, 8 (3.3%) had symptoms of water intoxication. In addition, approximately 70% to 80% of these polydipsic patients were diagnosed as having a chronic schizophrenic disorder. These researchers suggested that the incidence of water intoxication might be higher than the literature indicated. Okura and Morii (1986) conducted a similar study in Japan, where they found that among 225 inpatients in a public hospital, there were 7 (3.1%) identified with compulsive water drinking; of these, 6 had water intoxication.

Because polydipsia is believed to be an antecedent to episodes of water intoxication, prevalence of polydipsia in psychiatric institutions has been surveyed by several research teams. Blum, Tempey, and Lynch (1983) reported the prevalence of polydipsia to be 17.5% in their study of 241 male patients hospitalized in a Veterans Administration hospital. Another study of state psychiatric inpatients by Evenson, Jos, and Mallya (1987) reported the prevalence of polydipsia as 6.2%; of the 2,202 patients evaluated, 137 were identified with polydipsia. Using a suggested conservative water intoxication prevalence rate of 3%, these findings would suggest that during any point in time, anywhere from 480 to 2,760 inpatients in federal and state hospitals alone may be experiencing a water intoxication episode.

The wide variation in prevalence rates of polydipsia in psychiatric inpatients might be explained by the different methodologies used in the studies. For instance, in some studies (Evenson et al., 1987; Jose & Perez-Cruet, 1979; Okura & Morii, 1986), the subjects were identified by staff only as excessive water drinkers, and only these patients were confirmed after review of medical records. Another example of different methodology, with a different reported incident rate, was the Blum et al. (1983) study. They included only patients who were screened for urine specific gravity.

Their higher incident rate (17.5%) might suggest that patients may be chronically polydipsic but still not identified as such by staff.

Another possible explanation for the wide variation in the prevalence rate of polydipsia in psychiatric inpatients is that many of the earlier studies were retrospective. Some studies were generated from autopsy-like examination of the patient's medical records—sometimes even years after the patient's death—and left no opportunity to find any data that might be missing, except perhaps through speculation. It is possible, however, that a more accurate projection of prevalence of water intoxication could be found if more suspicious deaths were reviewed using the autopsy-like review mentioned earlier.

Because some studies in the literature concur regarding the prevalence of water intoxication in patients in psychiatric hospitals, while other studies report a wide variation in the prevalence rate, careful analysis of parts of the protocols and research design, especially regarding the criteria for inclusion of subjects in the study, is important. While questions have been raised about study methodologies, attention to congruence among population variables, instruments used for data collection, data collected, and statistics used in analysis must also be given serious consideration. Another possible reason for variability of prevalence rates is the paucity of replication of studies.

DISORDERED WATER BALANCE IN PERSONS WITH MENTAL ILLNESS

There are many differences between the water intoxication experience in persons with psychiatric disorders and those with other disorders, such as SIADH. In the psychiatric population, an episode of water intoxication is often not a onetime occurrence; it may represent one of many instances. There is also a compulsion to drink leading to the polydipsia and a repetitive daily pattern of drinking fluids that interferes with any other activity. In some persons the drive to drink fluids is so strong that they go to great lengths to satisfy the need, including drinking from showers and toilet bowls; they even drink their own urine. The rest of this chapter will focus on this phenomenon in those persons with a mental illness.

BACKGROUND

Observation of the antecedents leading to water intoxication led to many years of speculation that water intoxication in the psychiatric population was only a psychologically based phenomenon. In the early 1940s investigators began theorizing that polydipsia in psychiatric patients was a distinct illness with no biological-psychological interrelatedness. This initial view grew from the belief that the etiology of water intoxication in psychiatric patients was due to excessive water ingestion and was different from medical illnesses with similar symptoms, such as SIADH and diabetes insipidus (DI). Carter and Robbins (1947) supported this initial distinction when they found that urine responses to hypertonic saline infusions were normal in patients with mental disorders but not in those with diabetes mellitus. However, only nine subjects were included in the study, a small sample by today's standards.

In 1958, Barlow and deWardener attempted to further delineate patients with compulsive water drinking from those with DI and renal disease. While they found that some psychiatric patients had abnormal antidiuretic hormone secretion, they were unable to clearly identify diagnostic differences in physiological functioning. Barlow and deWardener (1959) concluded that compulsive water drinking was probable only if one or all of the following physiological factors occurred: (1) there was an absence of renal disease, (2) there were intermittent polydipsia and polyuria, (3) there were associated gross psychological disturbances, or (4) there was evidence of ADH secretion. Langgard and Smith (1962) and Sahadevan and Bayliss (1965) also attempted to delineate the pathophysiological differences among DI, SIADH, and polydipsia leading to water intoxication in psychiatric patients; they presented evidence from two psychiatric cases each that the etiology of water intoxication seemed to be simply excessive water ingestion without any evidence of inappropriate release of ADH.

According to observations, both patients with DI and psychiatric patients with polydipsia ingested excessive volumes of oral fluids and excreted large amounts of urine with low urine osmolality. But laboratory findings indicated that the serum sodium levels, osmolality, and blood urea nitrogen (BUN) levels were high in patients with DI and low in psychiatric patients with polydipsia. The higher levels in patients with DI were thought to be caused by excessive renal fluid loss and subsequent dehydration, while the lower levels in psychiatric patients were explained as extracellular fluid expansion. The lower levels in psychiatric patients were thought to be due only to excessive ingestion of water (Barter & Schwartz, 1967; Saruta et al., 1982).

In a comparison of patients with polydipsia and those diagnosed with SIADH, it was found that the serum sodium levels, osmolarity, and BUNs were low in both, but in SIADH patients, the extracellular fluid expansion was thought to be due to excessive renal water retention and not to excessive water intake, as with psychiatric patients with polydipsia. As a result of comparing the laboratory findings of patients with these different diagnoses, Mendelson and Deza (1976) suggested that the SIADH patients' concentrated urine was due to inappropriately secreted antidiuretic hormone, while the psychiatric patients' diluted urine was due to high volume throughout.

As research progressed in this area, later findings did not support clear distinctions between polydipsia in psychiatric patients and in those with DI and SIADH. Fricchione, Kelleher, and Ayyala (1987) described a patient with chronic schizophrenia who also was diagnosed with DI and polydipsia. The physiological distinction was further confused by numerous other reports—as early as 1963 by Hobson and English and as late as 1985 by Singh, Padi, Bullard, and Freeman—of patients diagnosed with SIADH and associated with massive water ingestion. Review of the results of these studies suggests that impaired excretory mechanisms influenced by the ADH may also play a role in the psychogenesis of water intoxication of psychiatric patients. Analysis of investigations by Raskind, Weitzman, Orenstein, Fisher, and Courtney (1977) and Emsley, Potgieter, Taljaard, Joubert, and Gledhill (1989) supported this view.

In the 1980s investigators started studying fluid disturbance in persons with long-term mental illnesses. It was first established that diurnal weight gain (the daily pattern of body weight fluctuation) could be used as a predictor of serum sodium levels and thus as an indirect measure of fluid imbalance (Delva & Crammer, 1988; Goldman & Luchins, 1987; Koczapski et al., 1987; Vieweg et al., 1989, 1988a, 1988b). Then the Vieweg group at the University of Virginia began to reconceptualize the problem from "water intoxication" to a syndrome of "disordered water balance." These investigators surveyed 93 persons with chronic psychosis, most of whom had schizophrenia; only 7 of them had been identified as being subject to water intoxication, but the study revealed an abnormal diurnal weight gain in over 60% of their subjects (Vieweg et al., 1989). When those with schizophrenia were studied, 70% had abnormal diurnal weight gain. They concluded that abnormal diurnal weight gain is common in persons with chronic psychosis, indicating that water dysregulation in people with severe and persistent mental illnesses is greater than was originally thought. Boyd (1990) speculated that if these rates for water dysregulation were considered over the possible projected federal and state hospitalized patients at that time, the figures could be staggering—anywhere from 16,000 to 92,000 patients may be chronically hyponatremic and experiencing chronic fluid imbalance.

TERMINOLOGY

The terminology used over the years reflects the struggle with trying to understand this phenomenon. Carter and Robbins (1947), and later Leiken and Caplan (1967), first used the term *psychogenic polydipsia* to describe excessive water ingestion leading to water intoxication in psychiatric patients. Sahadevan and Bayliss (1965) and Wyngaarden and Smith (1985) used the terms *primary polydipsia, compulsive water drinking, hyperdipsia,* and *hysterical polydipsia.* These terms were popular when it was believed to be only a psychological problem.

As the complexity of the problem was beginning to be recognized, however, it was named according to its symptoms. Excessive water ingestion, leading to a state of intoxication, was referred to as *self-induced water intoxication in schizophrenia* (SIWIS) and *self-induced water intoxication in psychosis* (SIWIP). Vieweg et al. (1988b) used the terms *psychosis, intermittent hypernatremia,* and *polydipsia* (PIP) to describe a syndrome that pertained to patients who generally resided in state mental hospitals and suffered complications, including generalized seizures, coma, and death secondary to hyponatremia.

Other terms that began to appear in the literature attempted to identify phases or stages of the problem, thereby explaining, studying, and suggesting treatment for water intoxication. Johnson, Breshahan, and Chan (1985) viewed this phenomenon as a psychiatric-physiologic dichotomy. They preferred to use the term *primary polydipsia* when describing abnormal drinking behavior caused by psychiatric or neurophysiological mechanisms in the absence of the need for fluids, and *secondary polydipsia* to describe an unusually large intake of water in response to increased need from abnormal loss (diabetes insipidus or mellitus) or other internal causes of thirst such as dry mouth from medication. Vieweg and colleagues used the term *disordered water balance,* thereby describing their understanding of the underlying problem. This term has not, however, become universal. Rather, in a recent review article, the terms polydipsia and water intoxication were still used (deLeon et al., 1994).

When the many different terms appearing in the literature to describe water intoxication are considered, it is interesting to note the lack of agreement about what this syndrome, and the various components of the syndrome, should be named. Perhaps this lack of agreement about terminology relates in some ways to the inability to address this syndrome from a biological-psychiatric perspective. Interestingly, there is one sentence related to water intoxication in the *Diagnostic and Statistical Manual of Mental Disorders—IV*: "Some individuals with Schizophrenia drink excessive amounts of fluid ("water intoxication") and develop abnormalities in urine specific gravity or electrolyte imbalances" (American Psychiatric Association, 1994, p. 280). In this chapter the term *disordered water balance* will be used to describe the syndrome of psychosis; *intermittent hyponatremia, polydipsia,* and *water intoxication* will be used to describe the medical emergency of hyponatremia.

OSMOLALITY AND SODIUM BALANCE REGULATION

Complex regulatory mechanisms in fluid and electrolyte balance are involved in determining the amount of water that is retained or secreted. Because the overriding problem in disordered water balance is hyponatremia, a review of the normal mechanisms for maintaining osmolality and a normal sodium concentration is presented.

One of the most important functions of the kidney is to control osmolality (concentration of solutes) of body fluids. Approximately four fifths of the total osmolality of the interstitial fluid and plasma is caused by sodium and chloride ions. When the osmolality falls too low and fluids become dilute, nervous and hormonal feedback mechanisms cause the kidney to excrete a great excess of water in the urine. This causes a dilute urine, but removes fluids from the body and results in an increase in fluid osmolality. When the osmolality is too great, the kidneys excrete an excess of solutes and concentrated urine, thereby reducing the body fluid osmolality. Osmolality and sodium concentration are inextricably related because the sodium ions in the extracellular fluids play the dominant role in determining the extracellular fluid osmolality. The sodium ions of the extracellular fluid determine either directly or indirectly over 90% of the osmotic pressure of the extracellular fluid. The osmolality of the extracellular fluid averages almost exactly 300 mOsm/L, and the sodium ion concentration averages 142 mEq/L. These rarely change more than ±3% in a day, indicating how tightly controlled they are. This control is achieved using three separate systems that operate in close association to regulate extracellular osmolality: (1) osmoreceptor-antidiuretic hormone system, (2) the thirst mechanism, and (3) the salt appetite mechanism (Guyton, 1991).

OSMORECEPTOR-ANTIDIURETIC HORMONE SYSTEM

The antidiuretic hormone (ADH), also called vasopressin, is the signal that tells the kidney to excrete a dilute or a concentrated urine. When body fluids are too concentrated, the posterior pituitary gland secretes large amounts of ADH, which allows the kidney to excrete large amounts of solutes but to conserve water (Guyton, 1991). In the absence of ADH, the kidney excretes large amount of dilute urine. This hormone is responsible for fluid retention by promoting water reabsorption from both the distal tubules and collecting ducts of the kidneys. When too much water is ingested or infused, osmoreceptors, found in the vicinity of the arteries supplying the hypothalamus, sense the increased osmotic pressure and transmit nerve impulses to the supraoptic nucleus of the hypothalamus. The nerve fibers from the hypothalamus to the posterior pituitary gland carry a message that there is a surplus of water in the body; then the antidiuretic hormone, which is normally secreted into the blood by the supraoptico-hypophyseal axis of the hypothalamus and neurohypophysis, is suppressed and less water is reabsorbed by the kidney tubules. In this way, more urine is produced and normal osmolality maintained.

When no ADH is secreted, the water is not reabsorbed by the kidney tubules; as a result, five to ten times the amount of normal urine is excreted, and the extracellular fluid becomes progressively more concentrated (Zerbe, Stropes, & Roberson, 1980). This is the case in diabetes insipidus. On the other hand, when large amounts of ADH are secreted, too much water is reabsorbed, causing small amounts of concentrated urine (400 to 500 ml) to be produced (i.e., less than one third of the normal volume). This water is conserved, extracellular fluid becomes dilute, and hyponatremia occurs.

When a person drinks a large amount of water, water diuresis occurs approximately 45 minutes after drinking. The delay in onset of diuresis occurs because of the time it takes for the water to be absorbed from the gastrointestinal tract and the time required for destruction of the ADH that has already been released by the pituitary gland prior to drinking the water (Guyton, 1991). Under normal conditions, the body can filter, reabsorb, and excrete a liter an hour of ingested fluids and maintain adequate osmolality.

THE THIRST MECHANISM

Thirst, the conscious desire for water, is equally important in regulating body water, osmolality, and sodium concentration because the amount of water in the body at any one time is determined by the balance between intake and output of water. Thirst is the primary regulator of the intake of water. The thirst center includes the area along the anteroventral wall of the third ventricle (also promotes antidiuresis) and small areas that are located anterolaterally in the preoptic hypothalamus. These cells function as osmoreceptors to activate the thirst mechanism. Additionally, an increase in osmotic pressure of the cerebrospinal fluid in the third ventricle has essentially the same effect to promote drinking.

After drinking water, thirst is immediately relieved, even before the water has been absorbed from the gastrointestinal tract. This relief is only temporary, and if the water does not enter the gastrointestinal tract after 15 minutes or more, thirst reappears. Once the stomach and the upper portion of the gastrointestinal tract are extended by water, another short period of temporary relief occurs until the fluid is absorbed and distributed throughout the body. The value of this mechanism is that a person will stop drinking before the body is overloaded with water, thereby allowing time for the water to be absorbed.

When the sodium concentration rises approximately 2 mEq/L above normal, the drinking mechanism is "tripped"; the person then reaches a level of thirst that is strong enough to activate the necessary motor effort to cause drinking. The person ordinarily drinks precisely the required amount of fluid to bring the extracellular fluids back to normal. Therefore, the major feedback mechanism for control of sodium concentration is the ADH-thirst mechanism.

SALT APPETITE MECHANISM

Sodium is reabsorbed as a part of the glomerular filtrate in the proximal tubules and loops of Henle returning the sodium back to the plasma. Sodium reabsorption is highly variable and depends on the concentration of aldosterone, a hormone secreted by the adrenal cortex. Three different factors are known to stimulate this secretion of aldosterone: (1) increased angiotensin II in the blood, (2) increased extracellular fluid potassium ion concentration, and (3) decreased extracellular fluid sodium ion concentration. The first and the third are important for the control of sodium excretion by the kidneys.

When the extracellular fluid volume falls too low, the arterial pressure decreases and the reflex stimulation of the sympathetic nervous system increases. Both of these reduce blood flow through the kidneys and excite the secretion of renin, which in turn causes the formation of angiotensin I. Angiotensin I is later converted to angiotensin II, which has a direct effect on the zona glomerulosa cells to increase the secretion of aldosterone. Additionally, a decrease in extracellular fluid sodium ion concentration also seems to have a direct weak stimulatory effect on aldosterone secretion, but it is much less potent than the effect of angiotensin II.

Under normal conditions, aldosterone is relatively unimportant in determining sodium ion concentrations. Even though aldosterone increases the quantity of sodium in the extracellular fluid, an increase in the reabsorption of water along with the sodium usually prevents a rise in sodium concentration. There is, however, an increase in total quantity of extracellular fluid. An increase in the extracellular fluid volume eventually leads to an increase in arterial pressure, and the increase in arterial pressure leads to increased glomerular filtration rate. The rapid flow of filtrate then overrides the excessive reabsorptive effect of the aldosterone and thereby almost nullifies the effect of aldosterone on extracellular fluid sodium concentration (Guyton, 1991).

ETIOLOGY, PATHOPHYSIOLOGY, AND CONTRIBUTING FACTORS

ETIOLOGY

The etiology of disordered water balance is unknown. It is no longer believed that ingestion of excessive fluids is caused by psychological problems. Many now believe that the neurobiological changes that occur in persons with long-term mental illnesses lead to the emotional, behavioral, and cognitive manifestations of disordered water balance. Hypothalamic (Ferrier, 1985) and hippocampal disturbances (Luchins, 1990) and a combination of both (Vieweg et al., 1988b) have been suggested. However, it is unclear whether these changes are iatrogenic responses or part of the mental disorder itself.

Related areas of research addressing different parts of the sodium regulation system in both human and animal studies include some recent studies that focus on ADH and angiotensin. The antidiuretic hormone was studied in 15 patients with schizophrenia or schizoaffective disorder and 15 controls following ingestion of 20 ml/kg of water (Ohsawa et al., 1993). In the patient group, ADH was secreted even when plasma osmolality was low, but the sensitivity to ADH was lower than in the controls. It was hypothesized that the volume expansion caused by inappropriate ADH secretion stimulated atrial natriuretic peptide (ANP), which contributed to the hyponatremia.

Animal studies show that angiotensin II is an important dipsogenic in animals. For example, it is known that chronic D_2 dopamine receptor blockade increases angiotensin II-induced thirst in animals. In humans, some conditions with abnormal thirst are associated with increased angiotensin function, and increased peripheral responses to angiotensin II have been documented. It is reasoned that chronic D_2 blockade with typical neuroleptics may increase sensitivity to angiotensin II and induce thirst. This is supported by recent case reports of improvement of polydipsia with clozapine, which has negligible D_2 blocking action (Verghese, deLeon, & Simpson, 1993). However, use of psychotropic medications cannot fully explain the phenomenon. One problem with a strictly pharmacological explanation is that polydipsia and water intoxication were reported prior to the discovery of current psychotropic medication.

A number of excessive water ingestion studies have considered possible contributing iatrogenic factors, including: (a) administration of psychotropic medications (DeSoto, Griffith, & Katz, 1985; Husband, Mai, & Carruthers, 1981; Sandifer, 1983); (b) withdrawal of psychotropic drugs (Shen & Sata, 1983; 1984); and (c) electroconvulsive shock therapy (ECT) (Jos, Evenson, & Mallya, 1986; Narang, Chaudhury, & Wig, 1973; Shah, Wig, & Chaudhury, 1973). In most cases there was some effect identified by the researchers. Analysis of the drug and ECT studies suggests that, for the most part, these studies examined the effect of a specific drug such as chlorpromazine and thiothixene on the antidiuretic hormone, arginine vasopressin (AVP). The problem with drawing any conclusions regarding the correlational relationships between the administration of psychotropic medications and vasopressin is that the relationship between the antidiuretic hormone and disordered water balance is still not understood.

The need for further research into the iatrogenic factors of psychotropic medications is suggested from the conflicting results of the Shen and Sata (1983) study; when medications—including thiothixene, lithium carbonate, chlorpromazine, amitriptyline, fluphenazine, and haloperidol—were administered to patients, their water drinking behavior became worse. Six patients in their study received psychotropic medication reduction and five patients had episodes of compulsive water drinking occurring within a week following reduction of neuroleptic dosages. Six episodes of compulsive drinking were stopped within 24 hours by doubling the dosage of the neuroleptic. While this later study suggests that the illness itself may influence excessive water drinking and water intoxication, a study by Goldman and Janecek found an initial worsening of polydipsia when neuroleptics were withdrawn (1989). The results of these studies point to the elusive nature of this phenomenon and to an obvious need for more research in this area.

POSSIBLE DEMOGRAPHIC AND/OR TREATMENT FACTORS

Some investigators have attempted, mainly unsuccessfully, to identify demographic or treatment factors that may be associated with excessive water ingestion or its progression into water intoxication. Roberge et al. (1984) and Resnick and Patterson (1969) proposed that water intoxication might occur more frequently in females, but Evenson et al. (1987) showed the prevalence to be only slightly higher in women (60%) than in men. Boyd (1990) suggested that this may reflect the population distribution of the study rather than an increased prevalence of water intoxication in females, pointing to the Blum et al. (1983) study that was conducted in an all-male institution. Review of records of identified patients who experienced excessive fluid ingestion while inpatient research subjects at the National Institute of Mental Health Neuropsychiatric Research Hospital (NIMH-NRH) revealed a prevalence rate of 70% for males that was more than twice the 30% rate for females (Interview with clinical nursing staff, 1989).

OTHER POSSIBLE CORRELATING FACTORS

Researchers have looked at other factors as having a possible correlation with water intoxication. It has long been known that cigarette smoking caused increased elevation of plasma vasopressin (Rowe, Kilgore, & Robertson, 1980). Vieweg et al. (1986) were unable to show that cigarette consumption is related to water intoxication, but Allon, Allen, Deck, and Clark (1990) implicated cigarettes as the cause of renal impairment in two persons with schizophrenia who developed severe hyponatremia with inappropriately concentrated urine. The Vieweg group argued that the Allon et al. findings were misinterpreted and were not applicable to persons with the typical symptoms of polydipsia and hyposthenuria (Vieweg, Veldhuis, Leadbetter, Hundley, & Shutty, 1991).

Use of alcohol and other substances has also been studied for iatrogenic effects. Ripley, Millson, and Koczapski (1989) found in their study that alcohol abuse was more common among 17 schizophrenic male inpatients with self-induced water intoxication than among 17 matched schizophrenic control inpatients. One factor, identified from this study and of note for future studies in this area, is that the alcohol abuse had begun 8 to 22 years before the diagnosis of water intoxication. However, these findings are contradicted by Cooney, who found no association between alcohol abuse and compulsive water drinking in patients and their families (1991). Nevertheless, multisubstance intoxication has been noted in many patients with schizophrenia (Koczapski, Ledwidge, Predes, Kogan, & Higenbottam, 1990). Clearly more work is needed in this area.

In summary, the etiology of disordered water balance in persons with mental illness is unknown, although there is some initial support for an underlying neurobiological dysfunction that affects the ADH-thirst and the salt appetite mechanisms. For example, animal studies are beginning to link dopamine receptors with polydipsia. Since the etiology is unknown and may very well be multidimensional, the clinical manifestations become very important in planning treatment.

CLINICAL FEATURES OF DISORDERED WATER BALANCE

As with other areas of this elusive syndrome, clinical descriptions of polydipsia and hyponatremia in psychiatric patients vary. However, review of the literature does provide several general features. Lapierre, Berthot, Gurvitch, Rees, and Kirch (1990) point out that "the syndrome tends to develop in patients with chronic schizophrenic disorders, especially among those patients who have a 5- to 15-year history of psychosis" (p. 89).

What also continues to elude researchers regarding water intoxication is why obvious excessive water drinking does not produce hyponatremia and water intoxication in all schizophrenic patients. They continue to ask why some patients can drink large volumes of fluid without lowering their serum sodium and experiencing adverse effects, while a small subpopulation cannot. What the reports do indicate, however, is that for patients who develop the disordered water balance, symptoms often range from subtle signs to lethal complications. Table 15–1 provides a listing of some frequent indicators for both polydipsia and hyponatremia.

A three-stage process has been suggested as a way of categorizing a progression of clinical manifestations. It includes (1) *simple polydipsia* with accompanying polyuria, which is thought to occur after 5 to 10 years of the psychosis; (2) *water intoxication,* with the onset after 5 to 10 years of polydipsia; and (3) *physical complica-*

TABLE 15–1. INDICATORS OF POLYDIPSIA AND HYPONATREMIA AMONG PSYCHIATRIC PATIENTS

Signs and Symptoms of Polydipsia
Excessive fluid consumption and/or fluid-seeking behavior
Polyuria
Dramatic or rapid weight fluctuations
Incontinence
Suggesting laboratory values
    Low serum BUN
    Low urine specific gravity

Signs and Symptoms of Hyponatremia Associated with Polydipsia
Mental status disturbance
    Confusion, disorientation
    Restlessness, irritability
    Psychosis (may develop or become more prominent)
Neurological disturbances
    Headaches
    Blurred vision
    Seizures
    Stupor, coma
Gastrointestinal disturbances
    Nausea, vomiting, diarrhea
Musculoskeletal disturbances
    Muscle cramps, twitches, tremors
Suggestive laboratory values
    Low serum sodium
    Low serum osmolality

From Berthot, B. D., Gurvitch, M., Rees, I., Kirch, D. G., & Lapierre, E. D. (1990). Polydipsia and hyponatremia in psychiatric patients: Challenge to creative nursing care. *Archives of Psychiatric Nursing, 4*(2), 87–92.

tions secondary to ingestion of large quantities of fluids over several years (deLeon et al., 1994). During stage 1, the polydipsia is the primary manifestation, and it may be episodic. At this point, patients may not be identified as having water dysregulation problems. During the second phase, the symptoms of water intoxication appear and are associated with the intermittent polydipsia, afternoon hyponatremia, and nocturnal diuresis. During the third stage, the complications secondary to chronic ingestion of water can develop, such as osteoporosis with pathological fractures and dilation of urinary and gastrointestinal tracts. Other complications may include cardiac failure, malnutrition, hernias, and permanent brain damage. While not everyone follows this progression, it is a way of conceptualizing the syndrome. Still, research is needed to determine whether most patients actually experience these stages, although there is agreement in the literature that the following clinical manifestations are typical of persons with this syndrome.

COGNITIVE FEATURES

Cognitive changes occur in patients with disordered water balance. Cognitive impairment was demonstrated in 16 persons with schizophrenia with disordered water balance when compared to 16 matched subjects with no evidence of water dysregulation (Emsley, Spangenberg, Robers, Taljaard, & Chalton, 1993). The patients with disordered water balance tended to obtain poorer scores than the controls on neuropsychological tests, including the Wechsler Memory Scale Visual Reproduction and Trail Marking Test, Part A. These differences were not attributed to differences in the duration of the illness, premorbid IQ, medication or electroconvulsive therapy received, or manifestations of symptoms.

Another University of Virginia Medical Center research group demonstrated deterioration in cognitive functioning as hyponatremia became more severe. When comparing cognitive functioning during hyponatremia (serum sodium <130 mmol/L) and during normonatremia (serum sodium >135 mmol/L), the groups found that during hyponatremia there were significant deficits involving complex information processing skills such as mental flexibility and verbal fluency. However, short-term memory was intact, and no deficits in sustained attention or visual-motor scan were observed (Shutty, Briscoe, Sautter, & Leadbetter, 1993).

The existence of cognitive impairments in persons with disordered water balance also was supported by the results of the Mini-Mental State Examination (MMSE) (Schnur, Wirkowski, Reddy, Decina, & Mukherjee, 1993). Subjects with water dysfunction performed significantly worse on the MMSE than did a comparison group. The differences could not be attributed to demographic characteristics, medication effects, tardive dyskinesia, or to a history of hyponatremic seizures. The MMSE was performed when the patients were not hyponatremic and at the time when their serum sodium levels were normal.

It is unclear whether the cognitive impairment is associated with those persons who have disordered water imbalance, or if the impairment is actually caused by the chronic state of hyponatremia. The findings of the Emsley group study (1993) support the association of disordered water balance with structural brain damage but do not support evidence of a lesion in a discrete area of the brain. The low performance throughout the group points to a more global impairment. Another explanation for the results could be that cognitive impairment is a consequence of disordered water imbalance as a result of many episodes of water intoxication. The cerebral edema that develops following hyponatremia causes the encephalopathy associated with neurological disturbance, which may lead to irreversible brain damage.

BEHAVIORAL FEATURES

POLYDIPSIA

The classic behavioral manifestation associated with disordered water balance is stereotypic, repetitive polydipsia. There are numerous reports of polydipsia describing patients who easily and rapidly consume 4 to 10 liters of fluid over a 24-hour period (Blum et al., 1983; Jose & Perez-Cruet, 1979; Shah & Greenberg, 1993), but there are few studies describing the actual polydipsic behavior. Bremner and Regan report a cross-sectional survey of the drinking behavior of 31 patients who, in the opinion of the nurses, drank 5 liters or more daily (1991). Another study examined the drinking patterns of persons with schizophrenia while on and off medication and compared them to volunteers with no history of mental illness who were asked to keep a diary of their fluid intake (Lawson et al., 1992). In this carefully designed study, the amount, time, and item drunk were assessed by pairs of trained nursing staff or psychologists for 48 to 62 hours. Patients were required to drink from cups of predetermined volumes when using the water fountain, and meals consisted of clear fluid and solid foods. All coffee was decaffeinated. The patients with schizophrenia tended to drink 2.5 liters a day, which was significantly higher than the normal controls. Further, fluid intake was significantly higher when the patients were unmedicated. It should be noted, however, that the two groups did not differ in terms of the number of episodes of drinking, but in the amount ingested.

One interesting aspect of the polydipsia is the compulsive nature of the drinking. It has even been suggested, following successful treatment of one patient with fluoxetine, that this behavior is a variant of obsessive-compulsive disorder (Deas-Nesmith & Brewerton, 1992). These patients are clearly driven to drink. When asked what happens that makes them want to drink, they will often respond that they "just have to have it."

POLYURIA

Polyuria associated with polydipsia is more an inconvenience than a real behavioral problem. The amount excreted is relative to the amount ingested and can easily be 3 to 5 liters in a 24-hour period. When diuresis occurs, several liters may be excreted at one time. Further, an urgency and incontinency may occur. Many patients are incontinent at night, causing frequent bedding changes and a pervasive urine odor in their rooms. The incontinency can present a social problem if family members do not want these patients to stay with them. When one patient was asked what could help him with his water problem, his reply was, "a rubber sheet."

EMOTIONAL FEATURES

Patients with disordered water balance often are easily provoked to anger, irritable, and emotionally labile, particularly as they become hyponatremic. While there are few reports in the literature about the emotional aspect because it is difficult to determine if the emotions are a function of the hyponatremia or the psychiatric disorder, clinically, as patients become hyponatremic, their psychiatric symptoms are more likely to be exacerbated. Therefore, if hostility is a symptom of a patient, then hostility will most likely be expressed during a hyponatremic state.

A feeling of euphoria has also been reported following ingestion of large amounts of water. In one case study, a young woman reported she experienced enjoyable feelings of being "a little dizzy, funny and high, like after a beer," which enabled her to fall asleep (Lee, Chow, & Koo, 1989). This woman drank up to 20 liters a day in a short period of time in order to have a more forceful effect and achieve an altered state of consciousness, in spite of the abdominal bloating, diarrhea, nausea, and sometimes vomiting. This feeling of euphoria may partially explain the attraction of drinking water to patients who are confined to long-term care treatment centers, which tend to be tightly controlled and environmentally sterile. Clinical experience has shown that patients do seem to use drinking water as a way of dealing with stressful situations and report a feeling of calmness after consuming large amounts of water (see Case Study 2).

CASE STUDY 2

Susan was diagnosed as having schizoaffective disorder in her late teens. She was hospitalized for her illness for many years but also experienced short periods of successful adjustment in the community. She was treated with many different psychotropics and also received several series of electroconvulsive therapy. She had her first episode of water intoxication in her middle twenties and it became her major problem.

A typical day for Susan began with breakfast and several cups of coffee. She would usually attend treatment activities in the morning and become loud, confused, and suspicious by afternoon. By dinner, she would be accusing the staff of taking her belongings and would often end up assaulting another patient.

At age 40, she agreed to try to follow a target weight procedure and was placed on a protocol. Initially, it was not uncommon for her weight to vary 10 to 12 pounds in one day. By exerting control over her intake, she stabilized her diurnal weight variation. Through identifying antecedents to the periods of weight gain, she realized that she would begin drinking when she was stressed. She used the water as a way of self-medication for stress reduction. As she gained insight into her behavior, she gradually substituted relaxation techniques for water ingestion.

She was discharged from the hospital into a group home and has been able to live in the community for 2 years with occasional hospitalizations.

PHYSIOLOGICAL MANIFESTATIONS

SERUM SODIUM LEVELS

Most of the physical manifestations of disordered water balance are related to lowered serum sodium levels. Lapierre et al., (1990) also point out that a decrease in serum sodium concentration warns of a more serious progression of the disorder. Lawson, Karson, and Begelow (1985) reported that significant clinical symptoms tended to appear when the serum sodium concentration drops below the normal range of 135 to 148 mEq/L. This finding was later confirmed in a study conducted by Illowski and Kirch (1988).

While it is important for the nurse to be aware of warning indicators of polydipsia and hyponatremia, an additional number of symptoms listed in Table 15–1 may indicate the onset of hyponatremia. As early as 1938, Barahal reported that among schizophrenic patients, psychosis may become more prominent. This finding was supported by the research of Jose and Perez-Cruet in 1979 and Blum et al. in 1983. Studies by Vieweg et al. (1985a) and Mareth (1988) indicate that when the sodium level drops below 120 mEq/L, seizures and coma are more likely to occur. The latter (Mareth, 1988) concluded from his study that all these clinical features vary with the degree of water intoxication and with the rapidity of serum sodium changes, and that among some of these patients, the onset of seizures may be the first signal of hyponatremia.

However, the serum sodium level of persons with disordered water balance may vary considerably from the normal population. Koczapski and Millson (1989) studied individual variation in serum sodium values of eight hospitalized men with disordered water balance for 12 months and found that morning sodium values varied greatly among patients, ranging from 125 to 147 mEq/L. Afternoon values were consistently lower, ranging from 119 to 139 mEq/L, along with an increase in patient weight. Symptoms of water intoxication occurred infrequently. When present, however, intoxication symptoms appeared to be related to the amount of *change* in serum sodium values with each patient rather than to the actual sodium *values*. For example, one patient had a usual morning serum sodium level of 147 mEq/L and developed slurred speech and ataxia when his afternoon serum sodium level fell to 135 mEq/L. He was stuporous when his sodium level fell to 131 mEq/L. On the other hand, another patient usually had a morning sodium level of 125 mEq/L and was mildly euphoric with afternoon serum sodium levels as low as 112 mEq/L. This patient's level returned to his baseline by the following morning without fluid restriction. He had never had seizures.

URINARY DILUTION

Urinary dilution, a typical indicator of disordered water balance that can be easily determined by urine specific gravities of below 1.008, is thought to occur because the ingestion of a large amount of fluid overloads the kidney. Blum et al. (1983) and Vieweg, Rowe, David, and Spradlin (1984) suggested that hyposthenuria, a urine specific gravity of 1.008 or less, is a useful marker for polydipsia-hyponatremia in its early stages. Indeed, in the early 1930s, abnormal urinary dilution was generally noted in persons with schizophrenia by investigators seeking a physiological basis for schizophrenia. Hoskins and Sleeper (1933) did extensive physiologic testing on a large sample of inpatients at Worcester State Hospital in Massachusetts. They found that there were remarkable differences in the results of urine volumes in schizophrenic patients compared with normal control subjects. They concluded that schizophrenic patients not only excreted an average urine volume twice that of normal controls, but they also showed larger than normal variation in their pattern of excretion. While the etiology of the polyuria was unclear, in 1935 Sleeper performed water load and water deprivation tests and was able to demonstrate that the polyuria resolved with control of polydipsia and that diabetes insipidus was not present.

Lapierre et al. (1990) pointed out how important it is for the nurse to remember that rapid urinary dilution may follow a large consumption of fluids. Estimating daily urine volume is difficult because accurate measures of output are almost impossible to obtain; however, using spot measures of urine dilution has been validated as an accurate indicator of urine volume (Vieweg et al., 1986; Koczapski & Millson, 1989; Goldman et al., 1990). These authors found that early morning and late afternoon urine creatinine concentrations, adjusted for body weight, are highly correlated to measured 24-hour urine volumes. Goldman et al. (1990) found that a 4:00 p.m. urine creatinine sample alone provided almost as much information as the two measurements.

THIRST

Because one of the mechanisms involved in maintaining normal osmolality is thirst, studies on thirst in individuals with disordered water balance might reasonably be expected. However, this is not the case. Thirst is reported clinically by patients when asked why they drink. Some do respond that they drink because they are thirsty. Since, however, evidence suggests that these patients do not actually drink more frequently than others, but longer, the question of the adequacy of their thirst mechanism is raised. This may well be an area of future investigation.

OTHER PHYSICAL MANIFESTATIONS

Electroencephalographic (EEG) changes during water intoxication have been documented (Okura et al., 1990). It was shown that during a state of hyponatremia (serum sodium <127.4 mEq/L), there are definitely EEG changes; they are probably related to the cerebral edema associated with hyponatremia, intercompartmental potassium shift, and generalized hypo-osmolality. Intravenous high osmolality saline improved the hyponatremia and the EEG eventually returned to normal. These authors recommend recording EEG changes in order to monitor and confirm the outcome of water intoxication.

NURSING MANAGEMENT

The nursing management of persons with disordered water balance leading to water intoxication is challenging and complex. There are two general aims in the nursing care of those with fluid imbalance. The first is the prevention of water intoxication; the second is helping the individual who is impaired with a severe and persistent mental illness develop self-monitoring skills and intervention strategies that control fluid balance.

ASSESSMENT

It is important to identify individual antecedents that lead to water intoxication. Any person who has had a long-term mental illness should be considered a candidate for this problem. The characteristic behavior pattern, of course, is frequent, compulsive drinking of fluids, followed by polyuria. However, for many patients the symptoms are not obvious. Because persons with this problem have not actually been shown to drink more often than other patients—rather, they probably drink more at one time—polydipsia may not be obvious. Additionally, disordered water balance is not just a problem of ingestion of fluids; it is also a problem of retention. In reality, some persons who do not drink more than normal may be unable to excrete normally.

There is a wide range of symptoms that are indicative of disordered water balance. Snider and Boyd (1991) have categorized symptoms according to severity in physiological, behavioral, and cognitive indicators, and they recommend this approach as a useful guide for nursing staff and families (see Table 15–2). Emotional changes are not included in the symptoms because of the difficulty in differentiating the emotional changes that result from hyponatremia from those of the mental disorder. This categorization of symptom severity has yet to be tested.

One of the best assessment techniques, as well as an intervention strategy, is a target weight procedure, a method for monitoring diurnal weight variation. This procedure involves establishing a baseline weight, calculating a target weight, and then weighing the patient throughout the day. If the patient's weight is above the target weight, the individual has abnormal diurnal weight variation and could develop seizures. Since diurnal weight has been shown to be an accurate indication of serum sodium level, monitoring weight is a method of assessing for hyponatremia state. Delva and Crammer (1988) found that with a 7% increase above basal weight, the plasma sodium decreased to a level below 125 mEq/L.

The first target weight procedure was reported by Goldman and Luchins (1987), who established baseline weights and simultaneous serum sodium concentration levels; these were obtained twice for 2 weeks. A baseline mean weight and a mean

TABLE 15–2. DISORDERED WATER BALANCE LEADING TO WATER INTOXICATION

SEVERITY	PHYSIOLOGICAL	BEHAVIORAL	COGNITIVE
Mild	Increased diurnal weight gain Urine specific gravity normal (1.011–1.025) Serum sodium normal (135–145 mEq/L)	Notable trips to water fountain or drinking more than average amount of fluids Notable trips to restroom 4 to 5 times in 8-hour period	Able to hold appropriate conversation for extended periods of time Verbal expression intact Motivation high As rationale, possibly gives explanation of dry mouth secondary to taking medication
Moderate	Urine specific gravity = 1.010–1.003 Increased diurnal weight gain Possible puffiness of face and/or orbital edema Periodic urinary incontinence during night	Periods of unexplained restlessness, including periods of highness or hypervigilance Seen carrying cups of fluids around frequently Signs of alertness shown during a.m. and deterioration during p.m.	Responds fairly well to limit setting Concentration level at least 30 to 45 minutes Able to verbalize understanding and repeat instructions back Demonstrates ability to engage in meaningful sequential conversation but intermittently shows evidence of delusions or blocking Able to verbalize realistic plans of life situation
Severe	Possible evidence of chronic stomach and/or bladder dilation Urine specific gravity = 1.003–1.000 Frequent signs of nausea and vomiting Possible history of major motor seizure Possible change in blood pressure or pulse Polyuria Polydipsia Urinary incontinence during day/night	Hypovigilance Frequent yelling and/or arguments with staff If smoker, increased smoking in association with increased fluid consumption Presence of chronic psychosis History of multiple admissions Periodic exaggerated behavior Demonstrates compulsive repetitive nature associated with fluids	Poor response to verbal interventions Impaired attention span (20 minutes or under) Impaired recall ability Inappropriate and nonreality-based thinking frequently exhibited Motivation level low—history of noncompliance Cognitive limitation Lack of interest in learning Possible discrepancy between chronological age and developmental level Impaired ability to reason Frequent inaccurate interpretation of environment Egocentricity

From Snider, K., & Boyd, M. A. (1991). When they drink too much: Nursing interventions for patients with disordered water balance. *Journal of Psychosocial Nursing and Mental Health Services, 28*(7), 10–16.

serum sodium concentration were then calculated and used to predict a target weight that would be roughly equivalent to a plasma sodium level of 125 mEq/L. Patients were weighed three times a week and whenever nurses suspected water intoxication. If the weight exceeded the target weight, a serum sodium level was drawn. If the serum sodium level was below the established level, interventions were begun. Koczapski and colleagues (1987) also reported successful use of weight monitoring throughout the day.

The use of serum sodium levels as validation of hyponatremia in the target weight procedure becomes problematic, however, because of the individual variability of serum sodium, the intrusive nature of venipuncture, and the lack of available laboratory facilities in many long-term care facilities. In fact, it was recently shown that a target weight procedure can be successfully applied without the intrusiveness of frequent venipunctures (Boyd et al., 1992). In the St. Louis State Hospital Target Weight Procedure (STWP), the baseline weight is initially determined as an early morning weight prior to dressing, after voiding, and before any oral intake. The target weight is calculated to be 105% of the baseline weight. For example, a person weighing 150 pounds at 6 AM has a target weight of 157.5 pounds. The target weight is established at 105% of the baseline weight rather than the 107% recommended by Delva and Crammer because of the likelihood that the baseline weight was elevated due to urinary retention and interstitial edema. Individuals are weighed at regular intervals throughout the day. The usual times (6 and 11 AM, and 2, 4, 7, 9, and 11 PM) are sometimes individualized, however, depending on the patient's activities. If an individual's diurnal weight variation is monitored using the STWP for 2 to 4 weeks, it is possible to determine whether there is an abnormal diurnal weight variation indicating the presence of disordered water balance. If the individual stays under the target weight, there is probably no fluid imbalance and the individual can successfully excrete fluids. The time of 2 to 4 weeks is needed in order to account for life-style changes and other biological cycles such as menstruation.

Other assessment data that can be used are serum sodium levels, which should be obtained at the time of the highest weight. If the serum sodium level falls below the normal range of 135 to 145 mEq/L, the person should be considered as potentially having a problem. However, this level should be interpreted in relation to the patient's serum sodium level at the time of the lowest weight in order to determine the true meaning of the sodium level.

Urinary dilution is another means of assessing the status of the fluid balance. Urine specific gravity, which is an indicator of urinary dilution and an indirect measure of fluid balance, is easily and inexpensively measured on the hospital unit or at home with the chemstrips that have a specific gravity measure. While it has been shown that persons with disordered water balance typically have hyposthenuria of 1.008 or less, low urine specific gravities are not good indicators of approaching intoxication. As a matter of fact, if the weight is increasing and the urine specific gravity remains normal, it is more likely that hyponatremia is becoming more severe. When the fluid is finally excreted and diuresis occurs, very dilute urine would indicate a return to a more normonatremic state.

Several tools have been used to assess behavior changes associated with hyponatremia (Boyd et al., 1992; Bugle, Andrew, & Heath, 1992). However, reliability and validity have not been established. At this point, the biological markers of abnormal diurnal weight gain, hyposthenuria, and below-normal serum sodium levels are the best indicators of disordered water balance.

Once the presence of fluid dysregulation is established, maintaining an individual on the target weight procedure is the best way to determine whether water intoxication is imminent. The more the person's weight exceeds the established target weight, the more likely hyponatremia is developing. Other indicators include confusion, restlessness, slurred speech, periorbital edema, distended abdomen, excessive perspiration, vomiting, and tremors. If a patient becomes stuporous or develops seizures, immediate medical attention is needed.

PREVENTION OF WATER INTOXICATION

Hyponatremia can be easily prevented by using a target weight procedure. The advantage of the target weight procedure is that it is easily implemented, there are no intrusive measures, and the 5% target weight gives the individual time to prohibit intake before becoming dangerously intoxicated. In order to maximize patient cooperation, the procedure needs to be carefully explained so that the patient understands the reason for the frequent weights and why fluid will be restricted if the target weight is exceeded. If an individual is at or over the target weight, he or she should be restricted from drinking fluids until diuresis occurs and the weight is below target weight. Usually, patients cooperate and are able to refrain from drinking more fluids, especially if they are temporarily restricted to the unit where they can be observed.

However, one of the characteristics of this problem is compulsive water-seeking behavior, and clinical experience indicates that water restriction is sometimes easier said than done. Some facilities actually have water intoxication treatment units that allow the staff to regulate the amount of available water by turning off water fountains, locking bathroom doors, and eliminating access to fluid receptacles. Patients are then prevented from accessing fluids by environmental control. These techniques are useful in preventing water intoxication but are not especially useful in helping individuals gain control over the fluid intake through self-monitoring. In many parts of the country, severely restricting the client's environment in this way is antithetical to treatment philosophy. Prim (1988) reported success with planning interventions by modifying a patient's focal stimuli and providing structured activities in an attempt to divert a patient's attention. Another technique that has been used to temporarily restrict fluid intake is assignment of one staff member to a patient (similar to suicide precaution). As a last resort, chemical or mechanical restraints can be used in some cases.

Investigators such as Goldberg (1981), Rendell et al. (1978), and Zubenko, Altesman, Cassidy, and Barreira (1984) have described behavioral interventions that address the medical treatment of disordered water balance; others discuss the psychopharmacological treatment of the underlying psychosis (Goldman & Luchins, 1985; Vieweg et al., 1988b). Yet few authors have addressed the aspects of studying behavioral interventions, and little is offered in the way of nursing interventions.

Behavioral treatment has focused on preventing water intoxication of those with a known history of excessive water consumption, for example, by restricting a mentally retarded female's access to water through behavior modification (McNally, Calamari, Hansen, & Kaliher, 1988), operating a water intoxication ward designed for managing and monitoring water ingestion (Ashby, 1987), and developing individual care plans within the context of the Roy Adaptation Model (Prim, 1988). McNally et al. (1988) and Prim (1988) demonstrated success in single-case studies. Success was defined in both studies as reduction in water ingestion and in episodes of water intoxication. Ashby (1987) described the protocol that was used on the water intoxication ward but did not report patient outcomes. Indeed, the literature on any type of behavioral protocol that was useful when intervening with these patients

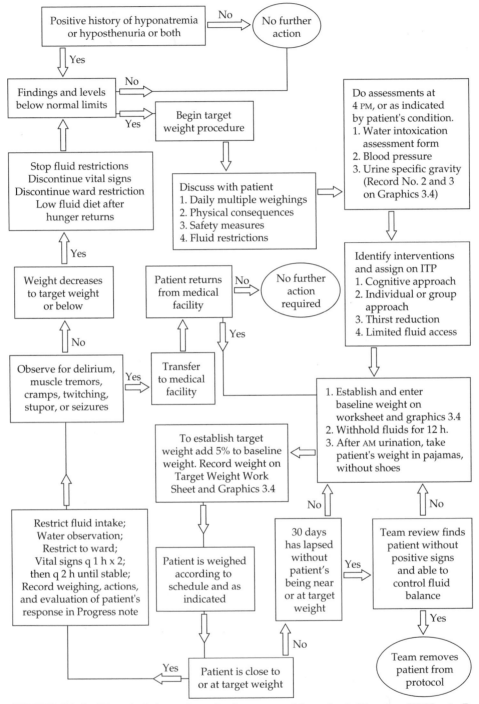

FIGURE 15–1. Water imbalance/intoxication protocol flow chart. (Courtesy W. Harris, B. Cobb, M. A. Boyd, Water Intoxication CQI Team, St. Louis State Hospital, St. Louis, Missouri, September 1994.)

was sadly lacking in descriptions of patient outcomes or (perhaps even more important) of sustained outcomes.

CONTROL OF FLUID BALANCE

Preventing water intoxication is actually only a small part of the nursing management of persons with disordered water balance. Persons with disordered water balance need to learn about the problem, what it means for them, and how they can monitor and control their fluid balance. In most facilities, a multidisciplinary approach works best. Because the nurse is responsible for coordinating care over 24 hours and this problem has a biological-psychological interrelationship, the nurse is ultimately the one who provides the clinical leadership for the care of these persons. In the inpatient or residential setting, a protocol may be useful in guiding treatment. The flow chart depicted in Figure 15–1 is an example of a multidisciplinary approach to the care of the patient with disordered water balance.

Until a person can adjust the drinking behavior to excretory function, the individual should follow a target weight procedure. By using this procedure, individuals can prevent hyponatremia and begin to learn how to monitor their own fluid balance. For example, some patients willingly weigh themselves, record the weight, and make a judgment about the amount of fluids that they can ingest. Ideally, all patients should be taught how to weigh themselves and monitor their weight. Patients can be discharged to apartments and group living situations with their personal scales.

Psychoeducation modules using a small group format can be used to teach patients about disordered water balance and what they can do to control their fluid balance (Snider & Boyd, 1991; Cosgray, Davidhizar, Giger, & Kreisl, 1993). Approaching the problem of water imbalance as a side effect of a mental illness and emphasizing that no one is to blame relieves the clients of any guilt that they are doing something wrong. Using patients' weight records for a teaching tool can help them analyze their drinking behavior and identify their "peak drink times." One patient found that he would exceed his target weight only on the weekends after he talked with a family member. Another patient found that she exceeded her target weight in the morning after her shower. She admitted that she was drinking from the shower. In both cases, it was possible to help the patients substitute other more appropriate activities.

Individuals with disordered water balance can develop strategies based on fluid regulation. Careful assessments of antecedents leading to water ingestion are important. With a time lag between ingestion and excretion, patients can be encouraged to avoid drinking until they have voided. If thirst is a problem, then hard candies or chewing gum may be useful. If stress is the precipitant of excessive ingestion, stress reduction techniques may be appropriate.

NURSING EDUCATION—CURRICULUM IMPLICATIONS

While education is a key factor as a preventive measure for these patients and their care providers, so also is education a key factor for nurses working with this patient population. Given what we know about the phenomenon of water imbalance and intoxication, there are some important and immediate recommendations for changes needed in undergraduate and graduate nursing education. If early detection is imperative, water intoxication needs to be taught in pathophysiology and again reinforced in the psychiatric–mental health nursing course at the undergraduate level. Because nursing is moving to a biological-psychological approach, undergraduate students must know normal functioning of the brain, especially the limbic system, and the fluid use and excretory functions of the body. Only then can they build on this foundation with the knowledge about abnormal changes, or patho-physiology, in these functions.

Nurses must also know how to assess for this disorder. They must know what the warning signs are, not only for early detection but also for progress. In some cases, such as emergency rooms, a patient in an advanced state of water intoxication may be the only stage of this disorder that nurses witness. They must become knowledgeable about nursing interventions that are effective in the clinical and psychosocial management of these patients. They must know how to plan for caring for these patients and how to use nursing diagnoses to focus their care. They must know how to provide effective education for these patients and their care providers. In addition, at the undergraduate stage of their education, nurses must start to ask the questions that will guide nursing research in developing improved assessment skills and tools, more effective interventions with measurable outcomes, and improved quality of life for these patients.

At the graduate level, students should be provided opportunities for expanding their knowledge base and enhancing their skills in the area of water imbalance. In a psychiatric–mental health nursing program, they not only need a sound theory base in the biological aspects; they must also learn to help individuals who are disabled by a mental disorder to change habitual, compulsive behavior and learn self-monitoring skills. Cognitive-behavioral models may be used as a basis for enhancement of self-monitoring skills. Patient education about water imbalance is especially important. The concepts underlying the disorder are fairly complex and not easily comprehended. Therefore, the advanced practice nurse has an important role in devising teaching techniques that can be used in the clinical settings by case managers and staff nurses.

Interventions need to be developed that can help patients monitor their fluid balance. One patient who had been participating in an educational module on water intoxication explained to an undergraduate nursing student new to a psychiatric unit exactly what his problem was: "You see, if I go over my target weight, my electrolytes will get messed up, and I could have a seizure and drop dead right there." He also explained how he stayed below his target weight. "Sometimes, when the nurses aren't looking, I just put the water in my mouth and then spit it out. That way I won't weigh too much." He had figured out his own strategy for maintaining his fluid balance, and it worked for him much of the time. A graduate student could help develop a reinforcement program for his maintenance strategies and assist him in developing others.

RESEARCH AGENDA

It was a decade ago that the first articles about water intoxication appeared in the nursing literature (Prim, 1988; Watson, 1985). These were reports of single-case studies that included helpful, but limited, care plans for particular patients. Recently, articles in the nursing literature on water intoxication have provided readers with analyses of past medical and nursing studies, discussion of the multiple and often confusing terms used to name this syndrome, and recommendations for research and practice (Baier & Gaertner, 1991; Baier, Robinson, DeShay, & Snider, 1989; Boyd, 1990; Cosgray, Hanna, Davidhizar, & Smith, 1990; Lapierre et al., 1990; Snider & Boyd, 1991). What is readily apparent from these articles is that astute observations and quick interventions by nurses are very effective in preventing water intoxication from progressing and in stabilizing the patient to his or her pre-water-intoxicated state. But what is noticeably lacking is nursing research concerning this clinical phenomenon. It seems apparent that disordered water balance is an elusive syndrome that is a fertile topic for nursing research, as it interfaces with both the behavioral and biomedical sciences. The elusiveness of water intoxication is, and can continue to be, dispelled by developing, implementing, and evaluating a research agenda set forth for nurses in this area.

The complexity of the fluid balance phenomenon generates many research questions applicable to a variety of theoretical and methodological approaches. The biological questions relate to etiology of the disorder and the long-term physiological effects of chronic fluid imbalance. Neurophysiologists continue struggling to understand the underlying etiological factors; meanwhile, the clinical manifestations and their implications are fertile nursing research areas. The relationship of urinary dilution to hyponatremia remains unclear. The effect of fluid restriction on hyponatremia also is unclear. Does fluid restriction impact the hyponatremic state and prevent long-term physiological side effects of chronic fluid imbalance? The actual progression of water imbalance from a state of occasional hyponatremic episodes to chronic water intoxication is also speculation at this point. Once investigations begin, many more questions will be raised.

Most of the studies that have been done have not addressed any gender differences. The area of neurohormonal changes and their relationship to diurnal weight gain according to gender needs to be addressed. Is the normal diurnal weight gain pattern different in females than in males? If target weight procedures are used as a method of fluid balance control, should the impact of the menstrual cycle be considered? Does the menstrual cycle significantly impact fluid retention in females, making them more susceptible to episodes of water intoxication? Do females differ in their clinical picture from males, and how do they compare to the general population?

Studies using the biological explanations as a basis for developing behavioral questions need to be generated. For example, if the urge to drink is not under voluntary control, what behavioral interventions can be developed to help patients resist their urge to drink? This line of research would be comparable to other investigations into understanding underlying emotional and psychological components of any chronic illness condition. However, these investigations will be further complicated by the effect of a severe mental illness that impairs cognitive functioning. Additionally, a side effect of antipsychotic medication is often a dry mouth, which only increases thirst and further complicates the interpretation of results.

There are very few explanations of how patients who actually do consume excessive amounts of fluids explain their drinking behavior. Most of these reports are serendipitous findings that were not systematically collected. For some, drinking fluids may be a way of handling stress; for others, it may be a compulsion. Studies of patients' perceptions of their need for fluids would be useful in developing an understanding of the experience of the need to drink. For these studies, a qualitative methodology would yield data that could be useful in designing interventions that are meaningful to patients.

CONCLUSION

Water imbalance and water intoxication are very real problems of persons with a long-term mental illness. The integration of the biological and psychosocial aspects of the problem is critical for care of these persons. With proper monitoring of fluid balance and helping clients gain control over the balance between fluid ingestion and excretion, it is possible to significantly improve their ability to control their symptoms.

REFERENCES

Allon, M., Allen, H., Deck, L., & Clark, M. (1990). Role of cigarette use in hyponatremia in schizophrenic patients. *American Journal of Psychiatry, 147*(8), 1075–1077.

American Psychiatric Association. (1994). *Diagnostic and statistical manual of mental disorders* (4th ed.). Washington, DC: Author.

Ashby, Y. (1987). Planned change: The development of a program for the management of self-induced water intoxication. *Canadian Journal of Psychiatric Nursing, 28,* 12–14.

Baïer, M., & Gaertner, J. (1991). Target weight procedure: Preventing water intoxication. *Journal of Psychosocial Nursing, 29,* 5–9.

Baier, M., Robinson, M., DeShay, E., & Snider, K. (1989). Issues in the nursing management of patients with water intoxication. *Archives of Psychiatric Nursing, 3,* 338–343.

Barahal, H. (1938). Water intoxication in a mental case. *Psychiatric Quarterly, 12,* 767–771.

Barlow, E., & deWardener, H. (1959). Compulsive water drinking. *Quarterly Journal of Medicine, 28,* 235–258.

Barter, R., & Schwartz, W. (1967). The syndrome of inappropriate secretion of antidiuretic hormone. *American Journal of Medicine, 42,* 790-806.

Bewley, T. (1964). Acute water intoxication from compulsive water drinking. *British Medical Journal, 2,* 864.

Blotcky, M., Grossman, I., & Looney, J. (1980). Psychogenic water intoxication: A fatality. *Texas Medicine, 76*(1), 58–59.

Blum, A., Tempey, F., & Lynch, W. (1983). Somatic findings in patients with psychogenic polydipsia. *Journal of Clinical Psychiatry, 44,* 55–56.

Boyd, M. (1990). Polydipsia in the chronically mentally ill: A review. *Archives of Psychiatric Nursing, 3,* 166–175.

Boyd, M., Williams, L., Evenson, R., Eckert, A., Beaman, M., & Carr, T. (1992). Target weight procedure for disordered water balance in long-term care facilities. *Journal of Psychosocial Nursing, 30*(12), 22–27.

Bremner, A., & Regan, A. (1991). Intoxicated by water: Polydipsia and water intoxication in a mental handicap hospital. *British Journal of Psychiatry, 158,* 244–250.

Bugle, C., Andrew, S., & Heath, J. (1992). Early detection of water intoxication. *Journal of Psychosocial Nursing, 30,* 31–34.

Carter, A., & Robbins, J. (1947). The use of hypertonic saline infusions in the differential diagnosis of diabetes insipidus and psychogenic polydipsia. *Journal of Clinical Endocrinology, 7,* 753–766.

Chinn, T. (1974). Compulsive water drinking. *The Journal of Nervous and Mental Disease, 158*(1), 78–80.

Cooney, J. (1991). Compulsive water drinking, water intoxication and alcohol abuse. *Irish Journal of Psychological Medicine, 8,* 22–25.

Cosgray, R., Hanna, V., Davidhizar, R., & Smith, J. (1990). The water intoxicated patient. *Archives of Psychiatric Nursing, 5,* 308–312.

Cosgray, R., Davidhizar, R., Giger, J., & Kreisl, R. (1993). A program for water-intoxicated patients at a state hospital. *Clinical Nurse Specialist, 7*(2), 55–61.

Deas-Nesmith, D., & Brewerton, T. (1992). A case of fluoxetine-responsive psychogenic polydipsia: A variant of obsessive-compulsive disorder? *The Journal of Nervous and Mental Disease, 180*(5), 338–339.

deLeon, J., Verghese, C., Tracy, J., Josiassen, R., & Simpson, G. (1994). Polydipsia and water intoxication in psychiatric patients: A review of the epidemiological literature. *Biological Psychiatry, 35,* 408–419.

Delva, N., & Crammer, J. (1988). Polydipsia in chronic psychiatric patients: Body weight and plasma sodium. *British Journal of Psychiatry, 152,* 242–245.

DeSoto, M., Griffith, S., & Katz, E. (1985). Water intoxication associated with nephrogenic diabetes insipidus secondary to lithium: Case report. *Journal of Clinical Psychiatry, 46,* 402–403.

Emsley, R., & Taljaard, F. (1987). Self-induced water intoxication: A case report. *South African Medical Journal, 74*(2), 80-81.

Emsley, R., Potgieter, A., Taljaard, F., Joubert, R., & Gledhill, R. (1989). Water excretion and plasma vasopressin in psychotic disorders. *American Journal of Psychiatry, 146,* 250–253.

Emsley, R., Spangenberg, J., Robers, M., Taljaard, F., & Chalton, D. (1993). Disordered water homeostasis and cognitive impairment in schizophrenia. *Biological Psychiatry, 34,* 630–633.

Evenson, R., Jos, C., & Mallya, A. (1987). Prevalence of polydipsia among public psychiatric patients. *Psychological Reports, 60,* 803–807.

Ferrier, I. (1985). Water intoxication in patients with psychiatric illness. *British Medical Journal, 291*(6509), 1594–1595.

Fricchione, G., Kelleher, S., & Ayyala, M. (1987). Coexisting central diabetes insipidus and psychogenic polydipsia. *Journal of Clinical Psychiatry, 48,* 75–76.

Goldberg, M. (1981). Hyponatremia. *Medical Clinics of North America, 65,* 251–269.

Goldman, M., & Janecek, J. (1989). Neuroleptics do not worsen hyponatremia in hyponatremic psychotics. *Schizophrenia Research, 1,* 1711–1715.

Goldman, M., & Luchins, D. (1985). Demeclocycline improves hyponatremia in chronic schizophrenics. *Biological Psychiatry, 20,* 1149–1155.

Goldman, M., & Luchins, D. (1987). Prevention of episodic water intoxication with target weight procedure. *American Journal of Psychiatry, 144*(3), 365-366.

Goldman, M., Marks, R., Blake, L., Petkovic, M., Hedeker, D., & Luchins, D. (1990). Estimating daily urine volume in psychiatric patients: Empiric confirmation. *Biological Psychiatry, 31*(12), 1228–1231.

Guyton, A. (1991). *Textbook of medical physiology* (8th ed.). Philadelphia: Saunders.

Hobson, J., & English, J. (1963). Self-induced water intoxication: Case study of a chronically schizophrenic patient with psychological evidence of water retention due to inappropriate release of antidiuretic hormone. *Annals of Internal Medicine, 58,* 324–332.

Hoskins, R., & Sleeper, R. (1933). Organic function in schizophrenia. *Archives of Neurological Psychiatry, 30,* 123–140.

Husband, D., Mai, F., & Carruthers, G. (1981). Syndrome of inappropriate secretion of antidiuretic hormone in a patient treated with haloperidol. *Canadian Journal of Psychiatry, 26,* 196–197.

Illowsky, B., & Kirch, D. (1988). Polydipsia and hyponatremia in psychiatric patients. *American Journal of Psychiatry, 145,* 675–683.

Johnson, R., Breshahan, D., & Chan, D. (1985). Polydipsia in psychiatric patients [Letter to the editor]. *American Journal of Psychiatry, 142,* 885.

Jos, C. (1984). Generalized seizures from self-induced water intoxication. *Psychosomatics, 25*(2), 153–157.

Jos, C., Evenson, R., & Mallya, A. (1986). Self-induced water intoxication: A comparison of 34 cases with matched controls. *Journal of Clinical Psychiatry, 47*(7), 368–370.

Jose, C., & Evenson, R. (1980). Antecedents of self-induced water intoxication. *The Journal of Nervous and Mental Disease, 168*(8), 498–500.

Jose, C., & Perez-Cruet, J. (1979). Incidence and morbidity of self-induced water intoxication in state mental hospital patients. *American Journal of Psychiatry, 136,* 221–222.

Keating, J., Schears, F., & Dodge, P. (1991). Oral water intoxication in infants: An American epidemic. *American Journal of Diseases in Children, 145,* 985–990.

Khamnei, A. (1983). Acute water intoxication from compulsive water drinking. *IRSC Journal of Medical Science, 11,* 520.

Klonoff, D., & Jurow, A. (1991). Acute water intoxication as a complication of urine drug testing in the workplace. *Journal of the American Medical Association, 265*(1), 84–85.

Koczapski, A., Ibraheem, S., Ashby, Y., Paredes, J., Jones, B., & Ancill, R. (1987). Early diagnosis of water intoxication by monitoring diurnal variations in body weight. *American Journal of Psychiatry, 144*(2), 1626.

Koczapski, A., Ledwidge, B., Predes, J., Kogan, C., & Higenbottam, J. (1990). Multisubstance intoxication among schizophrenic inpatients: Reply to Hyde. *Schizophrenia Bulletin, 16*(3), 373–375.

Koczapski, A., & Millson, R. (1989). Individual differences in serum sodium levels in schizophrenic men with self-induced water intoxication. *American Journal of Psychiatry, 146*(12), 1614–1615.

Langgard, J., & Smith, O. (1962). Self-induced water intoxication without predisposing illness. *New England Journal of Medicine, 266,* 378–381.

Lapierre, E., Berthot, B., Gurvitch, M., Rees, I., & Kirch, D. (1990). Polydipsia and hyponatremia in psychiatric patients: Challenge to creative nursing care. *Archives of Psychiatric Nursing, 4,* 87–92.

Lawson, W., Karson, C., & Begelow, L. (1985). Increased urine volume in chronic schizophrenia patients. *Psychiatry Research, 14,* 323–331.

Lawson, W., Roy, S., Parent, M., Herrera, J., Karson, C., & Bigelow, L. (1992). Fluid intake patterns in schizophrenia and normal controls. *Progress in Neuro-Psychopharmacology and Biological Psychiatry, 16*(1), 39–44.

Lee, S., Chow, S., & Koo, L. (1989) Altered state of consciousness in a compulsive water drinker. *British Journal of Psychiatry, 154,* 556–558.

Leiken, S., & Caplan, H. (1967). Psychogenic polydipsia. *American Journal of Psychiatry, 123,* 1573–1576.

Luchins, D. (1990). A possible role of hippocampal dysfunction in schizophrenic symptomatology. *Society of Biological Psychiatry, 28,* 87–91.

Mareth, T. (1988). Hyponatremia and schizophrenia: A case presentation. *Military Medicine, 153,* 40–41.

McNally, R., Calamari, J., Hansen, P., & Kaliher, C. (1988). Behavioral treatment of psychogenic polydipsia. *Journal of Behavior Therapy and Experimental Psychiatry, 19,* 57–61.

Mendelson, W., & Deza, P. (1976). Polydipsia, hyponatremia, and seizures in psychotic patients. *The Journal of Nervous and Mental Disease, 162,* 140–143.

Narang, R., Chaudhury, R., & Wig, N. (1973). Effect of electroconvulsive therapy on the antidiuretic hormone level in the plasma of schizophrenic patients. *Indian Journal of Medical Research, 61*(5), 766–770.

Ohsawa, H., Kishimoton, T., Shimayoshi, N., Matsumura, K., Tahara, K., Kitera, K., Higashirua, Y., Matsumoto, H., Hirai, M., & Ikasw, G. (1993). Atrial natriuretic peptide and arginine vasopressin secretion in schizophrenic patients. *Acra Psychiatrica Scandinavica, 88*(2), 130–134.

Okura, M., & Morii, S. (1986). Polydipsia, polyuria, and water intoxication observed in psychiatric inpatients. *Tokushima Journal of Experimental Medicine, 33,* 1–5.

Okura, M., Okada, K., Nagamine, I., Yamaguchi, H., Karisha, K., Ishimoto, Y., & Ikuta, T. (1990). Electroencephalographic changes during and after water intoxication. *The Japanese Journal of Psychiatry and Neurology, 44*(4), 729–734.

Peh, L., Devan, G., & Low, B. (1990). A fatal case of water intoxication in a schizophrenic patient. *British Journal of Psychiatry, 156,* 891–894.

Prim, J. (1988). Water intoxication and psychosis syndrome. *Journal of Psychosocial Nursing, 26,* 16–18.

Rae, J. (1976). Self-induced water intoxication in a schizophrenic patient. *Canadian Medical Association Journal, 114,* 438.

Raskind, M. (1974). Psychosis, polydipsia, and water intoxication. *Archives of General Psychiatry, 30,* 112–114.

Raskind, M., Weitzman, R., Orenstein, H., Fisher, D., & Courtney, N. (1977). Is antidiuretic hormone elevated in psychosis? A pilot study. *Biological Psychiatry, 13,* 385–390.

Rees, B., & Leach, D. (1975). The social inhibition of micturition (paruresis): Sex similarities and differences. *Journal of American College Health Association, 23,* 203–205.

Reimann, I., & Frolich, J. (1981). Risks of simultaneous tocyctic treatment with beta adrenergic and PG inhibiting agents. *Zeitschrift Geburtshilfe Perinatol, 185,* 305–312.

Rendell, M., McGrane, D., & Cuesta, M. (1978). Fatal compulsive water drinking. *Journal of the American Medical Association, 240,* 2557.

Resnick, M., & Patterson, C. (1969). Coma and convulsion due to compulsive water drinking. *Neurology, 19,* 1125–1126.

Ripley, T., Millson, R., & Koczapski, R. (1989). Self-induced water intoxication and alcohol abuse. *American Journal of Psychiatry, 146,* 102–103.

Roberge, R., Gernsheimer, J., Sparano, R., Tartakoff, R., Morgenstern, M., Rubin, K., Senekjian, D., Andrade, R., & Matther, V. (1984). Psychogenic polydipsia: An unusual cause of hyponatremic coma and seizure. *Annals of Emergency Medicine, 13*(4), 274–276.

Rowe, J., Kilgore, A., & Robertson, G. (1980). Evidence in man that cigarette smoking induces vasopressin release via an airway-specific mechanism. *Journal of Clinical Endocrinology and Metabolism, 51*(1), 170–172.

Rowntree, L. (1923). Water intoxication. *Archives of Internal Medicine, 32,* 157–174.

Sahadevan, M., & Bayliss, V. (1965). Compulsive water drinking: A report of two cases. *Journal of the Association of Physicians in India, 13,* 755–757.

Sandifer, M. (1983). Hyponatremia due to psychotropic drugs. *Journal of Clinical Psychiatry, 44,* 301–303.

Saruta, T., Fujimaki, M., Ogihara, T., Saito, I., Konishi, K., & Kondo, K. (1982). Evaluation of the reninangiotension system in diabetes insipidus and psychogenic polydipsia. *Nephrology, 132,* 14–17.

Schnur, D., Wirkowski, E., Reddy, R., Decina, P., & Mukherjee, S. (1993). Cognitive impairments in schizophrenic patients with hyponatremia. *Biological Psychiatry, 33,* 836–838.

Shah, P., & Greenberg, W. (1993). Polydipsia with hyponatremia in a state hospital. *Hospital and Community Psychiatry, 43*(5), 509–511.

Shah, D., Wig, N., & Chaudhury, R. (1973). Antidiuretic hormone levels in patients with weight gain after chlorpromazine therapy. *Indian Journal of Medical Research, 61*(5), 771–776.

Shen, W., & Sata, L. (1983). Self-induced water intoxication and hyper-dopaminergic state [Letter to the editor]. *American Journal of Psychiatry, 141*(10), 1305–1306.

Shen, W., & Sata, L. (1984). Hypothalamic dopamine receptor supersensitivity? A pilot study of self-induced water intoxication. *The Psychiatric Journal of the University of Ottawa, 8*(3), 154–158.

Singh, S., Padi, M., Bullard, H., & Freeman, H. (1985). Water intoxication in psychiatric patients. *British Journal of Psychiatry, 146,* 127–131.

Shutty, M., Briscoe, L., Sautter, S., & Leadbetter, R. (1993). Neuropsychological manifestations of hyponatremia in chronic schizophrenic patients with the syndrome of psychosis, intermittent hyponatremia and polydipsia (PIP). *Schizophrenia Research, 10*(2), 125–130.

Sleeper, F. (1935). Investigation of polyuria in schizophrenia. *Journal of Psychiatry, 91,* 1019–1031.

Snider, K., & Boyd, M. (1991). When they drink too much: Nursing interventions for patients with disordered water balance. *Journal of Psychosocial Nursing, 28,* 10–16.

Tarnow-Mordi, W., Shaw, J., Liu, D., Gardner, D., & Flynn, F. (1981). Iatrogenic hyponatremia of the newborn due to maternal fluid overload: A prospective study. *British Medical Journal, 283,* 639–642.

Verghese, C., deLeon, J., & Simpson, G. (1993). Neuroendocrine factors influencing polydipsia in psychiatric patients: An hypothesis. *Neurophychopharmacology, 9,* 157–166.

Vieweg, W., David, J., Rowe, W., Peach, J., Veldhuis, J., Kaiser, D., & Spradlin, W. (1985a). Psychogenic polydipsia and water intoxication—Concepts that have failed. *Biological Psychiatry, 20,* 1308–1320.

Vieweg, W., David, J., Rowe, W., Peach, J., Veldhuis, J., & Spradlin, W. (1986). Correlation of cigarette-induced increase in serum nicotine levels with arginine vasopressin concentrations in the syndrome of self-induced water intoxication and psychosis (SIWIP). *Canadian Journal of Psychiatry, 31*(2), 108–111.

Vieweg, W., David, J., Rowe, W., Wampler, G., Burns, W., & Spradlin, W. (1985b). Death from self-induced water intoxication among patients with schizophrenic disorders. *The Journal of Nervous and Mental Disease, 173*(3), 161–165.

Vieweg, W., Godleski, L., Graham, P., Barber, J., Goldman, F., Kellog, E., Bayless, E., Glick, J., Hundley, P., & Yank, G. (1988a). Abnormal diurnal weight gain among long-term patients with schizophrenic disorders. *Schizophrenia Research, 1,* 67–71.

Vieweg, W., Godleski, L., Shannon, C., Ranade, N., Kelly, W., Cook, K., Morris, P., Hundley, P., & Yank, G. (1989). Diurnal weight gain among patients with mental retardation. *American Journal on Mental Retardation, 93*(5), 558–565.

Vieweg, W., Rowe, W., David, J., & Spradlin, W. (1984). Hyposthenuria as a marker for self-induced water intoxication and schizophrenic disorders. *American Journal of Psychiatry, 141,* 1258–1260.

Vieweg, W., Rowe, W., David, J., Sutker, L., & Spradlin, W. (1984). Evaluation of patients with self-induced water intoxication and schizophrenic disorders (SIWIS). *The Journal of Nervous and Mental Disease, 172*, 552–555.

Vieweg, W., Veldhuis, J., Leadbetter, R., Hundley, P., & Shutty, M. (1991). Cigarette use and hyponatremia in schizophrenic patients [Letter to the editor]. *American Journal of Psychiatry, 148*(5), 688–689.

Vieweg, W., Weiss, N., David, J., Rowe, W., Godleski, L., & Spradlin, W. (1988b). Treatment of psychosis, intermittent hyponatremia, and polydipsia (PIP) using lithium and phenytoin. *Biological Psychiatry, 23*, 25–30.

Watson, C. (1985). Water intoxication. *Nursing Times, 2*, 40–42.

Wyngaarden, J., & Smith, L. (Eds.). (1985). *Cecil textbook of medicine.* Philadelphia: Saunders.

Zerbe, R., Stropes, L., & Roberson, G. (1980). Vasopressin function in the syndrome of inappropriate antidiuresis. *Annual Review of Medicine, 31*, 315–327.

Zubenko, G., Altesman, R., Cassidy, J., & Barreira, P. (1984). Disturbances of thirst and water homeostasis in patients with affective illness. *American Journal of Psychiatry, 141*, 436–437.

CHAPTER

16

INTEGRATING THE BEHAVIORAL AND BIOLOGICAL SCIENCES

IMPLICATIONS FOR PRACTICE, EDUCATION, AND RESEARCH

Angela Barron McBride, PhD, RN, FAAN, and Joan Kessner Austin, DNS, RN, FAAN

ABSTRACT

This integrative chapter summarizes the major themes evident in the commissioned chapters—the need for focused assessments and interventions; the extent to which nursing care can be organized in terms of reregulation in the face of hyperarousal; and the importance of explanation patterns and drug therapy to self-regulation. Implications of these themes for practice, education, and research are articulated. The principal implication is that psychiatric–mental health nursing is more consonant than ever before with the profession as a whole.

The task of this chapter is to reflect back on the 14 commissioned chapters to ascertain what they collectively suggest is our agenda for the future. Most chapters began by focusing on a medical diagnosis or vulnerable population, but in articulating the extent to which nursing functions on the interface between the behavioral and the biological sciences, they made clear some new themes that may be expected to dominate at least the next decade of psychiatric–mental health nursing. No emerging conceptualization is more pronounced than the nurse's role in the patient's self-regulation. While this is not a totally new emphasis given nursing's traditional promotion of self-help, the regulatory function of nursing takes on new meaning when considered in terms of growing evidence of the ramifications of neurochemical imbalance.

Nakagawa-Kogan sounded this theme most persistently as she outlined the wide range of possible targets for management—social environmental events, the central nervous system, behavioral and end-organ responses. While the pathways from distress to neuroendocrine arousal to immunologic and end-organ changes remain to be fully specified, nursing's possible role in helping individuals respond constructively (i.e., establishing goals and measures of success, reasserting where possible a sense of control, utilizing social support, explaining the experience in a growth-enhancing fashion, offering biofeedback training) is clearly taking shape. In the process, older nursing roles such as mother surrogate or global change agent are giving way to the role of coach or teacher, and the ethics is shifting away from doing good or doing unto others as one would wish for oneself to facilitating the patient in achieving desired self-change, usually one behavior at a time.

FOCUSED ASSESSMENTS AND INTERVENTIONS

An emphasis on self-regulation signals a major shift away from global interventions (e.g., general insight therapy) that are applied to all patients regardless of type of mental health problem. The approach is now on very focused interventions based on detailed assessments, including assessments of specific symptoms and the effectiveness of strategies being used to manage them. There is also a fundamental change in attitudes toward and interactions with patients' families. Families are no longer blamed for causing the mental illness but are taught about the condition and engaged in patient-family-nurse partnerships in which all take active roles in treatment.

If the nurse takes as her or his prime directive the facilitation of the patient's self-management, this necessarily involves the nurse in a series of activities—comprehensive assessments, drug therapy so that neuroendocrine arousal can be reregulated, the examination of ineffective self-treatment and functioning, behavior modification, cognitive restructuring, and symptom management. When described this way, commonalities between nursing as a whole and the specialty of psychiatric–mental health nursing are clear, for they both are concerned with promoting self-help and homeostasis while maximizing functional ability and quality of life.

Almost all the chapters provided examples of the circumscribed assessments necessary to a full understanding of the dysregulation and functional strengths an individual or family might possess. In assessing information processing, Fox and Kane made use of the Wisconsin Card Sort and the Halstead Category Test; in monitoring prodromal symptoms, they mentioned the Early Signs Questionnaire, Problem Appraisal Scale, and Functioning Inventory for Psychotic Disorder as helpful. Beeber outlined a range of scales for assessing depression and related factors. The Symptom Check List-90R was mentioned by Nakagawa-Kogan and others as a valid and reliable instrument for estimating limbic arousal. Austin described ways to assess family functioning as well as biological matters (e.g., seizure severity, side effects of medications, seizure description). Burgess and Hartman pointed out that the ratio of norepinephrine to cortisol is a biological benchmark for PTSD. Killeen and Bongarten noted that the dexamethasone suppression test was of use in gauging suicide attempts in adult patients.

Collectively, these chapters make clear the importance of formal measurement to nursing assessments for pinpointing problems, designing interventions, and evaluating progress toward desired outcomes. The need for formal assessments is especially important with the current emphasis on quality of care and cost-effectiveness of interventions. While the nursing process has traditionally encouraged careful assessment and evaluation, these steps have typically involved the application of expert clinical knowledge in interview situations rather than standardized appraisals using paper-and-pencil instruments, calibrated feedback mechanisms, mirror/photographic images, or analogue techniques. Formal measurement will never replace informal appraisals in clinical situations, but it has distinct advantages in providing baseline measurements, encouraging more systematic appraisals, helping patients understand where they fall in terms of norms, and focusing attention on specific strengths and limitations rather than on global matters (so helpful when seeking reimbursement for services rendered). Individualized assessment tools also play an important role in helping patients and their families track progress in symptom management and in identifying triggers for improvement or deterioration.

The implications of formal measurement for practice, education, and research are enormous. Because nurses work on the interface between the behavioral and the biological sciences, they must begin to develop some common understandings of the standardized instruments and techniques to be generally used in assessing major risk factors and areas of functioning. For example, why not adopt specific instruments for assessing limbic arousal and monitoring prodromal symptoms? Probably the area where nurses have been most active in using standardized instruments to guide specific interventions has been psychogeriatric care (Abraham, Currie, Neese, Yi, & Thompson-Heisterman, 1994).

There is also a need for nurses to develop new instruments as more is learned about the manifestations of neurobiological dysfunction. New instruments are also needed because many existing ones provide estimates of global functioning (e.g., Global Assessment Scale) and fail to provide specific information on which to base interventions. Examples of instruments needed are those for measuring patients' unique symptoms (e.g., specific thoughts, feelings, behavior, or sensations) that signify beginning stages of hyperarousal, for measuring symptoms of excess or deficits in the neurotransmitters, and for measuring existing use of coping strategies before dealing with cognitive deficits. Nurses need to know how to assess patients' readiness for self-care because a certain level of cognitive function is needed before patients can respond to cognitive approaches. The emphasis in instrumentation should be on measuring functional ability and quality of life because they are the domain of nursing.

The regular use of instruments to assess patients in nursing practice will have implications for nursing education. All the chapters highlighted assessment instruments that were appropriate for each population. At the undergraduate level, nursing students should be expected to become familiar with existing ways of appraising depression, anxiety, self-esteem, sleep patterns, social adjustment, and similar concepts. They also need to learn about the importance of assessment using individualized scales developed to measure each patient's unique set of symptoms. At the graduate level, students should be expected to be knowledgeable about ways to estimate concepts of concern to specific populations, including those that will be used to measure patient outcomes following interventions. At both levels, nurses need to learn more about the proper administration of instruments and use of tools for rating observed behaviors so that valid and reliable data may be obtained.

The consequences for research will be extensive because nurse scientists need to take the lead both in developing new scales and in assuring that the major instruments used have sound psychometric properties and cross-cultural relevance. It is particularly important that assessments of a nonnverbal nature be developed, too (e.g., controlled use of light to see if a person suspected of having seasonal affective disorder responds discernibly to that stimulus). The use made of drawings by Burgess and Hartman in their work is an example of how nonverbal assessments can be effective. Wolfe (1994) has urged nurses to incorporate pharmacological challenge studies into their practice to examine behavioral and neuroendocrine responses (e.g., using caffeine as a challenge agent in understanding patients with panic disorder). Once nurses incorporate formal measurement into their repertoire regularly, it becomes possible to consider the development of a minimum data set for the specialty. What information could be aggregated across individuals or settings that might be used either to estimate institutional effectiveness or to pursue secondary analyses of matters that concern vulnerable populations?

Systematic evaluation of patient outcomes and nursing care should be mindful of indicators of quality *and* cost effectiveness. The nurse should also be prepared to distinguish between efficacy (what works under relatively ideal conditions) and effectiveness (what works under relatively average conditions). This distinction has ramifications for the complementary relationship between research (concerned largely with efficacy) and practice (concerned largely with effectiveness).

The goal is neither to turn nurses into psychologists with their traditional professional reliance on paper-and-pencil testing nor to encourage nurses to become more like psychiatrists with their growing use of drug titers, cortisol levels, and brain imaging. While psychiatric–mental health nurses are generally conversant with the assessments used by these fields, it is increasingly clear that our own professional purview—that is, promoting functional ability and quality of life—will require of us the development of new and innovative ways of behavior mapping, especially along the vulnerable points in an illness trajectory, for the purpose of helping patients address various imbalances.

Assessment, however, is not just an activity of nurses but of their patients, too. Key to self-regulation is the development of the assessment abilities of patients and their families. New measurement strategies are needed to help patients carry out self-monitoring and assess their progress toward symptom management. Can they be encouraged to become more attuned to the patterning of their behavior? Can they monitor their mood changes, responses to stressors, and shifts in sleep, exercise, appetite, elimination, and libido for the purpose of better understanding what triggers dysfunction and what forestalls difficulties developing? When patients and their families are most troubled, they cannot see any solution to their problems. The more they can see their behavior as clues and themselves as detectives decoding these clues, the more they may realize that they themselves may hold the key to helpful strategies that can be implemented with the assistance of the nurse. For example, the identification of prodromal symptoms such as nervousness and sleep problems that indicate vulnerability to relapse is a promising area of inquiry. Stressing the importance of body-listening is itself a way of enabling patients to regain some sense of personal control.

Several authors in this book referred to teaching patients self-monitoring so they could identify early symptoms of problems. For example, Simmons-Alling advocated teaching patients to recognize and respond to early mood changes to help increase their sense of control over bipolar mood disorders. In other chapters, families were encouraged to monitor the environment of the patient. For example, Austin recommended that families keep seizure diaries to identify stimuli that elicited seizures in their children. Buckwalter and Hall suggested that caregivers monitor the environment for triggers that increased anxiety and decreased functioning in patients with Alzheimer's disease. Other psychiatric nurses are recommending that monitoring be used for patients with schizophrenia. For example, Murphy and Moller (1993) help patients and their families identify beginning relapse symptoms, triggers related to relapse, and strategies for successful coping to prevent relapse. There are two areas of self-monitoring that deserve special attention in practice, education, and research: assessment of hyperarousal and cognitive explanation patterns of events.

HYPERAROUSAL

One of the major themes in many of the chapters is the extent to which hyperarousal is evident. Hyperarousal refers to a generalized, diffuse overactivation of the autonomic nervous system, especially the sympathetic division (Wilson & Mathew,

1993). Hardin described hyperarousal in children who had experienced catastrophic stress; Stuart and Laraia identified hyperarousal as a major symptom in panic disorder; and Burgess and Hartman included hyperarousal as one of the three hallmark symptoms of posttraumatic stress disorder. Moreover, Killeen and Bongarten pointed out that hyperarousal has been found in adults with depression, even though it is contrary to what might be expected, and there is some evidence of increased noradrenergic function in major depressive disorder in children (Rogeness, Javors, & Pliszka, 1992). Indeed, physiologic hyperarousal can sometimes present as hypoarousal.

Several neuroanatomical areas are involved in hyperarousal, including the cerebral cortex, aspects of the limbic system (hippocampus, amygdala, and hypothalamus), the locus coeruleus, and raphe nuclei. The locus coeruleus, which is located in the brain stem and has projections to most parts of the brain, functions much as a thermostat or general regulator of the level of arousal (Perry & Pate, 1994; Schrift, 1994). The hypothalamus is responsible for the immediate response to stress that results in increases in sympathetic activity and the release of stress hormones (norepinephrine, epinephrine, and cortisol). Potential causes of hyperarousal are (1) the locus coeruleus is more active and reactive than normal, (2) the hippocampus and amygdala are overly sensitive to normal impulses, and (3) the hypothalamus is hypersensitive and sends signals to stimulate the sympathetic division (Shekhar, 1994).

A single traumatic event or persistence of a threat can affect the locus coeruleus and lead to an increase in the baseline level of arousal (Perry & Pate, 1994). Because the hippocampus and amygdala affect emotion, learning, and memory, these functions can be adversely affected by a serious trauma, such as rape, and can result in the loss of memory for the event as described so well by Burgess and Hartman. There is growing evidence that the effects of trauma can be much more pervasive than can be accounted for by a conditioning model (Pitman, Orr, & Shalev, 1993). Long-term hyperarousal such as that found in posttraumatic stress disorder can lead to the development of learning deficits (Charney et al., 1994).

Chronic hyperarousal can be brought about by kindling, a phenomenon discussed by several authors as neuronal reactivity, or emotional scarring whereby encoded memory leaves the individual susceptible to low doses of stimuli. Flashbacks or reexperiencing of the stressful event, which were described in the chapters by Hardin and by Burgess and Hartman, are likely to be a result of increased sensitization to stimuli as a result of kindling. In addition, kindling may help explain the finding mentioned in the chapter by Beeber that persons who have been depressed are at an increased risk for a subsequent depression. It should be noted that kindling has even been used to explain multiple chemical sensitivity syndrome—another example of heightened reactivity (Bell, Miller, & Schwartz, 1992).

Self-monitoring for arousal needs to be taught in conjunction with adaptive coping strategies that reduce hyperarousal. It is important for patients' families to learn strategies for adaptive coping because it appears that extinction of the increased sensitivity to stimuli results not from erasure of the original painful memory but from new learning (Charney et al., 1994). Furthermore, it is essential that patient learning of adaptive coping strategies precede the teaching of self-monitoring in patients who are hypervigilant about bodily symptoms, such as those with panic disorder as mentioned by Stuart and Laraia in their chapter. In some patients hyperarousal will need to be reduced with appropriate medication before they will be able to benefit from the teaching of self-monitoring and self-management of symptoms. Before any teaching, it is important to assess possible learning deficits because a certain degree of cognitive functioning is necessary before patients can respond to cognitive therapy (Sood & Koziol, 1994). Learning deficits and information processing problems such as those described by Fox and Kane can have a negative effect on the ability of the patient to learn new coping behaviors.

Suggestions by Nakagawa-Kogan and Stuart and Laraia to use deep breathing as a means of lowering arousal and encouraging stimulation of the parasympathetic system suggest that the relaxation response could become a major mechanism for the nurse to use in reducing hyperarousal. Patients might begin by becoming more attuned to the extent to which their breathing is shallow and full of gasps and sighs, then go on to practice how they can reduce their arousal through deep breathing, consequently reducing their anxiety and fear. Deep breathing, because it is under volitional control and can block sympathetic system activity, can be used generally as a technique for counteracting hyperarousal.

EXPLANATION PATTERNS

The other area of self-listening that should be encouraged, given all the authors' references to cognitive restructuring as an important therapeutic technique, is explanation patterns. Patients must become aware of the extent to which they typically explain their behavior or situation in a manner that is *not* ego enhancing—for example, owning failure but not success, ruminating, overgeneralizing, discounting what is positive or neutral. Psychiatric nurses have long used reframing techniques to help patients see their situations in a way that encourages new behaviors, for example, redefining a problem as a challenge or describing change as full of possibilities not just as a loss of the familiar. The more the nurse's role is assisting the patient's self-regulation in the face of hyperarousal or emotional scarring, the more important cognitive restructuring becomes. Reframing limits rumination, which itself can be conceptualized as a sort of cognitive "kindling."

In assisting the patient's self-regulation, the nurse must work to help the individual examine less effective efforts to reestablish homeostasis, for example, using alcohol and other drugs, craving sweets and other satiating foods, pumping up with caffeine, sleeping away the day, smoking, using sex to confirm self-worth, risk-taking to obtain the adrenalin rush. The reason issues of comorbidity were mentioned in so many of the chapters is that patients regularly self-treat using such strategies to calm themselves or make themselves feel more alive. The advantage of describing such activities as attempts at self-regulation is that it makes sense of such behaviors. Instead of regarding such behaviors as self-destructive, with the resultant unproductive blaming, they may be more amenable to change if understood as attempts to re-establish a sense of well-being, even though they typically cause more problems than they solve. The task then is to help patients cope more effectively—a stance that allows the patient to take some pride in having already tried to cope, albeit ineffectively.

Inappropriate self-treatment cannot be mentioned without some acknowledgment of the effects it can have nutritionally. Alcohol and other drug addictions often co-exist with dietary deficiencies. Niacin and thiamine are the two vitamins most likely to be compromised by excess alcohol consumption, and they influence the production of neurotransmitters; thus the interrelationships between and among self-medication, brain function, and behavior are even more complicated than apparent at first glance (Harper-Jaques & Reimer, 1992). Since food is frequently used to regulate mood and energy levels, a better understanding of these self-treatment strategies might uncover useful information, too.

Much of what has been suggested about hyperarousal and explanation patterns has not been systematically researched, even though there are encouraging pockets of information that suggest additional clinical experiments. For example, Kelsey's

(1993) discussion of reactivity habituation to psychological stress suggested several ways to counteract hyperarousal that might be employed by nurses, for example, limiting exposure to particular stressors with the same neural overlap and increasing time between exposure to stressors. Lazarus (1991) suggested two relevant principles that might guide interventions: (a) emotions shape thoughts and actions, and they can be transformed by relaxation, meditation, deconditioning, and biofeedback; and (b) thoughts shape emotions and actions, and they can be changed through cognitive restructuring. He, however, also reminded us that environment can shape thought, emotion, and action, as do the authors of the chapters on schizophrenia and Alzheimer's disease where stimulus reduction is urged. To limit excess disability given information-processing difficulties, the nurse can provide an environment that encourages routines and minimizes stressors, demands, and stimuli. White and Haack were also very mindful of the effect of the environment on thought, emotion, and action in their chapters.

DRUG THERAPY

Facilitating re-regulation necessarily involves the nurse in drug therapy to deal with chemical imbalances. Many of the authors described the importance of various medications to their areas of study. For example, Stuart and Laraia reviewed four categories of drugs important to panic disorder and other psychiatric problems—tricyclic antidepressants (TCAs), monoamine oxidase inhibitors (MAOIs), high-potency benzodiazepines (BZs), and selective serotonin reuptake inhibitors (SSRIs).

So important is this subject to nursing that in 1992, the American Nurses Association and NIMH funded the Psychiatric–Mental Health Nursing Psychopharmacology Project, overseen by a task force that included three chapter authors—Michele T. Laraia (Chair), Linda S. Beeber, and Susan Simmons-Alling. The outcome was a monograph that spells out considerations for nursing practice that could be used to shape study in that area. That booklet also outlines the overall neuroscience content needed by psychiatric nurses: neuroanatomy, genetic/familial correlates, systems of neuroregulation, psychoendocrinology, psychoimmunology, normal biological rhythms, psychobiological dysfunctions, biological theories of major psychiatric disorders, brain imaging in diagnosis of mental illness, and physiological indices of mental illness (Keltner & Callwood, 1994).

There is growing evidence that multimodal interventions—drug therapy in conjunction with other treatments—are most effective over time (Eckman et al., 1992; Lieberman & Corrigan, 1993; Sood & Koziol, 1994). The authors generally acknowledged that that is the case and elaborated on the advantages of using drug treatment to stabilize the patient so that cognitive restructuring and other behavioral strategies can be implemented. What combination of strategies works for what patients at what stages of the disease process remains to be explored.

Drug therapy cannot be discussed without some consideration of other means to correct a chemical imbalance without resorting to medication. There is mounting evidence of a link between mood and motor activity. Exercise that involves repetitive motions (e.g., jogging, bicycling) increases the activity of serotonin neurons and may help reduce the symptoms of some depressions (Jacobs, 1994). Looked at this way, some obsessive-compulsive behaviors, such as pacing, can be understood as a form of self-medication. The relationship between motor activity and serotonin suggests that the nurse might creatively encourage the therapeutic effects of breathing exercises, dancing, or even rhythmic leg bouncing.

IN CONCLUSION

The emphasis in this chapter has been on the nurse-patient relationship, but one of the themes in the commissioned chapters was on the nurse's role in accomplishing the previously described coaching/teaching through other people, for example, assistive personnel, family members. This is an area where considerable elaboration is in order. Indeed, Kimmel (1994) found the education of the paraprofessional staff on a psychiatric unit to be a neglected topic in the literature. If the nurse is to facilitate self-help and to coach or teach others, a number of questions need to be answered: How do nurses encourage effectiveness in others when those individuals lack an extensive knowledge base? What audiovisual/reading materials prepared by NIMH and other federal agencies and consumer groups can be helpful in symptom management? Can electronic networks function as self-help groups?

This chapter was not meant to be exhaustive but to signal some major changes taking place in the specialty that are likely to shape practice, education, and research in the future. Practice is increasingly being conceptualized as coaching the patient in the process of self-regulation. Education is being asked to incorporate neuroscience content into the curriculum and to teach students how to facilitate patients through other people. Research must be concerned with accurate assessments and the design and testing of clinical interventions (e.g., utilizing relaxation/biofeedback together with cognitive restructuring; tailoring environments in terms of functional strengths and limitations).

Most of the emphasis in this book has been on handling existing conditions, but there is a rich agenda that nurses should assume in promoting self-regulation prophylactically. It is important that psychiatric–mental health nursing become proactive and seek to prevent the development of mental illness. While it might not be cost-effective for nurses to engage in large-scale community interventions, they could begin to develop specific interventions for persons who are at risk for the development of mental health problems. For example, Austin identified children with chronic illness to be at risk for behavior problems, especially if the condition affected the brain. Hardin identified persons experiencing catastrophic stress to be at risk, and Beeber identified persons who had already experienced a major depression to be at risk for a subsequent one. These are just some of the persons who might benefit from health-promoting interventions. Strategies that have been suggested include teaching adaptive coping strategies (e.g., use approach strategies rather than avoidance strategies; emphasize self-enhancing explanations), strengthening self-competence, and increasing the vulnerable person's sense of personal control. Because the perception of powerlessness is a major source of psychopathology (Swift, 1992), not to mention a self-fulfilling prophecy, health-promoting interventions should be aimed at the empowerment of individuals through the development of their decision-making and problem-solving skills (Dunst, Trivette, & Deal, 1988).

Facilitating self-regulation is an organizing concept broad enough to suggest health promotion, disease management, and rehabilitation strategies. It is also a way of thinking about psychiatric–mental health nursing that is consonant with every other aspect of nursing. The emphasis on nursing's role in hyperarousal, which can sometimes appear masked as hypoarousal, has consequences beyond one nursing specialty. Counterproductive reactance is a concern in all clinical situations (Kang & McCarthy, 1994). Developments in neurobiology are not robbing psychiatric nurses of a therapeutic role in helping patients develop insight into their own behaviors. The meaning of that insight is changing, away from a narrow notion of the importance of psychological history to a rich and complex understanding of biopsychosocial influences (Abraham, Fox, & Cohen, 1992). The more influences there are on behavior, the more the patient has to work with in considering ways to change. This repertoire of expanding possibilities has energized implications for nursing practice, education, and research, too.

REFERENCES

Abraham, I. L., Currie, L. J., Neese, J. B., Yi, E. S., & Thompson-Heisterman, A. A. (1994). Risk profiles for nursing home placement of rural elderly: A cluster analysis of psychogeriatric indicators. *Archives of Psychiatric Nursing, 8,* 262–271.

Abraham, I. L., Fox, J. C., & Cohen, B. T. (1992). Integrating the bio into the biopsychosocial: Understanding and treating biological phenomena in psychiatric–mental health nursing. *Archives of Psychiatric Nursing, 6,* 296–305.

Bell, I. R., Miller, C. S., & Schwartz, G. E. (1992). An olfactory-limbic model of multiple chemical sensitivity syndrome: Possible relationships to kindling and affective spectrum disorders. *Biological Psychiatry, 32,* 218–242.

Charney, D. S., Southwick, S. M., Krystal, J. H., Deutch, A. Y., Murburg, M. M., & Davis, M. (1994). Neurobiological mechanisms of PTSD. In M. M. Murburg (Ed.), *Catecholamine function in posttraumatic stress disorder* (pp. 131–158). Washington, DC: American Psychiatric Press.

Dunst, C., Trivette, C., & Deal, A. (1988). *Enabling and empowering families.* Cambridge, MA: Brookline Books.

Eckman, T. A., Wirshing, W. C., Marder, S. R., Lieberman, R. P., Johnston-Conk, K., Zimmerman, K., & Mintz, J. (1992). Technique for training schizophrenic patients in illness self-management: A controlled trial. *American Journal of Psychiatry, 149,* 1549–1555.

Harper-Jaques, S., & Reimer, M. (1992). Aggressive behavior and the brain: A different perspective for the mental health nurse. *Archives of Psychiatric Nursing, 6,* 312–320.

Jacobs, B. L. (1994). Serotonin, motor activity and depression-related disorders. *American Scientist, 82,* 456–463.

Kang, D.-H., & McCarthy, D. O. (1994). The effect of psychological stress on neutrophil superoxide release. *Research in Nursing and Health, 17,* 363–370.

Kelsey, R. M. (1993). Habituation of cardiovascular reactivity to psychological stress: Evidence and implications. In J. Blascovich & E. S. Katkin (Eds.), *Cardiovascular reactivity to psychological stress and disease* (pp. 135–153). Washington, DC: American Psychological Association.

Keltner, N. L., & Callwood, G. B. (1994). Neurosciences: Developing a basic foundation for psychiatric nurses. In *Psychiatric mental health nursing psychopharmacology project* (pp. 22–24). Washington, DC: American Nurses Association.

Kimmel, L. H. (1994). Educating the paraprofessional staff on the psychiatric unit. A neglected topic. *Journal of Psychosocial Nursing, 32*(6), 23–27.

Lazarus, R. S. (1991). *Emotion and adaptation.* New York: Oxford University Press.

Lieberman, R. P., & Corrigan, P. W. (1993). Designing new psychosocial treatments for schizophrenia. *Psychiatry, 56,* 238–249.

Murphy, M. F., & Moller, M. D. (1993). Relapse management in neurobiological disorders: The Moller-Murphy Symptom Management Assessment Tool. *Archives of Psychiatric Nursing, 7,* 226–235.

Perry, B. D., & Pate, J. E. (1994). Neurodevelopment and the psychobiological roots of posttraumatic stress disorders. In L. F. Koziol & C. E. Stout (Eds.), *The neuropsychology of mental disorders* (pp. 129–146). Springfield, IL: Thomas.

Pitman, R. K., Orr, S. P., & Shalev, A. Y. (1993). Once bitten, twice shy: Beyond the conditioning model of PTSD. *Biological Psychiatry, 33,* 145–146.

Rogeness, G. A., Javors, M. A., & Pliszka, S. R. (1992). Neurochemistry and child and adolescent psychiatry. *Journal of American Academy of Child and Adolescent Psychiatry, 31,* 765–781.

Schrift, M. J. (1994). Mood disorders: Limbic system influences on behavior. In L. F. Koziol & C. E. Stout (Eds.), *The neuropsychology of mental disorders* (pp. 94–105). Springfield, IL: Thomas.

Shekhar, A. (1994). Personal communication.

Sood, A., & Koziol, L. F. (1994). The integration of psychopharmacological treatment with psychotherapy. In L. F. Koziol & C. E. Stout (Eds.), *The neuropsychology of mental disorders* (pp. 220–241). Springfield, IL: Thomas.

Swift, C. F. (1992). Empowerment: The greening of prevention. In M. Kessler, S. E. Goldston, & J. M. Joffe (Eds.), *The present and future of prevention* (pp. 99–111). Newberry Park, CA: Sage.

Wilson, W. H., & Mathew, R. J. (1993). Cerebral blood flow and metabolism in anxiety disorders. In R. Hoehn-Saric & D. R. McLeod (Eds.), *Biology of anxiety disorders* (pp. 1–59). Washington, DC: American Psychiatric Press.

Wolfe, B. E. (1994). The use of challenge studies in biobehavioral nursing research. *Archives of Psychiatric Nursing, 8,* 145–149.

CHAPTER

17

A Final Word About Career Development

Angela Barron McBride, PhD, RN, FAAN

ABSTRACT

The final chapter makes the point that the agenda outlined in the previous chapter will never be realized unless individuals within the specialty facilitate the career development of generations to come. Full career development is described in terms of four stages, and there is particular emphasis placed on the importance of research career development. A questionnaire consisting of 100 items is appended to help readers assess their own progress in this direction.

It is appropriate that this book end with some comment on career development because psychiatric nursing's agenda for the future will never come to pass if those of us in the specialty do not have *full* careers and at least some of us do not have *research* careers. Relatively few nurses have historically had full careers, meaning that few have moved beyond becoming personally competent to mentoring others within their home institution and then advising other institutions. As I noted in the first chapter, psychiatric and mental health nurses have generally been effective in moving the profession as a whole in certain directions, but they have tended to value clinical competence more than research expertise, and so relatively few have set out to have full research careers.

FULL CAREER DEVELOPMENT

Full career development is necessary for our loftiest caregiving values to be achieved. More often than not, all the talk about careerism these days seems to focus superficially on dressing for success, resumé preparation, self-presentation at job interviews, and career ladders. To some extent, the apparent self-absorption of careerists would seem to be antithetical to the "other" orientation that seems more appropriate to the care ethic. The truth of the matter is that full career development never loses sight of service to others as *the* goal.

Care (1984), an ethicist himself, considers a career to be a long-term investment through which service to others *and* self-actualization may both be achieved. The belief that service to others can best be achieved if the provider's developmental needs for learning, affirmation, and collegiality are attended to permeates the values system of all professions. A career in this view is characterized by lifelong work, strong commitment, a desire to benefit the public, expectations of personal growth, increasing levels of authority and responsibility, an overlap between personal and professional values, and the obligation to nurture subsequent generations.

Full development implies that an individual will go through all career stages (Dalton, Thompson, & Price, 1977; McBride, 1985, 1992). Stages are the favorite heuristic device used by developmentalists for conceptualizing movement from one set of expectations or themes to another set. Career development can be described as moving from getting prepared (stage 1), to demonstrating personal competence (stage 2), to facilitating others within the home institution (stage 3), and eventually to serving as an advisor to other institutions and within the profession (stage 4). In this sequence, the professional does not regard personal competence as the end point but assumes the obligation of using her or his own expertise to mentor others, to influence the home setting so that the best practice can be realized, and ultimately to shape the health care system in general.

When I was making the decision to enter nursing, my role models were all nurses who did their jobs very well, but they did not have a career orientation. They were doing in the present what they had essentially done in the past. One revolution that has occurred in my professional lifetime has been the commitment of increasing numbers of nurses to having full careers. This means that it is not enough to be skilled yourself but that you also have an obligation to use your expertise in service to your setting and your field. Being personally effective is an accomplishment worthy of praise, but only when these personal achievements are publicly scrutinized in the literature, at professional meetings, or in demonstration projects is debate encouraged and the knowledge base of the field expanded. Policies are shaped by such public debate; it is difficult to imagine an individual being regarded as an authority on a subject without a publication record, for a bibliography has become a shorthand statement of expertise (McBride & Lovejoy, 1995).

There are many advantages to thinking in terms of career stages. Such a model counters the notion that any one professional should be all things to all people at a given point. In the early career stages the task is to become prepared to practice independently and interdependently. This is not a time when the individual should worry about making public policy; that is an obligation that one can assume effectively only after having achieved a measure of expertise. Once having achieved personal competence, however, one must consider assuming more of an obligation to empower others and to be involved in strategic planning. You spend, I think, a certain number of years learning what to do, only to spend your remaining professional years learning how to marry knowing what to do with how to get it done. The latter calls for new skills that go well beyond the skills configuration of the novice, for example, developing a tolerance for ambiguity as you respond to changing circumstances; building interdisciplinary and consumer coalitions; communicating what is best at your home institution so that others will want to join forces to work for a common purpose.

RESEARCH CAREER DEVELOPMENT

No aspect of full career development is more important than research career development. The nurse scientist bears major responsibility for taking the lead in knowledge development, subsequent dissemination of findings to the field, and the incorporation of effective practices into clinical guidelines and curricula. A commitment to knowledge development involves the researcher in setting in motion a *program* of study in a definable area to answer a series of questions relevant to the field, which will ultimately, one hopes, improve the health of the public. The scholarly focus should be broad enough for a professional lifetime and narrow enough to keep up with the literature. In developing a program of study the researcher should be influenced by the factors important to setting any scholarly priorities—scientific integrity, public benefit, and presence of an infrastructure on which to build (Dutton & Crowe, 1988).

When I first began my own scholarly career, any nurse who was involved in research was regarded as exceptional. Most of the research published was an abbreviated version of a master's thesis or doctoral dissertation rather than research conducted in life after graduation. The emphasis was on conducting research, not on developing a relevant program of study, so there was less concern that a series of studies be in the same area. The doctorally prepared nurse was regarded as a finished product, and no one talked about the advantages of a postdoctorate. All of that has changed, as we have begun to articulate stages in a research career.

PREPARATION

The first stage of preparation involves both formal education and socialization experiences. At the undergraduate level, the prospective researcher should learn basic statistics and research methods and how to think critically and conceptually; see how all courses make use of classic studies in communicating information; and have an opportunity to interact with established researchers through independent studies and honors projects. At the graduate level, the prospective researcher should expand her/his inquiry skills (by taking courses in the philosophy of science, statistics, and methods); conduct research and disseminate the findings; apply for funding as appropriate; and develop a research focus. At the postdoctoral level, the researcher typically spends 2–3 years orchestrating a program of research with a senior mentor in that area of study, while extending her/his dissertation work further and publishing the results.

It is important to consider socialization experiences, too. Working as a research assistant is essential if one is planning a research career because of all the informal learning—coding data for eventual analysis; interviewing respondents; finding out how to handle unanticipated problems; running computer programs; interpreting data. In that experience, the research mentor is likely to provide important tips on which professional organizations to join and journals to purchase both within nursing and across disciplines in order to stay abreast.

PERSONAL COMPETENCE

The second career stage involves the researcher in working toward and achieving the status of principal investigator (PI). The PI of a funded project has withstood peer review of her/his credentials, ideas, and methods; her/his work is found to be substantive and on the cutting edge. On the way to PI status, the researcher may form alliances with colleagues in the same general area, obtain both intramural and external career development awards (McBride & Friedenberg, 1989), assemble a research team, attend to the politics of clinical sites, and develop skills as a reviewer. This is the period when the individual is most likely to be publishing and presenting findings as first author. With experience, the researcher inevitably develops a more complicated sense of what her/his program of research should include, for example, adding variables in light of the biopsychosocial model shaping the study.

MENTORING

In the third career stage, the researcher assumes responsibility for mentoring fledgling researchers and for providing leadership in the home institution for strategic planning around research development. The researcher may be ready now to apply for a program grant or an institutional research training grant in order to coordinate common interests or facilitate the education of doctoral students. As the researcher's reputation builds, the person is likely to be in demand as a peer reviewer for conference abstracts, grant proposals, and journal articles. Being chosen as a member of a regular study section by one of the agencies within the National Institutes of Health is an indication that one's research has become known nationally. As a mentor, it is likely that presentations and publications will increasingly involve others as co-authors so they can begin to build a track record.

ADVISING

In the fourth stage, the researcher may be asked to serve as a consultant to other researchers or research-minded organizations. At this level the person may be involved in consensus efforts, for example, evaluating research to create clinical practice guidelines for the Agency for Health Care Policy and Research (Clinton, McCormick, & Besteman, 1994). Writing at this stage becomes more integrative as the person is sought out for state-of-the-science presentations/publications (e.g., writing a chapter in the *Annual Review of Nursing Research*) or decides to author or edit a book synthesizing personal research and related work of colleagues or students. Invitations to serve on the advisory council of a federal funding agency or similar institution usually come at this stage.

• • •

At the end of this chapter is a questionnaire, "Playing the Nursing Research Game," which has been used successfully to enable nurses to assess how they are proceeding in their own research career development. The items were originally reviewed by six very established researchers for relevance and comprehensiveness; in use, the instrument's coefficient alpha (KR-20) was found to be .96. The instrument is correlated with educational level (.65) and academic rank (.68). Since that questionnaire was based on the distinctions just made in describing four possible career stages, it may be helpful to the reader who wishes to evaluate her/his own progress and to set future goals.

This discussion of research career development cannot end without some comment regarding the problems that will be likely to attend the individual wishing to conduct research on the interface between the behavioral and biological sciences. Since the behavioral sciences and the biological sciences are not likely to be taught in the same school, the individual will have to seek out interdisciplinary programs and mentors, use "minor" requirements to flesh out the material not available in the "major," select collaborators whose skills are complementary, and learn to make a virtue of the benefits to be derived from working on the interface when applying for career development opportunities.

Because nursing programs are currently biased toward the behavioral sciences in their models/theories, the prospective researcher should go out of her/his way to obtain needed background in the biological sciences. It should be noted, however, that the behavioral sciences are themselves taking steps to recombine specialty areas, for example, the emergence of cognitive neuropsychology (Margolin, 1992). Whatever difficulties the nurse scientist experiences in acquiring the background necessary to explore questions on the interface between the behavioral and biological sciences are likely to be worth it because of the clinical promise of such combinations and the public interest in such subject matter.

IN CONCLUSION

Psychiatric nursing's future agenda cannot be met without a critical mass of nurse scientists capable of developing our knowledge base. Research is especially needed in new areas, such as patient self-regulation, that are at the behavioral and biological interface. Self-regulation is fast becoming a major concern of all nurses and their patients. Enduringly successful outcomes require self-care skills, which in turn cannot come to pass without the patient and her/his family understanding some of the factors that influence the health problem itself: willingness to change, recurrence, and relapse. It is interesting that Kilburg (1991) uses self-regulation as the organizing framework for career development, too, because the professional is similarly concerned with growing and changing to reach full potential.

Constitutional physiological reactivity has been linked to behavioral patterns since the time of Pavlov, but new discoveries in this, "the decade of the brain," have made these links seem richer and more promising than ever before to nurses and other health care professionals. These links need to be systematically studied for what they reveal about health promotion, disease prevention, and rehabilitation—nursing's agenda for the 21st century. And these studies will only be realized if psychiatric nurse researchers are nurtured to develop the skills base from which to proceed.

REFERENCES

Care, N. S. (1984). Career choice. *Ethics, 94,* 283–302.

Clinton, J. J., McCormick, K., & Besteman, J. (1994). Enhancing clinical practice. The role of practice guidelines. *American Psychologist, 49,* 30–33.

Dalton, G. W., Thompson, P. H., & Price, R. L. (1977). The four stages of professional careers— A new look at performance by professionals. *Organizational Dynamics, 6*(1), 19–42.

Dutton, J. A., & Crowe, L. (1988). Setting priorities among scientific initiatives [Views]. *American Scientist, 76,* 599–603.

Kilburg, R. R. (1991). The art of self-regulation. In R. R. Kilburg (Ed.), *How to manage your career in psychology* (pp. 19–37). Washington, DC: American Psychological Association.

Margolin, D. I. (Ed.). (1992). *Cognitive neuropsychology in clinical practice.* New York: Oxford Press.

McBride, A. B. (1985). Orchestrating a career. *Nursing Outlook, 33,* 244–247.

McBride, A. B. (1992). Balancing career and personal development. In N. L. Wiegand (Ed.), *A second century of leadership. Papers from the centennial celebration* (pp. 93–110). Ann Arbor: University of Michigan School of Nursing.

McBride, A. B., & Friedenberg, E. (1989). Research opportunities at the National Institute of Mental Health. *Image: Journal of Nursing Scholarship, 21,* 251–253.

McBride, A. B., & Lovejoy, K. B. (1995). Requesting and writing effective letters of recommendation: Some guidelines for candidates and sponsors. *Journal of Nursing Education, 34,* 95–96.

17-1

PLAYING THE NURSING RESEARCH GAME

Nurses are increasingly interested in orchestrating research careers. This questionnaire is meant to help nurses assess how far they have progressed. The steps requisite to research productivity can be seen as a "game" in the sense of accumulating a series of experiences that net one important points on the way to success. The word "game" is not meant to be disrespectful, but to make self-assessment fun. The scoring instructions distinguish four levels of accomplishment, but are meant to be suggestive rather than definitive. Bear in mind that even the most accomplished researcher is not likely to be able to get a perfect score because all have had different opportunities.

Read each item and give yourself one point for each "yes" answer. Add your total number of points out of a possible 100, and calculate where you are in the nursing research game.

1. As an undergraduate, did you take a research, methods, or statistics course?
   Yes _____ No _____

2. Did you get involved in doing any research (formally or informally) as part of your undergraduate program?
   Yes _____ No _____

3. Are you able to use a word processor in preparing manuscripts?
   Yes _____ No _____

4. Have you ever read a research article and incorporated the findings into your thinking?
   Yes _____ No _____

5. Do you regularly read any professional journals?
   Yes _____ No _____

6. Do you subscribe to any research journals, for example, one in nursing which has the word "research" in its title?
   Yes _____ No _____

7. Do you regularly attend professional meetings as a way of keeping up?
   Yes _____ No _____

8. Are you an active member of any organization devoted specifically to promoting research?
   Yes _____ No _____

9. Do you buy books to develop your knowledge (and a personal library) in some area(s) of research interest?
Yes _____   No _____

10. Do you know whether "Grateful Med" is a rock group or a resource for reviewing the literature?
Yes _____   No _____

11. Do you collect copies of instruments for future research use?
Yes _____   No _____

12. Can you be "critical" and point out strengths and limitations in published research reports?
Yes _____   No _____

13. Do you know how to evaluate the quality and outcomes of your clinical practice?
Yes _____   No _____

14. Did you complete a master's study or thesis?
Yes _____   No _____

15. Did you formally present and/or publish the findings of your master's study or thesis?
Yes _____   No _____

16. Did you ever interview for a job and ask about the organization's commitment to research and/or scholarship?
Yes _____   No _____

17. Have you ever participated as a subject in a study of any sort?
Yes _____   No _____

18. Have you ever been involved in collecting or analyzing data for someone else's study?
Yes _____   No _____

19. Have you ever been paid for working formally as a research assistant on some project?
Yes _____   No _____

20. Do you know how to analyze data using descriptive statistics and/or ethnographic techniques?
Yes _____   No _____

21. Do you know how to analyze data using inferential statistics?
Yes _____   No _____

22. Do you know how to code data in preparation for its entry into a computer?
Yes _____   No _____

23. Can you read a computer printout of data?
Yes _____   No _____

24. Have you ever written a full research proposal (as a class assignment or otherwise)?
Yes _____   No _____

25. Have you ever as principal investigator sent a research proposal to some local or regional funding agency?
    Yes _____   No _____

26. Have you ever as principal investigator sent a research proposal to some national or international funding agency?
    Yes _____   No _____

27. Have you ever rewritten a research proposal that was previously disapproved or unfunded?
    Yes _____   No _____

28. Have you been involved in developing policies or protocols for a clinical agency based on published research?
    Yes _____   No _____

29. Have you ever as the principal investigator had a research project funded locally or regionally?
    Yes _____   No _____

30. Have you ever as principal investigator had a research project funded nationally or internationally?
    Yes _____   No _____

31. Have you earned a doctorate?
    Yes _____   No _____

32. Was your doctoral training or dissertation research supported by some grant for which you had to submit a proposal?
    Yes _____   No _____

33. Was your dissertation research published?
    Yes _____   No _____

34. Have you obtained postdoctoral research training?
    Yes _____   No _____

35. Have you ever been selected to present your research locally or regionally as a result of a **refereed** review process?
    Yes _____   No _____

36. Have you ever been selected to present your research nationally or internationally as a result of a **refereed** review process?
    Yes _____   No _____

37. Do you have research goals for the next three years?
    Yes _____   No _____

38. Do you know what the initials IRB stand for?
    Yes _____   No _____

39. Do you know what the initials NINR stand for?
    Yes _____   No _____

40. Have you ever formally evaluated your teaching or practice (i.e., collected some systematic data on the impact you have had)?
    Yes _____   No _____

41. Have you ever published your research locally or regionally as a result of a **refereed** review process?
Yes _____ No _____

42. Have you ever published your research nationally or internationally as a result of a **refereed** review process?
Yes _____ No _____

43. Are you an active member of an interdisciplinary research-oriented organization concerned with scholarship in your area of study, for example, National Council on Family Relations, American Public Health Association, Society for Research in Child Development?
Yes _____ No _____

44. Does the list of **refereed** publications (excluding abstracts) in your curriculum vitae cover a full printed page or more?
Yes _____ No _____

45. Does the list of **refereed** publications (excluding abstracts) in your curriculum vitae cover three full printed pages or more?
Yes _____ No _____

46. Have you ever published an integrative review of literature in an area of research (e.g., for *Annual Review of Nursing Research*)?
Yes _____ No _____

47. Have you ever gotten an unsolicited invitation to speak on your research/scholarship at a scholarly meeting?
Yes _____ No _____

48. Do you get invited to keynote regional and/or national conferences for the purpose of speaking on your research/scholarship?
Yes _____ No _____

49. Have you been a reviewer for the awarding of local and/or regional research grants?
Yes _____ No _____

50. Have you been a reviewer for the awarding of national and/or international research grants?
Yes _____ No _____

51. Have you been invited to serve on an expert panel by a national organization (e.g., NINR, AHCPR, professional associations) to establish research priorities?
Yes _____ No _____

52. Have you been invited to serve as a member of a regular study section reviewing research grants for a federal funding agency (NINR, NCI, NIMH, etc.)?
Yes _____ No _____

53. Have you been invited to serve as a member of the advisory council for a federal funding agency concerned with setting policy for research grants (NINR, NCI, NIMH, etc.)?
Yes _____ No _____

54. Have you served as a reviewer for a professional journal?
Yes _____   No _____

55. Have you ever served as a reviewer for a research journal, for example, one in nursing which has the word "research" in its title?
Yes _____   No _____

56. Have you served as an editor or on the editorial board of a professional journal?
Yes _____   No _____

57. Have you served as an editor or on the editorial board of a research journal, for example, one in nursing which has the word "research" in its title?
Yes _____   No _____

58. Do you have a complete, up-to-date curriculum vitae?
Yes _____   No _____

59. Do you have an up-to-date biographical sketch (1–2 pages) in the research-oriented format required by NIH for grant applications?
Yes _____   No _____

60. Have you had the experience of supervising paid personnel working on your research projects?
Yes _____   No _____

61. Have you ever discussed the policy implications of your research with legislators and/or other policymakers?
Yes _____   No _____

62. Have you ever formally reported back your findings to a clinical agency that was the site of your data collection?
Yes _____   No _____

63. If someone said, "What is the focus of your *program* of research?" could you answer the question?
Yes _____   No _____

64. Have you ever conducted a study which built on your own previously published research?
Yes _____   No _____

65. Have you had a research mentor?
Yes _____   No _____

66. Have you served as a research mentor?
Yes _____   No _____

67. Have you formally incorporated research into your own teaching?
Yes _____   No _____

68. Have you supervised undergraduate research or helped undergraduates with research projects?
Yes _____   No _____

69. Have you supervised master's-level research or served as a member of a doctoral student's dissertation committee?
Yes _____   No _____

70. Have you chaired a doctoral student's dissertation committee?
    Yes _____   No _____

71. Have you served as mentor to a postdoctoral fellow?
    Yes _____   No _____

72. Have you helped a student to obtain monies for her/his own research?
    Yes _____   No _____

73. Have you served on a committee concerned with research utilization?
    Yes _____   No _____

74. Have you served on a committee concerned with research development?
    Yes _____   No _____

75. Do you have a network of colleagues in the same research area whom you can call on to write letters of support or to serve as consultants for your work?
    Yes _____   No _____

76. Have you made use of consultants not located at your home institution in your research?
    Yes _____   No _____

77. Have you published on research development and/or research utilization?
    Yes _____   No _____

78. Have you ever made a formal presentation on research development and/or research utilization at a professional meeting?
    Yes _____   No _____

79. Have you helped others to obtain local or regional funding for their research?
    Yes _____   No _____

80. Have you helped others to successfully obtain national or international funding for their research?
    Yes _____   No _____

81. Have you helped others to get their research findings published?
    Yes _____   No _____

82. Have you helped others to get their research findings published in a research journal, for example, one in nursing which has the word "research" in its title?
    Yes _____   No _____

83. Have you taken more computer, statistics, or methods courses than you were required to take for your last degree?
    Yes _____   No _____

84. Have you ever obtained a continuation grant from a federal funding agency?
    Yes _____   No _____

85. Have you ever obtained a program/center grant, or one to develop institutional research training from a federal funding agency?
    Yes _____   No _____

86. Have you been asked by non-nurses to discuss nursing research and/or your area of study at a scholarly meeting?
    Yes _____   No _____

87. Have you been asked to advise a professional organization, hospital, or school regarding its program of research/scholarship?
    Yes _____   No _____

88. Have you been honored locally and/or regionally for your program of research (e.g., awards, distinguished lectureships)?
    Yes _____   No _____

89. Have you been honored nationally and/or internationally for your program of research (e.g., awards, distinguished lectureships)?
    Yes _____   No _____

90. Have you been honored locally/regionally for your research development and/or research utilization efforts?
    Yes _____   No _____

91. Have you been honored nationally/internationally for your research development and/or research utilization efforts?
    Yes _____   No _____

92. Do scholars from other universities and/or countries visit you to discuss your research/scholarship?
    Yes _____   No _____

93. Have you been asked to serve as a paid consultant to local and/or regional research projects?
    Yes _____   No _____

94. Have you been asked to serve as a paid consultant to national and/or international research projects?
    Yes _____   No _____

95. Have instruments you developed (or co-developed) been used by other researchers?
    Yes _____   No _____

96. Has your research been cited in the professional literature as methodologically noteworthy, to be used as a conceptual underpinning for a new piece of research, and/or to be used as a basis for practice?
    Yes _____   No _____

97. Do you regularly get requests for reprints of your articles?
    Yes _____   No _____

98. Have others replicated your research, then published the results?
    Yes _____   No _____

99. Are many non-nurse researchers familiar with your research?
    Yes _____   No _____

100. Do you have the sense that your research program is actually developing knowledge, that is, your studies (and those of your students or colleagues) are connected and building toward a general goal?
    Yes _____   No _____

SCORING INSTRUCTIONS

The 100 items are generally organized to demonstrate career movement from developing one's own expertise to facilitating the research of others. Items also reflect the development of a program of research and its subsequent dissemination and utilization.

Calculate your score by giving yourself one point for each "yes" answer, and ascertain where you are in playing the nursing research game.

0–25 points   You are a novice and need basic skills and formal learning experiences. Take advantage of the research opportunities that come your way.

26–50 points   You need to develop advanced skills and to do a better job of focusing your research and disseminating your scholarship.

51–75 points   You are already becoming known for your scholarly accomplishments.

76–100 points   Full professorships and, eventually, distinguished professorships await you.

INDEX

Note: Page numbers in *italics* refer to illustrations; page numbers followed by t refer to tables.

ISBN 0-7216-4038-9